1996
YEAR BOOK OF
MEDICINE®

Statement of Purpose

The YEAR BOOK Service

The YEAR BOOK series was devised in 1901 by practicing health professionals who observed that the literature of medicine and related disciplines had become so voluminous that no one individual could read and place in perspective every potential advance in a major specialty. In the final decade of the 20th century, this recognition is more acutely true than it was in 1901.

More than merely a series of books, YEAR BOOK volumes are the tangible results of a unique service designed to accomplish the following:

- to *survey* a wide range of journals of proven value
- to *select* from those journals papers representing significant advances and statements of important clinical principles
- to provide *abstracts* of those articles that are readable, convenient summaries of their key points
- to provide *commentary* about those articles to place them in perspective

These publications grow out of a unique process that calls on the talents of outstanding authorities in clinical and fundamental disciplines, trained literature specialists, and professional writers, all supported by the resources of Mosby, the world's preeminent publisher for the health professions.

The Literature Base

Mosby and its Editors survey more than 1,000 journals published worldwide, covering the full range of the health professions. On an annual basis, the publisher examines usage patterns and polls its expert authorities to add new journals to the literature base and to delete journals that are no longer useful as potential YEAR BOOK sources.

The Literature Survey

The publisher's team of literature specialists, all of whom are trained and experienced health professionals, examines every original, peer-reviewed article in each journal issue. More than 250,000 articles per year are scanned systematically, including title, text, illustrations, tables, and references. Each scan is compared, article by article, to the search strategies that the publisher has developed in consultation with the 270 outside experts who form the pool of YEAR BOOK editors. A given article may be reviewed by any number of editors, from one to a dozen or more, regardless of the discipline for which the paper was originally published. In turn, each editor who receives the article reviews it to determine whether or not the article should be included in the YEAR BOOK. This decision is based on the article's inherent quality, its probable usefulness to readers of that YEAR BOOK, and the editor's goal to represent a balanced picture of a given field in each volume of the YEAR BOOK. In addition, the editor indicates when to include figures and tables from the article to help the YEAR BOOK reader better understand the information.

Of the quarter million articles scanned each year, only 5% are selected for detailed analysis within the YEAR BOOK series, thereby assuring readers of the high value of every selection.

The Abstract

The publisher's abstracting staff is headed by a physician-writer and includes individuals with training in the life sciences, medicine, and other areas, plus extensive experience in writing for the health professions and related industries. Each selected article is assigned to a specific writer on this abstracting staff. The abstracter, guided in many cases by notations supplied by the expert editor, writes a structured, condensed summary designed so that the reader can rapidly acquire the essential information contained in the article.

The Commentary

The YEAR BOOK editorial boards, sometimes assisted by guest commentators, write comments that place each article in perspective for the reader. This provides the reader with the equivalent of a personal consultation with a leading international authority—an opportunity to better understand the value of the article and to benefit from the authority's thought processes in assessing the article.

Additional Editorial Features

The editorial boards of each YEAR BOOK organize the abstracts and comments to provide a logical and satisfying sequence of information. To enhance the organization, editors also provide introductions to sections or individual chapters, comments linking a number of abstracts, citations to additional literature, and other features.

The published YEAR BOOK contains enhanced bibliographic citations for each selected article, including extended listings of multiple authors and identification of author affiliations. Each YEAR BOOK contains a Table of Contents specific to that year's volume. From year to year, the Table of Contents for a given YEAR BOOK will vary depending on developments within the field.

Every YEAR BOOK contains a list of the journals from which papers have been selected. This list represents a subset of the more than 1,000 journals surveyed by the publisher and occasionally reflects a particularly pertinent article from a journal that is not surveyed on a routine basis.

Finally, each volume contains a comprehensive subject index and an index to authors of each selected paper.

The 1996 Year Book Series

Year Book of Allergy, Asthma, and Clinical Immunology: Drs. Rosenwasser, Borish, Gelfand, Leung, Nelson, and Szefler

Year Book of Anesthesiology and Pain Management: Drs. Tinker, Abram, Chestnut, Roizen, Rothenberg, and Wood

Year Book of Cardiology®: Drs. Schlant, Collins, Engle, Gersh, Kaplan, and Waldo

Year Book of Chiropractic®: Dr. Lawrence

Year Book of Critical Care Medicine®: Drs. Parrillo, Balk, Calvin, Franklin, and Shapiro

Year Book of Dentistry®: Drs. Meskin, Berry, Kennedy, Leinfelder, Roser, Summitt, and Zakariasen

Year Book of Dermatologic Surgery®: Drs. Swanson, Glogau, and Salasche

Year Book of Dermatology®: Drs. Sober and Fitzpatrick

Year Book of Diagnostic Radiology®: Drs. Federle, Clark, Gross, Latchaw, Madewell, Maynard, and Young

Year Book of Digestive Diseases®: Drs. Greenberger and Moody

Year Book of Drug Therapy®: Drs. Lasagna and Weintraub

Year Book of Emergency Medicine®: Drs. Wagner, Dronen, Davidson, King, Niemann, and Roberts

Year Book of Endocrinology®: Drs. Bagdade, Braverman, Horton, Kannan, Landsberg, Molitch, Morley, Nathan, Odell, Poehlman, Rogol, and Ryan

Year Book of Family Practice®: Drs. Berg, Bowman, Davidson, Dexter, and Scherger

Year Book of Geriatrics and Gerontology®: Drs. Beck, Burton, Rabins, Reuben, Roth, Shapiro, and Whitehouse

Year Book of Hand Surgery®: Drs. Amadio and Hentz

Year Book of Hematology®: Drs. Spivak, Bell, Ness, Quesenberry, Wiernik, and Blume

Year Book of Infectious Diseases®: Drs. Keusch, Barza, Bennish, Klempner, Skolnik, and Snydman

Year Book of Infertility and Reproductive Endocrinology: Drs. Mishell, Lobo, and Sokol

Year Book of Medicine®: Drs. Bone, Cline, Epstein, Greenberger, Malawista, Mandell, O'Rourke, and Utiger

Year Book of Neonatal and Perinatal Medicine®: Drs. Fanaroff and Klaus

Year Book of Nephrology, Hypertension, and Mineral Metabolism: Drs. Coe, Curtis, Favus, Henderson, Kashgarian, Luke, and Myers

Year Book of Neurology and Neurosurgery®: Drs. Bradley and Wilkins

Year Book of Neuroradiology: Drs. Osborn, Eskridge, Grossman, Hudgins, and Ross

Year Book of Nuclear Medicine®: Drs. Gottschalk, Blaufox, McAfee, Wackers, and Zubal

Year Book of Obstetrics and Gynecology®: Drs. Mishell, Herbst, and Kirschbaum

Year Book of Occupational and Environmental Medicine®: Drs. Emmett, Frank, Gochfeld, and Hessl

Year Book of Oncology®: Drs. Simone, Bosl, Cohen, Glatstein, Ozols, and Tallman

Year Book of Ophthalmology®: Drs. Cohen, Augsburger, Eagle, Flanagan, Grossman, Laibson, Maguire, Nelson, Rapuano, Sergott, Tasman, Tipperman, and Wilson

Year Book of Orthopedics®: Drs. Sledge, Cofield, Dobyns, Griffin, Poss, Springfield, Swiontkowski, Wiesel, and Wilson

Year Book of Otolaryngology–Head and Neck Surgery®: Drs. Paparella and Holt

Year Book of Pain: Drs. Gebhart, Haddox, Jacox, Janjan, Marcus, Rudy, and Shapiro

Year Book of Pathology and Laboratory Medicine: Drs. Mills, Bruns, Gaffey, and Stoler

Year Book of Pediatrics®: Dr. Stockman

Year Book of Plastic, Reconstructive, and Aesthetic Surgery®: Drs. Miller, Cohen, McKinney, Robson, Ruberg, and Whitaker

Year Book of Podiatric Medicine and Surgery®: Dr. Kominsky

Year Book of Psychiatry and Applied Mental Health®: Drs. Talbott, Ballenger, Breier, Frances, Meltzer, Schowalter, and Tasman

Year Book of Pulmonary Disease®: Drs. Bone and Petty

Year Book of Rheumatology®: Drs. Sergent, LeRoy, Meenan, Panush, and Reichlin

Year Book of Sports Medicine®: Drs. Shephard, Drinkwater, Eichner, Torg, Col. Anderson, and Mr. George

Year Book of Surgery®: Drs. Copeland, Bland, Deitch, Eberlein, Howard, Luce, Seeger, Souba, and Sugarbaker

Year Book of Thoracic and Cardiovascular Surgery®: Drs. Ginsberg, Wechsler, and Williams

Year Book of Ultrasound®: Drs. Merritt, Carroll, and Fleischer

Year Book of Urology®: Drs. DeKernion and Howards

Year Book of Vascular Surgery®: Dr. Porter

1996 The Year Book of MEDICINE®

Editors
Roger C. Bone, M.D.
Martin J. Cline, M.D.
Franklin H. Epstein, M.D.
Norton J. Greenberger, M.D.
Stephen E. Malawista, M.D.
Gerald L. Mandell, M.D.
Robert A. O'Rourke, M.D.
Robert D. Utiger, M.D.

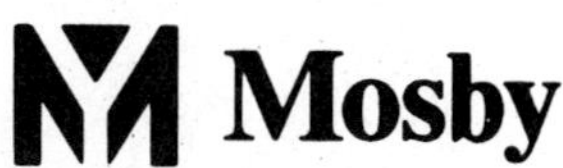

St. Louis Baltimore Boston Carlsbad Chicago Naples New York Philadelphia Portland
London Madrid Mexico City Singapore Sydney Tokyo Toronto Wiesbaden

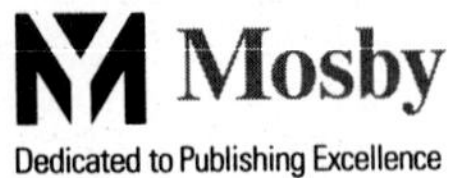

A Times Mirror
Company

Vice President and Publisher, Continuity Publishing: Kenneth H. Killion
Director, Editorial Development: Gretchen C. Murphy
Assistant Developmental Editor, Continuity: Kathleen L. Wallace
Acquisitions Editor: Linda Steiner
Illustrations and Permissions Coordinator: Lois M. Ruebensam
Manager, Continuity–EDP: Maria Nevinger
Project Manager, Editing: Tamara L. Smith
Senior Project Manager, Production: Max F. Perez
Freelance Staff Supervisor: Barbara M. Kelly
Director, Editorial Services: Edith M. Podrazik, R.N.
Information Specialist: Kathleen Moss, R.N.
Senior Marketing Manager: Eileen M. Lynch
Marketing Specialist: Lynn D. Stevenson

1996 EDITION

Printed in the United States of America
Composition by Reed Technology and Information Services, Inc.
Printing/binding by Maple-Vail

Mosby–Year Book, Inc.
11830 Westline Industrial Drive
St. Louis, MO 63146

Editorial Office:
Mosby–Year Book, Inc.
200 North LaSalle Street
Chicago, IL 60601

International Standard Serial Number: 0084-3873
International Standard Book Number: 0-8151-7269-9

Editorial Board

Contributing Editors

Dialysis
Robert S. Brown, M.D.
Associate Professor of Medicine, Harvard Medical School; Clinical Chief, Renal Unit, Beth Israel Hospital, Boston
Transplantation
Terry Strom, M.D.
Professor of Medicine, Harvard Medical School; Director, Division of Clinical Immunology, Beth Israel Hospital, Boston

Publisher's Preface

Publication of the 1996 YEAR BOOK OF MEDICINE marks the end of an era at Mosby–Year Book, Inc. With the release of this edition, we say goodbye to Roger C. Bone, M.D., Robert A. O'Rourke, M.D., and Franklin Epstein, M.D. We extend them our heartfelt thanks for their tireless dedication to the YEAR BOOK OF MEDICINE. The expertise they provided to their respective sections ensured this publication's broad appeal. It has been a pleasure to work with them, and we wish them much success in all of their future publishing endeavors.

At this time, we would like to welcome Thomas L. Petty, M.D., from the HealthONE Center for Health Sciences in Denver, Colorado, William Frishman, M.D., from the Albert Einstein College of Medicine and the Montefiore Medical Center in the Bronx, New York, and Saulo Klahr, M.D., from The Jewish Hospital of St. Louis in Missouri. We look forward to working with these distinguished experts.

Table of Contents

Journals Represented

Mosby and its Editors survey more than 1,000 journals for its abstract-and-commentary publications. From these journals, the Editors select the articles to be abstracted. Journals represented in this YEAR BOOK are listed below.

Age and Ageing
American Heart Journal
American Journal of Cardiology
American Journal of Clinical Pathology
American Journal of Emergency Medicine
American Journal of Epidemiology
American Journal of Hypertension
American Journal of Infection Control
American Journal of Kidney Diseases
American Journal of Medicine
American Journal of Nephrology
American Journal of Respiratory and Critical Care Medicine
American Journal of the Medical Sciences
American Surgeon
Annals of Allergy
Annals of Internal Medicine
Annals of Oncology
Archives of Internal Medicine
Archives of Pathology and Laboratory Medicine
Arthritis and Rheumatism
Artificial Organs
Blood
Blood Marrow Transplantation
British Journal of Cancer
British Journal of Haematology
British Journal of Surgery
British Journal of Urology
British Medical Journal
Chest
Circulation
Clinical Endocrinology
Clinical Infectious Diseases
Clinical Nephrology
Clinical Radiology
Clinical Science
Critical Care Medicine
Diabetes
European Heart Journal
European Journal of Endocrinology
European Journal of Haematology
European Respiratory Journal
Experimental Hematology
Gastroenterology
Gene Therapy
Gut
Hepatology
Hypertension
Journal of Bone and Mineral Research

Journal of Clinical Endocrinology and Metabolism
Journal of Clinical Investigation
Journal of Clinical Microbiology
Journal of Clinical Oncology
Journal of Experimental Medicine
Journal of Infectious Diseases
Journal of Medical Virology
Journal of Occupational and Environmental Medicine
Journal of Otolaryngology
Journal of Reproductive Medicine
Journal of Rheumatology
Journal of Thoracic and Cardiovascular Surgery
Journal of Urology
Journal of the American College of Cardiology
Journal of the American Geriatrics Society
Journal of the American Medical Association
Journal of the National Cancer Institute
Kidney International
Lancet
Leukemia
Mayo Clinic Proceedings
Medicine
Metabolism
Nephrology, Dialysis, Transplantation
Nephron
New England Journal of Medicine
Obstetrics and Gynecology
PACE - Pacing and Clinical Electrophysiology
Pediatric Infectious Disease Journal
Pediatric Nephrology
Quarterly Journal of Medicine
Radiology
Science
Surgery
Transplantation

Standard Abbreviations

The following terms are abbreviated in this edition: acquired immunodeficiency syndrome (AIDS), cardiopulmonary resuscitation (CPR), central nervous system (CNS), cerebrospinal fluid (CSF), computed tomography (CT), deoxyribonucleic acid (DNA), electrocardiography (ECG), health maintenance organization (HMO), human immunodeficiency virus (HIV), intensive care unit (ICU), intramuscular (IM), intravenous (IV), magnetic resonance (MR), imaging (MRI), and ribonucleic acid (RNA).

Note

To facilitate the use of the YEAR BOOK OF MEDICINE as a reference tool, all illustrations and tables included in this publication are now identified as they appear in the original article. This change is meant to help the reader recognize that any illustration or table appearing in the YEAR BOOK OF MEDICINE may be only one of many in the original article. For this reason, figure and table numbers will often appear to be out of sequence within the YEAR BOOK OF MEDICINE.

PART ONE

INFECTIOUS DISEASES

GERALD L. MANDELL, M.D.

Introduction

I have included 5 selections under the heading of Pediatric Infectious Diseases. There are several reasons for this. Many "pediatric" infections, such as varicella, polio, otitis media, and epiglottitis, are seen in adults. In addition, the organisms passed around by children frequently infect adults, and it is thought that much of the present-day resistance to antibiotics seen with *Pneumococcus* organisms is the result of frequent use of antibiotics for common infections in infants and children.

Common things are still common, and it is interesting that we continue to learn more about such common infections as otitis, pedal ulcers, and appendicitis. The potential therapeutic excitement generated a few years ago by major trials for sepsis therapies has waned. The field is still active, however, and the new players are the increase in cases and the better understanding of streptococcal toxic shock; these issues are addressed in the Sepsis chapter. Nosocomial infections are a moving target, and it seems that every time that there is an advance we encounter a new variety. Under the title of Miscellaneous Infections are discussed such important conditions as endocarditis, meningitis, and cytomegalovirus vasculitis. The big story in infectious disease continues to be AIDS and HIV infection and related opportunistic infections. Probably the most exciting information in this chapter relates to the data that strongly implicate an etiologic agent for Kaposi's sarcoma. Hepatitis C virus is now recognized as the most common cause of chronic hepatitis in the United States, and several interesting articles are presented. Headlines in infectious diseases are now focused on new and emerging infections, and a large chapter discusses some interesting new developments. Finally, although this has not been a breakthrough year for new therapies, several are available and are discussed in the Therapy chapter.

Gerald L. Mandell, M.D.

1 Pediatric Infections

Introduction

Some good news and some bad news fill this chapter. The success of *Hemophilus influenzae* type B vaccine continues to be documented and now includes prevention of epiglottitis. We are still faced with the problems of some "old" pathogens, such as *Pneumococcus* and group A *Streptococcus*.

Gerald L. Mandell, M.D.

Transmission of Multidrug-Resistant Serotype 23F *Streptococcus pneumoniae* in Group Day Care: Evidence Suggesting Capsular Transformation of the Resistant Strain In Vivo

Barnes DM, Whittier S, Gilligan PH, Soares S, Tomasz A, Henderson FW
(Univ of North Carolina, Chapel Hill; Rockefeller Univ, New York)
J Infect Dis 171:890–896, 1995 119-96-1–1

Introduction.—The appearance of multidrug-resistant (MDR) pneumococci has increased dramatically during the past 2 decades, although the antibiotic-resistant viruses had been identified only sporadically in the United States until 1989 and 1990, when these organisms began to occur more frequently in isolates. By 1991, MDR pneumococci had been isolated in patients from at least 19 states. Organisms of serotypes 23 and 6 made up most of these organisms at that time. In a research day care center in North Carolina, molecular tests were used to determine whether the MDR 23F serotype was related to a 23F isolate recovered in Cleveland.

Methods.—Between May 1990 and December 1991, 14 of 52 children were involved in an outbreak of nasal carriage of MDR serotype 23F organism. Nasopharyngeal secretions were obtained monthly on a routine basis and subjected to antibiotic susceptibility testing and molecular studies. Electrophoresis of penicillin-binding proteins and pulsed-field gel electrophoresis were used to determine the genetic backgrounds of the bacterial isolates.

Results.—Fourteen children had colonization with high-level MDR pneumococci of the serotype 23F strain similar to a serotype 23F serotype identified in Spain in the early 1980s. One of these children was shown subsequently to have an MDR serotype 14 organism, which was very similar to the circulating MDR serotype 23F strain. This finding indicated a possible serotype transformation. Pulsed-field gel electrophoresis profiles obtained after *Smal*I digestion of chromosomal DNA from the resistant isolates indicated that the organisms were also similar to both those identified in a Cleveland day care center and those found earlier in Spain. Penicillin-binding–protein patterns of the MDR serotype 23 and 14 isolates were also similar.

Conclusions.—These results strongly suggest that the day care setting may promote transmission of MDR pneumococcal strains. Because exposure to colonization among children occurs routinely, the opportunity for colonization with different serotypes is likely enhanced in this environment.

▶ We have known for some time that the day care incubator is an important engine for the propagation of antibiotic-resistant bacterial strains. This report focuses on a new and somewhat frightening wrinkle. An MDR *Pneumococcus* organism changed its capsular type (or serotype) from 14 to 23F. Obviously, there are 2 potential mechanisms whereby this could occur. One is that the genetic information for resistance could have moved from 1 capsular type organism to another. This mechanism was thought to be unlikely, because the resistance genes appeared not to be closely linked on the bacterial chromosomes, thereby making the likelihood of transfer extremely low. On the other hand, there is precedent for transformation of pneumococcal serotypes in the laboratory and in animals. In fact, a 1944 paper by Avery, MacLeod, and McCarty[1] established DNA as the substance that carried the message that coded for the pneumococcal capsular type, thus establishing the foundation for present-day molecular biology. The importance of the study by Barnes et al. relates to the ability of resistance genes to be found in different pneumococcal serotypes. Therefore, one can imagine that vaccination based on likely serotypes would be attacking a moving target; resistant serotypes could, and probably do, change over time.

G.L. Mandell, M.D.

Reference

1. Avery OT, MacLeod CM, McCarty M: Studies on the chemical nature of the substance inducing transformation of pneumococcal types. *J Exp Med* 79:137–157, 1994.

Intramuscular Injections Within 30 Days of Immunization With Oral Poliovirus Vaccine: A Risk Factor for Vaccine-Associated Paralytic Poliomyelitis

Strebel PM, Ion-Nedelcu N, Baughman AL, Sutter RW, Cochi SL (Ctrs for

Disease Control and Prevention, Atlanta, Ga; Ministry of Health, Bucharest, Romania)
N Engl J Med 332:500–506, 1995 119-96-1-2

Background.—Children in Romania have an unusually high rate of vaccine-associated poliomyelitis. In Romania, febrile illness in infants is commonly treated with antibiotic injection. The association between IM injections and the onset of poliovirus infection was investigated in Romanian children who had paralytic polio.

Method.—Thirty-one children who had polio were included in the cohort group; 18 had been vaccinated for poliomyelitis, and 13 had acquired the disease by contact. A control group of age-matched children was evaluated for comparison. Sociodemographic and medical record data were collected. The dates of administration of the oral polio vaccine (OPV) and the diphtheria and tetanus toxoids and pertussis vaccine were noted. The risk of paralysis associated with injection in relation to the date of vaccination and the attributable risk in the population were calculated. Statistical analysis was performed with use of the Wilcoxon rank-sum statistic.

Results.—The onset of paralysis occurred after 1 dose of OPV in 94% of the vaccinated children. Children with acquired disease were less likely than controls to have been vaccinated. All children with vaccine-associated polio had received at least 1 IM injection during the month before onset of paralysis, compared with 66% of the controls. The highest risk occurred in vaccinated children who received 10 or more injections during that time. Injections given after OPV was administered were associated with a very high risk of polio infection, whereas injections given before or simultaneously with OPV had no significant effect. Administration of penicillin G was strongly associated with paralysis. The minor polio illness occurred in 32% of the study cohort. The attributable risk in the population for an injection given within 30 days of paralysis onset was 86%.

Discussion.—Intramuscular injection appears to be related causally to vaccine-related paralytic poliomyelitis in Romanian children. The timing and type of injection also affects the risk. To reduce the incidence of paralysis in this group of children, IM-injectable antibiotics should be replaced with oral or IV preparations.

► Children who received OPV were 17 times as likely to have paralytic disease if they also received IM injections. Wild-type polio has now been eradicated from the Americas, but rare paralytic disease caused by other enteroviral infections and, in rare instances, by vaccine strains still exists. This study reinforces a recommendation that IM injections be avoided for 30 days after OPV administration. It is important to emphasize that subcutaneous diphtheria and tetanus toxoids and pertussis vaccine did not increase the risk of paralysis. Romania, where the study was carried out, is somewhat of an anomaly because large amounts of IM antibiotics, especially penicillin G, are used there. In this country, the newly proposed recommendation to precede oral polio immunization with killed (Salk) vaccine should greatly reduce the instance of vaccine-strain illness.

G.L. Mandell, M.D.

Group A Streptococcal Necrotizing Fasciitis Complicating Primary Varicella: A Series of Fourteen Patients

Brogan TV, Nizet V, Waldhausen JHT, Rubens CE, Clarke WR (Univ of Washington, Seattle)

Pediatr Infect Dis J 14:588–594, 1995 119-96-1-3

Background.—Group A *Streptococcus* necrotizing fasciitis may be occurring with increasing frequency. The successful management of this life-threatening infection depends on rapid diagnosis and treatment. The clinical course and treatment of 14 children who had group A *Streptococcus* necrotizing fasciitis as a complication of varicella were reviewed.

Methods.—The charts of 10 boys and 4 girls, aged 6 months to 10 years, who had group A *Streptococcus* necrotizing fasciitis and varicella during 16 months were reviewed. Information was obtained on the patients and the clinical course, symptoms, therapies, and outcome.

Results.—The children had varicella exanthem for a median of 3 days before the secondary symptoms developed. Initial symptoms of necrotizing fasciitis most frequently included erythema, focal pain, temperature higher than 38.5°C, and localized swelling. Diagnosis was delayed in 8 patients who were discharged with other diagnoses. After proper diagnosis and admission, all patients were given parenteral antibiotics before surgery; therapy included clindamycin and a penicillin. Definitive diagnosis was achieved in all patients with surgical exploration, in which a full thickness incision, including the muscle fascia, was used. All necrotic tissue was débrided surgically. Fasciotomies were performed if symptoms suggested a compartment syndrome. Two patients required skin grafting. Tissue cultures from all patients were positive for group A *Streptococcus*; 2 patients had positive blood cultures. Complications in 5 patients included hypotension, tachycardia, and oliguria, which were managed with fluid and ionotropic support. Twelve patients also received 2–6 treatments of adjunctive hyperbaric oxygen therapy at 12-hour intervals; the treatments were associated with reduced erythema and swelling in 6 patients. The length of stay was 6–28 days.

Conclusions.—The outcome was excellent, even in the 8 patients in whom diagnosis was delayed. Surgery is the basis of both diagnosis and treatment of group A *Streptococcus* necrotizing fasciitis. The benefits of other therapeutic modalities are difficult to assess. Further study should examine the role of clindamycin and hyperbaric oxygen therapy. Primary care physicians should be familiar with the signs of group A *Streptococcus* necrotizing fasciitis and its association with primary varicella.

▶ There are several interesting aspects of this paper to discuss. First, chickenpox is not always a benign disease. The increasing incidence of severe streptococcal disease complicating chickenpox is another reason to recommend immunization for all children who have not had chickenpox.

The patients did well, and there were no deaths. This is a potentially lethal disease, and the authors applied aggressive therapy that should be examined. Consensus and experience tells us that antibiotics, surgery, and fluid support are the mainstays of therapy. In animal models, clindamycin is more effective than penicillin, and the most frequent recommendation made is to combine clindamycin and penicillin. I know of no data that demonstrate the efficacy of hyperbaric oxygen in this condition. Many clinicians would use IV immunoglobulin, because of its potential activity in neutralizing group A streptococcal toxins that can function as superantigens. There are no convincing data of its efficacy.

G.L. Mandell, M.D.

Acute Epiglottitis in Children: Results of a Large-Scale Anti-*Haemophilus* Type B Immunization Program

Wurtele P (Centre Hospitalier Honoré Mercier, Saint Hyacinthe, Québec)

J Otolaryngol 24:92–97, 1995 119-96-1–4

Introduction.—In 1988, a PRP-D anti–*Haemophilus influenzae* type B (anti-HiB) vaccine was introduced into the vaccination schedule of children aged 18 months in Quebec. A significant reduction in the occurrence of acute epiglottitis was observed. Since 1992, new vaccines (PRP-T, HbOC, PRP-OMPC) have been given to infants at age 2 months. The impact of both anti-HiB vaccination programs on the incidence rates of acute epiglottitis in children in Quebec was evaluated.

Methods.—All pertinent data on the incidence of pediatric epiglottitis from 1984 to 1993 were retrieved from the Med-Echo system, an extensive provincial database system in Quebec. The results for 1992 represented the combined effect of the PRP-D vaccine and the new vaccines.

Results.—The incidence rate for the entire pediatric population (children aged 0–19 years) in Quebec decreased from 5.7 per 100,000 children/year in 1986–1987 to 1.7 per 100,000 children/year in 1992–1993. The incidence rate in the nonvaccinated population (children aged 7–19 years) remained stable. The changes in the global pediatric population were limited to preschool children. The vaccines effected a progressive decrease in the incidence of acute epiglottitis (Fig 1). Fifteen children in the group aged 0–6 years had acute epiglottitis during 1993 compared with a yearly average of 97 children during 1984–1987. This rate corresponds to 15.4% of the former level.

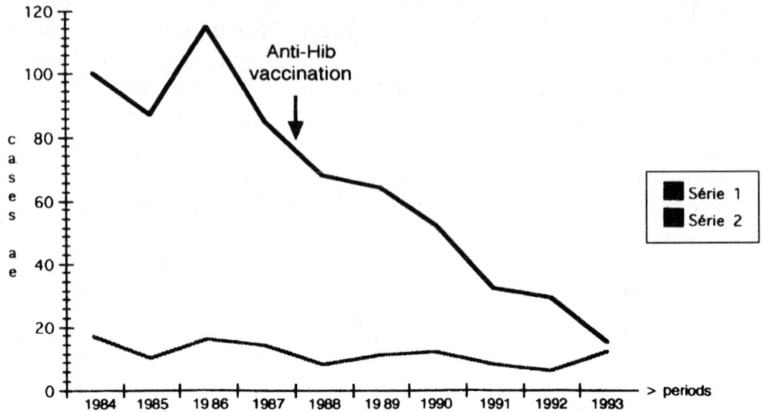

FIGURE 1.—Line 1 depicts the positive impact of the anti–*Haemophilus influenzae* type B vaccination on preschoolers (age, 0–6 years). Line 2 shows that the incidence of the disease among school children and adolescents is fairly stable (age, 7–19 years). (Courtesy of Wurtele P: Acute epiglottitis in children: Results of a large-scale anti-*Haemophilus* type B immunization program. *J Otolaryngol* 24:92–97, 1995.)

Conclusions.—The efficacy of the anti-HiB immunization program in preventing acute epiglottitis was estimated to be 86.4%. Acute epiglottitis continues to be a life-threatening illness, however, which justifies the need for unceasing vigilance.

▶ This article contains more wonderful data concerning the efficacy of immunization against *H. influenzae* type B. Prior studies documented the marked decrease in incidence of meninigitis; this study shows a similar effect (Fig 1) for epiglottitis. Remember that nontypeable strains, for which the vaccine gives no protection, represent the second most common cause of otitis media, bronchitis, and pneumonia in adults.

G.L. Mandell, M.D.

High Incidence of *Haemophilus influenzae* in Nasopharyngeal Secretions and Middle Ear Effusions as Detected by PCR

Ueyama T, Kurono Y, Shirabe K, Takeshita M, Mogi G (Oita Med Univ, Japan)
J Clin Microbiol 33:1835–1838, 1995 119-96-1–5

Introduction.—A sensitive and specific method for detecting bacteria in middle ear effusions (MEEs) is necessary to determine the relationship between bacterial infection and the pathogenesis of otitis media with effusion (OME). The P6 protein (a 16.6-kD outer membrane protein of *Haemophilus influenzae*) has been shown to be a potential vaccine component in preventing infections caused by *H. influenzae*. Newly designed oligonucleotide probes were used in dot blot hybridization tests to differentiate the P6 gene DNA of *H. influenzae* from that of *H. parainfluenzae*.

2 Common Infections

Introduction

Although the first article in this section discusses otitis media, it has strong implications for other pneumococcal infections. In this day of molecular biology and gene therapy, it is fascinating to read a paper (Abstract 119-96-2–2) in which "probing for bone" is the diagnostic breakthrough.

Gerald L. Mandell, M.D.

Comparison of PCR Assay With Bacterial Culture for Detecting *Streptococcus pneumoniae* in Middle Ear Fluid of Children With Acute Otitis Media

Virolainen A, Salo P, Jero J, Karma P, Eskola J, Leinonen M (Natl Public Health Inst, Helsinki; Univ of Helsinki)

J Clin Microbiol 32:2667–2670, 1994 119-96-2–1

Introduction.—Methods of gene amplification, such as polymerase chain reaction (PCR), are increasingly used to diagnose microbial infections. Pneumolysin is a species-specific protein toxin produced intracellularly by all clinically relevant pneumococcal strains. To improve the etiologic diagnosis of acute otitis media (AOM), a newly developed PCR assay was used for the first time to detect pneumolysin DNA in middle ear fluid (MEF) samples in children who had AOM.

Methods.—A total of 180 MEF samples from 125 children who had 125 episodes of AOM were analyzed with the use of the newly developed pneumococcal PCR for *Streptococcus pneumoniae.* The results were compared with those of bacterial culture. For pneumococcal PCR assay, DNA from MEF samples was extracted by phenol-chloroform. A 348–base-pair region of the pneumolysin gene was amplified by the outer primers, and a 208–base-pair region was amplified by the inner primers.

Results.—Among the 180 MEF samples, *S. pneumoniae* was cultured in 33 (18%), and pneumolysin PCR was positive for 51 (28%). Only 2 of 21 PCR-positive, *S. pneumoniae* culture–negative samples were positive for other otitis media pathogens. Of the 33 *S. pneumoniae* culture–positive

MEF samples, 30 (91%) were positive by PCR; the other 3 samples showed no evidence of inhibitors of the amplification reaction, and all pneumococcal strains isolated from these samples contained pneumolysin DNA. By combining MEF culture and PCR results, 54 MEF samples (30%) had evidence of pneumococcal etiology.

Conclusion.—Pneumolysin PCR is a sensitive and specific new method to study pneumococcal involvement in MEF samples from children who have AOM. The results are available the next day, which is 1 day earlier than by routine culture of *S. pneumoniae*. However, PCR assay is more expensive, and culture is still needed to obtain strains for antimicrobial susceptibility testing and for serotyping of *S. pneumoniae*. At this time, pneumolysin PCR cannot be used routinely but can be helpful in research.

▶ In studies of patients with community-acquired pneumonia, pneumococcal antigen–detection assays usually double the number of cases attributed to infection with this organism. These studies suggest that the same ratio holds in otitis media. The authors found that culture detected *Pneumococcus* in 18% of MEF samples, and PCR increased that number to 30%.

A portion of the pneumolysin gene appeared to be a good choice for PCR. Although the role of pneumolysin in the pathogenesis of *Pneumococcus* is unclear, this protein is found in all strains that cause disease. We do not really know why the *Pneumococcus* is so fastidious and so difficult to grow even in a modern microbiology laboratory, but that is the case. This article adds support to the concept that pneumococcal disease of the lung, sinus, and middle ear is twice as common as the culture indicates.

G.L. Mandell, M.D.

Probing to Bone in Infected Pedal Ulcers: A Clinical Sign of Underlying Osteomyelitis in Diabetic Patients

Grayson ML, Gibbons GW, Balogh K, Levin E, Karchmer AW (Harvard Med School, Boston)

JAMA 273:721–723, 1995 119-96-2–2

Introduction.—In pedal infections, the differentiation between soft-tissue infection alone and infection complicated by osteomyelitis is often difficult. The presence of bone in the depths of infected pedal ulcers in patients who have diabetes may be indicative of osteomyelitis. Exposed, but not visible, bone in the ulcer can be accurately identified by gently probing the ulcer base with a sterile, blunt probe during the initial wound evaluation. The relationship between the presence of palpable bone by probing and the presence of osteomyelitis was examined prospectively.

Study Design.—Seventy-five hospitalized patients with diabetes who had 76 infected foot ulcers were included. A sterile, blunt, stainless steel probe was used to examine the ulcer for the presence of palpable bone, described as a rock-hard, often gritty structure at the ulcer base without the apparent presence of any intervening soft tissue.

TABLE 1.—Comparison of Diagnostic Techniques in the Identification of Pedal Osteomyelitis in Patients With Diabetes

Investigation	Source	Sensitivity, %	Specificity, %	Positive Predictive Value, %
Probe to bone	Current study	66	85	89
Plain radiograph	References10–13, 17	28–93	50–92	74–87
Technetium-99m bone scan	References 10–14, 17–19	68–100	18–79	43–87
Indium-111 leukocyte scan	References 10, 12, 14, 15, 18, 19	45–100	67–89	75–85
Magnetic resonance imaging	References 13–15, 20	29–100	78–89	50–93

Note: Reference articles may be found in original tearsheet article.

(Courtesy of Grayson ML, Gibbons GW, Balogh K, et al: Probing to bone in infected pedal ulcers: A clinical sign of underlying osteomyelitis in diabetic patients. *JAMA* 273;721–723, 1995.)

Results.—Osteomyelitis, defined histopathologically and/or clinically, was diagnosed in 50 foot ulcers (66%) and was excluded in 26. Bone was palpable by probing in 33 ulcers (66%) that had contiguous osteomyelitis, compared with only 4 ulcers that did not; the difference was significant. As an indication of underlying osteomyelitis, palpable bone on probing the ulcer base had a sensitivity of 66%, a specificity of 85%, a positive predictive value of 89%, and a negative predictive value of 56% (Table 1).

Conclusion.—Palpation of bone in the depths of infected pedal ulcers in patients who have diabetes is strongly correlated with the presence of underlying osteomyelitis. If bone is palpated with gentle probing, evaluation may proceed directly to microbiological and histologic confirmation of osteomyelitis, either by percutaneous needle biopsy or open débridement, without performing roentgenographic and radionuclide tests. Probing for bone should be part of the routine initial assessment of infected pedal ulcers in patients who have diabetes.

► What a simple, elegant concept! One of the major problems in treating patients with pedal ulcers (most frequently seen in patients who have diabetes) concerns the differentiation between soft tissue infection and bone infection. The most common clinical scenario is a deep, soft tissue ulcer in the foot of a patient who has diabetes with an x-ray film that does not show obvious bony involvement. The x-ray film is a relatively insensitive predictor of bone involvement. Karchmer and colleagues found that blunt-probe tactile contact with bone is a very strong indicator of the presence of osteomyelitis. Table 1 indicates that although this technique is not very sensitive, it is highly specific and has a high positive predictive value. Positive bone probe tests will often be an indication for a bone biopsy, so that the microbiology of the bony infection can be ascertained with accuracy.

G.L. Mandell, M.D.

Randomized Controlled Trial of Appendicectomy Versus Antibiotic Therapy for Acute Appendicitis

Eriksson S, Granström L (Karolinska Inst, Danderyd, Sweden)

Br J Surg 82:166–169, 1995 119-96-2–3

Objective.—Although the concept of conservative antibiotic treatment for acute appendicitis is not new, it is still controversial. There have been no prospective, randomized trials of this therapy. The results of antibiotic and surgical treatment were compared in patients who had acute appendicitis in a randomized pilot trial.

Methods.—Forty patients who had acute appendicitis were included. All were admitted to the hospital with abdominal pain that lasted less than 72 hours. They were selected randomly to receive antibiotic treatment, which included 2 days of IV antibiotics followed by 8 days of oral treatment, or surgery. The IV antibiotic treatment consisted of 2 g of cefotaxime every 12 hours and 800 mg of tinidazole daily; oral treatment included 200 mg of ofloxacin twice daily and 500 mg of tinidazole twice daily. Patients in the antibiotic group who had suspected recurrent appendicitis were treated surgically.

Results.—One patient in the antibiotic group required surgery 12 hours after admission because of peritonitis that resulted from perforated appendicitis. The remaining 19 were discharged after 2 days; 7 of the 19 were readmitted within 1 year because of recurrent appendicitis. All underwent surgery, which confirmed the diagnosis of appendicitis. In these patients, including 1 who had perforated appendicitis, the diagnostic accuracy was 85%.

Conclusions.—For patients who have acute appendicitis, antibiotic treatment is as effective as surgery, with less pain and less need for analgesia. The rate of recurrent appendicitis, however, is high. Larger studies are needed to confirm the superiority of antibiotics.

► I have vague memories of old World War II movies in which the corpsman (or perhaps the cook) in a submarine performed an appendectomy via radio instructions. Too bad antibiotics were not available in the early part of the war. I would like to highlight the authors' conclusion: "Antibiotic treatment of patients with acute appendicitis was as effective as surgery. The patients had less pain and required less analgesia, but recurrence rate was high." This was a relatively small study, with only 20 patients in each group. Note that in addition to typical history and clinical signs, increase in white blood cell count and positive findings by ultrasonography were required. The authors administered tinidazole (which is similar to metronidazole) plus cefotaxime. Recurrent infection was the major drawback of antibiotic therapy, occurring in 7 of 21 patients who received antibiotics. I would like to think of appendicitis in ways that we think of other infections, i.e., antibiotic therapy would be expected to be curative except in those patients in whom there is necrosis or significant formation of pus. Modern imaging techniques will probably help in this analysis.

G.L. Mandell, M.D.

3 Sepsis

Introduction

After reading the paper concerning streptococcal superantigen (Abstract 119-96-3–2), refer back to Chapter 1 for these infections seen in children with chickenpox (Abstract 119-96-1–3).

Gerald L. Mandell, M.D.

Efficacy and Safety of Monoclonal Antibody to Human Tumor Necrosis Factor α in Patients With Sepsis Syndrome: A Randomized, Controlled, Double-Blind, Multicenter Clinical Trial

Abraham E, for the TNF-α MAb Sepsis Study Group (Univ of Colorado, Denver)

JAMA 273:934–941, 1995 119-96-3–1

Background.—The mortality rate associated with septic shock remains high in the United States, despite the development of new antimicrobial therapies. Neutralization of tumor necrosis factor–α (TNF-α) with TNF-α monoclonal antibody (TNF-α MAb) may decrease the mortality rate in patients who have sepsis syndrome. The efficacy and safety of TNF-α MAb evaluated in a prospective, double-blind trial.

Method.—Patients who had sepsis syndrome for less than 12 hours were assigned to either the shock or the nonshock group. They were selected randomly to receive a single dose of 15 mg of TNF-α per kg, 7.5 mg of TNF-α per kg, or a placebo. Nine hundred seventy-one patients received an IV infusion of the study drug. Data were evaluated with the use of pairwise comparisons and Cochran-Mantel-Haenszel χ^2 tests.

Results.—Among patients in the nonshock group, TNF-α MAb showed no efficacy. Those in the shock group who received TNF-α MAb showed a trend toward a reduced mortality rate. No decrease in mortality rate occurred in placebo and TNF-α patients. There was no significant difference in mortality rate between patients in the shock group who received placebo and who received TNF-α MAb treatment.

Discussion.—Therapy with TNF-α MAb appears to reduce the mortality rate in patients who have sepsis syndrome and shock.

▶ I am afraid that this is yet another negative study for therapy of sepsis syndrome. The authors' key finding is that no overall decrease in mortality rate resulted from TNF-α MAb. However, as in many studies in which immunomodulators were used in sepsis syndrome, there was a suggestion that a subgroup benefited from therapy. This subgroup concept has tantalized investigators and biotechnical companies.

The challenge is to prospectively identify a group of patients that will gain significant benefit from this and similar therapies. It has been suggested that these subgroups can be identified by measurements of cytokine profiles. Hopefully, these assays could be done in a very short period in patients selected for therapy. Thus, MAb to TNF-α joins antibodies to endotoxins and interleukin-1 receptor antagonist as therapies that were promising but which showed no overall benefit in patients with sepsis syndrome.

G.L. Mandell, M.D.

▶ The variety of pharmacotherapeutic approaches that are in development or in some phase of a clinical trial attest to the complexity of sepsis, sepsis syndrome, and septic shock. In biotechnology alone there are compounds for bacterial lipopolysaccharide (LPS) neutralization, polyvalent LPS, lipid A analogue, and anticytokine approaches that include murine and humanized TNF monoclonal antibodies, interleukin-1 (IL-1) inhibitors, bradykinin antagonists, platelet-activating factor inhibitors, immunostimulants, and antiadhesion molecule antibodies.[1] Proinflammatory cytokines such as IL-1 and TNF are known to have a central role in inflammatory responses; monoclonal antibodies to TNF-α and soluble TNF receptor can block various acute and chronic responses of inflammatory disease in animal models,[2] and the availability of anticytokine antibodies has made the therapeutic use of antibodies in human disease practical.[3] Trials of murine anti–TNF-α monoclonal antibodies have reported some transient improvement but, also, side effects that investigators believed could limit usefulness.[4, 5]

Abraham has pointed out that the difficulty in affecting outcome in patients with sepsis may be less a reflection of the potency of new therapies than an indication of the complex pathophysiologic processes of sepsis.[6] Some investigators have said that anticytokine therapeutics are much more complex than was first believed.[7] This abstracted study by Abraham et al. represents work going forward on the basis of what is currently known about the role of elaborated cytokines in sepsis syndrome. Progress is in the form of small steps, but it continues.

R.C. Bone, M.D.

References

1. Highfield PE: Sepsis: The more the murkier. *Biotechnology* 12:828, 1994.
2. Lee JC, Laydon JT, McDonnell PC, et al: A protein kinase involved in the regulation of inflammatory cytokine biosynthesis. *Nature* 372:739–746, 1994.

3. Wherry JC, Pennington JE, Wenzel RP, et al: Tumor necrosis factor and the therapeutic potential of an anti-tumor necrosis factor antibody. *Crit Care Med* 21:436S–440S, 1993.
4. Fisher CJ, Opal SM, Dhainaut J-F, et al: Influence of an anti-tumor necrosis factor monoclonal antibody on cytokine levels in patients with sepsis. *Crit Care Med* 21:318–327, 1993.
5. Vincent JL, Bakker J, Morecaux G, et al: Administration of anti-TNF antibody improves left ventricular function in septic shock patients: Results of a pilot study. *Chest* 101:810–815, 1992.
6. Abraham E, Raffin TA: Sepsis therapy trials: Continued disappointment or reason for hope (editorial). *JAMA* 271:54–65, 1994.
7. NIH Conference: Selected treatment strategies for septic shock based on proposed mechanisms for pathogenesis. *Ann Intern Med* 120:771–783, 1994.

Selective Depletion of Vβ-Bearing T Cells in Patients With Severe Invasive Group A Streptococcal Infections and Streptococcal Toxic Shock Syndrome

Watanabe-Ohnishi R, Low DE, McGeer A, Stevens DL, Schlievert PM, Newton D, Schwartz B, Kreiswirth B, Ontario Streptococcal Study Project, Kotb M (Univ of Tennessee, Memphis; VA Med Ctr, Memphis, Tenn; Mount Sinai Hosp, Toronto; et al)

J Infect Dis 171:74–84, 1995 119-96-3–2

Introduction.—Reports of severe infection with group A *Streptococcus* have increased recently. Because of clinical features similar to those seen with staphylococcal toxic shock syndrome (TSS), these infections have been termed streptococcal toxic shock–like syndrome. Streptococcal toxins, found in isolates from patients who have streptococcal TSS, are related to bacterial proteins known as superantigens. These superantigens interact with the variable β region of the T-cell receptor (TCR Vβ). To date, however, there has been no direct evidence for the role of streptococcal superantigens in streptococcal TSS and severe group A streptococcal infections. The role of superantigens in streptococcal TSS was determined by correlating streptococcal TSS, Vβ profile, and group A streptococcal toxins.

Methods.—Twenty patients who had documented or suspected gram-positive coccal infections were studied. Expression of TCR Vβ in peripheral blood mononuclear cells was analyzed with the use of reverse-transcriptase polymerase chain–based technique. Peripheral mononuclear cells were also analyzed for evidence of apoptosis.

Results.—Group A streptococcal infection was confirmed in 15 patients. Six of these cases were streptococcal TSS and 7 were invasive and 2 were noninvasive group A streptococcal infection. Five cases of invasive group A streptococcal infection were considered severe, and 2 were not severe. One additional patient had a highly probable group A streptococcal infection. Compared with healthy control individuals, patients who had severe group A streptococcal infection showed no evidence of Vβ overexpression. Patients who had streptococcal TSS and severe invasive group A streptococcal infection, however, showed a significant reduction in the percentage of expression of 3 Vβ families: Vβ1 (2.25 vs. 6.7 for controls), Vβ5.1 (0.88 vs. 3.8 for controls), and Vβ12 (0.83 vs. 2.4 for controls). No significant differences in expression of Vβ were found between patients who had nonsevere group A streptococcal infections and control individuals. In 1 patient with severe toxic shock in whom no isolate could be identified, all 3 Vβ products showed depletion. Evidence for apoptosis was found in peripheral blood mononuclear cells from 8 of 9 patients who had documented or suspected severe group A streptococcal infection.

Discussion.—A streptococcal superantigen appears to be involved in the pathogenesis of severe group A streptococcal infections. This streptococcal superantigen had a specificity for 3 Vβ products—Vβ1, Vβ5.1, and Vβ12—and differed from the in vitro Vβ specificity of known streptococcal superantigens, which indicated the presence of a novel superantigen.

▶ The most attractive hypothesis to explain the severe and often fatal illness associated with *Streptococcus pyogenes* infections implicates superantigens. Several streptococcal toxins can function as superantigens. A superantigen has the ability to interact with a TCR in such a way as to bypass the normal antigen binding site. Therefore, superantigens can activate large numbers of T cells and induce immune hyperactivity with release of inflammatory cytokines, thereby resulting in a severe sepsis syndrome. Superantigens do not stimulate all T cells but, rather, preferentially stimulate human TCR Vβ. In animals, T-cell clones interacting with superantigens are frequently reduced in number, thus supporting the concept that depletion of certain clones of T cells is a "footprint" of a superantigen. The therapeutic implication of superantigen disease lies in the possibility that antibody to the superantigen (which may be found in normal pools of immunoglobulin) would prevent the superantigen from activating T cells. This is an unproved hypothesis.

G.L. Mandell, M.D.

4 Nosocomial Infections

Introduction

This field of research requires never-ending vigilance. Nosocomial infections are a moving target, as indicated by these selections.

Gerald L. Mandell, M.D.

Postoperative Infections Traced to Contamination of an Intravenous Anesthetic, Propofol
Bennett SN, McNeil MM, Bland LA, Arduino MJ, Villarino ME, Perrotta DM, Burwen DR, Welbel SF, Pegues DA, Stroud L, Zeitz PS, Jarvis WR (Centers for Disease Control and Prevention, Atlanta, Ga; Texas Dept of Health, Austin)
N Engl J Med 333:147–154, 1995 119-96-4–1

Introduction.—In May and June of 1990, the Centers for Disease Control and Prevention (CDC) were informed of a sudden and simultaneous onset of postoperative infections of the bloodstream, surgical sites, or other sites that involved a variety of organisms at hospitals in 4 states. The outbreaks were traced to the use of propofol, a newly introduced anesthetic agent. This sterile, white, nonpyrogenic, oil-based IV anesthetic was manufactured in the United States and approved by the Food and Drug Administration. It has been used since 1989 in the induction and maintenance of anesthesia. The results of investigations in 7 hospitals were reported.

Methods.—A case-control or cohort study was performed at each hospital. The operating room and anesthesia practices were reviewed, the surgical procedures were observed, written questionnaires were administered, and infection control policies were reviewed. All available isolates from each patient, the environment, and hospital personnel were sent to the CDC for identification.

Results.—Forty-nine of 62 patients who met case definitions underwent surgery during an epidemic period. The attack rate was significantly higher during the epidemic period than in the period preceding it. The epidemic periods lasted from 2 to 65 days (median, 11 days). Postoperative infectious complications were significantly associated with the receipt of propofol at all the hospitals investigated. Specific anesthesiologists and nurse-anesthetists were epidemiologically associated with postoperative infections. Lapses in aseptic technique by anesthesia personnel were reported or observed. The following etiologic agents were isolated: *Staphylococcus aureus, Candida albicans, Moraxella osloensis, Enterobacter agglomerans,* and *Serratia marcescens.* The cultures of unopened ampules of propofol from hospitals were negative. Ampules used at the time of outbreaks were not available in most hospitals for analysis. At 2 hospitals, propofol syringes were available for culture. They were positive with organisms identical to those of case patients who received propofol from the syringes.

Conclusions.—Patients who received propofol for general anesthesia or sedation should be watched carefully for infection or fever. Any acute febrile episode in patients who received propofol should be reported to the state health department. Lipid-based medications support rapid bacterial growth at room temperature and must be handled with strict aseptic techniques.

▶ This lipid-based anesthetic turned out to be a fertile culture medium for microbes. Breaches in technique that would not have resulted in infection with other agents were amplified with this agent and resulted in a multicenter outbreak. There are several important messages in this article. First, be alert for instances of unexplained fever and infection and try to determine the connecting thread. Second, lipid-based medications are inherently more dangerous regarding risk of infection than are non–lipid-based medications. Single-use vials are an effective preventive strategy.

G.L. Mandell, M.D.

Nasal Carriage of *Staphylococcus aureus* as a Major Risk Factor for Wound Infections After Cardiac Surgery

Kluytmans JAJW, Mouton JW, Ijzerman EPF, Vandenbroucke-Grauls CMJE, Maat AWPM, Wagenvoort JHT, Verbrugh HA (Univ Hosp, Rotterdam, The Netherlands; Univ Hosp, Utrecht, The Netherlands)

J Infect Dis 171:216–219, 1995 119-96-4–2

Purpose.—In patients who undergo thoracic surgery, sternal wound infections can lead to significant morbidity and mortality. At the study institution, most of these infections result from *Staphylococcus aureus.* Cross-infection does not seem to be an important mode of transmission, which suggests that many infections are caused by endogenous *S. aureus* strains. Nasal carriage of *S. aureus* was studied as a risk factor for poststernotomy surgical wound infections.

Methods.—The case-control study included 1,980 consecutive patients who underwent sternotomy for cardiac surgery from 1988 through 1990. All patients had nasal swabs taken for microbiological study on the day before surgery. The case group included 40 patients who had a sternal wound infection in which cultures yielded *S. aureus*. Their findings were compared with those of 120 control patients matched by proximity of the operation date.

Results.—Ninety percent of the sternal wound infections were deep. The significant risk factors for *S. aureus* sternal wound infection were preoperative nasal carriage of this organism, present in 53% of case patients vs. 13% of control patients; insulin-dependent diabetes mellitus, present in 10% of case patients vs. none of the control patients; and younger age, with a mean of 59 years in case patients vs. 64 years in control patients. The crude odds ratio for preoperative nasal carriage was 9.6. Median length of postoperative stay was 40 days in case patients vs. 10 days in control patients, and mortality rate was 10% vs. .8%.

Conclusions.—Preoperative nasal carriage of *S. aureus* is a significant and independent risk factor for sternal wound infection with this organism. The risk attributable to nasal carriage is 86%. Further studies are needed to evaluate the efficacy of perioperative elimination of nasal carriage in reducing surgical wound infection rates.

▶ In patients who have postoperative staphylococcal infections, our first instincts might be to wonder which health care provider was the culprit. Was it the surgeon, the surgical nurse, the attendants, or the anesthesiologist? This is not altogether irrational, because data suggest that staphylococcal infection is usually acquired directly from humans rather than from contaminated surfaces or fomites. In this report, the authors document beautifully that the human who transmitted the infection was the patient himself. They found an impressive association of nasal carriage of *S. aureus* with wound infection after cardiac surgery, with an odds ratio of 9.6 in case patients compared with controls. Phage typing in all 10 cases in which the preoperative nasal isolate could be compared with the causative organism in the wound indicated that the isolates were identical.

Older studies have documented the association of nasal carriage of *S. aureus* with higher rate of postoperative *Staphylococcus* infections. The obvious next step is to eliminate nasal carriage, probably with a topical agent such as mupirocin, and see what this does to the rate of staphylococcal infection. Of note, these patients with wound infection were all given prophylactic antibiotics, and their infection rate was almost 2% for *S. aureus*.

G.L. Mandell, M.D.

The Risk for Transmission of *Mycobacterium tuberculosis* at the Bedside and During Autopsy

Templeton GL, Illing LA, Young L, Cave MD, Stead WW, Bates JH (John L McClellan VA Hosp, Little Rock, Ark; Univ of Arkansas, Little Rock; Arkansas Dept of Health, Little Rock)

Ann Intern Med 122:922–925, 1995 119-96-4-3

Introduction.—Hospital personnel present at autopsy can be at considerable risk for acquiring tuberculosis, despite the low risk for infection among health care workers who care for patients with tuberculosis before death.

> *Case Report.*—Man, 57, was admitted with a diagnosis of postural hypotension secondary to autonomic dysfunction; dehydration contributed to his weakened, cachectic condition. His medical history included anemia; adenocarcinoma of the prostate, which was treated with radical prostatectomy and radiation; and abuse of alcohol and tobacco. No recognizable infection was present, and the patient showed no signs of recurrent malignancy. He was successfully treated for a urinary tract infection on hospital day 6. Ten days later, the patient became dyspneic and less responsive. Findings included ascites, pulmonary infiltration, and pleural effusions, which were thought to be caused by congestive heart failure or hepatic cirrhosis. Intradermal skin tests for tuberculosis did not produce a reaction at 48 hours. The patient died on hospital day 21, and a postmortem examination was done.

Findings.—At autopsy, hundreds of tubercle bacilli were found in the lung, hilar lymph nodes, spleen, peritoneum, kidneys, testes, brain, and vertebral bodies. Cultures of all tissues and of the blood and ascitic fluid obtained 5 days before death were positive for *Mycobacterium tuberculosis*. An epidemiologic investigation was then initiated. Because tuberculosis was not suspected, no respiratory precautions had been taken by the 47 health care workers who came in contact with the patient. None of the 40 workers in this group who did not react had converted to positive on tuberculin testing 8 weeks after the patient's death. Among the 10 hospital personnel in the autopsy room, however, all 5 nonreactors converted from negative to positive and were treated with rifampin and/or isoniazid. Isolates from the patient and the 2 autopsy personnel with positive induced sputum results had identical DNA fingerprints.

Discussion.—During the autopsy, the air was contaminated inordinately with tubercle bacilli because of the extent of disease dissemination. Tuberculosis had run an acute course, instead of the usual chronic progression. The 2 individuals who had positive cultures of induced sputum were among the 4 workers who spent the most time (2–3 hours) in the autopsy room.

► Tuberculosis is one of the classic airborne diseases. Patients are usually not considered to be at great risk as transmitters of infection if they do not have pulmonary or airway involvement and cough. Therefore, it was somewhat of a surprise to me to see the very high rate of infectivity in an autopsy suite. A partial explanation appears to be the use of an oscillating bone saw, which apparently is an efficient aerosolizer of microbes. It was very interesting to note that on the wards that did not have isolation precautions, there were no instances of transmission, even after a 21 day hospitalization, as contrasted with the autopsy room infectivity rate of 100%.

G.L. Mandell, M.D.

Recommendations for Preventing the Spread of Vancomycin Resistance: Recommendations of the Hospital Infection Control Practices Advisory Committee (HICPAC)

The Hospital Infection Control Practices Advisory Committee (Ctrs for Disease Control and Prevention, Atlanta, Ga)

Am J Infect Control 23:87–94, 1995 119-96-4–4

Introduction.—From 1989 through 1993, hospitals in the United States reported a rapid increase in the incidence of infection and colonization with vancomycin-resistant enterococci (VRE). Patients in ICUs significantly contributed to the overall increase, but a trend was also noted among patients who were not in ICUs. Public health concerns led to meetings in 1993 and 1994, convened by the Centers for Disease Control and Prevention (CDC) and attended by representatives from the American Hospital Association and various medical societies. Recommendations of the Hospital Infection Control Practices Advisory Committee of the CDC were presented.

Recommendations.—Hospitals were urged to develop a comprehensive strategic plan to prevent, detect, and control infection and colonization with VRE. Five main elements were recommended for inclusion in the institution-specific plans: prudent use of vancomycin, continuing education programs, establishment of the microbiology laboratory as the first line of defense against spread of VRE in the hospital, aggressive control measures to limit nosocomial spread of VRE, and routine antimicrobial susceptibility testing, together with confirmation and reporting of VRE infection or colonization to the CDC and state health department.

All hospitals and other health care delivery services should develop a comprehensive plan regarding the use of antimicrobial agents to educate the medical staff. Guidelines regarding the proper use of the agent also should be developed. Specific examples of situations in which vancomycin is appropriate or should be discouraged were provided. In addition, detailed recommendations were offered concerning the role and practices of the microbiology laboratory, including screening procedures. Prevention and control were stressed, and isolation precautions were advised to prevent patient-to-patient transmission of VRE.

Discussion.—The recent increase in the incidence and colonization of VRE poses several problems, including the lack of available antimicrobials for treatment of VRE infection and the potential for vancomycin-resistance genes to be transferred to other gram-positive microorganisms. Although most enterococcal infections have been attributed to endogenous sources within the individual patient, recent reports show that patient-to-patient transmission can also occur. Prevention and control of VRE will require the coordinated efforts of various hospital departments and all personnel involved in patient care.

▶ The spread of vancomycin resistance has frightened many of us. Currently, the only significant strains of vancomycin-resistant gram-positive bacteria that cause infections in hospitals have been enterococci. Infections with these organisms can be very difficult to treat, and various experimental regimens are being investigated. Enterococci are less virulent pathogens than many other gram-positive bacteria, and infections have been limited in large part to hospitalized patients with severe impairments in host defense. The spread of vancomycin resistance to highly virulent organisms, such as *Pneumococcus* or *Staphylococcus aureus,* is a frightening prospect. We are already challenged with pneumococcal and staphylococcal infections in which vancomycin is the only consistently effective antibiotic.

The CDC has put together this outline to prevent the development and spread of vancomycin resistance. Several points should be emphasized. When organisms are susceptible to β-lactam antibiotics, such as penicillin and cephalosporins, and to vancomycin, then therapy should be initiated with β-lactam agents for 2 reasons. First, the data suggest that the β-lactams are more rapidly bactericidal and more effective clinically. Second, use of vancomycin increases the potential for development of resistance. Antibiotic-associated colitis therapy should be initiated with oral metronidazole. Vancomycin should be reserved for failures or especially severe cases. Routine prophylaxis with vancomycin should not be used.

G.L. Mandell, M.D.

5 Miscellaneous Infections

Introduction

This potpourri of selections addresses viral, fungal, and bacterial infections, and an unusual reaction to infection (vasculitis).

Gerald L. Mandell, M.D.

Infective Endocarditis in Patients With Negative Blood Cultures: Analysis of 88 Cases From a One-Year Nationwide Survey in France

Hoen B, Selton-Suty C, Lacassin F, Etienne J, Briançon S, Leport C, Canton P (Centre Hospitalier Universitaire de Nancy, France; Hôpital Cardiologique, Lyon, France; Centre Hospitalier Universitaire Bichat, Paris)

Clin Infect Dis 20:501–506, 1995 119-96-5–1

Background.—In up to 10% of cases of infective endocarditis (IE), patients will have a negative blood culture. To determine the clinical features and reasons for this finding, 88 cases of blood culture–negative IE were examined and compared with blood culture–positive IE cases.

Method.—Patients responded to a detailed questionnaire concerning this medical history. Questions regarding previous heart disease, existence of prosthetic valves, current IE episode, and previous positive blood cultures were included. Each case was evaluated with the use of von Reyn's criteria. When evaluation of 620 cases revealed a blood culture–negative rate of 15%, all medical charts of patients who had a negative blood culture were reviewed for additional information. At least 1 blood culture was found positive in 82% of cases, and all blood cultures were found negative in 88 cases (14%). These 88 cases were compared with blood culture–positive cases of IE. Data were interpreted with the use of the Mann-Whitney U test, Pearson's χ^2 test, and Fisher's exact test.

Results.—Prosthetic valve replacement occurred in 32% of patients who had a negative blood culture. High-grade fever (> 39°C) occurred in 13 patients; medium-grade fever in 57; low-grade or no fever (< 38°C) in 17. The mean number of blood cultures performed was 9 ± 4 for the 88 patients, but 42 (48%) had received antibiotic therapy before blood for culture was drawn. Seven patients who had not received antibiotic therapy before blood was drawn had high IgG and IgA titers to *Coxiella burnetti.* The in-hospital mortality rate was higher in patients who had authentic negative blood cultures. Thirteen patients died, for an overall mortality rate of 15%. Patients who had a negative IE blood culture tended to have a prosthetic valve, more left-sided involvement, and more surgery.

Discussion.—Some of the blood culture–negative cases in this series may have resulted from noninfective inflammatory endocarditis. Patients who have suspected IE should not undergo antibiotic therapy before blood cultures are drawn, and large volumes of blood for culture should be drawn over a long interval.

► One of the perennial questions in the field of infectious diseases relates to causative organisms in patients suspected of having IE in whom the blood cultures are negative. This very nice study gives us a modern, although partial, answer. Of their 88 patients with presumed endocarditis (620 total cases and 14% with negative blood cultures), the causative organism is identified only in 15. In 7, the causative organism was considered to be Q fever; in 2 others it was chlamydial infection. Perhaps more important were the 5 cases in which surgically removed valves were cultured. Three of these yielded coagulase-negative *Staphylococcus;* 1 a *Streptococcus* species; 1, a *Corynebactium* species; and 1; a *Propionibacterium* species. Thus, the clinical answer to the question is that once you have ruled out certain unusual organisms by serologic technique (*Chlamydia, Coxiella, Legionella, Bartonella*), you should treat for unusual gram-positive pathogens.

The recommendation of vancomycin plus gentamicin (usually with the addition of high-dose penicillin) makes sense. Note that nearly half the patients with blood culture–negative endocarditis received antibiotic therapy before blood cultures. This strongly suggests that many of these patients had infection with common organisms that were suppressed but not eliminated.

G.L. Mandell, M.D.

Diagnosis of Histoplasmosis by Antigen Detection During an Outbreak in Indianapolis, Ind

Williams B, Fojtasek M, Connolly-Stringfield P, Wheat J (Indiana Univ, Indianapolis; Wishard Mem Hosp, Indianapolis, Ind; Veterans Affairs Hosp, Indianapolis, Ind)

Arch Pathol Lab Med 118:1205–1208, 1994 119-96-5–2

Introduction.—*Histoplasma capsulatum* var *capsulatum* antigen detection has been used for the diagnosis of histoplasmosis. The sensitivity of the test for the diagnosis of various manifestations of histoplasmosis was reevaluated during a recent outbreak of the disease.

Methods.—Patients who underwent *H. capsulatum* var *capsulatum* antigen testing and had compatible clinical findings of histoplasmosis were identified retrospectively. Four clinical groups were identified: patients who had disseminated histoplasmosis and AIDS, patients who had disseminated histoplasmosis but did not have AIDS, patients who had chronic pulmonary histoplasmosis, and patients who had self-limited syndromes. Laboratory methods used for diagnosis of histoplasmosis included positive cultures or fungal stains, positive immunodiffusion or complement fixation tests with titers at least 1:8, or positive tests for blood or urine *H. capsulatum* var *capsulatum* antigen.

Results.—Of 252 patients who had positive test results for histoplasmosis, 195 were eligible for the study. One hundred eight patients had disseminated histoplasmosis, 70 had self-limited syndromes, 14 had chronic pulmonary histoplasmosis, and 3 had asymptomatic infection. Ninety-seven patients who had disseminated histoplasmosis, 5 who had self-limited syndromes, 4 who had chronic pulmonary histoplasmosis, and 1 who had asymptomatic histoplasmosis were immunosuppressed. Antigen tests were more sensitive in patients who had disseminated histoplasmosis, with 92% (99/108) of patients positive for antigen compared with 21% of patients who had chronic pulmonary histoplasmosis and 39% who had self-limited syndromes. Serologic testing was positive for 71% (57/80) of patients who had disseminated histoplasmosis, 100% of those who had chronic pulmonary histoplasmosis, and 98% of those who had self-limited syndromes. Culture results were positive in 85% (90/106) of patients who had disseminated histoplasmosis, 85% of those who had chronic pulmonary histoplasmosis, and 15% of those who had self-limited syndromes.

Discussion.—The *H. capsulatum* var *capsulatum* antigen test was most sensitive in the diagnosis of disseminated histoplasmosis and less sensitive for the detection of chronic pulmonary and self-limited syndromes of histoplasmosis. The test also had a slightly higher sensitivity for patients who had AIDS compared with nonimmunosuppressed patients who had disseminated histoplasmosis. Serologic testing for both the chronic pulmonary and self-limited forms of histoplasmosis and culture of respiratory secretions for pulmonary infections appear to be the more sensitive means of testing for diagnosis.

► Dr. Joseph Wheat and colleagues from Indiana University are to be congratulated on the development of a highly useful clinical test for histoplasmosis. Selection of this article allows us to examine the outbreak in Indianapolis but, perhaps of broader interest, it allows us to review the efficacy and indications for the diagnostic test. Approximately half the patients in this cluster also had AIDS. The authors did not convince me that this was a true outbreak, i.e., data for years before and after the study were not included, but that quibble may be a semantic one. There were a lot of cases of histoplasmosis.

Important points to emphasize are that the Wheat test is an antigen-detection test and, thus, is not dependent on the host immune response. As would be anticipated in an antigen-detection test, patients with the most severe (disseminated) disease had the highest rate of positivity, and those with both AIDS and disseminated disease had the highest rates of positivity (95%). Urine was a more reliable source of antigen than was serum. The authors quote unpublished data to state that 75% of patients with severe acute pulmonary disease will have antigen in their serum or urine. Antigen tests are highly specific. Asymptomatic patients with positive tests for antigen have not been identified. In patients with self-limited disease, the antigen positivity is low, and diagnosis of histoplasmosis should be based on biopsy, culture, and serologic studies.

G.L. Mandell, M.D.

Serogroup C Meningococcal Outbreaks in the United States: An Emerging Threat

Jackson LA, Schuchat A, Reeves MW, Wenger JD (Ctrs for Disease Control and Prevention, Atlanta, Ga)

JAMA 273:383–389, 1995 119-96-5–3

Objective.—Outbreaks of disease caused by serogroup C *Neisseria meningitidis* have been reported from many areas of the United States in recent years. Information on all such outbreaks occurring from 1980 through mid-1993 was sought by using MEDLINE, by reviewing the records of the Centers for Disease Control and Prevention, and by questioning state health department authorities, infectious disease experts, and the manufacturer of meningococcal vaccine.

Definition.—An outbreak was defined as the occurrence of at least 3 cases of serogroup C meningococcal disease within 3 months either in a community or within a school or other institution. The minimum attack rate accepted was 5/100,000 population.

Findings.—Twenty-one outbreaks were recorded, but only 5 were reported in the medical literature. Eleven outbreaks occurred in schools or institutions, whereas 10 occurred in the community. School cases tended to be clustered closely in time, in contrast to community cases. In 5 outbreaks, additional cases occurred after a vaccination program was instituted. Both the number of outbreaks and the extent of vaccination campaigns tended to increase over time. In 11 of 13 instances, all isolates from a given outbreak were identical.

Implications.—Outbreaks of serogroup C meningococcal disease are becoming more prevalent in the United States, and vaccination efforts are increasing to a corresponding degree. Effective vaccination campaigns rely on early and accurate recognition of outbreaks.

► Sporadic meningococcal disease with multiple outbreaks is still a problem in this country. Meningococcal vaccine, which is a quadravalent polysaccharide vaccine that is protective against serogroups A, C, Y, and W135, is not routinely used. Its efficacy is poor in children younger than 2 years of age (who have a high risk of meningococcal disease), and immunity from vaccination appears to be limited. In addition, the overall rates of meningococcal disease are low. Immunization is recommended in response to certain outbreaks. Of note, more than half the cases of meningococcal disease in this country are caused by serogroups not covered in the available vaccine, especially group B. There is no good explanation as to why group C outbreaks are becoming more common. Close contacts of patients with meningococcal disease should receive preventive therapy with rifampin. Adults should be given 600 mg every 12 hours in 4 dosages. Children should be given 10 mg/kg every 12 hours in 4 dosages. For adults, ciprofloxacin in a single dose of 750 mg is also effective.

G.L. Mandell, M.D.

Can Respiratory Syncytial Virus and Influenza A Be Distinguished Clinically in Institutionalized Older Persons?

Wald TG, Miller BA, Shult P, Drinka P, Langer L, Gravenstein S (Univ of Wisconsin, Madison; State Lab of Hygiene, Madison, Wis; Wisconsin Veterans Home, King)

J Am Geriatr Soc 43:170–174, 1995 119-96-5-4

Background.—Respiratory syncytial virus (RSV), the most common cause of lower respiratory tract illness in infants and young children, has also been associated with a clinically significant, influenza-like illness in residents of long-term care facilities and nursing homes. When an outbreak of illness occurs in a nursing home population, it is important to determine whether the cause is RSV or influenza because the routes of transmission and treatments differ. Concurrent outbreaks of RSV and influenza were studied to determine whether the 2 diseases can be distinguished clinically.

Methods.—The outbreaks occurred during the winter of 1991–1992 in a rural Wisconsin nursing home. A prospective surveillance study for the prevention of influenza was being conducted when RSV illnesses were detected. A total of 287 illnesses developed in 215 individuals during the study.

Findings.—The organisms isolated were influenza A/Victoria-like in 32 patients, RSV in 9, and herpes simplex virus in 6. The disease conditions caused by influenza A and RSV were similar: No single upper respiratory symptom was diagnostic for either virus. The patients who had influenza were more likely to have extrarespiratory symptoms. There was no difference in median duration of illness.

Conclusions.—The clinical illnesses associated with influenza A and RSV infection are similar. If cultures are not taken, patients who have RSV infection may be assumed to have influenza. Comparison of individual symptoms cannot distinguish between the 2 diseases, although patients who have RSV infection have more frequent extrarespiratory involvement. Through analysis of the frequency of these symptoms and the use of rapid antigen detection kits, it may be possible to use amantadine more effectively and apply more specific infection control methods when outbreaks of respiratory illness occur in nursing homes.

▶ The answer to the title question is no. Although the number of patients in the study, especially those with RSV, was small, there were some trends that were suggestive but not significant. For example, fever was seen more commonly in the influenza patients (90%) as compared with the RSV patients (57%), whereas gastrointestinal symptoms were noted in 38% of the influenza patients and in none of the RSV patients. This report emphasizes that RSV is not just a pediatric disease but is a relatively common cause of respiratory illness in nursing homes.

G.L. Mandell, M.D.

Cytomegalovirus Vasculitis: Case Reports and Review of the Literature

Golden MP, Hammer SM, Wanke CA, Albrecht MA (New England Deaconess Hosp, Boston; Harvard Med School, Boston)

Medicine 73:246–255, 1994 119-96-5–5

Introduction.—Infection with cytomegalovirus (CMV) can manifest as several clinical syndromes. Patients most at risk for active infection include neonates, allograft recipients, and those with immunosuppression. The virus also appears to have specificity for vascular endothelium, which results in local vasculitis and tissue damage. Gastrointestinal lesions, meningoencephalitis, pneumonitis, and skin ulcerations can result from CMV-associated vasculitis. Reported cases of CMV vasculitis were described, and the literature was reviewed.

Patients and Findings.—A review of the records from a single institution of patients who had CMV isolated from vascular tissue revealed 4 well-documented cases of CMV vasculitis. A diagnosis of vasculitis was based on pathologic findings of vascular involvement with necrosis, luminal compromise, and tissue damage. Vasculitis was found only in conjunction with CMV-infected endothelial cells, which indicated that the initial event was infection with CMV. Three of 4 cases described intestinal lesions; 1 of these patients, who was HIV positive, died. The fourth case described an HIV-positive patient who had a history of opportunistic infections, including CMV retinitis and viral colitis positive for herpes simplex virus and CMV. Pathologic examination after lung biopsy revealed CMV pneumonitis with vasculitis and vessel-wall necrosis. After initial response to ciprofloxacin and ganciclovir, CMV hepatitis, worsening of CMV retinitis, sepsis, and pneumonia developed; the patient eventually died of intracranial bleeding. Autopsy revealed CMV retinitis and encephalitis. Although there was no histologic evidence of CMV on examination of lung tissue, CMV inclusions in abnormal vessels with tissue damage implicated CMV as a primary pathogen. A review of the literature found the gastrointestinal tract, CNS, and skin to be the 3 organs most commonly involved in CMV-associated vasculitis. Eight of 16 patients described in the literature had died.

► Vasculitis has long been associated with infectious agents. Rocky Mountain spotted fever represents an acute, severe vasculitis caused by endothelial invasion by the infecting microbe. Other types of vasculitis are thought to be caused by immune mechanisms, such as the vasculitis associated with hepatitis C infection. The cases of CMV vasculitis described in this study appear to be the result of direct invasion of the endothelial cells by the virus. Cytomegalovirus infection is ubiquitous but quiescent in most of us. Immunosuppression frequently results in CMV disease, and CMV vasculitis is an uncommon type of CMV disease. One cannot help but think that most of the long list of eponymous vasculitities described in textbooks eventually will be found to involve infectious agents.

G.L. Mandell, M.D.

Viridans Streptococcal Bacteraemia in Patients With Neutropenia

Richard P, Del Valle GA, Moreau P, Milpied N, Felice M-P, Daeschler T, Harousseau J-L, Richet H (Hôtel-Dieu, Nantes, France; Faculté de Chirurgie Dentaire, Nantes, France)

Lancet 345:1607–1609, 1995 119-96-5–6

Background.—Viridans streptococcal bacteremia is common in patients who have neutropenia and is associated with a 10% to 15% mortality rate. The risk factors for viridans streptococcal bacteremia in this patient population were investigated in a case-control study.

Methods and Findings.—Twenty-five patients who had neutropenia and viridans streptococcal bacteremia were compared with a control group of 64 randomly selected patients who had neutropenia but did not have the bacteremia. The 2 groups were hospitalized at the same time. The patient group included 15 women and 10 men (median age, 47 years). The groups were similar in age, sex, duration and nature of hematologic disease, severity and duration of neutropenia, exposure to invasive procedures, and mucositis occurrence. Independent risk factors for streptococcal bacteremia were exposure to repeated chemotherapy or cytarabine. The use of carboxyureidopenicillins and a stay in laminar airflow rooms had a protective effect. In a different cohort of 49 patients, all 7 patients who had bacteremia had recovery of oral streptococci with the same ribotype as blood isolates.

Conclusions.—The oral mucosa appears to be the entry portal for viridans streptococci, thereby causing bacteremia in patients who have neutropenia. The use of first-line antibiotic regimens directed against gram-positive species may be appropriate in patients at high risk, especially those repeatedly exposed to aggressive chemotherapy. Alternatively, local oral prophylaxis may be cost-effective for preventing streptococcal infections.

► The term viridans streptococci describes a group of related organisms, including *Staphylococcus mitis, S. oralis,* and *S. sanguis.* The viridans streptococci are the most common cause of bacterial endocarditis. Other infections caused by these organisms were unusual until recent years, when they were found to be important pathogens for patients with neutropenia. It has been assumed that systemic prophylaxis with agents that had poor gram-positive activity would increase the risk of these infections, and that probably is true. Therefore, prophylaxis with a fluoroquinolone is effective in reducing gram-negative infections but may result in a relative increase in gram-positive infections, including those caused by viridans streptococci. This report, however, is different in that the prophylactic regimen used included oral vancomycin, polymyxin, and tobramicin. This regimen would be expected to be active against many gram-positive organisms.

G.L. Mandell, M.D.

6 HIV and Related Infections

Introduction

There still has been no big breakthrough in prevention or treatment of HIV infections, although the selections in this chapter illustrate some small victories.

Gerald L. Mandell, M.D.

Multiple False Reactions in Viral Antibody Screening Assays After Influenza Vaccination

Simonsen L, Buffington J, Shapiro CN, Holman RC, Strine TW, Grossman BJ, Williams AE, Schonberger LB (Ctrs for Disease Control and Prevention, Atlanta, Ga; American Red Cross, Washington DC; Natl American Red Cross, Rockville, Md)

Am J Epidemiol 141:1089–1096, 1995 119-96-6–1

Background.—In December 1991, blood centers in the United States reported an unusual increase in blood donations that tested falsely reactive for antibodies to 2 or more of several viruses, including HIV type 1, human T-cell lymphotrophic virus type I (HTLV-I), and hepatitis virus. Because many of these donations were from individuals who had recently received influenza vaccination, the vaccine may have caused this problem. The events that led to this increase were investigated in a large-scale, case-control study.

Methods and Findings.—One hundred one affected donors and a control group of 191 matched individuals were included. Recent vaccination with any brand of influenza vaccine was significantly correlated with a multiple false positive test result. A history of recent acute illness and of allergies was also associated with multiple false positive results. In a review of monthly rates of multiple reactive donations between May 1990 and December 1992, the seasonal cluster of multiple false positive donations was linked with the use of viral screening test kits that were thought to react nonspecifically to donor IgM. No increase in multiple false positive donations was noted during the 1992 to 1993 influenza vaccination season after the HIV-1 and hepatitis C virus tests were replaced, but the number of donations falsely reactive for HTLV-I nearly doubled, which demonstrated that false reactivity was not associated exclusively with the 1991–1992 influenza vaccine. When affected donors were retested, the duration of HTLV-I and hepatitis C virus false reactivity was found to range from 3 to 6 months.

Conclusions.—The receipt of 1991–1992 influenza vaccine was strongly correlated with multiple false positive results in viral antibody screening tests at that time. No single brand caused this dramatic increase. The cluster of multiple false positive donations most likely resulted from the test kits used, not from the influenza vaccine.

► A false positive HIV test result can be a disconcerting episode to say the least. The conclusion of the investigators was that although influenza immunization was related to the false positive results, it was not caused by a "fault" of the influenza vaccine. The proposed mechanism involved an increase in IgM antibodies to influenza immunization, which falsely reacted to the tests for HTLV-1 and hepatitis C used at that time. When the tests were replaced with more modern tests, the false positive results disappeared.

G.L. Mandell, M.D.

Detection of Herpesvirus-Like DNA Sequences in Kaposi's Sarcoma in Patients With and Those Without HIV Infection

Moore PS, Chang Y (Columbia Univ, New York)
N Engl J Med 332:1181–1185, 1995 119-96-6–2

Introduction.—Unique DNA sequences associated with Kaposi's sarcoma in patients who have AIDS have been identified. It is not certain whether these sequences suggest a new human herpesvirus. The presence of these herpesvirus-like DNA sequences was determined in tissue samples from patients who had AIDS-associated Kaposi's sarcoma, patients who had classic Kaposi's sarcoma, and HIV-seronegative homosexual men who had Kaposi's sarcoma.

Methods.—Tissue specimens were obtained from lesions and uninvolved skin at the time of biopsy. Control skin samples were obtained during elective plastic surgery from patients who did not have Kaposi's sarcoma or AIDS. Control samples of peripheral-blood mononuclear cells were obtained from healthy, HIV-seronegative donors. A polymerase chain reaction analysis for $KS330_{233}$ was done on all DNA samples.

Results.—Sarcoma tissue was available from 11 patients who had AIDS-associated Kaposi's sarcoma, 6 patients who had classic Kaposi's sarcoma, and 4 HIV-seronegative homosexual men who had Kaposi's sarcoma. Ten patients who had AIDS-associated Kaposi's sarcoma were either homosexual or bisexual. The other man reportedly was infected through heterosexual activities. Five patients who had classic Kaposi's sarcoma were men who reported no homosexual activity or drug use and were seronegative for HIV at biopsy. All patients who had AIDS-associated Kaposi's sarcoma had depressed CD4+ T-cell counts, compared with normal counts in the other 2 groups. Tissue samples were positive for $KS330_{233}$ in 10 of 11 samples from patients who had AIDS-associated Kaposi's sarcoma, all 6 samples from patients who had classic Kaposi's sarcoma, and all 4 samples from HIV-seronegative homosexual men who had Kaposi's sarcoma. Tissue samples of uninvolved skin were positive for $KS330_{233}$ in 3 of 14 patients who had Kaposi's sarcoma; 13 of these patients had lesions positive for $KS330_{233}$. One of 21 control samples was positive for $KS330_{233}$. A second evaluation with the polymerase chain reaction of the positive control sample was negative.

Conclusion.—The herpesvirus-like DNA sequence may have an etiologic role in the development of Kaposi's sarcoma in patients who have and those who do not have HIV infection. Because these DNA sequences are also found in lesions from women and heterosexual men who have Kaposi's sarcoma, male homosexual activity cannot be the exclusive mode of transmission.

Human Herpesvirus-Like Nucleic Acid in Various Forms of Kaposi's Sarcoma

Huang YQ, Li JJ, Kaplan MH, Polesz B, Katabira E, Zhang WC, Feiner D, Friedman-Kien AE (New York Univ Med Ctr; North Shore Univ Hosp, Manhasset, NY; State Univ of New York Health Science Ctr, Syracuse; et al)
Lancet 345:759–761, 1995 119-96-6–3

Introduction.—Previous studies have reported detection of DNA sequences of what appears to be a new human gamma-herpes–like virus in patients who have AIDS-associated Kaposi's sarcoma. Various forms of Kaposi's sarcoma were examined with the use of polymerase chain reaction (PCR) for the occurrence of the DNA sequences of this herpeslike virus.

Methods.—Thirty specimens of Kaposi's sarcoma, including 10 from African endemic cases, 12 AIDS-associated samples from the United States, and 8 classic Kaposi's sarcoma specimens, were collected. Control specimens were obtained from 12 biopsies of uninvolved skin from the patients who had AIDS and from 10 biopsies of normal skin from HIV-negative patients who underwent plastic surgery. Two samples from Africa were HIV-1–positive, and 2 were HIV-2–positive. Fresh tissues or 5-μm sections of formalin-fixed, paraffin-embedded specimens were used for extraction of DNA. Only specimens that showed an amplified *p53* gene by PCR were included for further study.

Results.—With the use of a primer pair specific for the herpesvirus-like DNA in the PCR reaction, the predicted 233–base-pair band was detected in all 12 AIDS-associated Kaposi's lesions, 7 of 8 classic lesions, and 7 of

10 African specimens. The herpesvirus-like DNA was identified in both positive and negative specimens for HIV-1 and HIV-2. Samples from 2 patients who had AIDS-associated Kaposi's sarcoma, but none of the samples of normal skin from individuals who were HIV-1 negative, demonstrated the herpesvirus-like DNA. Varied patterns of shifted bands observed at single-strand conformational polymorphism analysis and by direct sequencing suggest that the nucleic-acid variations differed among samples. Alterations in nucleic acid were least common in the specimens of classic Kaposi's sarcoma.

Conclusion.—The unique herpeslike virus detected in these investigations may have a role in the pathogenesis of different forms of Kaposi's sarcoma. Because the tumor is most prevalent in homosexual men and is rarely seen in patients infected with HIV by heterosexual sex, IV drug use, or blood transfusion, AIDS-associated Kaposi's sarcoma may be a sexually transmitted disease independent of HIV.

▶ That Kaposi's sarcoma is much more frequent in homosexuals with AIDS in comparison with IV drug abusers with AIDS has suggested that the neoplasm is caused by an agent other than HIV. These important studies (Abstracts 119-96-6–2 and 119-96-6–3) implicate a herpeslike virus as the etiologic agent for Kaposi's sarcoma associated with AIDS, the classic Kaposi's sarcoma (elderly men of Mediterranean, Middle Eastern, or Eastern European origin), and homosexual men who are HIV negative. If this is a sexually transmitted herpesvirus, it is hard to understand the association of classic Kaposi's sarcoma with elderly men of a certain ethnic group. The technique involved probing for a 233–base-pair sequence, which had previously been found in Kaposi's sarcoma in patients with AIDS. The finding of this sequence in the 3 different types of Kaposi's sarcoma is highly suggestive that the agent is causative and not merely an opportunistic pathogen.

G.L. Mandell, M.D.

Herpesvirus-Like DNA Sequences in Patients With Mediterranean Kaposi's Sarcoma

Dupin N, Grandadam M, Calvez V, Gorin I, Aubin JT, Havard S, Lamy F, Leibowitch M, Huraux JM, Escande JP, Agut H (Pitié Salpêtrière Hosp, Paris; Tarnier Hosp, Paris)

Lancet 345:761–762, 1995 119-96-6–4

Introduction.—The frequent occurrence of Kaposi's sarcoma in patients who have HIV infection, along with its association with other immunodeficiency syndromes, suggests that a sexually transmitted infectious agent may cause this malignancy. Skin biopsy specimens from 5 patients who had Mediterranean Kaposi's sarcoma and 4 who had AIDS-associated Kaposi's sarcoma were examined by polymerase chain reaction (PCR) for the presence of herpesvirus-like sequences.

Methods.—Biopsy specimens of lesions and adjacent skin from the 9 patients were analyzed without knowledge of the underlying disease. The patients who had Mediterranean Kaposi's sarcoma were negative for HIV antibodies by enzyme-linked immunosorbent assay. In addition, 6 specimens from HIV-seronegative patients who did not have Kaposi's sarcoma were examined for DNA sequences.

Results.—The amplification of β-globin gene DNA was positive in all 9 samples from patients who had Mediterranean or AIDS-associated Kaposi's sarcoma, which suggests the absence of major PCR inhibitors in DNA samples. All lesions also exhibited herpesvirus-like sequences, as did all but 1 of the samples of clinically normal skin adjacent to the Kaposi's lesions. As expected, HIV-1 provirus DNA was not detected in any samples from the HIV-1–negative patients who had Mediterranean Kaposi's sarcoma. Four Kaposi's lesions and 3 normal skin samples from the HIV-positive patients yielded HIV-1 provirus DNA. For both patient groups, the quantity of herpesvirus-like DNA was consistently higher in Kaposi's lesions than in normal skin, whereas the proviral HIV load was identical in all skin samples from patients who had AIDS. Tissue from a control group of patients who did not have Kaposi's sarcoma showed neither HIV-1 provirus nor herpesvirus-like DNA.

Conclusion.—Herpesvirus-like DNA sequences were detected both in HIV-negative patients who had Mediterranean Kaposi's sarcoma and in patients who had AIDS-associated Kaposi's sarcoma. The lesions in these 2 groups exhibited a higher load of herpesvirus-like DNA than did normal adjacent skin. These findings strongly argue for the existence of an infectious agent closely related to gamma-herpesvirus in the pathogenesis of Kaposi's sarcoma.

► The authors of this article report more patients with Kaposi's sarcoma associated with AIDS and Mediterranean Kaposi's sarcoma who have the herpesvirus-like sequence. Of interest, the investigators found that the virus is present in uninvolved skin. The latter finding supports the concept that the virus is not merely a superinfector of the tumor.

G.L. Mandell, M.D.

Suspected *Pneumocystis carinii* Pneumonia With a Negative Induced Sputum Examination: Is Early Bronchoscopy Useful?

Huang L, Hecht FM, Stansell JD, Montanti R, Hadley WK, Hopewell PC (Univ of California, San Francisco)

Am J Respir Crit Care Med 151:1866–1871, 1995 119-96-6–5

Background.—Pneumonia caused by *Pneumocystis carinii* is a frequent indicator of AIDS. Specimens for microscopic evaluation usually are obtained through sputum induction or bronchoscopy with bronchoalveolar lavage (BAL). The value of bronchoscopy in light of a negative induced sputum analysis was determined.

Methods.—All analyses of sputum inductions in patients who had known or suspected *P. carinii* infection during a 4-year period were reviewed. Specimens were obtained through bronchoscopy, BAL, or trans-

TABLE 1.—Pathogens and Potential Pathogens From 602 Bronchoscopic Evaluations Performed After a Negative Sputum Examination for *Pneumocystis Carinii*

	Bronchoscopies		Coexistent *P. carinii*	
	(*n*)	(*% of total*)	(*n*)	(*% of diagnosis*)
Pathogen				
Pneumocystis carinii	192	31.9		
Kaposi's sarcoma	93	15.4	25	26.9
Mycobacterium tuberculosis	28	4.7	2	7.1
Cryptococcus neoformans	9	1.5	3	33.3
Histoplasma capsulatum	6	1.0	2	33.3
Coccidioides immitis	3	< 1.0	1	33.3
Legionella species	3	< 1.0	1	33.3
Strongyloides stercoralis	2	< 1.0	0	
Nocardia asteroides	1	< 1.0	0	
Toxoplasma gondii	1	< 1.0	0	
Total	338		34	
Potential pathogen				
M. avium complex	84	14.0	67	79.8
Aspergillus species	58	9.6	11	19.0
Mycobacterium kansasii	6	1.0	2	33.3
Mycobacterium xenopi	2	< 1.0	1	50.0
Bordetella pertussis	1	< 1.0	1	100.0
Total	151		82	

(Courtesy of Huang L, Hecht FM, Stansell JD, et al: Suspected *Pneumocystis carinii* pneumonia with a negative induced sputum examination: Is early bronchoscopy useful? *Am J Respir Crit Care Med* 151:1866–1871, 1995.)

bronchial biopsy and were processed according to standard laboratory protocol. The records of patients who had a negative sputum analysis for *P. carinii* and did not undergo subsequent bronchoscopy were also analyzed. Outcomes were determined at follow-up as a function of treatment.

Results.—Induced sputum examination was positive in 46.6% of patients. Bronchoscopy after a negative induced sputum examination produced a diagnosis 50% of the time. Tuberculosis and other infections caused by mycobacteria were cultured frequently, but fungi were cultured rarely. Other diagnoses included pneumonia with *Cryptococcus neoformans* and tracheobronchial Kaposi's sarcoma (Table 1). No serious complications, such as hemorrhage or pneumothorax, occurred. Bronchoscopy was not performed if another diagnosis was made, the patient died, or the patient refused. After a negative result with BAL, empiric treatment for *P. carinii* was discontinued.

Discussion.—If a patient has suspected pneumonia caused by the opportunist *P. carinii*, early bronchoscopy with BAL is advisable after a negative induced sputum analysis for the organism.

▶ The specificity of induced sputum for making a diagnosis of *P. carinii* pneumonia is excellent and probably approaches 100%. However, the sensitivity is variable. In this San Francisco General Hospital study, induced sputum examination was positive for *P. carinii* in 800 of 1,716 episodes of suspected *P. carinii* pneumonia, for a 46.6% positivity rate. Of those patients with negative sputum examinations, 31.9% were found to be positive on bronchoscopy with BAL. Not all patients had bronchoscopy after negative sputum examination. The authors calculate a sensitivity of induced sputum for detecting *P. carinii* pneumonia of 75% to 80%. Therefore, a patient with a positive sputum examination usually does not require bronchoscopy, but a patient with a negative sputum examination does.

G.L. Mandell, M.D.

A Randomized Trial Comparing Fluconazole With Clotrimazole Troches for the Prevention of Fungal Infections in Patients With Advanced Human Immunodeficiency Virus Infection

Powderly WG, for the NIAID AIDS Clinical Trials Group (Washington Univ, St Louis, Mo)

N Engl J Med 332:700–705, 1995 119-96-6–6

Introduction.—Among patients who have HIV infection, serious fungal infections, such as cryptococcal meningitis, are common. The orally active triazole antifungal agent fluconazole is effective in the long-term suppression of many fungal infections. Its effectiveness as a method of primary prophylaxis, which remains unclear, was evaluated prospectively.

Methods.—Four hundred twenty-eight patients who had advanced HIV infection were enrolled. All patients were also participants in a randomized trial of primary prophylaxis against *Pneumocystis carinii* pneumonia. The patients were selected randomly to receive either fluconazole, 200 mg/day, or clotrimazole in 5 daily 10-mg troches. The patients' status was followed for a median of 35 months.

Results.—Invasive fungal infections developed in 4% of patients in the fluconazole group compared with 11% of those in the clotrimazole group. After adjustment for the CD4+ cell count, the relative hazard was 3.3. Seventeen of 32 invasive fungal infections were cryptococcosis. All but 2 of these cases occurred in the clotrimazole group, for an adjusted relative hazard of 8.5. Fluconazole was more effective for patients who had CD4+ cell counts of 50/mm^3 or less. Esophageal candidiasis was also less frequent in the fluconazole group, with an adjusted relative hazard of 5.8. The rate of confirmed and presumed oropharyngeal candidiasis was 6 cases per 100 person-years of follow-up in the fluconazole group vs. 38 cases in the clotrimazole group. There was no significant difference in survival.

Conclusions.—For patients who have advanced HIV infection, prophylactic fluconazole reduces the frequency of fungal infections, including cryptococcosis, esophageal candidiasis, and superficial infections. The benefits of fluconazole are greatest for patients who have a CD4+ lymphocyte count of 50/mm^3. Compared with clotrimazole troches, however, prophylactic fluconazole does not reduce the overall mortality rate.

► It was disappointing to see that fluconazole prophylaxis, as compared with clotrimazole troches, did not reduce the mortality rate. However, fungal infections, including cryptococcosis, esophageal candidiasis, oral thrush, and vaginitis, can all have a severely negative impact on the quality of life.

Fluconazole was very effective in reducing the incidence of these conditions. Four potential negative factors are cost of therapy, development of resistance to fluconazole, fluconazole toxicity, and fluconazole interactions with other agents. None of these factors were significant in the study, but the potential for harm must be continually evaluated. The authors indicate that 11,756 doses of fluconazole were given to prevent each case of invasive fungal infection. According to the Wiley International Dictionary of Medicine and Biology, a troche is a trochiscus, a morsulus, a rotulais, a lozenge. More people understand lozenge, but the medical literature insists on using troche.

G.L. Mandell, M.D.

A Randomized Trial of Three Antipneumocystis Agents in Patients With Advanced Human Immunodeficiency Virus Infection

Bozzette SA, for the NIAID AIDS Clinical Trials Group (Univ of California, San Diego)

N Engl J Med 332:693–699, 1995 119-96-6–7

Background.—Several chemoprophylactic regimens can prevent *Pneumocystis carinii* pneumonia and enhance survival in patients who have advanced HIV infection. Each of these regimens, including trimethoprim-sulfamethoxazole, aerosolized pentamidine, and dapsone, has advantages and disadvantages. The 3 regimens were studied for their effectiveness in preventing first episodes of *P. carinii* pneumonia in patients who had HIV infection.

Methods.—The open-label trial included 843 patients who had HIV infection and a CD4+ cell count of less than 200/mm^3. All patients received zidovudine. In addition, they were selected randomly to receive initial chemoprophylaxis with trimethoprim-sulfamethoxazole, dapsone, or aerosolized pentamidine. For patients in whom intolerance developed, these agents were followed by a specified sequence of other drugs.

Results.—The 36-month cumulative risk of *P. carinii* pneumonia was 18% with trimethoprim-sulfamethoxazole, 17% with dapsone, and 21% with aerosolized pentamidine. There was little or no difference for patients whose CD4+ cell count was 100/mm^3 or more at baseline. For patients who had lower CD4+ cell counts, however, the risk was 19% with trimethoprim-sulfamethoxazole and 22% with dapsone, compared with 33% for aerosolized pentamidine. Treatment failure was least likely in patients who received trimethoprim-sulfamethoxazole and more likely in those who received 50 mg vs. 100 mg of dapsone. The rate of toxoplasmosis was less than 3%. Fewer than one fourth of patients assigned to the 2 systemic therapies were still taking their assigned drug and dose at the end of the study. All 3 groups had a median survival of approximately 39 months. The mortality rate from *P. carinii* pneumonia was only 1%.

Conclusions.—The 3 chemoprophylaxis techniques studied have similar effectiveness in preventing *P. carinii* pneumonia in patients who have advanced HIV disease. For patients who have CD4+ lymphocyte counts of less than 100/mm^3, it is best to start with trimethoprim-sulfamethoxazole or high-dose dapsone than with aerosolized pentamidine. To optimize therapy for these patients, it might be better to try to limit intolerance to trimethoprim-sulfamethoxazole or to reserve this chemoprophylactic approach for the most vulnerable patients.

► This is yet another article that shows the superiority of trimethoprim-sulfamethoxazole over aerosolized pentamidine for prophylaxis of *P. carinii* pneumonia in patients infected with HIV. The differences were magnified in those patients at greatest risk, i.e., those with fewer than 100 CD4 cells. In patients who are intolerant of trimethoprim-sulfamethoxazole, use dapsone, 50 mg, twice daily. The recent US Public Health Service/Infectious Disease Society of America guidelines for the prevention of opportunistic infections in persons infected with HIV[1] recommend 1 double-strength tablet daily, but 1 double-strength tablet 3 times a week is also effective. The data are good that this regimen decreases the incidence of toxoplasmosis, and it appears that it also decreases the incidence of infection caused by *Pneumococcus* and *Haemophilus influenzae.*

G.L. Mandell, M.D.

Reference

1. US Public Health Service and Infectious Disease Society of America: Guidelines issued for prevention of opportunistic infections in persons with HIV. *Am Fam Physician* 52:1922, 1924–1927, 1995.

Clearance of HIV Infection in a Perinatally Infected Infant

Bryson YJ, Pang S, Wei LS, Dickover R, Diagne A, Chen ISY (Univ of California, Los Angeles)

N Engl J Med 332:833–838, 1995 119-96-6–8

Background.—Some seronegative children born to HIV-positive mothers have transiently positive viral markers. Such cases have usually been dismissed as laboratory mistakes. A child who was identified as HIV-1 infected after birth, but whose infection appears to have cleared completely, was reported.

Case Report.—Male infant, (weight 2.3 kg), born at 36 weeks' gestation, was delivered vaginally to a woman aged 33 years (gravida 4, para 2, abortus 2). During early pregnancy, the mother had sexual relations with a former IV drug user. In the fourth month of her pregnancy, asymptomatic HIV-1 infection was diagnosed. The infant did not receive blood products and was not breast-fed. He was examined frequently and has remained asymptomatic. His growth and development have been normal, and he is now 5 years old and attending kindergarten.

His complete blood cell counts, blood chemistries, immunoglobulin levels, CD4 T-cell subgroups, and CD4/CD8 ratios have been normal. Cultures of peripheral-blood mononuclear cells for HIV-1 were negative at birth and on day 33 and positive on days 19 and 51. Quantitative plasma culture at 51 days was also positive by DNA polymerase chain reaction. Tests for plasma p24 antigen and HIV-1 IgA dot assays were negative. At 1 year of age, he became negative for HIV antibody, as determined by enzyme linked immunosorbent assay and Western blot assay. Many cultures, polymerase chain reactions of peripheral-blood lymphocytes, and the enzyme linked immunosorbent assay for HIV antibody have remained negative. He has no laboratory or clinical evidence of HIV infection.

Discussion.—The data document the apparent clearing of HIV-1 from an infant who was perinatally infected. Clearance of HIV infection can occur and may be underrecognized. Early cellular immune responses, as measured by the proliferation of interleukin-2 to HIV-specific peptide antigens, may be associated with the absence of infection. Careful study of such infants should provide insights into the pathogenesis of HIV and help explain why more than 70% to 80% of infants born to HIV-1 infected mothers do not become infected.

► Earlier in the AIDS pandemic, I remember an excited phone call from a colleague who told me that a child under his care had "cured" himself of HIV disease. In retrospect, what had happened was the now well-known phenomenon of transient antibody positivity after birth. In a noninfected infant, this maternal antibody gradually disappears over time, and the child becomes HIV-antibody negative. These children were not infected.

In contrast, this report documents a patient who was infected with HIV, as defined by positive viral cultures and a positive DNA polymerase chain reaction. The child was never treated for his infection. Is this more common than we know? If this child had not had cultures, it would have appeared as a case of an antibody at birth that later cleared, indicating noninfection. Understanding the clearance of the virus in this child may be crucial in the battle against HIV infection. So far there are no answers, although the obvious suspects are the child's immune system and, perhaps, a defective, less virulent virus.

G.L. Mandell, M.D.

Natural Protection Against HIV-1 Infection Provided by HIV-2

Travers K, Mboup S, Marlink R, Guèye-Ndiaye A, Siby T, Thior I, Traore I, Dieng-Sarr A, Sankalé J-L, Mullins C, Ndoye I, Hsieh C-C, Essex M, Kanki P (Harvard School of Public Health, Boston; Univ Cheikh Anta Diop, Dakar, Senegal; Inst of Social Hygiene, Dakar, Senegal)

Science 268:1612–1615, 1995 119-96-6-9

Background.—Although HIV-1 and HIV-2 share substantial genetic relatedness and virologic characteristics, HIV-2 infection is largely confined to West Africa and has a significantly lower rate of sexual and perinatal transmission and a longer asymptomatic period than HIV-1. Few studies have examined the interaction of these 2 viruses at the host or population level. Whether susceptibility to HIV-1 could be altered in individuals already infected with HIV-2 was determined in a cohort of commercial sex workers in Senegal.

Methods.—Researchers examined registered commercial sex workers, who gave informed consent for the study and provided sequential serum samples. Dual infection with HIV-1 and HIV-2 was confirmed by polymerase chain reaction (PCR) evidence of both viruses in DNA samples from peripheral blood mononuclear cells. The women were also regularly evaluated for sexually transmitted diseases. Those identified as seropositive for HIV-1 or HIV-2 were randomly matched on the basis of age, nationality, and number of years of registered prostitution to 2 randomly selected women who were seronegative for both viruses.

Results.—A total of 756 women, including 138 who were HIV-2 seropositive at entry and 618 who were HIV seronegative, were enrolled and evaluated prospectively. Forty-nine women who were seronegative initially seroconverted to HIV-2, and 61 seroconverted to HIV-1. Among the 187 women who were initially HIV-2 seropositive or who seroconverted to HIV-2 during the study (1985–1994), only 7 seroconverted to an HIV dual-reactive status. Both seronegative and seropositive groups showed a trend of increasing HIV-1 incidence rate. The incidence of sexually transmitted diseases was not lower in the HIV-2–seropositive group. This finding would have suggested that these women had adopted safer sex practices than women in the initially seronegative group.

Conclusion.—Analysis based on Cox's proportional hazards model indicated a significantly lower risk of infection with HIV-1 for women who were HIV-2 seropositive at study entry. This protective effect was independent of CD4+ cell count. Infection with HIV-1 did not appear to confer a protective effect against HIV-2. The protective effect associated with HIV-2 may be a result of cross-reactive immunity to epitopes conserved between the 2 viruses and suggests a new course of investigation in the development of an HIV-1 vaccine.

► William Jenner noted that milkmaids who had been infected with cowpox were protected from smallpox infection. A modified strain of *Mycobacterium bovis,* known as BCG, is currently used to provide some protection against infection with *Mycobacterium tuberculosis.* Is this another example of the same phenomenon? Human immunodeficiency virus 2 causes a milder, slower type of AIDS, but AIDS nonetheless. Obviously, this is not a good candidate for use as a vaccine, but perhaps the observations will be exploitable. Is there an epitope in HIV-2 that will be cross-reactive and protective against HIV-1? Note that the risk of HIV infection among commercial sex workers was 3 times higher for those who were not infected with HIV-2 as compared with those who were.

G.L. Mandell, M.D.

7 Hepatitis C

Introduction

Most of us have been observing this story since the beginning. We knew that there were cases of hepatitis that were neither A nor B, and we thought that this "non-A non-B" hepatitis was a mild post-transfusion disease. Now that there are biological markers for hepatitis C, we are starting to get a more complete picture of this serious illness.

Gerald L. Mandell, M.D.

Sexual Transmission of Hepatitis C Virus Among Patients Attending Sexually Transmitted Diseases Clinics in Baltimore: An Analysis of 309 Sex Partnerships

Thomas DL, Zenilman JM, Alter HJ, Shih JW, Galai N, Carella AV, Quinn TC (Johns Hopkins Univ, Baltimore, Md; Baltimore City Health Dept, Md; Natl Inst of Allergy and Infectious Diseases, Bethesda, Md)

J Infect Dis 171:768–775, 1995 119-96-7–1

Introduction.—Transmission of hepatitis C virus (HCV) through blood transfusions or contaminated needles is well recognized and accounts for the high rate of HCV among IV drug users and patients who have hemophilia. The extent to which sexual transmission of HCV without parenteral exposures has not been established, however, and remains controversial. Newly developed sensitive and specific assays, as well as viral nucleotide sequences for quantifying HCV RNA, were used to examine the evidence for sexual transmission of HCV.

Methods.—Antibody prevalence to HCV (anti-HCV), behavioral and laboratory-derived risk factors for anti-HCV, and quantity and homology of HCV RNA were evaluated in 1,039 patients who had a sexually transmitted disease and were not IV drug users. These patients represented 309 sex partnerships. All participants completed a detailed questionnaire and underwent a physical examination. Variables such as age, use of alcohol, and number of lifetime sex partners were categorized into 3 levels, and all data were analyzed and compared with serologic test results separately for each sex.

Results.—Antibody prevalence to HCV was found in 7% of males and 4% of females. Factors associated with anti-HCV included age, more lifetime sex partners, HIV infection, *Trichomonas* infection, smoking, and male homosexual exposure. Females whose sex partners were anti-HCV positive were 3.7 times more likely to have a positive test result than those whose partners were anti-HCV negative. Ribonucleic acid homology between anti-HCV–positive females and their male partners was higher than that among randomly selected patients (94% vs. 82%).

Conclusions.—The high rate of anti-HCV suggests that sexual transmission of HCV contributes to the proliferation of the virus in this primarily high-risk urban population. Further studies are needed to determine why rates of HCV are so high among residents of inner cities in the United States.

▶ Hepatitis C virus (responsible for the vast majority of what was previously known as non-A non-B hepatitis) is a very serious disease. More than 90% of patients infected stay permanently infected, and 50% of these patients go on to have chronic liver disease develop, with an end result of cirrhosis and/or hepatic carcinoma. The source of infection for most patients with HCV is unknown. This study reinforces the role of sexual transmission of HCV. For a second opinion, see Abstract 119-96-7–2, in which there was no transmission from women to men. Sexual transmission is probably relatively inefficient, as previous studies of monogamous couples indicated a very low rate of transmission from the infected to the noninfected person. It is possible that with exposure to multiple partners, only some of these partners are effective transmitters.

G.L. Mandell, M.D.

Transmission of Hepatitis C Virus to Children and Husbands by Women Infected With Contaminated Anti-D Immunoglobulin

Meisel H, Reip A, Faltus B, Lu M, Porst H, Wiese M, Roggendorf M, Krüger DH (Inst of Med Virology, Berlin; Humboldt Univ, Berlin; City Hosp Dresden, Germany; et al)

Lancet 345:1209–1211, 1995 119-96-7–2

Introduction.—Uncertainty still exists over the vertical and perinatal transmission of hepatitis C virus (HCV). To estimate the risk of children who acquire the infection from their mothers, the rate of vertical HCV transmission must be determined. The rate of horizontal transmission that occurs through sexual and social contact also may be important. The transmission of HCV to children and husbands of women who were infected from a single source was investigated.

Methods.—In Germany, an outbreak of HCV occurred because of a contaminated anti-D immunoglobulin preparation given to women after delivery to prevent rhesus incompatibility. The status of 231 children and 94 husbands of 74 women who had self-limited HCV and 86 women who had chronic HCV was followed 10–15 years to determine the transmission of HCV to children and husbands. None of the women had HBV or HIV, and all usually breast-fed their children.

Results.—Of the children born to mothers who had acute self-limited hepatitis, none were anti-HCV positive. Of the children born to mothers who had chronic HCV, only 3 were anti-HCV positive; however, neither chronic nor apparent hepatitis developed in these children. No HCV antibodies or HCV RNA was found in the serum samples obtained from the 94 husbands.

Conclusion.—The risk of perinatal, intrauterine, and family-contact transmission of HCV is very low. The spread of HCV in the population is not substantially transmitted vertically or sexually. The question of how the frequency of HCV infection is maintained in the population remains unresolved, as half the cases cannot be attributed to specific risk factors.

► This remarkable study is built on the experience of the 1978–1979 single-source outbreak of HCV infection that developed in women who received contaminated anti-D immunoglobulin. The study showed very infrequent transmission of HCV infection to the children born of these mothers and no sexual transmission from women to their husbands. Where do most patients acquire their infection? We still do not know.

G.L. Mandell, M.D.

Molecular Epidemiology of an Outbreak of Infection With Hepatitis C Virus in Recipients of Anti-D Immunoglobulin

Power JP, Lawlor E, Davidson F, Holmes EC, Yap PL, Simmonds P (St Finbarr's Hosp, Cork, Ireland; Edinburgh and South East Scotland Blood Transfusion Service; Univ of Oxford, England; et al)

Lancet 345:1211–1213, 1995 119-96-7-3

Introduction.—In 1977, it was found that the Irish Blood Transfusion Service Board had manufactured anti-rhesus D immunoglobulin (anti-D) with hepatitis C virus (HCV) RNA sequences. A national screening of women exposed to anti-D (57,000 to date) was conducted, and more than 900 were found to be anti-HCV positive. Virus typing and nucleotide-sequence analysis were described to determine whether recipients of the anti-D were infected from a common source.

Methods.—Variants infecting 100 women who received anti-D from 1 of the implicated batches were compared retrospectively with 39 epidemiologically unrelated individuals who had HCV infection to determine whether HCV was transmitted by anti-D. Phylogenetic analysis was conducted.

Results.—Consistent with a single-source outbreak, all 100 women were infected with a single genotype, whereas 3 different virus genotypes were found in the individuals infected by different routes. These individuals either had a blood donation or had risk factors other than administration of anti-D. Seventeen years after the transmission event, nucleotide sequences from a 222-base fragment from the NS-5 region of the genome amplified from stored aliquots of the batch from the Irish Blood Transfusion Service Board closely matched those found in the anti-D recipients.

Conclusion.—Genotyping assays and phylogenetic analysis of HCV sequences are valuable tools for documenting the spread of HCV transmission and investigating the epidemiology.

► This study documented the value of using nucleotide sequences from a fragment of the genome as an epidemiologic tool. One can separate those patients who acquired HCV from the contaminated anti-D from those who were infected by other means.

G.L. Mandell, M.D.

Frequent Patient-To-Patient Transmission of Hepatitis C Virus in a Haematology Ward

Allander T, Gruber A, Naghavi M, Beyene A, Söderström T, Björkholm M, Grillner L, Persson MAA (Karolinska Inst, Stockholm)

Lancet 345:603–607, 1995 119-96-7–4

Introduction.—Use of IV drugs and transfusion of blood products are the most common means of transmission of hepatitis C virus (HCV). For many cases of HCV infection, however, the source cannot be determined. Transmission of the virus may be related to numerous IV procedures or immunosuppression, either from disease states or drug therapy. The source of infection with HCV in a specific population of hospitalized patients was investigated by genotyping of the viral strains.

Methods.—Thirty-seven patients who had hematologic malignancies or disorders and HCV infection were included. None of the patients had HCV antibodies detectable on admission, and serum aminotransferases were normal. During hospitalization, patients underwent multiple IV procedures (blood sampling, drug administration, and transfusions). Polymerase chain reaction assays were used to detect HCV RNA and genotype HCV. Nucleotide sequencing was done on the hypervariable region of the E2 gene with the use of serum samples obtained near the time of onset of signs of hepatitis. Blood components administered near the time of onset of hepatitis were identified, and blood samples from donors were evaluated for HCV RNA with the polymerase chain reaction assay.

Results.—At least 160 nucleotides were determined for each patient with the use of nucleotide sequencing. Five clusters, which contained similar or identical strains of virus, were identified; clusters 1 and 2 accounted for 21 patients. For 15 patients who had type 1b HCV, a 94% or greater similarity in sequence was found among isolates analyzed. Two separate clusters were present in patients who had type 3a infection, which showed a similarity in sequence of 98.1% to 100%. For type 1a infection, 4 isolates had a similarity of 98.8% to 100%. Two type 1a isolates found after 1990 were identical. Donors tested were found to be negative for HCV RNA. Fifteen of 17 patients who received blood products that had been screened with anti-HCV testing were in cluster 1 or 2. One patient was in cluster 5. No staff members tested positive for HCV.

Conclusion.—Clusters 1 and 2 were the largest and represented the most recent cases of HCV infection. Additionally, some patients in these clusters had received blood products that were negative on HCV testing, and no blood donor was found to be positive for HCV. Because some patients who had similar or identical isolates were in the same ward during the same time periods, patient to patient transmission of HCV is thought to have occurred. This prevalence, which was higher than expected, suggests that this mode of transmission may be a common and overlooked means of spread of HCV.

► This very disturbing report from Sweden documents the acquisition of HCV in 37 patients treated for either malignancy or aplastic anemia. Even more disturbing is that 17 patients received only blood components that had been screened by second-generation tests for HCV. The viral isolates suggested that there were clusters, indicating patient-to-patient spread. I think we have to assume that the standards of practice at the Karolinska Institute are equivalent to those in the most advanced hospitals in the United States.

There are many mysteries associated with the acquisition of HCV, and the most perplexing of these is that at least half the patients with HCV infection have acquired it via a cryptic route, that is, there is no history of transfusion, IV drug abuse, or sexual activity with an infected partner. Could it be that the hospital environment magnifies these cryptic routes. The authors discussed the possibility that saliva, tears, tubes, and lesions of the oral and nasal mucous membranes are either sources or access routes for infection.

G.L. Mandell, M.D.

8 New, Emerging, and Unusual Infections

Introduction

We can define emerging infections as those that are newly identified or those whose incidence in humans has significantly increased during the past decade. Of course, rarely are the infections truly "new," such as in the case of AIDS. If you are really interested in emerging infections, I suggest that you get online with ProMED (no charge), which is a program for monitoring emerging diseases. You can contact this service through ProMED@USA.Healthnet.ORG.

Gerald L. Mandell, M.D.

Bartonella (Rochalimaea) quintana Endocarditis in Three Homeless Men

Drancourt M, Mainardi JL, Brouqui P, Vandenesch F, Carta A, Lehnert F, Etienne J, Goldstein F, Acar J, Raoult D (Hôpital Saint-Joseph, Paris; Hôpital Félix Houphouet-Boigny, Marseilles, France; Hôpital Louis Pradel, Lyons, France)

N Engl J Med 332:419–423, 1995 119-96-8–1

Background.—Bartonella quintana, an organism transmitted by the body louse, was the agent that caused trench fever in soldiers during World Wars I and II. This organism has reappeared and has been reported in HIV-infected and HIV-negative individuals who live in squalid conditions. *Bartonella* was isolated from 3 HIV-negative, alcoholic, homeless men who had endocarditis.

Case 1.—Man, 47, who had weight loss, fatigue, fever, chronic alcoholism, and a heart murmur, was treated with amoxicillin and gentamicin, followed by replacement of the mitral valve. Five of 8 blood cultures grew *B. quintana,* and the patient had high titers of *B. quintana* antibody. The patient was well 10 months after surgery.

Case 2.—Man, 41, who had fever, a history of chronic alcoholism and cigarette smoking, and aortic insufficiency, was treated for aortic vegetations with ofloxacin and netilmicin, followed by rifampin and pristinamycin. All blood cultures were negative. He had an aortic valve replacement and was well 6 months after surgery.

Case 3.—Man, 43, had congestive heart failure and fever. He had a history of alcoholism and cigarette smoking and a significant recent weight loss. Endocarditis was diagnosed and treated with ceftazidime and ofloxacin, followed by the addition of netilmicin. Both the aortic and mitral valves were replaced. All microbiological studies were negative. He had serologic titers for *Chlamydia* and *Bartonella* species. The patient died 4 months after surgery.

Discussion.—The 3 patients had titers of IgG antibodies against *Chlamydia pneumoniae,* which is likely caused by cross-reactivity against *B. quintana* and *Chlamydia* species. Because *Bartonella* is a proved etiologic agent of endocarditis, all strains of *Bartonella* should be considered in the differential diagnosis of culture-negative endocarditis.

▶ Just when we learned to spell *Rochalimaea,* that genus has effectively disappeared, and these organisms are now classified as *Bartonella.* It is fascinating that the disease described in alcoholic, homeless men is similar in some ways to severe trench fever. Our present understanding is that *B. quintana* causes trench fever and fever and endocarditis in lousy (those with lice) patients. *Bartonella henselae* appears to be the major, if not the only, cause of cat scratch disease and the major, if not the only, cause of bacillary angiomatosis. The authors emphasize that there is cross-reactivity between *Bartonella* and *Chlamydia* species and that some cases that were previously thought to be chlamydial infection may actually be *Bartonella* infection.

G.L. Mandell, M.D.

Pertussis Infection in Adults With Persistent Cough

Wright SW, Edwards KM, Decker MD, Zeldin MH (Vanderbilt Univ, Nashville, Tenn)

JAMA 273:1044–1046, 1995 119-96-8–2

Background.—The public, as well as some physicians, continues to believe that pertussis occurs only in children. There is increasing evidence, however, that adults have a key role in transmitting the disease and may even be the chief reservoir. Nevertheless, pertussis often is not considered when an adult with a persistent cough is seen in the emergency department. The frequency of pertussis was determined in adult patients seen in a university hospital emergency department.

Methods.—Seventy-five patients, aged 18 years or older, who had a cough that had been present for at least 2 weeks were included. Patient serum specimens from 67 patients who did not have respiratory symptoms were assayed for antibodies to pertussis toxin, and filamentous hemagglutinin. Nasopharyngeal specimens were cultured and subjected to direct fluorescent antibody testing for *Bordetella pertussis.* Criteria for pertussis included a positive culture; a fourfold change in pertussis toxin or filamentous hemagglutinin titer; and a single titer 2 SD or more above the geometric control mean.

Results.—Only 1 symptomatic patient had a positive direct fluorescent antibody test, and none were culture-positive for *B. pertussis*. Sixteen patients (21%), however, met serologic criteria for pertussis. They could not be identified from the clinical picture, history of exposure, or lymphocyte or white blood cell counts. One patient had serologic evidence of acute mycoplasma infection.

Conclusion.—Pertussis is not infrequent among patients who have persistent cough and are seen at an emergency department.

► In Nashville, Tennessee, 16 of 75 patients (21%) with chronic cough appeared to have pertussis infection. Several points should be emphasized. First, this finding is consistent with those of previous studies and should not surprise us, although most clinicians do not consider pertussis a likely cause of chronic cough. Second, cultures are highly insensitive, and none of the patients had positive cultures. The serology indicated recent or active infection. Third, lymphocytosis was not noted. Fourth, there were no clinical clues to separate patients with pertussis who had chronic cough from those without pertussis. Once the diagnosis is made, most physicians would treat the patients with erythromycin, although there are very few data that late in the disease it would alter the clinical course. Treatment will reduce carriage and transmission.

G.L. Mandell, M.D.

► Cough is a defense mechanism as well as a symptom, and the problem in diagnosis of persistent cough is to sort out the signs, symptoms and history to determine what is causing the patient to continue coughing. As Wright et al. note in their paper, pertussis is often not likely to be high on the index of suspicion if the patient is an adult.[1] Should pertussis be suspected, confirmation of the diagnosis may be elusive: a nasopharyngeal culture is not likely to be positive if the illness has persisted longer than two weeks;[2] previously immunized persons may have lower positive culture results; and any earlier antibiotic therapy, particularly with erythromycin, tetracycline or trimethoprim-sulfamethoxazole, may reduce positive culture results.[2] If the patient is in a household, school, or other institution with children[3] on a regular basis, the patient's history may be helpful.

The study by Wright et al. suggests that a single acute serologic specimen showing a fourfold increase in pertussis toxin or filamentous hemagglutinin titers may be diagnostic. The decision to implement antibiotic treatment may rest with the clinical decision of the physician, because using antibiotic therapy in adults late in the disease may not alter the course.[4] Preventive measures may be warranted for unvaccinated children in the household.

R.C. Bone, M.D.

References

1. Herwaldt LA: Pertussis in adults: What physicians need to know. *Arch Intern Med* 109:1510–1512, 1991.
2. Onorato IM, Wassilak SGF: Laboratory diagnosis of pertussis: The state of the art. *Pediatr Infect Dis* 6:145–151, 1987.
3. Long SS, Welkon CJ, Clark JL: Widespread silent transmission of pertussis in families. *J Infect Dis* 161:480–486, 1990.
4. Linneman CC, Nasenbeny J: Pertussis in the adult. *Annu Rev Med* 28:179–185, 1977.

Infection With a Babesia-Like Organism in Northern California

Persing DH, Herwaldt BL, Glaser C, Lane RS, Thomford JW, Mathiesen D, Krause PJ, Phillip DF, Conrad PA (Mayo Clinic and Found, Rochester, Minn; Natl Ctr for Infectious Diseases, Atlanta, Ga; Univ of California, San Francisco; et al)

N Engl J Med 332:298–303, 1995 119-96-8–3

Background.—Human babesiosis is a rare infection transmitted by tick bite. The zoonotic piroplasm WAI, a *Babesia*-like protozoan, was identified recently as a human pathogen. The case reports of 5 infected men, 4 of whom were from California and had undergone splenectomy, were presented. In addition, the seroprevalence of this organism was determined in 2 different northern California populations.

Case 1.—Man, 24, reported flulike symptoms after participating in field training exercises as a soldier at Fort Ord.

Case 2.—Man, 31, completed field training exercises and went camping before becoming ill with influenza-like symptoms.

Case 3.—Man, 36, lived in Sonoma county. He was bitten by a tick and died 1 day after hospitalization.

Case 4.—Man, 41, experienced flulike symptoms after a camping trip. He recovered after having disseminated intravascular coagulation, pulmonary edema, and renal insufficiency. Intraerythrocytic merozoites were found on a peripheral blood smear.

Case 5.—Man, 62, had a 6-week history of flu symptoms and weight loss. Infection with *Babesia microti* was confirmed serologically.

Methods.—Serologic titers were performed on each patient and on 51 healthy soldiers stationed at Fort Ord. A group of 115 healthy persons from a different California location was also tested. Follow-up specimens were obtained 10 months later from WAI-seropositive men. Serologic testing was performed with indirect immunofluorescent antibody methods. Piroplasm-specific ribosomal DNA was characterized.

Results.—A piroplasm-specific DNA product was identified in all 5 patients, and 3 of 4 had a markedly elevated WAI titer within 1 month of becoming ill. Elevated titers were found in 16% of the healthy soldiers and in 3.5% of the healthy individuals in the second group. The seroreactivity was specific for WAI.

Conclusion.—These cases suggest the discovery of a new species of piroplasms that can cause human babesiosis. The arthropod vector and the animal reservoir of infection have not yet been identified.

▶ Although babesiosis may occur in patients with an intact spleen, it is rarely recognized. It usually appears as a flulike illness that is self-limited. However, babesiosis in patients who have undergone splenectomy may cause severe and even fatal illness. In the United States, nearly all cases of babesiosis have been caused by *B. microti,* which is acquired from the bite of an infected tick, usually in the coastal areas and islands of New England and the Middle Atlantic states. *Ixodes scapularis* appears to be the major tick vector. This report is important because it identifies a *Babesia*-like organism that may represent a new species associated with this disease in the western part of the country. Although not proved, it is assumed that this organism is transmitted by tick bite, and this disease should be added to Rocky Mountain spotted fever, Lyme disease, granulocytic and monocytic erlichiosis, and babesiosis as tickborne diseases endogenous in the United States.

G.L. Mandell, M.D.

Long-Term Sequelae of *Helicobacter pylori* Gastritis

Kuipers EJ, Uyterlinde AM, Peña AS, Roosendaal R, Pals G, Nelis GF, Festen HPM, Meuwissen SGM (Free Univ Hosp, Amsterdam; Sophia Hosp, Zwolle, The Netherlands)

Lancet 345:1525–1528, 1995 119-96-8–4

Background.—Chronic gastritis may be an important risk factor for the development of gastric mucosal atrophy, intestinal metaplasia, and ultimately gastric cancer. The long-term effects of gastritis associated with *Helicobacter pylori* on the gastric mucosa was investigated in a group of patients who underwent repeated endoscopic biopsy sampling.

Methods.—The status of 49 patients who were *H. pylori*-negative and 58 who were positive was followed prospectively for a mean 11.5 years. The patients were selected randomly from a group of patients who had been referred for endoscopy of the upper gastrointestinal tract to investigate possible gastric pepsinogen A and C. Serum samples were collected at initial and follow-up visits, and the presence of *H. pylori* IgG antibodies was determined. Gastroscopies with biopsy sampling were also performed in all patients to assess *H. pylori* infection and histology.

Findings.—Atrophic gastritis and intestinal metaplasia developed in 2 patients (4%) who were uninfected and in 16 (28%) of those who were infected. Atrophy regression was documented in 4 patients (7%) who were infected. *Helicobacter pylori* infection was significantly correlated with the development of atrophic gastritis and intestinal metaplasia. The proportion of atrophic gastritis increased annually by 1.2%.

Conclusions.—Helicobacter pylori infection is an important risk factor for atrophic gastritis and intestinal metaplasia. These findings support the causal role of such infection in the development of gastric cancer.

▶ Because gastroenterologists (in contrast to infectious disease specialists) have been convinced only recently that *H. pylori* causes gastritis, it is fascinating to see a study with an 11.5-year follow-up. This prospective study confirms epidemiologic data that closely link *H. pylori* infections with atrophic gastritis, intestinal metaplasia, and gastric cancer. The good news is that, at least in some patients, treatment resulted in regression of the gastric atrophy.

G.L. Mandell, M.D.

Coxsackie B Virus Infection and Onset of Childhood Diabetes

Clements GB, Galbraith DN, Taylor KW (Ruchill Hosp, Glasgow, Scotland; Royal London Hosp)

Lancet 346:221–223, 1995 119-96-8–5

Introduction.—Viruses have been linked to the development of insulin-dependent diabetes mellitus (IDDM) on the basis of controversial findings of virus antibodies in human beings. Diabetes in animals can be caused by Coxsackie B4 viruses. Children from several centers in England, who had newly diagnosed juvenile-onset IDDM, were examined for enteroviral RNA in serum.

Methods.—Fourteen children, aged 1.4–6 years (mean age, 3.9 years) were included. Serum samples were obtained close to the time of diagnosis and were compared with the serum of 45 children matched for age, sex, date of specimen receipt, and, if possible, geographic area.

Results.—The rate of positivity with the polymerase chain reaction (PCR) for enteroviral sequences was 64% in the group with IDDM and 4% in the control group. There was a high degree of similarity in the PCR amplicons of patients with IDDM who had the Coxsackie B3 v irus (90% to 93%) and the Coxsackie B4 virus (91% to 95%). Many of the PCR products from patients who had IDDM shared sequence features. They also had similarities to 2 Coxsackie B4 sequences that have been collected from human beings and are diabetogenic in murine models.

Conclusions.—The sequences found in patients who had newly diagnosed IDDM were similar to the Coxsackie B3 and B4 virus types. This finding points to a causal relationship between B3 and B4 infection and the onset of diabetes.

▶ Type 1, or juvenile, diabetes is thought to occur via autoimmune attack of the islet cells triggered by infection in a genetically susceptible host. Coxsackie B virus is an enterovirus associated with asymptomatic infection, febrile illness (with or without respiratory symptoms), asymptomatic meningitis, encephalitis, pleurodynia and, rarely, paralysis.

G.L. Mandell, M.D.

A Case-Control Study of Hantavirus Pulmonary Syndrome During an Outbreak in the Southwestern United States

Zeitz PS, Butler JC, Cheek JE, Samuel MC, Childs JE, Shands LA, Turner RE, Voorhees RE, Sarisky J, Rollin PE, Ksiazek TG, Chapman L, Reef SE, Komatsu KK, Dalton C, Krebs JW, Maupin GO, Gage K, Sewell CM, Breiman RF, Peters CJ (Natl Ctr for Infectious Diseases, Atlanta, Ga, and Fort Collins, Colo; Indian Health Service, Albuquerque, NM; New Mexico Dept of Health, Santa Fe; et al)

J Infect Dis 171:864–870, 1995 119-96-8–6

Introduction.—A rare outbreak of hantavirus pulmonary syndrome (HPS) occurred in the southwestern United States in May 1993. Five distinct hantaviruses have been recognized, and each has a single rodent species as its primary reservoir. Humans contract the virus by inhaling aerolsolized rodent urine, feces, or saliva or particulates containing rodent excreta. Risk factors for HPS were identified in a case-control study. In addition, prevention strategies for possible future outbreaks were developed.

Methods.—Seventeen patients who had HPS were compared with 3 control groups, including members of patient households (household controls), members of neighboring households (near controls), and members of randomly chosen households at least 24 km away (far controls). Patients and controls were similar with regard to age, gender, and race.

Results.—More small rodents were trapped at case households than at near or far control households. After the number of rodents had been controlled, patients were found to hand plow and clean feed storage areas more often than household controls. They were also more likely than near controls to plant and more likely than far controls to clean animal sheds.

Conclusions.—The removal of rodents from human environments is the best method for prevention of hantavirus transmission. Preventing rodents from entering buildings and eliminating nesting sites, as well as removing potential food sources in the vicinity, will help control the problem. In addition, cleaning and agricultural activities should be done only after proper ventilation and disinfection procedures have been performed. Because this study does not address the issue of risk factors in open vs. closed spaces, further research is needed.

► Cases of pulmonary hantavirus are being reported from many states far from the original 4 corners outbreak. This case-control study highlights the associated risks, which are, in retrospect, obvious. Seroprevalence of healthy controls is very low in the endemic area, which suggests that most infection results in disease. The clinical clues to HPS are unexplained adult (often now called acute) respiratory distress syndrome with bilaterial pulmonary infiltrates on chest radiograph plus suggestive clues, such as an increased level of hematocrit, abnormal lymphocytes on smear, mild thrombocytopenia, and a history of exposure to rodents or rodent excreta.

G.L. Mandell, M.D.

Outbreak of Brucellosis at a United States Pork Packing Plant

Trout D, Gomez TM, Bernard BP, Mueller CA, Smith CG, Hunter L, Kiefer M (North Carolina Dept of Enviroment, Health, and Natural Resources; United States Dept of Agriculture, Atlanta, Ga; Natl Inst for Occupational Safety and Health, Atlanta, Ga, and Cincinnati, Ohio)

J Occup Environ Med 37:697–703, 1995 119-96-8–7

Introduction.—Brucellosis is caused by bacteria of the genus *Brucella.* Symptoms include fever, chills, headaches, sweats, myalgia, anorexia, arthralgia, weight loss, and undue fatigue. Even when treated with antibiotics, fatigue can last more than a month. In 1947, the number of cases of brucellosis peaked at 6,300; in 1992, 105 cases were reported. An outbreak of brucellosis was described among employees of a pork slaughter and processing plant.

Methods.—Eighteen reports of brucellosis were received in 1992 by the North Carolina Department of Environment, Health, and Natural Resources. All patients worked on the kill floor, where the swine are slaughtered and initial processing takes place. Two patients were hospitalized for their illness. All employees on the kill floor were asked to participate in a questionnaire and serologic survey. The industrial hygiene investigation included observation of work practices, categorization of processing activities, evaluation of ventilation systems and plant sanitation activities, and review safety and health training efforts.

Results.—One hundred fifty-four employees were included, and 30 had evidence of recent brucellosis. Sixteen of the 30 represented previously unrecognized cases. Potential risk factors included being nonwhite and having a history of being cut or scratched while working and of not washing hands with soap before breaks. Few workers wore the optional protective equipment of face shields and rubber gloves, but most used mandatory personal protective equipment, which consisted of hardhats, metal mesh gloves, arm guards, safety shoes, and hearing protection.

Conclusion.—Significant exposure to *Brucella* is occurring among packing plant workers in North Carolina, and the production workers in pork processing plants are at risk of contracting swine brucellosis. Hogs must be free of *Brucella* infection when sent for processing. The impact of the disease can be lessened with increased education among employees, use of appropriate personal protective equipment, and prompt medical evaluations for symptomatic employees.

► Brucellosis is an uncommon disease in the United States. Most cases can be traced to meat processing plants, and the greatest risk seems to be pork. At a recent infectious diseases conference at the University of Virginia, a puzzling patient with fever of unknown origin turned out to have brucellosis acquired from eating cheese in Portugal. Because of the graphic description of activities on the kill floor and in other sections of the plant, vegetarians will probably have their vegetarianism reconfirmed by reading this article.

G.L. Mandell, M.D.

The Infectivity of *Cryptosporidium parvum* in Healthy Volunteers

DuPont HL, Chappell CL, Sterling CR, Okhuysen PC, Rose JB, Jakubowski W (Univ of Texas, Houston; Univ of Arizona, Tucson; Univ of South Florida, Tampa; et al)

N Engl J Med 332:855–859, 1995 119-96-8–8

Background.—The coccidian parasite *Cryptosporidium parvum* is found in many animal species and is a common cause of diarrhea in nearly all human populations. Ingesting oocysts in drinking water may cause diarrheal disease in normal hosts. It is possible for *C. parvum* oocysts to contaminate even treated drinking water. The infective dose of *C. parvum* oocysts was determined.

Methods.—Twenty-nine healthy individuals whose sera did not contain anti-cryptosporidium–specific antibodies were included. The individuals received single doses in capsule form of 30 to 1 million oocysts obtained from a calf, and oocyst excretion was monitored for 8 weeks.

Results.—Fourteen of 16 individuals given 300 or more oocysts became infected. Only 1 of 5 who received 30 oocysts was infected, compared with all 7 who were given 1,000 or more oocysts (Table 3). The median infective dose was 132 oocysts. Enteric symptoms developed in 11 of 18 recipients who excreted oocysts. Seven of these individuals had diarrhea as well as abdominal pain, cramps and, in most cases, nausea, thereby qualifying for the diagnosis of clinical cryptosporidiosis. All patients recovered, and none of their household contacts had diarrhea.

Conclusion.—Ingestion of a relatively small number of *C. parvum* oocysts may cause cryptosporidiosis in healthy adults who lack serologic evidence of past infection.

► Cryptosporidiosis was first recognized as a disease associated with animal handlers. It was then noted to be a cause of severe and often intractible diarrhea in patients who have AIDS; most recently, very large outbreaks

TABLE 3.—Rate of Infection, Enteric Symptoms, and Clinical Crytosporidiosis, According to the Intended Dose of Oocysts

Intended Dose of Oocysts	No. of Subjects	Infection	Enteric Symptoms	Crypto-sporidiosis
			number (percent)	
30	5	1 (20)	0	0
100	8	3 (37.5)	3 (37.5)	3 (37.5)
300	3	2 (66.7)	0	0
500	6	5 (83.3)	3 (50)	2 (33.3)
≥1,000†	7	7 (100)	5 (71.4)	2 (28.6)
Total	29	18	11	7

Note: Linear regression analysis of the data yielded an r^2 of .983 and a mean infective dose (ID_{50}) of 132 oocysts.

* The intended dose was 1,000 oocysts in 2 patients, 10,000 in 3, 100,000 in 1, and 1 million in 1.

associated with contamination of municipal water systems have occurred in healthy individuals. This study documents the dose required for infectivity in normal volunteers. As indicated in Table 3, even 30 cysts infected 1 of 5 volunteers, and 300 cysts approached the infective dose for half the volunteers. Note also that many of the infected patients had no symptoms. Further studies are proposed to determine whether these asymptomatic infections are protective.

One could anticipate that immunosuppressed patients, such as those with HIV infection, would be infected with even smaller doses. This brings up an important public health dilemma. What number of cysts in drinking water should be acceptable? There are several problems. Microscopic enumeration of cysts doesn't allow one to determine whether the cysts are viable. Some bottled water companies in major cities, such as New York, have produced full-page advertisements stating that municipal drinking water is rarely cyst free and suggesting that everybody buy their product.

G.L. Mandell, M.D.

Outbreak of *Shigella sonnei* Infection Traced to Imported Iceberg Lettuce

Kapperud G, Rørvik LM, Hasseltvedt V, Høiby EA, Iversen BG, Staveland K, Johnsen G, Leitao J, Herikstad H, Andersson Y, Langeland G, Gondrosen B, Lassen J (Natl Inst of Public Health, Oslo, Norway; Norwegian College of Veterinary Medicine, Oslo; Norway; Food Inspection Service in Midt-Rogaland, Forus, Norway; et al)

J Clin Microbiol 33:609–614, 1995 119-96-8–9

Background.—A nationwide outbreak of *Shigella sonnei* gastroenteritis occurred in Norway in 1994. This outbreak was likely part of a larger outbreak that affected other European countries. The infection was traced to iceberg lettuce imported from Spain. The outbreak and the process of investigation were described.

Methods.—Each case patient was matched with 6 controls. Case and control patients completed a questionnaire about diarrheal illness in other family members, consumption of both domestic and imported food items, and trips abroad. Microbiological testing was done on patients and on iceberg lettuce. Isolates of *S. sonnei* underwent plasmid profile analysis, phage typing, and susceptibility testing. Data were interpreted with the use of univariate analysis and logistic regression.

Results.—*Shigella sonnei* was cultured from 110 patients, more than two thirds of whom were adults, who had not traveled abroad recently. Consumption of imported iceberg lettuce was strongly associated with the development of gastroenteritis. Although the number of cases decreased when imported lettuce was banned, *S. sonnei* was never isolated successfully from the suspected food source. High numbers of antibiotic-resistant fecal bacteria (*Escherichia coli*) were isolated from iceberg lettuce taken from the homes of patients. Nine of 13 isolates represented 2 closely related plasmid profiles. All isolates were susceptible to the 13 antimicrobial agents tested.

Discussion.—The widespread dissemination of antibiotic-resistant genes in addition to *Shigella* during this outbreak is of considerable concern. It is likely that consumers from several European countries other than Norway were exposed to antibiotic-resistant coliform bacteria.

► I am surprised that there have not been more reports documenting enteric infection resulting from imported produce. A large percentage of our salad materials are imported from south of the border, and the North American Free Trade Agreement will accelerate this. The authors make the point that, even without clinical disease, dissemination of antibiotic-resistance genes may occur from imported foods.

G.L. Mandell, M.D.

A Morbillivirus That Caused Fatal Disease in Horses and Humans

Murray K, Selleck P, Hooper P, Hyatt A, Gould A, Gleeson L, Westbury H, Hiley L, Selvey L, Rodwell B, Ketterer P (CSIRO Australian Animal Health Lab, East Geelong, Victoria, Australia; Centre for Public Health Sciences, Brisbane, Queensland, Australia; Queensland Health, Brisbane, Australia; et al)

Science 268:94–97, 1995 119-96-8–10

Background.—New and emerging animal diseases have been ascribed to nonhuman morbilliviruses, but no new human morbillivirus has been confirmed since measles was described 10 centuries ago.

Epidemiology.—Twenty-one horses in Australia had severe respiratory disease associated with high fever; 14 died or were killed in 1994. Severe, influenza-like illness developed in the trainer and a stablehand who had had contact with a pregnant mare that was affected 2 weeks before; the trainer died of marked interstitial pneumonia. Cytopathic changes were produced with homogenates of spleen and lung from 2 of the horses and with postmortem samples of lung, liver, spleen, and kidney from the patient who died. Febrile respiratory disease developed in inoculated horses, and viral nucleocapsids were found in lung homogenates from the recipient animals, as well as in their lungs, liver, kidneys, and lymph nodes.

Histopathology.—The horses that died in the field or experimentally had interstitial pneumonia with proteinaceous alveolar edema, hemorrhage, alveolar thrombosis and necrosis, and necrotizing changes in the walls of small blood vessels. Syncytial giant cells were found in the endothelium of pulmonary arterioles, capillaries, and, in experimental cases, parenchymal vessels. Cytoplasmic inclusions resembling nucleocapsids were found within syncytial giant cells.

Viral Studies.—Ultrastructural studies demonstrated a pleomorphic virus possessing an envelope, ranging from 38 to more than 600 nm in size.

Gold labeling studies indicated that the same virus had infected horses and human beings. None of the antisera tested, including those to morbilliviruses, neutralized the virus. The organism was not a paramyxovirus. Sequence analyses of part of the matrix protein gene identified it as a member of the genus *Morbillivirus*.

▶ This is the stuff of movies and books. Fortunately, there have been no further reports of disease in horses or humans. The authors are to be congratulated for a beautiful piece of work and an astounding series of technical accomplishments. What is even more remarkable is that the first cases were recognized in late September 1994, and the paper was submitted to *Science* on December 22, 1994. Wow! This outbreak is especially frightening, as measles, also a *Morbillivirus,* is spread via the respiratory route, and doomsday scenarios of emerging diseases target respiratory transmission as the most ominous. The authors recognized the epidemic in horses and human beings, cultured the virus, characterized the cytopathic effect, established the model of infection in horses, characterized the immune response to the virus, described the morphology of the virus, used molecular biological techniques to classify the virus, and created a phylogenetic tree.

G.L. Mandell, M.D.

9 Therapy

Introduction

The year 1995 was relatively quiet for the introduction of new antimicrobial agents, and this small section reflects that.

Gerald L. Mandell, M.D.

Itraconazole Treatment of Disseminated Histoplasmosis in Patients With the Acquired Immunodeficiency Syndrome

Wheat J, Hafner R, Korzun AH, Limjoco MT, Spencer P, Larsen RA, Hecht FM, Powderly W, and the AIDS Clinical Trial Group (Indiana Univ, Indianapolis; Albert Einstein College of Medicine, Bronx, NY; Natl Inst of Allergy and Infectious Diseases, Rockville, Md; et al)

Am J Med 98:336–342, 1995 119-96-9–1

Introduction.—The standard treatment for histoplasmosis in patients who have AIDS has been amphotericin B, an effective but poorly tolerated agent. A recent study involving a small number of patients reported that itraconazole, previously used as an effective maintenance treatment, might be of value as induction therapy for disseminated histoplasmosis. The efficacy and safety of itraconazole were assessed prospectively in a multicenter, open-label, nonrandomized trial.

Methods.—Patients who had AIDS and first episodes of disseminated histoplasmosis, but who did not have evidence of severe disease or CNS histoplasmosis, were included. Eligible patients received oral itraconazole, 300 mg twice daily for 3 days, then 200 mg twice daily for 12 weeks. Those who completed the induction phase successfully were offered maintenance therapy of 200 mg/day for at least 52 weeks. Patients were evaluated for response to treatment, adverse events, and clearance of positive cultures.

Results.—Fifty of 59 evaluable patients (85%) responded to itraconazole therapy. One patient died of a presumed pulmonary embolus within the first week of treatment, 5 withdrew because of progressive infection (4 during the first 2 weeks), 2 withdrew because of toxicity, and 1 was lost to follow-up. The 2 patients who withdrew because of toxicity had showed clinical improvement, and adverse events cleared in both after switching to amphotericin B. Fatigue resolved a median of 6 weeks after the start of treatment, and fever resolved at a median of 3 weeks. The median time to weight gain was 2 weeks. Fungemia cleared after a median of 1 week, and antigen levels of *Histoplasma capsulatum* var *capsulatum* were reduced at mean rates of 0.2 (urine) and 0.3 (serum) units per week.

Discussion.—Itraconazole was an effective, generally well-tolerated, and relatively low-cost therapy for patients who had AIDS and mild disseminated histoplasmosis. Clinical manifestations improved soon after the start of treatment and had resolved by week 8 in 90% of patients who responded. Resolution of fever and clearance of antigen, however, were slower with itraconazole than with amphotericin B. Patients who have more severe infections may benefit from initial treatment with amphotericin B followed by itraconazole after clinical improvement is achieved.

▶ Itraconazole now joins fluconazole and ketoconazole as oral drugs available for systemic fungal infections. Fluconazole appears to be highly effective for *Candida* infections and cryptococcal infections. Ketoconazole may be used for oropharyngeal or esophageal candidiasis, and itraconazole is very useful for the therapy of histoplasmosis. Amphotericin is still considered the drug of choice for patients who are acutely ill and those who have CNS disease. Itraconazole can then be used for follow-up therapy.

Dr. Wheat and colleagues from Indiana University have developed an antigen test for the diagnosis of histoplasmosis. It is highly specific and very sensitive for patients with disseminated disease (especially AIDS), and it appears to be useful in follow-up evaluation.

G.L. Mandell, M.D.

Emergence of Fluoroquinolone-Resistant Tuberculosis in New York City

Sullivan EA, Kreiswirth BN, Palumbo L, Kapur V, Musser JM, Ebrahimzadeh A, Frieden TR (New York City Dept of Health; Public Health Research Inst, New York; Baylor College of Medicine, Houston; et al)

Lancet 345:1148–1150, 1995 119-96-9–2

Introduction.—Fluoroquinolone has few adverse effects and broad-spectrum antibacterial activity. However, resistance to fluoroquinolones can develop rapidly. Patients who had fluoroquinolone-resistant tuberculosis were studied to determined the epidemiology, molecular genetics, and clinical outcomes.

Methods.—Between January 1991 and November 1993, 22 patients (median age, 41 years) who were infected with fluoroquinolone-resistant *Mycobacterium tuberculosis* were identified.

Results.—Resistance occurred in 16 patients because of inadequate or inappropriate treatment. Six of these patients had primary infection with fluoroquinolone-resistant organisms; in 5, the organisms were acquired nosocomially. In isolates from 21 patients, 7 distinct patterns of restriction-fragment length polymorphism were identified. Sixteen patients (all HIV-positive) died; 6 remained alive. Median survival for the HIV-infected patients who had fluoroquinolone-resistant tuberculosis was 165 days; median survival for the 2 HIV-seronegative patients was 821 days; and median survival for the 2 patients who had unknown HIV status was 517 days. None of the patients were following a regimen of directly observed therapy. All had received at least 3 antituberculosis drugs when resistance to fluoroquinolone emerged.

Conclusion.—In patients who have multidrug-resistant disease or intolerance to other antituberculosis drugs, fluoroquinolones should be restricted. Directly observed therapy should be prescribed for all patients who have multidrug-resistant tuberculosis.

▶ Fluoroquinolones, especially ofloxacin and ciprofloxacin, are frequently used as second- and third-line agents for the treatment of tuberculosis. This study documents rapid development of resistance to these agents and emphasizes the point that the drugs should be used only in those situations where they are needed and where it can be assured that the patient is taking at least 2 agents to which the strain is known to be susceptible. In most cases, the only way to be sure of this is to use the technique of "directly observed therapy," in which the patient actually swallows the drug under supervision.

G.L. Mandell, M.D.

Cost-Effectiveness of Interferon-α2b Treatment for Hepatitis B e Antigen–Positive Chronic Hepatitis B

Wong JB, Koff RS, Tinè F, Pauker SG (Tufts Univ, Boston; MetroWest Med Ctr, Framingham, Mass; V Cervello Hosp; Palermo, Italy)

Ann Intern Med 122:664–675, 1995 119-96-9–3

Background.—Recombinant α2b-interferon was approved recently for use in the treatment of chronic hepatitis B. Only some treated patients, however, lose viral serologic markers or, eventually, hepatitis B virus surface antigen. Much longer follow-up will be needed to determine the effects of α2b-interferon treatment on more definitive clinical end points, such as cirrhosis or hepatocellular carcinoma. Because the treatment is expensive and associated with short-term adverse effects, a decision analytic model was used to estimate the cost-effectiveness of α2b-interferon treatment for patients who have chronic hepatitis B and are positive for hepatitis B e antigen (HBeAg).

Methods.—A meta-analysis of 9 randomized, controlled trials and a cost-effectiveness analysis were used. The expected clinical and economic outcomes associated with changes in the serologic markers of hepatitis B viral replication were projected. For a total of 552 patients who had confirmed chronic hepatitis B infection and HBeAg positivity, lifetime incidence of cirrhosis and hepatocellular carcinoma, life expectancy, quality-adjusted life expectancy, and costs and marginal cost-effectiveness ratios from a societal perspective were considered.

Results.—Within 1 year of α2b-interferon treatment, the likelihood of becoming negative for HBeAg increased from 9% to 46%. The likelihood of becoming negative for hepatitis B surface antigen increased from 2% to 8%. For a patient aged 35 years, treatment with α2b-interferon was estimated to increase life expectancy by 3.1 years or by 3.4 quality-adjusted life-years. The analysis suggested that α2b-interferon would decrease projected lifetime costs, even if future savings were discounted. Even when the model was biased strongly in favor of standard care, the marginal cost-effectiveness ratio of interferon was no greater than $12,000 per life-year gained.

Conclusions.—For HBeAg-positive patients who have chronic hepatitis B, treatment with α2b-interferon should prolong life and reduce costs. Until the results of a clinical trial prove otherwise, the available data suggest that α2b-interferon treatment should be routine.

▶ When an article starts with "cost-effectiveness," my eyes usually glaze over and my head nods. This article was an exception. The authors carefully analyzed available data to give us some good estimates as to what we could expect with interferon-α2b therapy. At first glance, the advantage is not great, i.e., an increase in life expectancy of 3.1 years. However, the calculations indicate that the maximal cost per life-year gain is about $12,000, which is in a very favorable range and therefore recommends for the use of this intervention. The actual cost per year would probably be significantly lower, in the $4,000 to $6,00 range.

G.L. Mandell, M.D.

The Treatment of Scabies With Ivermectin

Meinking TL, Taplin D, Hermida JL, Pardo R, Kerdel FA (Univ of Miami, Fla)

N Engl J Med 333:26–30, 1995 119-96-9–4

Background.—Anecdotal reports and a few clinical studies suggest that scabies can be treated effectively with ivermectin, an oral anthelmintic agent used successfully for treating onchocerciasis and other filarial infestations. The effectiveness of ivermectin in treating scabies both in otherwise healthy and in HIV-positive patients was examined.

Methods.—Ivermectin was administered in a single oral dose of 200 µg/kg to 11 otherwise healthy patients and to 11 HIV-positive individuals, including 7 whose disease had progressed to AIDS. Severity of scabies ranged from mild to crusted lesions. Skin scrapings were examined for the mite at initiation and at 2 and 4 weeks after treatment. No other scabicides were used 1 month before treatment or during the study. Close contacts of the patients were treated with topical 5% permethrin cream to reduce chance of reinfestation.

Results.—At 4 weeks after treatment, all otherwise healthy patients were cured, as were 8 of the 11 HIV-positive patients. Of the remaining 3 patients, 2 were given a second dose 2 weeks after the first treatment and were cured by week 4. The remaining patient, who had AIDS, tuberculosis, and heavily crusted lesions, improved dramatically after a second dose at week 2 but still had crusts on her elbows at week 4. Live mites were recovered, and she was given a third dose of ivermectin along with total body 5% permethrin cream; 2 weeks later her case of scabies was cured.

Discussion.—There were no adverse effects, and pruritus diminished very soon after initial treatment. One patient became reinfested 2 months after treatment, which indicated that ivermectin has no residual activity against scabies 2 months after the initial dose. A single dose of 200 µg/kg appears to cure most cases of scabies, but crusted or other stubborn cases may require additional ivermectin and topical treatments.

► Dog owners know ivermectin as the 1-pill-per-month preventive agent for heartworm. The world of tropical medicine knows ivermectin as an amazingly successful single-dose treatment for river blindness (onchocerciasis), for which it was donated free of charge by Merck and Company. This recent study shows that a single oral dose was impressively effective for eradicating scabies. At this writing, ivermectin is available only from the Centers for Disease Control and Prevention for treatment of onchocerciasis.

G.L. Mandell, M.D.

PART TWO

THE CHEST

ROGER C. BONE, M.D.

Introduction

During the past 2 years, on these pages, I have recounted my experience of being handed a diagnosis of renal cancer. I felt this was appropriate because of the relationship of science to humanity and illness in our profession of medicine. I also wrote about these experiences on 2 occasions in the *Journal of the American Medical Association*.[1, 2]

After recovering from my operation, in which my right kidney and adrenal gland were removed, and living as a cancer survivor, I became more appreciative and reflective of the world around me. I found more time to devote to my family and friends and to enjoy a Beethoven symphony or a good novel or a fine dinner.

Recently, I learned that I have metastasis to both lungs and a positive bone scan. As a cancer survivor, I spent the past 2 years with the threat of this possibility. The reality is not easy to accept. There is denial, anger, and a sense of great loss.

I have to realize, however, that the observations I wrote on these pages are still true:

1. Good health is often taken for granted; however, it is the most precious commodity one possesses
2. One's spouse, children, family, and friends are the essential ingredients that allow one to endure an experience such as a serious and unexpected illness
3. When faced with death, one realizes the importance of God and one's relationship to God
4. The things one does throughout one's life that seem so urgent are, most of the time, not so important.

These observations have become a way of life for me.

In my previous essays, I quoted American writers Thornton Wilder and Henry David Thoreau, who both noted that most men and women lead frantic and desperate lives and seldom pause to reflect on their activities. I am glad that the initial diagnosis of cancer prepared me for the most feared of its complications: metastatic disease. I am most happy, however, that the initial diagnosis made me think anew about life and, therefore, consider the contemplative philosophies of both Wilder and Thoreau. One activity that brought me peace after the initial diagnosis was having quiet time, during which I just enjoyed being alone surrounded by nature—similar to, I imagine, Thoreau contemplating Walden Pond.

The day that my metastasis was confirmed was, of course, very traumatic considering the shock of the findings and the initial flurry about what should be done and how soon. Finally, I politely called a halt to all activity for the day. I told my staff and friends at work that I was simply going home to be with my family and sit and look at the river.

Which is what I did.

Our house sits on a rather steep bluff, and the Maumee River curves around a very wide bend below us. Our yard slopes gently to the edge of the bluff, then descends through grasses and wildflowers and bushes to the edge of the river. Birds and squirrels and chipmunks populate this slope of land. If you stand above the slope on a quiet day and gaze out at the river, you can hear the rustling of the animals in the grasses. Occasionally, there will be a bird's song.

It was a perfect October day, sunny, 70 degrees, with a gentle breeze. The wide blue river sparkled when stirred by the wind. On both sides of the river, the trees grew down to the edge. The trees were still mostly green, with only a hint of autumn reds and yellows.

The river's course flows in such a way that, at this time of the year, the sun seems to set exactly into the water. A great fire being extinguished by the cool river.

I sat on a lawn chair, my suit coat and tie on the green grass beside me. At that moment, time stopped. My life—past, present, and future—was compressed into that second of time.

Thoreau went to Walden Pond to search for his soul. There, in communion with nature, he found serenity and fulfillment. He recognized and recorded for us a state where one can come closest to the unity between nature and creation.

Thornton Wilder, nearly 100 years later in his play *Our Town,* emphasized that most of us are blind to the everyday wonders of the world. He dramatized that life can end quickly and without warning. The theme of his play is simple: Life is short; be certain to take the time to smell the roses. Over time, the seemingly trivial things do become more important. Wilder stated that at one moment you get married and, before you know it, that white-haired lady by your side is 70 years old and has eaten 50,000 meals with you.

Time slipped past again, and I looked up and saw my wife standing next to my chair with a glass of lemonade for me. Our daughter had just made a pitcher. I tasted the sweetness of the drink. The wind suddenly stirred the grass. A bird chirped. A small boat appeared far off in the river, making its way upstream.

I took my wife's hand, and we stayed there a moment longer looking at the world passing before us.

Life has been good to me.

The 1996 YEAR BOOK OF MEDICINE once again features the best of this year's research results, including studies of clinical and basic research. The Chest section is separated into 16 chapters that encompass the major clinical entities of pulmonary and critical care medicine. The significant events in pulmonary and critical care medicine that are presented in this year's edition include the following:

Asthma

- Self-management protocols and home peak expiratory flow rate monitoring, which were thought to improve asthma care, showed a compliance rate of only 40% (Abstract 119-96-10–1).

- Allergen immunotherapy is a highly effective treatment option in selected patients who have extrinsic ("allergic") asthma if the allergens can be identified (Abstract 119-96-10–2).
- High-dose systemic corticosteroids have no additional benefit compared with low-dose corticosteroids in the treatment of severe acute asthma (Abstract 119-96-10–3).

Chronic Obstructive Pulmonary Disease

- Significant improvement is seen with antibiotic therapy in patients who have exacerbations of chronic obstructive pulmonary disease (COPD) (Abstract 119-96-11–1).
- Significant improvement is seen in patients who have COPD after bilateral pulmonary volume reduction (Abstract 119-96-11–2).
- Alveolar-arterial oxygen gradient contributes to the predictive model in patients who have acute exacerbation of COPD and a high risk of death (Abstract 119-96-11–3).
- Measurements of ciliary beat frequency, numbers of outer and inner dynein arms, and ciliary orientation may be a better parameter in patients who have primary ciliary dyskinesia (Abstract 119-96-11–4).

Cystic Fibrosis

- Ibuprofen taken for 4 years significantly slowed the progression of lung disease in patients who had cystic fibrosis (Abstract 119-96-12–1).

Lung Cancer

- Males who are long-time smokers of mentholated cigarettes have an increased risk of lung cancer compared with female smokers (Abstract 119-96-13–1).

Pulmonary Vascular Disease

- Inhaled nitric oxide administered in low doses is as safe and effective as prostacyclin for assessing acute pulmonary vasodilator responsiveness in patients who have primary pulmonary hypertension (Abstract 119-96-14–1).
- The presence of factor V gene was associated with an increased risk of venous thrombosis, but it was not a risk factor for myocardial infarction or stroke (Abstract 119-96-14–2).
- Enoxaparin is more expensive than low-dose warfarin, but its cost-effectiveness in total hip replacement is comparable to that of other accepted interventions (Abstract 119-96-14–3).
- Heparin-induced thrombocytopenia and other events are more common in patients treated with unfractionated heparin than in those treated with low–molecular weight heparin (Abstract 119-96-14–4).

Respiratory Infection

- Identifying risk factors on admission to the hospital can predict the outcome of individuals who have pneumococcal pneumonia and bacteremia (Abstract 119-96-15–1).
- Strains of influenza A virus have RNA sequence–documented resistance to amantadine and rimantadine without exposure to either drug (Abstract 119-96-15–2).

Tuberculosis

- Tuberculosis infection can be transmitted in any closed environment, including a church (Abstract 119-96-16–1).
- Pulmonary tuberculosis should be suspected in patients with AIDS who have a very low CD4 count and an atypical radiographic pattern until it has been ruled out (Abstract 119-96-16–2).
- Measures for controlling infection effectively prevent nosocomial transmission of tuberculosis to health care workers (Abstract 119-96-16–3).

Interstitial Lung Disease

- A reduction of the forced expiratory volume in 1 second/forced vital capacity ratio and an increase in percentage of total lung capacity at the first examination are prognostic factors for pulmonary lymphangioleiomyomatosis (Abstract 119-96-17–1).
- Pulmonary tuberous sclerosis should be suspected in all patients who have lymphangioleiomyomatosis (Abstract 119-96-17–2).
- Alveolar hemorrhage is rarely a cause of lung injury and is usually associated with other causes of pneumonia (Abstract 119-96-17–3).
- Fibrotic tissue changes of idiopathic pulmonary fibrosis and, possibly, other chronic interstitial lung diseases may result from the local effects of interleukin-1 (IL-1) receptor antagonist protein (Abstract 119-96-17–4).

Occupational Lung Disease

- Occupational asthma caused by the use of latex gloves occurs in approximately 2.5% of hospital employees and should be considered a risk factor for respiratory health care personnel (Abstract 119-96-18–1).

Pleural Disease

- Thoracoscopy has its greatest diagnostic yield in older patients who have a history of malignancy and have a lymphocytic, hemorrhagic, high lactate dehydrogenase effusion (Abstract 119-96-19–1).
- Pleural fluid pH can be used as a predictor of complicated parapneumonic effusions (Abstract 119-96-19–2).

Sleep Apnea

- More than 10% of patients who have sleep apnea syndrome have an associated obstructive airway disease (Abstract 119-96-20–1).

Critical Care

- Barotrauma is an indication of severity of acute lung injury rather than a major cause of increased mortality (Abstract 119-96-21–1).
- Application of human factor engineering concepts to the study of the weak points of a specific ICU may help reduce the number of errors (Abstract 119-96-21–2).
- The best survival estimates combine an objective prognosis with a physician's clinical estimate (Abstract 119-96-21–3).
- Physicians weigh requests along with other factors, including possible medical futility, when determining whether to continue treatment for the critically ill patient (Abstract 119-96-21–4).
- Adrenal insufficiency should be suspected in patients who have septic shock and do not respond to conventional treatment (Abstract 119-96-21–5).
- The most comprehensive approach is to combine invasive pressure monitoring with transesophageal echocardiography estimates of intracardiac flow and volume in critically ill patients (Abstract 119-96-21–6).
- Appropriate respiratory care and infection control practices must be followed to avoid outbreaks of *Burkholderia cepacia* in mechanically ventilated patients when multiple-dose medication vials are used (Abstract 119-96-21–7).
- Gastric emptying in critically ill, sedated, and mechanically ventilated patients can be significantly improved by adding cisapride to a routine enteral feeding protocol (Abstract 119-96-21–8).
- Patients in the ICU who were given early enteral feeding supplemented with arginine, dietary nucleotides, and fish oil tolerated the food well and had a shorter hospital stay (Abstract 119-96-21–9).

Sepsis

- The natural history of the inflammatory response to infection can be described as a continuous progression from systemic inflammatory response syndrome to septic shock (Abstract 119-96-22–1).
- With current plasma assays for IL-1β, IL-1 receptor antagonist may be a more sensitive marker of human inflammation than IL-1β or tumor necrosis factor-α (Abstract 119-96-22–2).

Acute Respiratory Distress Syndrome

- A significant decrease in fatality rates is seen in patients younger than 60 years and in those who have sepsis syndrome as their risk for acute respiratory distress syndrome (ARDS) (Abstract 119-96-23–1).

- Oxygenation is primarily a function of mean airway pressure, and longer inspiratory times can be used as an alternative to applied positive end-expiratory pressure to increase this oxygenation (Abstract 119-96-23–2).
- The intensity and duration of inflammation, as reflected by plasma levels of cytokines, may determine the ultimate outcome in patients who have ARDS (Abstract 119-96-23–3).
- The beneficial effects of inhalation of nitric oxide can be observed in most patients who have severe ARDS. In some patients, however, it may fail to improve pulmonary gas exchange or to reduce pulmonary hypertension without obvious explanation (Abstract 119-96-23–4).

Mechanical Ventilation

- Nosocomial pneumonia in mechanically ventilated patients can be significantly reduced by using a simple method that decreases the chronic microaspirations through the cuff of endotracheal tubes (Abstract 119-96-24–1).
- High incidences of tricuspid regurgitation and vena caval backward flow indicate poor reliability of the thermodilution method for measurement of cardiac output when used in ventilated patients (Abstract 119-96-24–2).
- Extubation was achieved 3 times faster than mandatory ventilation when a once-daily trial of spontaneous breathing was used and twice as quickly as pressure support ventilation (Abstract 119-96-24–3).
- Upper airway narrowing at a more proximal site, such as the oropharynx or velopharynx, may be the cause of the increase in respiratory work (Abstract 119-96-24–4).
- The use of esophageal balloon technology provides data to help shorten the duration of mechanical ventilation (Abstract 119-96-24–5).

Transplantation

- To predict outcome in single lung transplant recipients in whom bronchiolitis obliterans develops, monitoring the forced expiratory volume in 1 second is useful (Abstract 119-96-25–1).

Roger C. Bone, M.D.

References

1. Bone RC: The taste of lemonade on a summer afternoon. *JAMA* 273:518, 1995.
2. Bone RC: Another "taste of lemonade." *JAMA* 274:1656, 1995.

10 Asthma

Objective Measurements of Compliance in Asthma Treatment

Chmelik F, Doughty A (Univ of Illinois, Rockford)

Ann Allergy 73:527–532, 1994 119-96-10–1

Background.—Self-management measures for asthma have attracted increasing interest as morbidity and mortality rates associated with asthma have increased. The use of peak expiratory flow rate (PEFR) meters has been suggested, but the extent to which patients will follow self-management guidelines and use these instruments to control their asthma remains uncertain. Compliance and accuracy were determined in a pilot study.

Methods.—Twenty consecutive patients, aged older than 6 years, who required the use of metered-dose inhalers on a daily basis were included. Metered-dose inhaler cartridges and a peak flow meter, the VMX Wright Mini-Log Peak Flow Recorder, were distributed. In the first week, patients followed their customary protocol and kept a diary of meter and inhaler use. An individualized self-management protocol was then written on the basis of the predicted or highest PEFR recorded in the baseline week. The frequency and dose of anti-inflammatory aerosol and the need for bronchodilator were based on recordings of flow rate. Readings of 25% of predicted (or specified) indicated the need for urgent care.

Results.—When diary entries were compared with the electronic memory of the flow meter, 3.6% of readings in the baseline week and 17% of those in the final week were too high. In 9% and 6% of cases, respectively, the peak flow readings were lower than the electronic record. In the baseline week, 3% of all readings were "phantom" reports of readings that were never done. The figure increased to 15% in the final week of the study. It was not uncommon for patients to record more medication use than what actually occurred. Overall PEFR values showed slight improvement during the 5-week study.

Implications.—Overall compliance with recommended self-management of asthma was only 40%, despite extensive educational efforts. Electronic monitoring of the PEFR and inhaler use can identify noncompliant patients at an early stage.

▶ Patient education has been the cornerstone of self-management programs directed at preventing asthma attacks or managing symptoms of asthma.[1] An essential element of effective patient education is teaching the patient how to self-monitor and why self-monitoring is important to ensure compliance.[2] Home PEFR monitoring and/or use of a written diary are used by most successful asthma self-management programs. Both methods have been found useful,[3] and both have been found to have limitations.[4] Objective measures of medication compliance include electronic monitoring, although this technology may not give a good picture of inhaled medication despite accurate counting of dispensed doses.[2]

That electronic monitoring may pick up PEFR errors and noncompliance, which, as the authors found, tend to increase with time, must be judged within the framework that noncompliance may be "intelligent."[2] That is, a patient may alter a regimen or protocol in response to a situation, not in an attempt to engage in risky behavior. Physicians who deal with these situations would hopefully be able to recognize when electronic monitoring has picked up a "risky noncomplier" vs. an "intelligent noncomplier" and make an appropriate decision regarding how best to return this patient to effective self-management.

R.C. Bone, M.D.

References

1. Wilson SR, Scamagas P, German DF, et al: A controlled trial of two forms of self-management education for adults with asthma. *Am J Med* 94:564–576, 1993.
2. Rand CD, Wise RA: Measuring adherence to asthma medication regimens. *Am J Respir Crit Care Med* 149:69S–76S, 1994.
3. Malo JL, l'Archeveque J, Trudeau C, et al: Should we monitor peak expiratory flow rates or record symptoms with a simple diary in the management of asthma? *J Allergy Clin Immunol* 91:702–709, 1993.
4. Kendrick AH, Higgs CMB, Whitfield MJ, et al: Accuracy of perception of severity of asthma: Patients treated in general practice. *BMJ* 307:422–424, 1993.

Is Allergen Immunotherapy Effective in Asthma: A Meta-Analysis of Randomized Controlled Trials

Abramson MJ, Puy RM, Weiner JM (Monash Med School, Melbourne, Australia; Alfred Hosp, Melbourne, Australia; St Vincent's Hosp, Melbourne, Australia)

Am J Respir Crit Care Med 151:969–974, 1995 121-96-10–2

Background.—The efficacy of allergen immunotherapy for asthma was determined in a meta-analysis of published randomized controlled trials. Data were gathered with the use of a computerized bibliographic search of investigative articles written only in English.

Method.—Data for asthmatic symptoms, medication requirements, lung function, and bronchial hyperreactivity were collected for patients who received placebo and those who received immunotherapy. One mold, 9 mite, 5 pollen, and 5 animal dander trials were included. The results were categorized as odds ratios for improvement or no change. Data were analyzed with the chi-square test, Mantel-Haenszel test, and χ^2 statistic.

Results.—For all studies, the odds ratios of improvement with immunotherapy were 2.7%; of reduction of medication, 4.2%; and of reduction in bronchial hyperreactivity, 13.7%. The mean effect for any immunotherapy on all continuous outcomes was 0.71, which corresponded to a mean predicted improvement in forced expiratory volume in 1 second of 7.1%.

Conclusion.—Allergen immunotherapy is an effective treatment option for patients who have extrinsic asthma if the allergen can be identified and certain stringent guidelines are followed.

▶ The term "meta-analysis" was first described in 1976 as "the analysis of the results of statistical analyses for the purpose of drawing general conclusions."[1] Since then, the use of meta-analyses has become widespread in many fields, including medicine. Although there were statistical techniques of combining information from several research studies, even as early as the 19th century,[2] the methodology called meta-analysis is fairly recent. More and more meta-analyses are appearing in the medical literature, and they may be regarded by many as superior to the traditional medical review article. Individual meta-analyses may be criticized for including studies of questionable quality; this criticism may often be legitimate, because the average trial is not of optimal quality, or it may be more of a complaint regarding unwelcome results.[3] Allergists who believe strongly in the efficacy of allergen immunotherapy in asthma may find the meta-analysis by Abramson et al. to be less supportive than a standard review article, but on the whole, the authors identified a highly specific clinical role for allergen immunotherapy within carefully drawn parameters of risk-benefit assessment, close monitoring of the patient, use of a specific and effective extract, and the ability to treat adverse effects. Not surprisingly, the authors stated a need for more large, multicenter randomized clinical trials in which standardized available allergen extracts are used.

R.C. Bone, M.D.

References

1. Glass GV: Primary, secondary, and meta-analyses of research. *Educ Res* 5:3–8, 1976.
2. Stigler SM: *The History of Statistics: The Measurement of Uncertainty Before 1900.* Cambridge, MA, Belknap Press of Harvard University, 1986.
3. Antman EM, Lau J, Kupelnick B, et al: A comparison of results of meta-analyses of randomized control trials and recommendations of clinical experts. *JAMA* 268:240–248, 1995.

High-Dose and Low-Dose Systemic Corticosteroids Are Equally Efficient in Acute Severe Asthma

Marquette C-H, Stach B, Cardot E, Bervar JF, Saulnier F, Lafitte JJ, Goldstein P, Wallaert B, Tonnel A-B (CHRU de Lille, France)

Eur Respir J 8:22–27, 1995 121-96-10–3

Introduction.—Systemic corticosteroids (CS) are widely used in the management of acute severe asthma, especially in patients who do not respond to therapy with intensive β_2-agonists. The optimal dose of CS has not been determined, however, and current recommendations show a considerable range. Because high doses of CS have potential hazards, the efficacy of low-dose methylprednisolone was compared with that of high-dose methylprednisolone in patients who had acute severe asthma.

Methods.—Eligible patients were 18–65 years of age and were admitted with an acute severe asthma attack. All were unresponsive to an intensive β_2-agonist regimen administered during a run-in period. Patients who had fever, a need for prompt ventilatory support, abnormal findings on chest radiograph, and certain medical conditions were excluded. Twenty-three patients were randomly selected in a double-blind manner to receive low-dose methylprednisolone, 1 mg/kg^{-1}, and 24 were selected to receive a high dose, 6 mg/kg^{-1}. Concurrent treatment was standardized. Serial bedside spirometry was used to evaluate response.

Results.—The 2 groups were similar in mean age, other demographic characteristics, history of asthma, and severity of the current attack. Significant improvement, as measured by forced expiratory volume in 1 second at 24 and 44 hours, was noted in both groups, and the difference in effects between low- and high-dose CS was not significant. Respiratory rates were similar on admission in the 2 groups, and decreased significantly and with the same magnitude with high- and low-dose CS. No patient had acute respiratory failure requiring mechanical ventilation, and all were discharged alive. The mean duration of hospitalization was similar for the low-dose (7.1 days) and high-dose (8.2 days) groups.

Conclusion.—High-dose CS is associated with the risk of serious adverse effects in patients who have severe acute asthma. Furthermore, no pharmacologic rationale supports the use of high doses in this setting. These findings confirm those of previous studies indicating that high doses of CS are no more beneficial than low doses in patients who have an attack of acute severe asthma.

► Reversal of airway inflammation is widely recognized as a primary objective of treatment for severe asthma, and CS are widely recommended as the agents of choice. Therapeutic rationale for use of CS is perhaps being established by studies that show a relationship between CS treatment and regulation of cytokine synthesis.[1] The use of CS in the management of severe acute asthma is recognized as being especially important in those patients who are refractory to intensive β-agonist therapy.[2] The recommended dose has varied widely, however, and Marquette et al. found in their literature review a trend toward increasing the dose. Their prospective, double-blind randomized trial reported here, however, did not support an increased dose. They note a recent review by McFadden,[3] in which the optimal dose of CS for treatment of severe asthma was found to remain an unresolved issue. Although the number of patients in the study by Marquette et al. was not large, the findings strengthen the argument to keep this issue open until more studies with large enough populations are carried out and published.

R.C. Bone, M.D.

References

1. Robinson D, Hamid Q, Ying S, et al: Prednisolone treatment in asthma is associated with modulation of the bronchoalveolar lavage cell interleukin-4, interleukin-5, and interferon-gamma cytokine gene expression. *Am Rev Respir Dis* 148:401–406, 1993.
2. National Asthma Education Program: *Expert Panel Report: Guidelines for the Diagnosis and Management of Asthma.* August, 1991. US Dept of Health and Human Services publication No. 91-3042.
3. McFadden ER: Dosages of corticosteroids in asthma. *Am Rev Respir Dis* 147:1306–1310, 1993.

11 Chronic Obstructive Pulmonary Disease

Antibiotics in Chronic Obstructive Pulmonary Disease Exacerbations: A Meta-Analysis

Saint S, Bent S, Vittinghoff E, Grady D (Univ of California, San Francisco; San Francisco Gen Hosp)

JAMA 273:957–960, 1995 119-96-11–1

Introduction.—Chronic obstructive pulmonary disease (COPD) is the fourth leading cause of death in the United States. Exacerbations of COPD are usually treated with antibiotics, despite clear evidence that such therapy is beneficial. The efficacy of antibiotics in patients who had exacerbations of COPD was examined in a meta-analysis of published randomized trials.

Methods.—Data were obtained from English-language studies published between 1955 and 1994 through a MEDLINE search of the terms "COPD," "chronic bronchitis," "exacerbation," and "antibiotic(s)." In addition, reference lists of articles published before 1966 and found in *Index Medicus* were scanned. Eligible studies included the following components: patients who had a presumed diagnosis of COPD and were thought to be having an exacerbation, a randomized design in which an antibiotic in the treatment group and placebo in the control group were used, at least 5 days of follow-up, and sufficient data to calculate an effect size (ES).

Results.—Of 230 studies found through a literature search, only 9 randomized trials met inclusion criteria. The overall summary ES of 0.22 suggested a small benefit for antibiotic treatment vs. placebo. Six studies that provided data on peak expiratory flow rate (PEFR) changes were analyzed separately and yielded a summary ES of 0.19 and a summary change in PEFR of 10.75 L/min, which favored the antibiotic-treated group. These results were not substantially altered by sensitivity analyses that used different outcomes and excluded 3 studies that based outcomes on number of exacerbations rather than on number of patients.

Conclusion.—Patients who had exacerbations of COPD and were given antibiotics showed a small but statistically significant improvement compared with patients given placebo. Although the antibiotic-associated improvement in PEFR was small, the change could be significant in severely ill patients who have low baseline PEFR.

▶ The role of bacterial infection in exacerbations of chronic bronchitis is still regarded as somewhat enigmatic.[1] Pathogenic bacteria can be cultured from the bronchi in a high percentage of patients who have chronic bronchitis, as they can from airways of patients who have other lung diseases, such as carcinoma and tuberculosis. The presence of bacteria may have a role in perpetuation of the disease and may also have a role in producing exacerbations.[2] In patients who consistently produce purulent sputum with cough, the diagnosis of an acute infection may be difficult.[3] Physicians may often empirically attribute an exacerbation to an organism commonly found in the airways of patients who have chronic bronchitis, e.g., *Haemophilus influenzae* or pneumococci, and they may select an oral antibiotic accordingly. The first-line oral antibiotics chosen by physicians include trimethoprim-sulfamethoxazole, amoxicillin-clavulanate, and erythromycin. Tetracycline has also been used for acute episodes and prophylactically.

As Saint et al. note, the overall benefit of oral antimicrobial therapy in exacerbations of chronic bronchitis has been questionable.[4] This meta-analysis of 9 studies published between 1957 and 1992 suggests that oral antibiotic therapy may have a small but clinically significant effect on improving PEFR, particularly in hospitalized patients. A definitive answer, however, may not be available without a large, well-designed, randomized, placebo-controlled trial.

R.C. Bone, M.D.

References

1. Murphy TF, Sethi S: Bacterial infection in chronic obstructive pulmonary disease: State of the art. *Am Rev Respir Dis* 146:1067–1083, 1992.
2. Leeder SR: Role of infection in the course of chronic bronchitis and emphysema. *J Infect Dis* 131:731, 1975.
3. Gump DW, Phillips CA, Forsyth BR, et al: Role of infection in chronic bronchitis. *Am Rev Respir Dis* 113:465–467, 1976.
4. Anthonisen NR, Manfreda J, Warren CPW, et al: Antibiotic therapy in exacerbations of chronic obstructive pulmonary disease. *Ann Intern Med* 106:196–199, 1987.

Bilateral Pneumectomy (Volume Reduction) for Chronic Obstructive Pulmonary Disease

Cooper JD, Trulock EP, Triantafillou AN, Patterson GA, Pohl MS, Deloney PA, Sundaresan RS, Roper CL (Washington Univ, St Louis, Mo)

J Thorac Cardiovasc Surg 109:106–119, 1995 119-96-11–2

Objective.—The effect of bilateral pneumonectomy in patients who had severe chronic obstructive pulmonary disease (COPD) was assessed. Whether the procedure could lessen thoracic distention and improve the mechanics of breathing was determined.

Methods.—Twenty patients who had COPD were included. All patients had significantly limited pulmonary function despite optimal medical treatment and had a distended thorax. Via a median sternotomy, 20% to 30% of the volume of each lung was excised with the use of a linear stapling device that could buttress the staple lines with strips of bovine pericardium. The strips also eliminated air leakage through the staple holes. The most severely affected parts of the lungs were selectively removed, but most patients had diffuse changes without bullae.

Results.—There have been no early or late deaths. Patients remained in the hospital an average of 15 days. Eleven patients had air leakage for longer than 1 week. Four of these patients underwent reexploration. During a mean follow-up of 6.4 months, forced expiratory volume in 1 second nearly doubled; forced vital capacity improved less markedly. Performance on the 6-minute walking test improved gradually after volume reduction. Dyspnea was substantially less troublesome after surgery. Patients could better engage in activities at work and at home.

Conclusion.—These preliminary findings indicate that bilateral pulmonary volume reduction may significantly improve the lives of selected patients who have marked COPD.

► Lung volume reduction surgery has become a "hot" surgical procedure for the treatment of emphysema (COPD). The potential candidates already form waiting lists for evaluation at the several centers where the procedure is done. Physicians are urgently questioned by patients regarding the availability of the operation. A difficulty for many physicians has been the paucity of data regarding this procedure in the medical and surgical literature. This report by Cooper et al. provides a rationale for the procedure, a comparative rationale for the bilateral approach vs. single-lung and thoracoscopic approaches, and data, albeit short-term, on 20 patients. The objective measures of improvement in spirometry, lung volume, and performance in the 6-minute walk test complement subjective measurements by patients.

The technique of Cooper et al.—sternotomy, bilateral pneumonectomy, stapling of the lobes, and use of bovine pericardium to buttress the staple line—is a "big" operation, as noted by the authors. Physicians who must advise patients regarding lung volume reduction surgery will be anxiously awaiting reports from groups that have opted for thoracoscopic, video-assisted procedures, as well as extended data from Cooper et al. Each of these groups is developing selection criteria for patients, and these are also much needed by physicians.

R.C. Bone, M.D.

Predicting Mortality of Patients Hospitalized for Acutely Exacerbated Chronic Obstructive Pulmonary Disease

Fuso L, Incalzi RA, Pistelli R, Muzzolon R, Valente S, Pagliari G, Gliozzi F, Ciappi G (Catholic Univ, Rome)

Am J Med 98:272–277, 1995 119-96-11-3

Introduction.—The reported mortality rates among patients hospitalized because of chronic obstructive pulmonary disease (COPD) have varied widely, from as low as 6% in some studies to 40% in others. These discrepancies could occur because of differences in baseline patient characteristics, therapeutic strategies, and weight of comorbidity. The factors that affect short-term prognosis in hospitalized patients who had acutely exacerbated COPD were identified.

Patients and Methods.—Five hundred ninety patients in whom COPD was diagnosed at a single institution from 1981 through 1990 were included. In all patients, COPD was the primary disease, and all were treated according to a standardized protocol. The patient records were analyzed, and 23 admission clinical and laboratory variables collected. Variables that significantly or nearly significantly correlated with outcome, age, and alveolar arterial oxygen gradient (PA-aO_2) were used as independent variables in a multivariate logistic regression analysis; death was the dependent variable.

Results.—The most common causes of COPD exacerbation were acute respiratory infection, poor drug or oxygen therapy compliance, and cardiac arrhythmias. Co-existing diseases included hypertension in 140 patients, diabetes mellitus in 65, and chronic renal failure in 45. Most patients had been treated with bronchodilators, diuretics, corticosteroids, and/or digitalis. The acute episode of COPD resulted in 85 deaths, for an in-hospital mortality rate of 14.4%. Patients who died were significantly older and had a greater PA-aO_2 compared with those who survived the episode. Mechanical ventilation was also associated with a higher mortality rate. Multivariate analysis identified 4 variables that independently predicted death: age, PA-aO_2 greater than 41 mm Hg, ventricular arrhythmias, and atrial fibrillation. When the 5-year periods of 1981–1985 and 1986–1990 were analyzed separately, age was an independent predictor of mortality in both periods; PA-aO_2 predicted death in the earlier years, and atrial fibrillation predicted death in the more recent period.

Conclusion.—Among patients who have a wide clinical spectrum of COPD, certain variables present at admission with an acute exacerbation identified those with a high risk of death. In addition to older age, ventricular arrhythmias, atrial fibrillation, and PA-aO_2 contributed to the predictive model.

► These authors suggest, on the basis of their retrospective study, that age plus factors of interaction between heart and lungs can be short-term predictors of mortality in a patient hospitalized for acute exacerbation of COPD. In addition, these predictors may be identifiable when the patient is admitted. The authors take care to recognize that the atrial fibrillation and ventricular arrhythmia identified as predictors of short-term mortality are not necessarily associated with co-existent heart disease; rather, they could be manifestations of the exacerbation of COPD on heart rhythm. It may be useful to note in this regard that history of myocardial infarction just missed reaching the significance level in the multivariate analysis. Fuso et al. also caution that PA-aO_2 values, as defined in their study, reflect only the derangement of gas exchange resulting from the exacerbation and not the severity of the COPD. What the authors, by implication, tell us to remember is that COPD is a "disease of the chest," not only a lung disease.

R.C. Bone, M.D.

Ciliary Defects in Healthy Subjects, Bronchiectasis, and Primary Ciliary Dyskinesia

de Iongh RU, Rutland J (Concord Hosp, New South Wales, Australia)

Am J Respir Crit Care Med 151:1559–1567, 1995 119-96-11–4

Introduction.—Normal limits of ciliary defects in a normal population need to be established to help clinically diagnose primary ciliary dyskinesia (PCD) and distinguish ciliary defects in patients or disease groups that do not have a structural basis for impaired mucociliary clearance. Quantitative methods were used to determine the ranges of ciliary microtubule defects, numbers of dynein arms, and the variation in ciliary orientation in a large group of healthy persons. The observed ranges were then used to identify and compare patients who had abnormalities of ciliary motility and ultrastructure with those who had respiratory disease symptoms consistent with clinical features of PCD.

Methods.—A research group of 61 healthy individuals and a group of 31 patients who had chronic recurrent upper and/or lower respiratory tract disease were evaluated for ciliary beat frequency and ciliary ultrastructure. There were 31 nonsmokers, 20 ex-smokers, and 11 smokers in the research group. Members of both groups underwent the following tests: ciliary motility and ultrastructure, with samples of epithelium obtained from the surface of the interior turbinate by nasal mucosal brushing; electron microscopic evaluation of ciliated epithelium; and quantification of ultrastructural parameters. The ultrastructural parameters included compound cilia, central and peripheral microtubule defects, inner and outer dynein arms, and ciliary orientation.

Results.—In the research group, there were no significant differences in between-group mean ciliary beat frequencies (CBF) or ciliary ultrastructure parameters, regardless of smoking history or age.

In patients who had respiratory tract disease, the mean CBF of patients who had bronchiectasis was within normal limits and similar to that of healthy individuals. The mean CBF of patients who had PCD was significantly less, however, compared with that of healthy individuals. In patients who had PCD, the cilia showed a range of ultrastructural defects, such as reduced numbers of dynein arms, including inner, outer, and both inner and outer dynein arms; eccentrically located central microtubules; extra single microtubules; displaced peripheral doublet microtubules; and compound cilia. Abnormal orientation of cilia and microtubule defects, such as absence of 1 or more peripheral doublets, supernumerary doublets, and absence of the "B" tubule in peripheral doublets were commonly seen in patients who had PCD. Compared with healthy individuals, patients who had PCD had significantly less mean inner and outer dynein numbers and greater mean incidences of central and peripheral microtubule defects and mean ciliary deviation.

The measurements of CBF in repeat investigations of 6 patients who had PCD were consistent with previous studies. Ultrastructural findings in 3 of 5 siblings of patients who had PCD showed similar ultrastructural ciliary defects. The other 2 siblings had similar findings with every feature except for numbers of inner dynein arms.

Conclusion.—Findings have facilitated the establishment of criteria that have been useful in the diagnosis of PCD. Measurements of CBF, numbers of outer and inner dynein arms, and ciliary orientation may be better parameters than measurements of the incidence of microtubule defects and compound cilia in identifying patients who have PCD.

► As our understanding of the genetic basis of disease continues to increase, there is a tendency to assume a mechanistic genotype-to-phenotype relationship in pathophysiology that appears to be genetically controlled. Classic papers on immotile cilia syndrome[1] and Kartagener's syndrome[2] noted the ciliary dysfunction that affected pulmonary function and motility of spermatozoa, albeit genetic control of axonemal structure in different parts of the body may be regulated by different genes.[3, 4]

In this abstracted paper, de Iongh and Rutland note that respiratory tract infection may be involved in some cases of PCD; whether a genetic "predisposition" to ciliary disorientation might exist is at least suggested in that ciliary disorientation is a consistent feature of PCD in some patients. This report provides quantitative data regarding the variations in incidence of ciliary defects in healthy individuals and in patients who have recurrent respiratory tract disease not caused by PCD, which is important for reliable differential diagnosis.

R.C. Bone, M.D.

References

1. Eliasson R, Mossberg B, Camner P, et al: The immotile cilia syndrome. *N Engl J Med* 297:1–6, 1977.
2. Pedersen M, Mygind N: Absence of axonemal arms in nasal mucosa in Kartagener's syndrome. *Nature* 121:494–495, 1976.
3. Lungarella G, Fonzi L, Burrini AG: Ultrastructural abnormalities in respiratory cilia and sperm tails in a patient with Kartagener's syndrome. *Ultrastruct Pathol* 3:319–323, 1982.
4. Jonsson MS, McCormick JR, Gillies GG, et al: Kartagener's syndrome with motile spermatozoa. *N Engl J Med* 307:1131–1133, 1982.

12 Cystic Fibrosis

Effect of High-Dose Ibuprofen in Patients With Cystic Fibrosis

Konstan MW, Byard PJ, Hoppel CL, Davis PB (Case Western Reserve Univ, Cleveland, Ohio)

N Engl J Med 332:848–854, 1995 119-96-12–1

Introduction.—In patients who have cystic fibrosis, an inflammatory reaction to chronic pulmonary infection contributes to destructive lung changes. Whether effective anti-inflammatory measures would slow the progress of lung disease in these patients was investigated.

Method.—Eighty-five children and adults who had cystic fibrosis and mild lung disease, defined as forced expiratory volume in 1 second (FEV_1) 60% or more of predicted, were included. The patients were randomly selected to receive either ibuprofen or an oral placebo twice daily for 4 years. The dose of ibuprofen was adjusted to maintain a peak plasma level of 50–100 μg/mL.

Results.—Average compliance approached 70% in both groups. The FEV_1 decreased significantly less rapidly in patients who received ibuprofen than in those who received placebo. Similar trends were noted for forced vital capacity and the ratio of residual volume to total lung capacity. Ibuprofen was most helpful in patients aged younger than 13 years when enrolled. Body weight was better maintained in patients who received ibuprofen, and chest radiograph scores decreased less in these patients. Comparable numbers of patients withdrew because of side effects.

Conclusion.—Continuous high-dose ibuprofen therapy effectively slows the progress of initially mild pulmonary disease in patients who have cystic fibrosis without causing serious side effects.

► As efforts increase to use newer knowledge of the basic defect in cystic fibrosis to develop therapies at the molecular and cellular levels, it is encouraging to read the report of Konstan et al. regarding an approach to control airway inflammation. Although the 4-year time frame of the study does not permit us to know the long-term outcomes of ibuprofen therapy, the shorter term results are optimistic for keeping younger patients in an improved condition for substantial periods. Some of these younger patients could potentially survive long enough to become candidates for advanced drug therapies. The cost of ibuprofen is also welcome for patients and their families who know the economic consequences of this chronic disease.

Konstan et al. have been working for some years on the investigation of ibuprofen as a nonsteroidal anti-inflammatory agent that inhibits the migration, adherence, swelling, and aggregation of neutrophils and thereby helps maintain normal pulmonary anatomy and function in patients who have cystic fibrosis.[1] Their work continues a line of investigation that pursued the use of corticosteroids to delay the progressive impairment in lung function of these patients.[2] Like Konstan et al., these investigators hypothesized that patients younger than 12 years of age would benefit most from a treatment that reduces structural damage caused by the inflammatory response to microbial invasion. The earlier anti-inflammatory line of investigation was halted because of unacceptable adverse effects of prednisone.[3] The trial by Konstan et al. demonstrates that ibuprofen therapy produces some adverse effects that may potentiate some existing symptoms (e.g., abdominal pain, which is nearly universal in these patients) or that may initiate symptoms that require close monitoring (e.g., conjunctivitis and epistaxis). The adverse effects required discontinuing ibuprofen in only a small number of patients, however.

The anti-inflammatory strategy in cystic fibrosis, as an augmentation of conventional therapy, deserves rapid investigation in more clinical trials.

R.C. Bone, M.D.

References

1. Konstan MW, Hoppel CL, Chai BL, et al: Ibuprofen in children with cystic fibrosis: Pharmacokinetics and adverse effects. *J Pediatr* 118:956–964, 1991.
2. Auerbach HS, Williams M, Kirkpatrick JA, et al: Alternate-day prednisone reduces morbidity and improves pulmonary function in cystic fibrosis. *Lancet* 2:686–688, 1985.
3. Rosenstein BJ, Eigen H: Risks of alternate-day prednisone in patients with cystic fibrosis. *Pediatrics* 87:245–246, 1991.

13 Lung Cancer

Mentholated Cigarette Use and Lung Cancer

Sidney S, Tekawa IS, Friedman GD, Sadler MC, Tashkin DP (Kaiser Permanente Med Care Program, Oakland, Calif, Univ of California, Los Angeles)

Arch Intern Med 155:727–732, 1995 119-96-13–1

Objective.—Although menthol combustion is known to produce carcinogenic benzo[a]pyrenes, few studies have related health risks to smoking mentholated cigarettes. The association between mentholated cigarette use and lung cancer were investigated prospectively.

Methods.—A total of 11,761 individuals, aged 30–89 years, who had smoked for at least 20 years were included. Follow-up for lung cancer averaged 8.7 years for individuals who smoked mentholated cigarettes (average age, 50.2 years) and 8.5 years for those who smoked nonmentholated cigarettes (average age, 51.9 years).

Results.—Younger individuals, black individuals, and women smoked more mentholated cigarettes. Lung cancer was diagnosed in 93 individuals who smoked mentholated cigarettes and 225 of those who smoked nonmentholated cigarettes. Years of smoking mentholated cigarettes was related to lung cancer in men but not in women. The relative risk of lung cancer in individuals who smoked mentholated cigarettes compared with those who smoked nonmentholated cigarettes was 1.45 in men and 0.75 in women.

Conclusion.—Men who smoked mentholated cigarettes had a 45% increase in the incidence of lung cancer compared with those who smoked nonmentholated cigarettes. Additional studies are needed to determine the causes of lung cancer owing to mentholation.

▶ The ability of the tobacco industry to identify specific markets for its products is a modern marketing success story and the bane of all who would try to find ways to help people stop smoking. If mentholated cigarettes are selectively smoked by relatively more blacks than whites, it would be rational to suppose that this is well known to the tobacco industry and that the industry does all it can to maintain and expand this market niche. It would also be rational to suppose that market research has led to the creation of metholated cigarettes targeted to this particular market.

The information provided in this study might be used by physicians in obtaining smoking histories from black patients. A history of smoking mentholated cigarettes, especially in a black male, could be a flag for possible increased risk for lung cancer. Longer duration of use of mentholated cigarettes would be an indication of even greater risk. The physician's clinical responsibility, however, should always be to encourage smoking cessation rather than brand switching. Mentholation is perhaps an added risk, but the high rate of cigarette smoking by blacks is the fundamental issue to be addressed.

R.C. Bone, M.D.

14 Pulmonary Vascular Disease

Inhaled Nitric Oxide as a Screening Vasodilator Agent in Primary Pulmonary Hypertension: A Dose-Response Study and Comparison With Prostacyclin

Sitbon O, Brenot F, Denjean A, Bergeron A, Parent F, Azarian R, Herve P, Raffestin B, Simonneau G (Hôpital Antoine Béclère, Clamart, France)

Am J Respir Crit Care Med 151:384–389, 1995 119-96-14–1

Objective.—Numerous agents have been used to measure the capacity of the lungs to vasodilate in patients who have primary pulmonary hypertension (PPH). Some agents, like prostacyclin, have potentially serious side effects. Although nitric oxide (NO) has demonstrated the ability to vasodilate pulmonary vessels selectively in a variety of hypertensive lung disease conditions, measurements of hemodynamic responses and tests of air-NO mixes were not explicit. The short-term hemodynamic effects of prostacyclin and incremental concentrations of air-NO mixtures were compared.

Methods.—Ten men and 25 women, aged 20–74 years, who had PPH were included. Hemodynamic evaluations, vasodilator responses, oxygen parameters, and drug tolerances were determined after treatment with an acute infusion of prostacyclin and with inhalation of 10, 20, 30, and 40 ppm of NO. A vasodilator response was defined as a decrease of 30% or more in total pulmonary pressure relative to the baseline value.

Results.—Thirteen patients had vasodilator responses to both agents, and 22 had responses to neither. The mean right atrial pressure was significantly higher in the nonresponders than in the responders. Otherwise, the vasodilator responses produced by prostacyclin and NO were similar. With both agents, changes in mean pulmonary pressure correlated with total pulmonary resistance. The maximum vasodilator response to NO was achieved at a concentration of 10 ppm; a combination of the 2 agents did not result in an additive response. Prostacyclin caused adverse reactions, including bradycardia and severe systemic hypotension. Nitric oxide had no systemic effects and caused no adverse reactions, although an increase in the level of methemoglobin was observed.

Conclusion.—Inhaled NO at low doses is as safe and effective as prostacyclin for assessing acute pulmonary vasodilator responsiveness in patients who have PPH. In addition, this method does not produce systemic effects.

► Sitbon et al. venture to say that inhaled NO can now be considered the gold standard screening agent in patients who have PPH and are being evaluated for vasodilator therapy. They qualify that optimistic statement by noting that long-term use of NO in these patients has yet to be evaluated. Inhaled NO as an air-NO mixture in their study was as effective as infused prostacyclin in the assessment of acute pulmonary vasodilator responsiveness. Unlike infused prostacyclin, the air-NO mixture at a concentration of 10 ppm NO in air did not cause side effects, such as cutaneous flushing or headache. The air-NO mixture did not induce any significant change in cardiac output. Thus, this mixture appears to be the better agent to screen patients who may benefit from chronic administration of a vasodilator. This method apparently does not result in any patients being missed in the screen: 37% of patients in this study responded to both inhaled NO and infused prostacyclin, and 63% responded to neither screening agent.

R.C. Bone, M.D.

Mutation in the Gene Coding for Coagulation Factor V and the Risk of Myocardial Infarction, Stroke, and Venous Thrombosis in Apparently Healthy Men

Ridker PM, Hennekens CH, Lindpaintner K, Stampfer MJ, Eisenberg PR, Miletich JP (Harvard Med School, Boston; Harvard School of Public Health, Boston; Washington Univ, St Louis, Mo)
N Engl J Med 332:912–917, 1995 119-96-14–2

Background.—A point mutation in the gene coding for coagulation factor V has been associated with a form of activated protein C that resists degradation and, therefore, may increase the risk of venous thrombosis. The mutation involves a substitution for guanine at nucleotide 1691. Whether healthy individuals are at increased risk was investigated.

Patients.—A total of 14,916 healthy men were enrolled in the Physicians' Health Study. The G1691A mutation was found in 374 participants who subsequently had myocardial infarction, in 209 who had strokes, and in 121 who had deep venous thrombosis and/or pulmonary embolism. The same number of enrollees who remained healthy served as a control group.

Findings.—The prevalence of the factor V mutation was 6.1% in men who had myocardial infarction and 4.3% in those who had strokes, which is not significantly different from the 6.0% rate in those who remained free of cardiovascular disease. The mutation was found, however, in 11.6% of men in whom venous thrombosis or pulmonary embolism developed during follow-up. The adjusted relative risk of thrombosis or embolism in heterozygous patients was 2.7, and the risk of primary venous thrombosis was 3.5. The increased relative risk occurred chiefly in older men. The mutation was found in 25.8% of men older than 60 years of age who had primary venous thrombosis.

Conclusion.—The G1691A mutation of the factor V gene is the most common inherited factor known to predispose to venous thrombosis.

► Protein C is a vitamin K–dependent glycoprotein-serine-protease-zymogen that circulates in the blood in a proenzyme state. In the presence of co-factor protein S, another factor VIII glycoprotein, protein C selectively inactivates factors V and VIII and enhances tissue plasminogen activator by inactivating tissue plasminogen activator inhibitor.[1] Recent investigations of the protein C system described resistance to activated protein C; resistance was seen in some patients who had venous thromboembolism, particularly those who had positive family histories and were relatively young when seen initially.[2] The co-factor subsequently found to be responsible for resistance to activated protein C was a form of factor V that was procoagulant but resistant to degradation by activated protein C;[3] the resistance has been identified as a point mutation in the gene coding for factor V.[3, 4]

In this study, Ridker et al. show that the factor V mutation is prevalent among men older than 60 years of age who have a first episode of venous thrombosis. This finding, however, is contrary to the earlier observation that presentation typically is seen in men younger than 40 years of age.[2] Ridker et al. raise the possibility that, because it is now known that 6% of the male population in the United States is genetically at increased risk for venous thromboembolism, the persons at risk should be identified for singular treatment.

R.C. Bone, M.D.

References

1. Clouse LH, Comp PC: The regulation of hemostasis: The protein C system. *N Engl J Med* 314:1298–1304, 1986.
2. Dahlback B, Carlsson M, Svensson PJ: Familial thrombophilia due to a previously unrecognized mechanism characterized by poor anticoagulant response to activated protein C: Prediction of a cofactor to activated protein C. *Proc Natl Acad Sci U S A* 90:1004–1008, 1993.
3. Bertine RM, Koeleman BPC, Koster T, et al: Mutation in blood coagulation factor V associated with resistance to activated protein C. *Nature* 369:64–67, 1994.
4. Dahlback B, Hildebrand B: Inherited resistance to activated protein C is corrected by anticoagulant cofactor activity found to be a property of factor V. *Proc Natl Acad Sci U S A* 91:1396–1400, 1994.

Cost-Effectiveness of Enoxaparin vs. Low-Dose Warfarin in the Prevention of Deep-Vein Thrombosis After Total Hip Replacement Surgery

Menzin J, Colditz GA, Regan MM, Richner RE, Oster G (Policy Analysis Inc, Brookline, Mass; Harvard Med School, Boston)

Arch Intern Med 155:757–764, 1995 119-96-14-3

Background.—Deep-vein thrombosis (DVT) is an important postoperative complication in patients undergoing total hip replacement surgery. Prophylaxis reduces thromboembolic risk more cost-effectively than screening or clinical diagnosis and treatment. Current concerns, however, revolve around which prophylaxis to use. Enoxaparin sodium, a low–molecular weight heparin, was recently approved for use in the United States. Its cost-effectiveness relative to that of low-dose warfarin sodium, which is used most frequently, remains to be determined. The cost-effectiveness of enoxaparin sodium in the prevention of DVT after total hip replacement surgery was compared with that of low-dose warfarin sodium.

Methods.—A decision-analytic model was used to compare 2 prophylactic strategies, enoxaparin sodium (30 mg given twice daily) and low-dose warfarin, with no prophylaxis. With the use of a hypothetical cohort of 10,000 patients undergoing hip replacement surgery, the expected number of patients who had confirmed DVT or pulmonary embolism, the expected number of thromboembolic deaths, and the expected costs of prophylaxis, diagnosis, and treatment were estimated for all 3 strategies. Data were obtained primarily from the published literature.

Results.—When compared with no prophylaxis, low-dose warfarin could be expected to reduce the numbers of patients who had confirmed DVT from approximately 1,000 to 420 per 10,000 patients. This strategy also would reduce the number of thromboembolic deaths from nearly 250 to 110, and the costs of care from approximately $530 to $330 per patient. Although prophylaxis with enoxaparin sodium could be expected to decrease further the number of patients with confirmed DVT to 250 and the number of thromboembolic deaths to 70, the costs of care would increase by approximately $50. The cost-effectiveness of enoxaparin relative to that of low-dose warfarin would be approximately $12,300 per avoided death.

Conclusions.—Although use of enoxaparin prophylaxis after total hip replacement surgery is associated with higher patient-care costs in comparison with low-dose warfarin, it can further reduce the risk of thromboembolism in individuals undergoing such surgery. Moreover, the cost-effectiveness of enoxaparin compares favorably with that of other commonly endorsed medical interventions. These findings may help facilitate decisions involving rational use of resources in the inpatient setting.

▶ The value of preventing catastrophic disease is unquestioned by nearly all physicians, but data to support such seemingly foregone conclusions do not always exist. This is the case when one considers the efficacy of DVT prophylaxis in preventing pulmonary embolism and thromboembolic death.[1] These authors inferred efficacy, as there are sparse data to show efficacy, of either enoxaparin or low-dose warfarin in preventing pulmonary embolism after total hip replacement.[2] Menzin et al. infer efficacy and construct tables showing the value in terms of relative costs of treating DVT rather than pulmonary embolism. The availability of a low–molecular weight heparin provides the clinician with a wider range of prophylactic choice in patients who undergo total hip replacement. The clinician must weigh the choices available in light of data available, i.e., the additional reduction of risk for DVT offered by enoxaparin against lower per-patient cost of low-dose warfarin.

R.C. Bone, M.D.

References

1. Goldhaber SZ, Morpugo M, WHO/ISFC Task Force on Pulmonary Embolism: Diagnosis, treatment, and prevention of pulmonary embolism: Report of the WHO/International Society and Federation of Cardiology Task Force. *JAMA* 268:1727–1733, 1992.
2. Prevention of venous thrombosis and pulmonary embolism: Consensus conference. *JAMA* 256:744–749, 1986.

Heparin-Induced Thrombocytopenia in Patients Treated With Low-Molecular-Weight Heparin or Unfractionated Heparin

Warkentin TE, Levine MN, Hirsh J, Horsewood P, Roberts RS, Gent M, Kelton JG (McMaster Univ, Hamilton, Ont, Canada)
N Engl J Med 332:1330–1335, 1995 119-96-14–4

Introduction.—Thrombocytopenia induced by heparin appears approximately 5 days after the start of heparin therapy. It is defined by the presence of heparin-dependent IgG antibodies and, paradoxically, can be complicated by thrombolic complications. Platelet counts and heparin-dependent IgG antibodies were analyzed in a randomized, double-blind, controlled investigation of patients who underwent elective hip surgery and received prophylaxis against venous thrombosis.

Methods.—Six hundred sixty-five patients were randomly selected to receive twice-daily subcutaneous injections of either low–molecular weight heparin or 7,500 units of unfractionated heparin beginning the day of surgery until 14 days after surgery, or until discharge. Platelet counts were obtained at baseline and daily. A subgroup of 387 patients was also tested for heparin-dependent IgG antibodies. Heparin-induced thrombocytopenia was defined as a decrease in the platelet count to below 150,000 per cubic millimeter at 5 or more days after the start of heparin therapy, and a positive test for heparin-dependent IgG antibodies.

Results.—Twelve patients had thrombocytopenia after receiving heparin therapy for 5 or more days. Nine of the 332 patients (2.7%) who received unfractionated heparin and none of the 333 who received low–molecular weight heparin had heparin-induced thrombocytopenia. Eight of the 9 patients who had heparin-induced thrombocytopenia had 1 or more thrombolic events. None of the patients who had heparin-induced thrombocytopenia experienced major or minor hemorrhagic events. A higher frequency of heparin-dependent IgG antibodies was detected in patients who received unfractionated heparin, compared with those who received low–molecular weight heparin (7.8% vs. 2.2%).

Discussion.—None of the patients treated with low–molecular weight heparin had heparin-induced thrombocytopenia or thrombolic events. By comparison, 9 patients who received unfractionated heparin had thrombocytopenia. Heparin-induced thrombocytopenia was a strong risk factor for venous thrombosis.

► The anomalous occurrence of thrombosis and associated pathology in patients who have thrombocytopenia has been a conundrum of heparin therapy.[1] Recent reports have done much to reveal the pathogenesis of heparin-induced thrombocytopenia[2] and to suggest the immunologic basis for predisposition of a heparin-challenged patient to thrombosis or disseminated intravascular injury.[2–4] The report by Warkentin et al. is welcome news for physicians and their patients who require heparin therapy, in that no patient in their trial had heparin-induced thrombocytopenia from low–molecular weight heparin. It appears likely that low–molecular weight heparin does not react with some procoagulants (e.g., factor IIa) with which unfractionated heparin is active. It is less capable than unfractionated heparin of activating resting platelets to release platelet factor 4, and it is less capable of binding to platelet factor 4.[5] The current high cost of low–molecular weight heparin in the United States may retard its use in some environments.

R.C. Bone, M.D.

References

1. Warkentin TE, Kelton JG: Heparin-induced thrombocytopenia. *Prog Hemost Thromb* 10:1–34, 1991.
2. Visentin GP, Ford SE, Scott JP, et al: Antibodies from patients with heparin-induced thrombocytopenia/thrombosis are specific for platelet factor 4 complexed with heparin or bound to endothelial cells. *J Clin Invest* 93:81–88, 1994.
3. Greinacher A, Potzsch B, Amiral J, et al: Heparin-associated thrombocytopenia: Isolation of the antibody and characterization of the multimolecular PF4-heparin complex as the major antigen. *Thromb Haemost* 71:247–251, 1994.
4. Kelton JG, Smith JW, Warkentin TE, et al: Immunoglobulin G from patients with heparin-induced thrombocytopenia binds to a complex of heparin and platelet factor 4. *Blood* 83:3232–3239, 1994.
5. Lane DA, Pejler G, Flynn AM, et al: Neutralization of heparin-related saccharides by histidine-rich glycoprotein and platelet factor 4. *J Biol Chem* 261:3980–3986, 1986 (erratum *J Biol Chem* 261:13387, 1986).

15 Respiratory Infection

Risk Factors for Adverse Outcome in Persons With Pneumococcal Pneumonia

Marfin AA, Sporrer J, Moore PS, Siefkin AD (Ctrs for Disease Control and Prevention, Morgantown, WVa; Kaiser-Permanente Med Group, Sacramento, Calif; New York City Dept of Health; et al)

Chest 107:457–462, 1995 119-96-15–1

Background.—Despite the use of antibiotics, rates of death among patients who have pneumococcal pneumonia remain high. Many investigators have tried to identify patients who do not benefit from antibiotic therapy and, therefore, contribute disproportionately to the high mortality. Risk factors for death and respiratory failure in patients who had penicillin-sensitive pneumococcal bacteremia and pneumonia were determined retrospectively.

Methods.—Data available at initial clinical assessment were analyzed for 102 adults consecutively hospitalized for treatment of pneumococcal pneumonia with bacteremia.

Findings.—Twenty-five patients died, and 17 survived mechanical ventilation for respiratory failure. A univariate analysis indicated that patients who had preexisting lung disease, initial body temperatures of less than 38°C, or nosocomial infections or those who were aged 48 years or older had a higher risk for adverse outcomes than patients who did not have these risk factors. Of the 25 patients who died, only 1 did not have these risk factors. The other 24 did not need intensive care. A multivariate logistic model including these risk factors would have predicted death or respiratory failure in 67% of the patients and better outcomes in 83%. Nosocomial infection was the greatest risk factor in a multivariate analysis (Table 2).

Conclusions.—Certain data available at hospital admission can be used to predict outcomes in patients who have pneumococcal pneumonia and bacteremia. Identifying these risk factors may enable earlier use of intensive care or more aggressive therapy. The greatest risk factor for death or respiratory failure, independent of age, was nosocomial infection.

► As physicians learn to be more adept at using the techniques of statistical modeling, studies such as this one will be more readily incorporated into clinical practice. The modeling of data from retrospective cohort review

TABLE 2.—Significant Risk Factors for Adverse Outcomes in 102 Patients With Pneumococcal Bacteremia and Pneumonia, From Univariate and Multivariate Logistic Regression Analyses

	Univariate Analysis		Multivariate Logistic Regression	
Risk Factor (No. of Persons)	Relative Risk	(95% CI)	Coefficient	Adjusted Odds Ratio (95% CI)
Age ≥ 48 yr (52)	2.7	(1.5–4.8)	1.194	3.3 (1.2–9.2)
Preexisting lung disease (24)	2.0	(1.3–3.0)	1.400	4.1 (1.3–13.0)
Temperature < 38°C (52)	2.1	(1.3–3.6)	1.376	4.0 (1.4–11.4)
Nosocomial infection (14)	2.5	(1.8–3.6)	2.848	17.3 (3.1–97.5)
Chronic obstructive pulmonary disease (18)	1.7	(1.0–2.6)	Did not contribute to the logistic model	
History of pulmonary tuberculosis (8)	2.3	(1.5–3.4)	Did not contribute to the logistic model	
Preexisting medical disease (61)	4.2	(1.6–10.6)	Did not contribute to the logistic model	

(Courtesy of Marfin AA, Sporrer J, Moore PS, et al: Risk factors for adverse outcome in persons with pneumococcal pneumonia. *Chest* 107:457–462, 1995.)

provides a mechanism for identifying patients who have penicillin-sensitive pneumococcal bacteremia and pneumonia and are at risk of respiratory failure and death, and for distinguishing these patients from those who are less likely to require early intensive care. Univariate analysis of the data showed that age older than 50 years is a major risk factor for death or respiratory failure caused by pneumococcal pneumonia—as it has been for decades.[1] Older age plus lower body temperature identified persons who were more likely to have an adverse outcome. The analysis suggested that the risk factor of low body temperature was independent of both older age and chronic illness. The high risk of mortality associated with nosocomial pneumococcal pneumonia in the multivariate analysis suggests the presence of more virulent serotypes with multiple resistance to antibiotics.

R.C. Bone, M.D.

Reference

1. Austrian R, Gold J: Pneumococcal bacteremia with especial reference to bacteremic pneumococcal pneumonia. *Ann Intern Med* 60:759–770, 1964.

Amantadine-Resistant Influenza A in Nursing Homes: Identification of a Resistant Virus Prior to Drug Use

Houck P, Hemphill M, LaCroix S, Hirsh D, Cox N (Health Care Financing Administration Region X, Seattle; Ctrs for Disease Control and Prevention, Atlanta, Ga; Washington State Dept of Health, Seattle; et al)

Arch Intern Med 155:533–537, 1995 119-96-15–2

Background.—Influenza A infection causes severe morbidity and mortality in elderly individuals, especially those in nursing homes. Amantadine hydrochloride and rimantadine hydrochloride have been used to treat and prevent such infection. Outbreaks of influenza A viruses in 3 nursing homes in Yakima County, Washington, in January 1992 were reported.

Methods and Findings.—An enzyme immunoassay and sequencing of the viral nucleic acid encoding the transmembrane domain of the M2 protein were used to analyze 10 influenza A viruses isolated during the outbreaks for resistance to amantadine and rimantadine. Five strains were resistant to amantadine. These 5 strains had the same mutation in the M2 protein—serine to asparagine in position 31. One resistant virus had been recovered before any amantadine had been used, and 1 was recovered within 48 hours of administration of the first drug.

Conclusions.—This is the first report of influenza A virus with RNA sequence–documented resistance to amantadine and rimantadine without exposure to either agent. It is also the briefest reported period between the initiation of amantadine treatment and isolation of a resistant influenza A virus strain. Surveillance for amantadine- and rimantadine-resistant influenza A is warranted, as the use of these agents is likely to increase.

▶ Amino acid changes in the M2 structural protein is the well-documented mechanism of amantadine-rimantadine resistance in influenza viruses. Having that knowledge in hand helps the clinician to at least understand how resistance develops to 2 drugs that will probably be increasingly used in nursing home and other long-term-care populations. Eventually, it may be the molecular biologist who will use this understanding to try to find a "way around" the resistance mechanism. The report by Houck et al. suggests that a vigorous search for a way around resistance could begin sooner than one might have anticipated. The appearance of 3 amantadine-resistant influenza strains at nursing home A before any known use of the drug and the apparent rapid appearance of resistance in a previously sensitive influenza strain at nursing home C are warning flags for any physician involved with patients such as these. The authors raise the possibility of laboratory contamination in these reported cases but believe the probability to be low. The use of amantadine-rimantadine as an adjunct to influenza vaccine, observing Centers for Disease Control and Prevention guidelines,[1, 2] seems to be the course to continue, but with heightened surveillance regarding resistance.

R.C. Bone, M.D.

References

1. Centers for Disease Control: Prevention and control of influenza: Recommendations of the Immunization Practices Advisory Committee (ACIP). *MMWR Morb Mortal Wkly Rep* 41:10–13, 1992.
2. Centers for Disease Control: Control on influenza A outbreaks in nursing homes: Amantadine as an adjunct to vaccine—Washington, 1989–90. *MMWR Morb Mortal Wkly Rep* 40:841–844, 1991.

16 Tuberculosis

Outbreak of Tuberculosis in a Church

Dutt AK, Mehta JB, Whitaker BJ, Westmoreland H (Upper Cumberland Chest Clinic, Cookeville, Tenn)

Chest 107:447–452, 1995 119-96-16–1

Background.—Prolonged exposure in a closed environment to a person who has active tuberculosis (TB) greatly increases the risk of infection. Such transmission has been reported in schools, jails, day care centers, and nursing homes. An outbreak involving the exposure of a large church congregation to an infection case was reported.

Methods and Findings.—The index case was a man, 48, who had abnormal findings on chest radiograph but in whom TB was undiagnosed for 4 years. Investigation with purified protein derivative (PPD) tuberculin test showed positive tuberculin reactions in 7 of 8 of the man's initial close contacts (88%) and in 12 of 46 of his co-workers (26%). A PPD survey of 184 of the 200 members of the patient's church showed positive reactions in 42%. Thirty percent of the members younger than 35 years of age were infected, which suggested transmission of infection. Including the index case, 8 cases of active TB were detected, for a case rate of 4.3% among the church members (Table 1). Bacteriologic findings were available in only 3 of these patients. Two patients had phage typing of organism identical to the index case, and the third had recrudescent TB disease. Of the remaining 5 patients who did not have bacteriologic confirmation, 2 had pleural TB and 2 had localized pulmonary nodules, which suggested primary infection progressing to disease. The fifth patient was a child who had progressive primary TB (Table 2).

Conclusions.—Tuberculosis infection can be transmitted in any closed environment, including a church. Physicians therefore must be conversant with TB control measures and preventive treatment guidelines to preclude unforeseen transmission of disease.

► Tuberculosis can be transmitted in any environment conducive to transmission, and a church that has relatively poor ventilation and probably poor mixing of lower with upper room air would be just such an environment. However, it would require a health care professional who had public health experience and an index of suspicion to link an outbreak of TB with a church as the mechanism of transmission. The authors appear to meet these

TABLE 1.—Active Cases of Tuberculosis Identified Among Church Members

Case No./Age, y/ Race/Sex	Date	Presentation	Diagnosis
Index case/48/W/M	4/86	Pulmonary infiltration	Sputum smear and culture positive, positive, PPD
1/63/W/F	7/86	Pleural	Clinical, positive PPD, previous PPD unknown but likely primary
2/6/W/F	7/86	Pleural	Pleural biopsy and positive AFB, not cultured, *PPD conversion*
3/2/W/F	2/87	Hilar adenopathy and pulmonary segmental collapse	Clinical, positive PPD, *PPD conversion*
4*/23/W/F	2/87	Pulmonary infiltration	Sputum smear and culture positive, *PPD conversion*, phase typing identical to index case
5/71/W/F	5/87	Pulmonary nodule	Excision biopsy, positive AFB, not cultured, positive PPD, previous PPD unknown but likely primary
6†/43/W/M	3/88	Pulmonary infiltration	Sputum smear and culture positive, positive PPD, previous PPD unknown, phage typing unlike index case, recrudescent disease
7/67/W/M	6/88	Pulmonary nodule	Excision biopsy, positive AFB, not cultured, positive PPD, previous PPD unknown but likely primary

*Index case and case 4: phage type 2 (7, 9, 12, 13).
†Case 6: phage type 1 (13).
Abbreviations: AFB, acid-fast bacilli; *PPD,* purified protein derivative.
(Courtesy of Dutt AK, Mehta JB, Whitaker BJ, et al: Outbreak of tuberculosis in a church. *Chest* 107:447–452, 1995.)

TABLE 2.—Final Results of Tuberculin Testing and Preventive Therapy in the Church, 1986–1988

		Initial Examination			Preventive Treatment					
			Tuberculin Test					Stopped		
Age Group yr	Total	Radiograph	Negative	Positive	Recom	Started	Completed	SGOT	SX	Yield Active* Cases
0 to 4	11	3	8	3	2	2	2			1
5 to 9	13	3	9	4	3	3	3			1
10 to 14	15	1	14	1	1	1	1			
15 to 19	10	3	6	4	4	4	4			
20 to 34	32	15	20	12	11	11	10		1	1
35 to 49	31	16	16	15	11	11	9	1	1	1
50 to 64	48	31	23	25	17	16	10	5	1	1
65+	24	16	11	13	3	2	1		1	2
Total	184	88	107	77	52	50	40	6	4	7

*Index case not included.

Abbreviations: Recom, recommended; *SX,* symptoms; *SGOT,* serum glutamate oxaloacetate transaminase.

(Courtesy of Dutt AK, Mehta JB, Whitaker BJ, et al: Outbreak of tuberculosis in a church. *Chest* 107:447–452, 1995.)

criteria: the region of Tennessee served by the chest clinic they staff had a TB case rate of 20.7 in 1988 compared with 12.5 for the state of Tennessee. The authors recognized the highly infectious nature of their index case and confirmed their suspicion by finding a large number of tuberculin reactors in the patient's family and workplace. They followed up on the tuberculin reactors identified among members of the patient's church and persisted in their investigation despite resistance from church leaders.

A clear message in their report is the failure of medical and public health protocols that set this outbreak in motion. Although the index patient had radiographic abnormalities and a positive tuberculin reaction in 1982, no preventive therapy was given, and the disease remained active. Over the next 4 years, many of the members of his family, his co-workers, and members of his church became infected. From 1982 to 1986, the patient's chest radiograph showed deterioration, but because cultures from sputum and bronchoscopy washings were negative, another opportunity for adequate therapy was missed. The authors make a strong point regarding private physicians in their region who apparently are not well educated regarding TB, despite the high case rate of TB. Ominously, it is just these physicians who must be depended on to "take up the slack" when state budgets for TB control programs are reduced.

R.C. Bone, M.D.

CD4 T Lymphocyte Count and the Radiographic Presentation of Pulmonary Tuberculosis: A Study of the Relationship Between These Factors in Patients With Human Immunodeficiency Virus Infection

Keiper MD, Beumont M, Elshami A, Langlotz CP, Miller WT Jr (Univ of Pennsylvania, Philadelphia)

Chest 107:74–80, 1995 119-96-16–2

Background.—The clinical and radiographic presentations of pulmonary infection and tumor in patients who have AIDS are variable. Associations between the radiographic presentation of pulmonary tuberculosis and CD4 T lymphocyte counts were investigated in patients infected with HIV to establish an empirical guideline for early diagnosis, treatment, and isolation of infected individuals.

Patients and Methods.—Thirty-five patients who were seropositive for HIV and had culture-verified pulmonary tuberculosis were identified from 3 urban hospitals. Chest radiographs, CD4 T lymphocyte counts, and clinical histories were analyzed retrospectively. On radiographs, the presence of patterns either characteristic or uncharacteristic of post-primary tuberculosis (representing typical and atypical patterns, respectively) were evaluated.

Results.—Atypical patterns of pulmonary tuberculosis were observed in 21 of 26 patients who had CD4 T lymphocyte counts less than 0.20×10^9 cells/L. Conversely, only 1 of 9 patients who had CD4 T lymphocyte counts greater than or equal to 0.20×10^9 cells/L showed an atypical

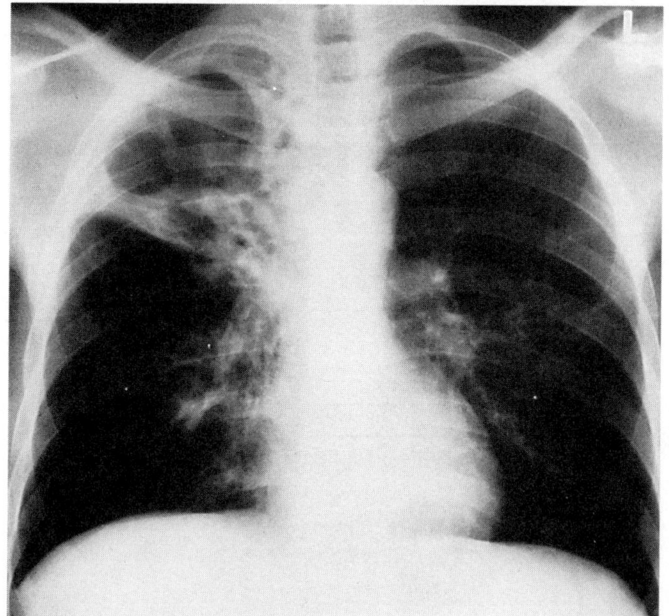

FIGURE 1.—Typical pattern with CD4 count of 0.20×10^9 cells/L. There is a cavitary right upper lobe opacity, typical of reactivation tuberculosis. (Courtesy of Keiper MD, Beumont M, Elshami A, et al: CD4 T lymphocyte count and the radiographic presentation of pulmonary tuberculosis: A study of the relationship between these factors in patients with human immunodeficiency virus infection. *Chest* 107:74–80, 1995.)

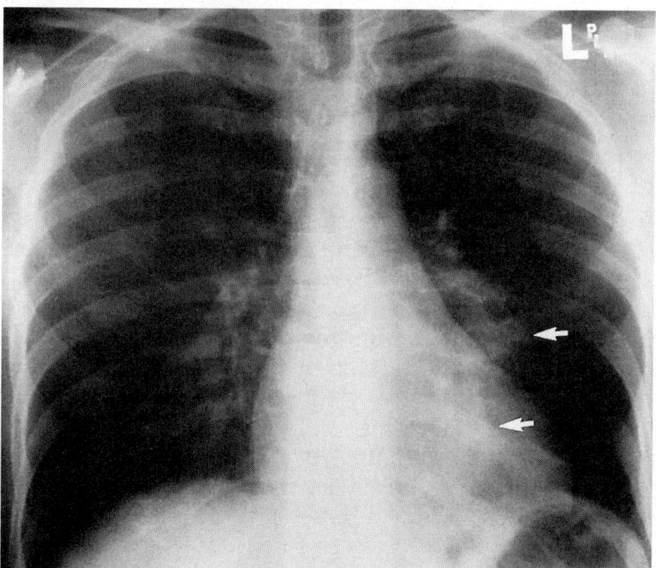

FIGURE 2.—Atypical pattern with low CD4 count of 0.01×10^9 cells/L. A focal alveolar opacity is seen in the left lower lobe (*arrows*), obscuring the inferior hilum. This pattern does not automatically implicate tuberculosis. (Courtesy of Keiper MD, Beumont M, Elshami A, et al: CD4 T lymphocyte count and the radiographic presentation of pulmonary tuberculosis: A study of the relationship between these factors in patients with human immunodeficiency virus infection. *Chest* 107:74–80, 1995.)

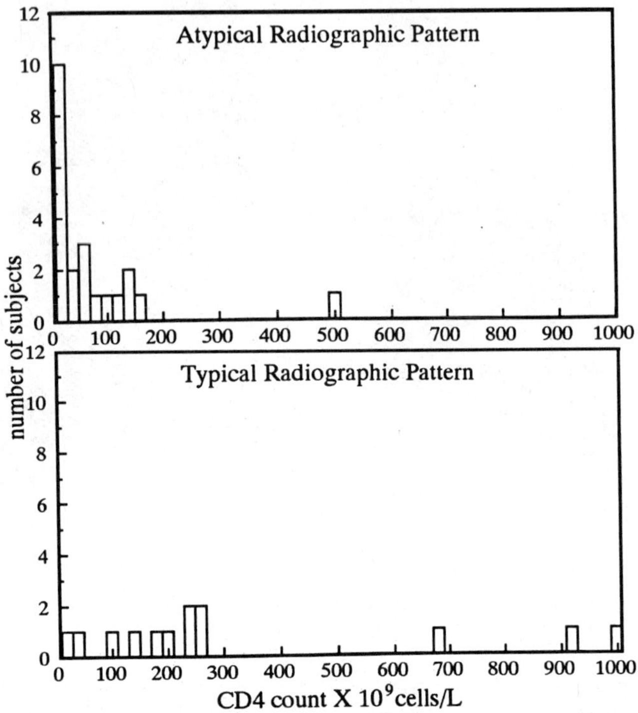

FIGURE 4.—Distribution of CD4 T-lymphocyte counts according to radiographic pattern. (Courtesy of Keiper MD, Beumont M, Elshami A, et al: CD4 T lymphocyte count and the radiographic presentation of pulmonary tuberculosis: A study of the relationship between these factors in patients with human immunodeficiency virus infection. *Chest* 107:74–80, 1995.)

pattern (Figs 1 and 2). The mean CD4 T lymphocyte count of 22 patients who had atypical radiographic patterns was 0.069×10^9 cells/L compared with 0.323×10^9 cell/L in 13 patients who had typical radiographic patterns. The between-group difference was statistically significant (Fig 4). Twenty-one patients who had atypical patterns of pulmonary tuberculosis were significantly immunocompromised. Atypical radiographic patterns consisted of diffuse and lower lobar opacities, pleural effusion, mediastinal adenopathy, intestinal nodules, and normal chest radiographs.

Conclusions.—Pulmonary tuberculosis should be suspected in patients with AIDS who have CD4 counts less than 0.20×10^9 cells/L and atypical radiographic patterns for pulmonary tuberculosis. Appropriate treatment and early isolation should be initiated in these patients until the diagnosis of pulmonary tuberculosis has been ruled out.

► Tuberculosis has become an opportunistic invader of great concern in patients who have AIDS, and the disease has proved no less difficult to diagnose than one would expect from this classically invasive organism. The radiographic picture can be equivocal as to whether the patient does or does not have a tuberculosis pattern. Keiper et al. retrospectively paired radiology with immunology to demonstrate a relationship of considerable potential clinical usefulness. In most of the 35 patients whose records were reviewed, a CD4 T lymphocyte count less than 0.20×10^9 cells/L and a culture-proven pulmonary tuberculosis had chest radiographic patterns atypical for reactivation tuberculosis. The authors recommend that this radiologic and immunologic pattern in a patient at risk for tuberculosis infection should cause the physician to have high suspicion and should be an indication to institute isolation and treatment until a diagnosis is confirmed or excluded.

R.C. Bone, M.D.

Preventing the Nosocomial Transmission of Tuberculosis

Blumberg HM, Watkins DL, Berschling JD, Antle A, Moore P, White N, Hunter M, Green B, Ray SM, McGowan JE Jr (Emory Univ, Atlanta, Ga)

Ann Intern Med 122:658–663, 1995 119-96-16–3

Background.—The increase in tuberculosis in the United States during the past decade has been linked to both the AIDS epidemic and nosocomial transmission of the infection in hospitals, prisons, and shelters. Patients who have unsuspected tuberculosis are clustered with immunocompromised patients, diagnosis is delayed in patients who have HIV infection and an atypical clinical picture, and the ongoing infectiousness of cases has not been recognized. The efficacy of expanded tuberculosis infection control measures was examined in a university-affiliated, inner-city hospital.

Methods.—The measures consisted of an expanded respiratory isolation policy, with isolation discontinued only after 3 consecutive negative acid-fast bacilli sputum smears were obtained. In addition, the Epidemiology and Infection Control Department increased its surveillance, health care worker education was expanded, and a tuberculosis infection control coordinator was hired. Ninety rooms were converted to negative-pressure rooms, and personal respiratory protection equipment replaced the standard surgical masks previously used by health care workers. Efficacy was evaluated by comparing the number of episodes of tuberculosis exposure and skin test conversion rates of health care workers before and after measures were introduced.

Results.—The number of episodes of tuberculosis exposure, which was defined as the number of patients who were not placed in respiratory isolation at admission but who subsequently were confirmed to have pulmonary tuberculosis during that admission or within 2 weeks of discharge, decreased from 4.4 to 0.6 per month after expanded infection control measures were introduced. The cumulative number of days per month that potentially infectious patients were not in isolation also decreased significantly, from 35.4 to 3.3. Tuberculin skin test conversion rates in health care workers, evaluated during a 2.5-year period, declined from 3.3% to 0.4%.

Conclusion.—Expanded procedures designed to prevent the nosocomial transmission of tuberculosis in this public inner-city hospital were successful. There was a marked reduction in episodes of tuberculosis exposure and tuberculin skin test conversions among health care workers. Although only 14% of patients placed in respiratory isolation had culture-confirmed tuberculosis, a policy of overisolation succeeded in appropriately isolating 95% of patients in whom tuberculosis was subsequently diagnosed. A high index of suspicion and careful screening for tuberculosis is a cost-effective method for hospitals that have limited resources.

▶ Institutional control measures for tuberculosis are analogous to home cooking: We have to keep rediscovering them to learn how good they really are. Administrative and engineering controls may be "old hat" but are quite effective in preventing nosocomial transmission of tuberculosis. Tuberculin skin testing of health care workers at 1-year intervals is among the control measures that have been effective; however, as at Grady Memorial Hospital, a 6-month mandatory testing cycle may be necessary to complement the rigorous controls needed at an urban hospital. Probably among the most neglected or poorly understood control measures are air-flow testing and isolation. A room designated for isolation of high-risk patients who have tuberculosis often does not meet the guidelines of the Centers for Disease Control and Prevention for negative air pressure and hourly changes in room air.[1]

Another group of investigators recently called attention to the risk for transmission of *Mycobacterium tuberculosis* in the autopsy room;[2] this group believed they observed one of the most infectious cases of tuberculosis ever encountered. The report by Blumberg et al. is a welcome, and necessary, reminder regarding the effectiveness of those "old hat" control measures for tuberculosis.

R.C. Bone, M.D.

References

1. Guidelines for preventing the transmission of *Mycobacterium tuberculosis* in health-care facilities. *MMWR Morb Mortal Wkly Rep* 43:1–132, 1994.
2. Templeton GL, Illing LA, Young L, et al: The risk for transmission of *Mycobacterium tuberculosis* at the bedside and during autopsy. *Ann Intern Med* 122:922–925, 1995.

17 Interstitial Lung Disease

Pulmonary Lymphangioleiomyomatosis: A Report of 46 Patients Including a Clinicopathologic Study of Prognostic Factors

Kitaichi M, Nishimura K, Itoh H, Izumi T (Chest Disease Research Inst, Kyoto, Japan; Kyoto Univ Hosp, Japan)

Am J Respir Crit Care Med 151:527–533, 1995 119-96-17–1

Background.—Pulmonary lymphangioleiomyomatosis (LAM) is rare and affects the lungs of women. It has been reported that affected individuals die of respiratory failure within 10 years after onset of symptoms. Few treatments have improved the course of the disease. Clinical and pathologic features of patients who had LAM were reported, and prognostic factors of the disease were clarified.

Methods.—The clinical features of 46 patients who had LAM were analyzed. These features included age of onset, date of first examination, date and method of diagnosis, history of lung disease and hormonal therapy, clinical and radiographic features, concurrent conditions, clinical course, serial lung function tests, and arterial blood gas analyses. Computed tomographic scans were reviewed, and response to treatment was evaluated.

Results.—Forty of 60 treatments could be evaluated, and 2 were considered effective. Of 42 patients who underwent pulmonary function tests, 12 (29%) showed airflow limitation, 11 (26%) showed a restrictive dysfunction, and 15 (36%) showed a combined restrictive and obstructive dysfunction (Table 1). A reduced forced expiratory volume in 1 second/forced vital capacity ratio was associated with poor prognosis 2–5 years after first examination; the differences were statistically significant. An increased percentage of predicted total lung capacity was associated with poor prognosis at 2, 3, and 5 years after first examination; the differences were statistically significant. Histologically, pulmonary lesions were either predominantly cystic or predominantly muscular. Patients who had predominantly cystic lesions tended to have a poor prognosis 2–5 years after biopsy. The open lung biopsy findings indicated that higher grades of abnormal areas were associated with poor prognosis 2–5 years after biopsy; the differences were statistically significant. Survival and higher

TABLE 1.—Clinical and Laboratory Findings in 46 Women With Lymphangioleiomyomatosis at First Examination

Age	34.8 ± 9.1 yr (range, 21–65 yr)
Smoking history: Nonsmokers 36 Smokers 3; Exsmokers 5 Unknown 2	
Symptoms	
Dyspnea,	
Resting	13/43 (30%)
Exertional	38/43 (88%)
Cough	25/41 (61%)
Chest pain	14/42 (33%)
Chyloptysis	0/40 (0%)
Hemoptysis	11/39 (28%)
Physical findings	
Clubbing	2/42 (5%)
Crackles	10/45 (22%)
Rhonchi	6/42 (14%)
Chylothorax	3/41 (7%)
Chylous ascites	2/41 (5%)
Chest radiography	
Normal	1/46 (2%)
Bilateral infiltrates	45/46 (98%)
Reticulonodular shadows	39/46 (85%)
Cysts or bullae	25/45 (56%)
Effusion	5/45 (11%)
Pneumothorax	18/46 (39%)
Hyperinflation	22/46 (48%)
Physiologic findings	
Normal range	4/42 (10%)
Obstructive (%VC ≥ 80% and FEV_1/FVC < 70%)	12/42 (29%)
Restrictive (%VC < 80% and FEV_1/FVC ≥ 70%)	11/42 (26%)
Combined restrictive and obstructive	15/42 (36%)
Increased %TLC (%TLC > 120% predicted)	7/23 (30%)
Decreased %TLC (%TLC < 80% predicted)	3/23 (13%)
Increased RV/TLC (RV/TLC > 45%)	19/35 (54%)
Decreased diffusing capacity	
(< 80% predicted)	30/31 (97%)
(< 45% predicted)	22/31 (71%)
Hypoxemia (Pa_{O_2} < 80 mm Hg)	35/43 (81%)

Abbreviations: FEV_1, forced expiratory volume in 1 second; *FVC*, forced vital capacity; *% TLC*, percent predicted total lung capacity; *VC*, vital capacity.

(Courtesy of Kitaichi M, Nishimura K, Itoh H, et al: Pulmonary lymphangioleiomyomatosis: A report of 46 patients including a clinicopathologic study of prognostic factors. *Am J Respir Crit Care Med* 151:527–533, 1995.)

grade cystic lesions were inversely correlated at 2, 4, and 5 years after biopsy; the differences were statistically significant.

Discussion.—This was the largest group of patients with LAM studied and the first report of prognostic factors of the disease. It is important to clarify such factors to determine the effects of treatments.

▶ The etiology of LAM remains unknown, but advances in diagnosis and treatment are made nevertheless. The rarity of the disease reduces the odds that most physicians, except those in large tertiary care centers, would be called on to use these advances in following the status of a patient with LAM from diagnosis to advanced stages. The patient would, of course, be female and most likely young to middle-aged, unless the disease was far advanced. The association between LAM and women in the reproductive years is well established but not understood.

The clinical features and laboratory findings at first examination should provide some clues to prognosis, as reported in this study of 46 patients. Detection of increase in percent predicted total lung capacity correlates with a poor prognosis at 2, 3, and 5 years after the first examination. This, together with the poor prognosis at 2 years associated with reduced forced expiratory volume in 1 second/forced vital capacity, reflects the obstructive nature of LAM pulmonary function patterns. This pattern also is reflected in the major clinical presentations at first examination: dyspnea, cough, pneumothorax, bilateral reticulonodular infiltrates, cysts or bullae, and hyperinflation. Open lung biopsy specimens typically reveal diffuse effacement of normal architecture by cystic spaces up to 2 cm in diameter and/or a smooth muscle proliferation. In this group of patients, the predominantly cystic lesions were associated with a poorer prognosis 2–5 years after biopsy. Although early treatment of LAM with some form of hormone therapy may be beneficial, the long-term outcomes remain to be clarified; until recently,[1] patients might be expected to die within 10 years of onset of symptoms. Patients in advanced stages may be considered for lung transplantation.[2, 3]

R.C. Bone, M.D.

References

1. Taylor JR, Ryu J, Colby TV, et al: Lymphangioleiomyomatosis: Clinical course in 32 patients. *N Engl J Med* 323:1254–1260, 1990.
2. Wellens F, Estenne M, de Francquen P, et al: Combined heart-lung transplantation for terminal pulmonary lymphangioleiomyomatosis. *J Thorac Cardiovasc Surg* 89:872–876, 1985.
3. Raffin TA, Taylor JR, Colby TV: Treatment of lymphangioleiomyomatosis. *N Engl J Med* 325:64, 1991.

Pulmonary Tuberous Sclerosis

Castro M, Shepherd CW, Gomez MR, Lie JT, Ryu JH (Mayo Clinic and Found, Rochester, Minn)

Chest 107:189–195, 1995 119-96-17–2

Background.—Pulmonary involvement in tuberous sclerosis complex (TSC), an autosomal dominant disorder, is rare, with a reported incidence of less than 1% of patients. Accordingly, this particular disease is not well characterized, and little is known about its natural course or treatment. The clinical presentation, pulmonary function tests, chest radiograph and CT findings, hormonal treatment response, and survival duration in patients who had pulmonary involvement in TCS were reviewed to provide a guide to treatment.

Patients and Findings.—Nine female patients were included. The average age at onset of symptoms was 16 years, and the average follow-up was

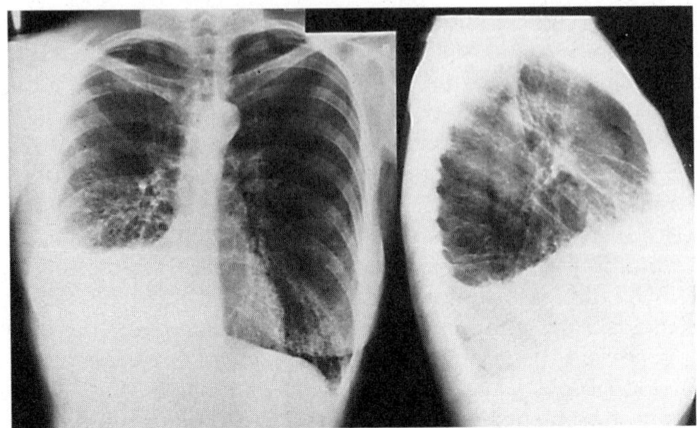

FIGURE 1.—Posteroanterior (*left*) and lateral (*right*) chest radiograph of a patient with pulmonary involvement in tuberous sclerosis complex, demonstrating bilateral interstitial infiltrates with cystic changes and chylothorax. (Courtesy of Castro M, Shepherd CW, Gomez MR, et al: Pulmonary tuberous sclerosis. *Chest* 107:189–195, 1995.)

17 years. Pulmonary involvement was not observed until an average age of 33 years, and there was an average delay of 8 years before proper diagnoses were obtained. Seizures, pneumothorax, dyspnea, and typical skin changes were commonly observed at initial examination, and obstruction to airflow and decreased single-breath diffusing capacity were frequent findings on pulmonary function tests. A characteristic feature on chest radiography and CT was diffuse interstitial infiltrates with cystic changes (Figs 1 and 2). The kidneys were involved in 8 patients, all of whom had renal angiomyolipomas (Fig 3). Two asymptomatic patients who had mild pulmonary involvement have remained stable without hormonal therapy. Five of 7 patients who had moderate-to-severe airway obstruction have

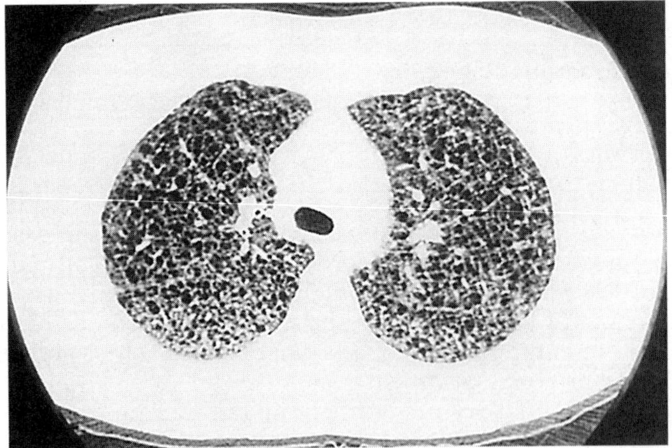

FIGURE 2.—High-resolution chest CT of a patient with pulmonary involvement in tuberous sclerosis complex, demonstrating numerous well-defined cysts outlined by thin walls. (Courtesy of Castro M, Shepherd CW, Gomez MR, et al: Pulmonary tuberous sclerosis. *Chest* 107:189–195, 1995.)

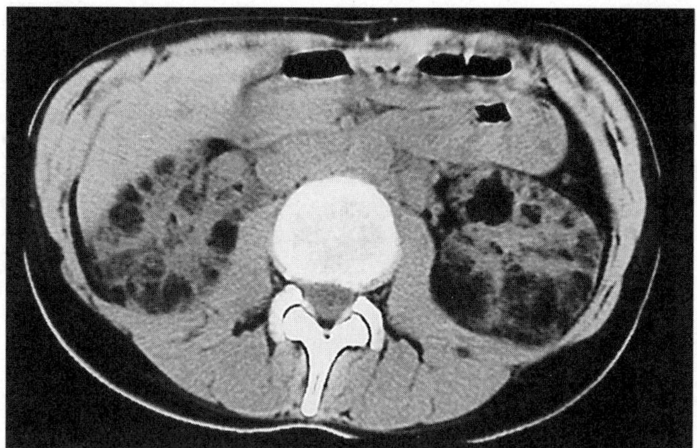

FIGURE 3.—Abdominal CT of a patient with pulmonary involvement in tuberous sclerosis complex, demonstrating bilateral renal angiomyolipomas. (Courtesy of Castro M, Shepherd CW, Gomez MR, et al: Pulmonary tuberous sclerosis. *Chest* 107:189–195, 1995.)

undergone hormonal therapy; 3 of these patients achieved a clinical response. The 2 patients who did not receive therapy died of progressive respiratory failure.

Conclusions.—Most patients who have pulmonary involvement in TSC have a slowly deteriorating clinical course. Although the data are limited, a trial of hormonal therapy is advised for patients who have symptomatic pain and for those who have worsening pulmonary function. In all patients who have a diagnosis of lymphangioleiomyomatosis, TSC should be suspected.

► This report from the Mayo Clinic represents a continuum of the fine work from physicians at that institution on lymphangioleiomyomatosis (LAM) and TSC.[1] Neither entity would commonly be seen in an internal medicine practice, and pulmonary complications are even more rare (2.3% of 388 patients who had TSC seen at Mayo Clinic between 1948 and 1991). Both because of relative rarity and because differentiation of LAM from TSC can be a difficult diagnostic challenge, the data derived from the records of the 9 patients who had TSC reported in this abstract are valuable for internists as well as pulmonologists who may be called on to diagnose and treat pulmonary complications arising from the proliferation of smooth muscle characteristic of this disease.

Radiography—flat plate and CT—helped detect pulmonary involvement in patients with or without respiratory symptoms. High-resolution CT was more sensitive in identifying pulmonary involvement in patients who had normal chest radiographic findings. The distinct presentation of TSC with pulmonary involvement includes a preponderance of female patients, in contrast to no sex predilection in patients who have TSC without known lung involvement, and onset of pulmonary symptoms in the third to fifth decade of life, in contrast to patients without lung involvement, who are usually first seen in infancy with neurologic manifestations.

Based on the results of treatment in some of the 9 patients, the authors recommend a trial of hormonal therapy in the pulmonary patient when the disease becomes symptomatic or when there is progressive deterioration on pulmonary function testing. Monthly IM methoxyprogesterone is the recommended initial hormonal treatment, with oophorectomy, tamoxifen, and leuprolide reserved as options.

R.C. Bone, M.D.

Reference

1. Shepherd CW, Gomez MR, Lie JT, et al: Causes of death in patients with tuberous sclerosis. *Mayo Clin Proc* 66:792–796, 1991.

Alveolar Hemorrhage: Diagnostic Criteria and Results in 194 Immunocompromised Hosts

De Lassence A, Fleury-Feith J, Escudier E, Beaune J, Bernaudin J-F, Cordonnier C (Hôpital Henri Mondor, Cíeteil, France; Hôpital Tenon, Paris)

Am J Respir Crit Care Med 151:157–163, 1995 119-96-17–3

Introduction.—Pulmonary complications, such as alveolar hemorrhage (AH), are a common cause of morbidity and mortality among immunocompromised patients. Since the 1970s, bronchoalveolar lavage (BAL) has been used to identify AH, although there is no single definition of AH using this technique. A simple method was devised to establish the diagnosis of AH from BAL data, based on the percentage of siderophages among the total alveolar macrophages recovered from BAL fluid. This method was compared with other diagnostic criteria for AH and correlated with clinical, biological, and histologic parameters.

Methods.—The results of 240 BALs performed in 194 immunocompromised patients were reviewed retrospectively. There were 161 male and 79 female patients (age range, 11–76 years). Prussian blue staining for macrophages was performed on each sample, and the Golde score was calculated for 47 randomly chosen samples.

Results.—The percentage of siderophages correlated well with the Golde score, with AH defined as a minimum of 20% siderophages (Fig 2). Alveolar hemorrhage was detected in 36% of these samples. It was significantly associated with thrombocytopenia, other abnormal coagulation parameters, renal failure, and a history of heavy smoking. Alveolar hemorrhage did not correlate with either the cause or the outcome of pneumonia. It was more frequent in patients who underwent cardiac transplant than in other immunocompromised patients.

Conclusions.—If at least 20% of total alveolar macrophages from BAL fluid are detected as siderophages, then AH can be diagnosed. This method is simple and reliable. In this population, AH appears to be more a symptom than a disease. It is correlated with coagulation disorders and renal insufficiency. It may be advisable, therefore, to correct these factors

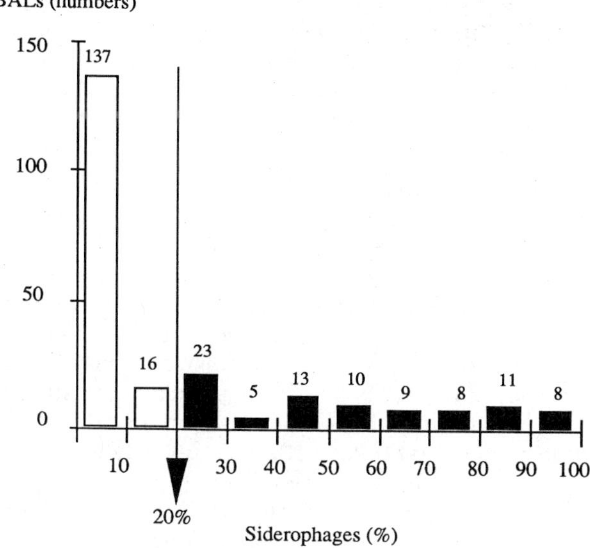

FIGURE 2.—Frequency with which various percentages of alveolar siderophages were observed in 240 bronchoalveolar lavages performed in immunocompromised patients. Alveolar hemorrhage (*filled columns*) was defined by a percentage of siderophages ≥ 20%. (Courtesy of De Lassence A, Fleury-Feith J, Escudier E, et al: Alveolar hemorrhage: Diagnostic criteria and results in 194 immunocompromised hosts. *Am J Respir Crit Care Med* 151:157–163, 1995.)

in immunocompromised patients, particularly in patients who undergo cardiac transplant and those who have a history of smoking. The benefits derived from such corrective measures should be investigated prospectively.

► It would be a truism to say that a pathologic condition that is difficult to diagnose is apt to be misdiagnosed or missed altogether. Nevertheless, such is the case, and the difficulty in diagnosis is increased when a standard diagnostic test is difficult to administer or to interpret. De Lassence et al. conclude that their method of diagnosing AH in immunocompromised patients, i.e., calculating the percentage of siderophages among the total alveolar macrophages recovered by BAL, is easier to use than the standard method of Golde score. The findings were found to correlate well with Golde score in a sample of 47 BAL samples.

The diagnostic meaning of the findings was often equivocal. The diagnosis of AH did not correlate well with either the cause or outcome of pneumonia in immunocompromised patients. In fact, AH was rarely found to be the cause of lung injury. Because thrombocytopenia, other coagulation disorders, and renal insufficiency were found to be correlated with a diagnosis of AH, the authors recommend that these 3 conditions be corrected in the setting of pulmonary disease, particularly in cardiac transplant patients, who were seen to be at higher risk for AH, and in heavy smokers in whom smoking history was statistically correlated with risk of AH.

R.C. Bone, M.D.

Increased Interleukin-1 Receptor Antagonist in Idiopathic Pulmonary Fibrosis: A Compartmental Analysis

Smith DR, Kunkel SL, Standiford TJ, Rolfe MW, Lynch JP III, Arenberg DA, Wilke CA, Burdick MD, Martinez FJ, Hampton JN, Whyte RI, Orringer MB, Strieter RM (Univ of Michigan, Ann Arbor)

Am J Respir Crit Care Med 151:1965–1973, 1995 119-96-17–4

Introduction.—The cause of idiopathic pulmonary fibrosis (IPF) remains unknown, and its prognosis is dismal. The chronic and destructive features of this disease include exaggerated reparative processes and interstitial fibrosis. In sufficient quantities, interleukin-1 receptor antagonist protein (IRAP) acts as a pure antagonist of interleukin-1 (IL-1) that can attenuate a variety of IL-1 actions in vitro and in vivo. A significant increase in the level of IRAP has been detected in patients who have sarcoidosis and may play a role in other pulmonary diseases. The potential role of IRAP in patients who have IPF was investigated.

Methods.—Tissue specimens were obtained by open lung biopsy from 18 patients who had suspected IPF. In addition, normal tissue was obtained from 20 patients who underwent thoracotomy for suspected primary bronchogenic carcinoma. Tissue samples were isolated and cultured for pulmonary fibroblasts. Patients in the study group also underwent bronchoalveolar lavage, and results were compared with those of 8 healthy, nonsmoking individuals in the research group. Paraffin-embedded tissue was processed for immunohistochemical localization of IRAP and IL-1β, and IRAP messenger RNA was localized by in situ hybridization.

Results.—The content of IRAP in bronchoalveolar lavage fluid from patients who had IPF was significantly greater compared with that from healthy, nonsmoking individuals. Patients with IPF also had significant increases in IL-1β, compared with control individuals. Although not significant, the IL-1β content was higher in smoking than nonsmoking patients who had IPF. The IRAP:IL-1β ratio was 10:1 in patients who had IPF compared with 5.8:1 in normal individuals. Homogenate levels of IRAP in patients who had IPF were significantly increased compared with normal tissue samples from patients undergoing resection for primary bronchogenic carcinoma. No significant difference in homogenate levels of IRAP was detected between smokers and nonsmokers who had IPF. Total homogenate content of IL-1β in patients who had IPF was significantly depressed compared with normal individuals. Patients who had IPF and smoked had twofold higher levels of IL-1β, compared with nonsmokers. The ratios of IRAP:IL-1β were 19:1 for patients who had IPF and 1.3:1 for normal individuals; no ratio differences were observed between smokers and nonsmokers who had IPF. Lung tissue homogenates in patients who had IPF were significantly elevated for transforming growth factor-β content compared with normal individuals. Patients who had IPF had greater values of transforming growth factor-β if they were smokers compared with values in nonsmokers. There were no significant differences between patients who had IPF and healthy individuals or between smoking and nonsmoking patients in the tumor necrosis factor-α content in tissue homogenates. Staining of normal lung tissue showed little antigenic IRAP or IL-1β. Staining in patients who had IPF, however, showed marked qualitative increases in IRAP staining, localized to hyperplastic type II pneumocytes lining the alveoli, macrophages, and fibroblasts. Positive staining of IRAP messenger RNA in IPF tissue resembled protein expression and was localized to hyperplastic type II pneumocytes and fibroblast cells. No differences in constitutive production of IRAP were detected between patients who had IPF and normal individuals.

Conclusion.—The fibrotic tissue changes in patients who have IPF may result from the local effects of IRAP. Pulmonary nonimmune cells may influence local tissue changes through the elaboration of IRAP.

▶ Studies from this laboratory recently showed that IRAP is significantly increased in sarcoidosis.[1] Extending that work in the framework of a hypothesis that IRAP may play a role in the tissue fibrosis of the interstitial lung diseases, Smith et al. show in this report that IRAP is increased in the bronchoalveolar lavage fluid of patients who have IPF as compared with fluid from normal individuals. The finding of increased IRAP in the alveolar space in IPF lung offers the puzzle that the cytokine environment in these lungs is less, rather than more, proinflammatory, i.e., IRAP attenuates IL-1 in both in vitro and in vivo models.[2] The cellular courses of the IRAP, demonstrated by immunohistochemistry, proved to be hyperplastic type II pneumocytes, interstitial fibroblasts, and resident macrophages. The authors hypothesize a continuum of events in IPF, perhaps beginning with a local inflammation, which results finally in failure of tissue repair and remodeling on an organic scale because of an as-yet-unidentified dysregulation of the immune response.

R.C. Bone, M.D.

References

1. Rolfe MW, Standiford TJ, Kunkel SL, et al: Interleukin-1 receptor antagonist expression in sarcoidosis. *Am Rev Respir Dis* 148:1378–1384, 1993.
2. Dinarello CA: Interleukin-1 and interleukin-1 antagonism. *Blood* 77:1627–1652, 1991.

18 Occupational Lung Disease

Prevalence of Occupational Asthma Due to Latex Among Hospital Personnel

Vandenplas O, Delwiche J-P, Evrard G, Aimont P, Van Der Brempt X, Jamart J, Delaunois L (Catholic Univ of Louvain, Yvoir, Belgium; Semilux Occupational Health Service, Libramont, Belgium; Clinique Saint-Luc, Namur, Belgium)

Am J Respir Crit Care Med 151:54–60, 1995 119-96-18–1

Background.—Latex can cause immediate hypersensitivity reactions, ranging from contact urticaria to severe anaphylaxis. Latex proteins may also act as airborne allergens, resulting in rhinitis and asthma. The prevalence of occupational asthma from latex gloves among health care providers was determined.

Methods.—Two hundred one nurses, 50 members of the cleaning staff, and 38 laboratory technologists in a primary care hospital were surveyed. A questionnaire and skin-prick tests with latex and common inhalant allergens were administered to 94% of these individuals. In the second part of the study, a histamine inhalation challenge was done on workers who were sensitive to latex.

Findings.—Thirteen workers (4.7%) showed skin reactivity to latex. All workers who had latex sensitivity reported glove-related urticaria. This reaction was associated with rhinoconjunctivitis in 12 workers and asthma in 5. None of the workers who had a negative skin-test result to latex had a history that suggested occupational asthma. The 12 workers who underwent a histamine inhalation challenge demonstrated significant bronchial hyperresponsiveness. Specific inhalation challenges with latex gloves performed on all 12 workers in the laboratory resulted in significant bronchial response to latex glove exposure in 7 (Fig 3). Four reactions were immediate, and 3 were dual.

Conclusions.—Occupational asthma caused by latex occurred in 2.5% of these hospital employees. The widespread use of latex gloves should be considered a significant risk to the respiratory well-being of health care workers.

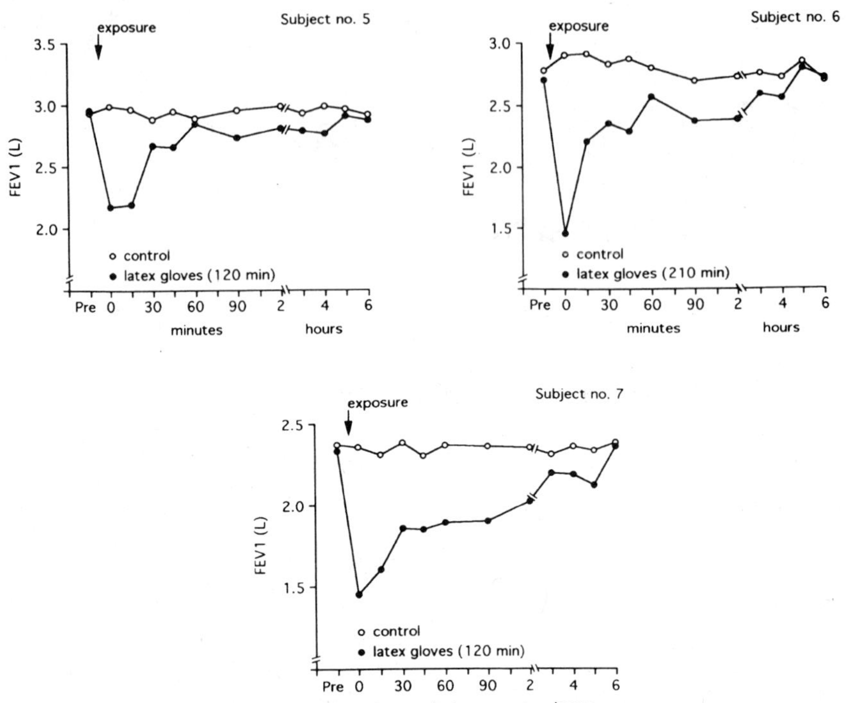

FIGURE 3.—Results of specific inhalation challenges with latex gloves in 3 patients. (Courtesy of Vandenplas O, Delwiche J-P, Evrard G, et al: Prevalence of occupational asthma due to latex among hospital personnel. *Am J Respir Crit Care Med* 151:54–60, 1995.)

▶ This study by Vandenplas et al. adds to an increasing body of data regarding the importance of the workplace in the etiology of asthma. Occupational asthma caused by latex was found in 2.5% of 273 hospital employees tested with a stepped protocol of questionnaire and skin-prick testing, assessment of nonspecific bronchial responsiveness, and specific inhalation challenges with latex gloves.

Malo and Chan-Yeung[1] have comprehensively addressed asthma in the workplace, including latex sensitivity among such entities as red cedar dust, crab proteins, and isocyanates. Physicians should be aware of the hospital as a source of occupational asthma, both for the well-being of employees and in history-taking when examining the adult patient who has asthma.

R.C. Bone, M.D.

Reference

1. Malo JL, Chan-Yeung M: Population surveys of occupational asthma, in Bernstein IL, Chan-Yeung M, Malo JL, Bernstein DI (eds): *Asthma in the Workplace.* New York, Marcel Dekker, 1993, pp 145–170.

19 Pleural Disease

The Impact of Thoracoscopy on the Management of Pleural Disease

Harris RJ, Kavuru MS, Mehta AC, Medendorp SV, Wiedemann HP, Kirby TJ, Rice TW (Cleveland Clinic Found, Ohio)

Chest 107:845–852, 1995 119-96-19–1

Introduction.—Thoracoscopy is reported to have a high diagnostic sensitivity, especially for malignant pleural disease. Many questions remain, however, regarding patient selection, timing of the procedure, and the effect on the management and outcome of pleural disease. The records of patients who underwent thoracoscopy for pleural disease were reviewed retrospectively.

Patients and Methods.—One hundred eighty-two consecutive patients, examined from 1987 through 1992, were included. The group was predominantly male (65%) and older than 50 years of age (80%). Sixty percent of the patients were former or current smokers. Thoracoscopy was performed for therapeutic purposes after a diagnosis had been established in 58 patients; in 154 patients, the procedure was undertaken to establish a specific chest diagnosis or to specify type of malignancy. Data collected included the results of pre- and post-thoracoscopy assessments, final diagnosis in chest, effect of thoracoscopy on diagnosis and treatment, complications, and outcome.

Results.—The final diagnoses were malignant disease in 54% of patients, benign disease in 32%, and idiopathic disease in 14%. Thoracoscopy had a diagnostic sensitivity of 100% for benign disease and 95% for malignant disease. Information that directly influenced treatment was obtained in 85% of patients. In most of these patients, further surgical or therapeutic procedures were undertaken or deferred on the basis of thoracoscopic findings. Perioperative complications were common (20%), and there was 1 thoracoscopy-related death. A significant association was noted between a combined history of malignancy, age older than 50 years, and exposure to carcinogens and the finding of malignancy at thoracoscopy. No preoperative radiographic findings or combination of findings increased the likelihood that benign or malignant disease would be diagnosed. A combined lymphocytic and hemorrhagic effusion, however, was associated with malignancy.

Conclusion.—Thoracoscopy increased the diagnostic yield for both benign and malignant disease in this series of patients, but with a high rate of complications. The procedure was of clinical value, as it influenced management of pleural disease in 85% of patients. Its greatest diagnostic yield was in patients who were older, had a history of malignancy, and had an effusion that was lymphocytic and hemorrhagic and had a high value of lactate dehydrogenase.

► A retrospective study, such as this one by Harris et al., is generally unable to recover a full picture of medical decision-making from patient charts. In this instance, for example, we do not know case by case why patients were selected for thoracoscopy. Although lack of this information does not necessarily weaken the findings of a study that was designed to be retrospective, it does serve as a reminder that patient selection must be a rigorous process.

In the tertiary-care setting, and with a generally older patient population, thoracoscopy demonstrated diagnostic usefulness for the evaluation of suspected malignancy in patients who had a lymphocytic, hemorrhagic effusion that had high lactate dehydrogenase value. Thoracoscopy was directly associated with changes in clinical management in a large majority of the patients. In this population, thoracoscopy increased the yield for malignant and benign disease when thoracentesis and closed pleural biopsy were nondiagnostic.

However, physicians who are outside a tertiary-care center and/or treat patients who have different characteristics must carefully consider which preoperative variables might be associated with finding malignancy by thoracoscopy. Reports on the complication rates of thoracoscopy also indicate dependence on characteristics of the patient, type of anesthesia, diagnostic indication, and operator experience.[1, 2] Also to be considered is the lack of agreement, based on available data, regarding the impact of thoracoscopy on final outcome in patients with advanced disease.

R.C. Bone, M.D.

References

1. Menzies R, Charbonneau M: Thoracoscopy for the diagnosis of pleural disease. *Ann Intern Med* 114:271–276, 1991.
2. Page RD, Jeffrey RR, Donnelly RJ: Thoracoscopy: A review of 121 consecutive surgical procedures. *Ann Thorac Surg* 48:66–68, 1989.

Pleural Fluid Chemical Analysis in Parapneumonic Effusions: A Meta-Analysis

Heffner JE, Brown LK, Barbieri C, DeLeo JM (Univ of Arizona Health Sciences Ctr, Tucson; NIH, Bethesda, Md)

Am J Respir Crit Care Med 151:1700–1708, 1995 119-96-19–2

Objective.—The need to drain the parapneumonic effusions that can occur in half the patients who have pleural pneumonia is controversial. Although detection of intrapleural pus with a positive Gram stain is an accepted indication for drainage, the diagnostic sensitivity is low. There is no general agreement on the use of other diagnostic criteria. The usefulness of pleural fluid pH, lactate dehydrogenase, and glucose for identifying parapneumonic effusions that require draining was assessed in a meta-analysis.

Methods.—Seven studies were included. The diagnostic accuracy of pleural fluid testing in distinguishing between complicated and uncomplicated effusions with the use of receiver operating characteristic analyses was determined. In addition, the validity of the studies was established, accuracies were compared, and generalizability of results was assessed.

Results.—Measuring the area under the curve (AUC) of the receiver operating characteristic plot showed that pleural fluid pH had the highest diagnostic accuracy (AUC = 0.92), followed by pleural fluid glucose (AUC = 0.84), and lactate dehydrogenase (AUC = 0.82). When patients who had purulent effusions were excluded, pleural pH fluid still had the highest diagnostic accuracy (AUC = 0.89). There were no investigator or clinician blinded studies, and follow-up periods were not specified. Pleural effusion collection techniques were described in 6 studies, and equipment was described in 5. Descriptions of patients, complaints, pathogens, and comorbid diseases were scant or lacking.

Conclusion.—From this analysis, the pleural fluid decision threshold should be 7.21 for patients at high risk to 7.29 for those at low risk. The studies validate the use of pleural fluid pH as a predictor of complicated parapneumonic effusions. The accuracy of fluid analyses could not be determined because of the lack of generalizable information or missing information. A generally accepted reference standard for complicated parapneumonic effusions needs to be developed.

► Physicians who are not familiar with the methodologic criteria for a meta-analysis in which diagnostic tests are evaluated may wish to review the methodology used by Heffner et al. for this study.[1] Meta-analysis may serve up unexpected results, particularly if the topic being scrutinized is one enshrined in dogma and standard texts. The meta-analysis reported in this abstract does not refute current teaching and practice, but it does call somewhat into question the data on which they are founded.

R.C. Bone, M.D.

Reference

1. Irwig L, Tosteson NA, Gatsonis C, et al: Guidelines for meta-analysis evaluating diagnostic tests. *Ann Intern Med* 120:667–676, 1994.

20 Sleep Apnea

Association of Chronic Obstructive Pulmonary Disease and Sleep Apnea Syndrome

Chaouat A, Weitzenblum E, Krieger J, Ifoundza T, Oswald M, Kessler R (Hôpital de Hautepierre, Strasbourg, France; Univ Hosp, Strasbourg, France)

Am J Respir Crit Care Med 151:82–86, 1995 119-96-20–1

Background.—Sleep apnea syndrome (SAS) is a relatively common disease, especially among men older than 40 years of age. Chronic obstructive pulmonary disease is also common, and the 2 conditions sometimes occur in the same patients. This association has been termed the overlap syndrome. The frequency of the overlap syndrome was examined prospectively in unselected patients who had a confirmed diagnosis of SAS.

Study Design.—Twenty-two women and 243 men (average age, 54 years) who had an established diagnosis of obstructive SAS on the basis of polysomnographic criteria were assessed between November 1983 and September 1991.

Findings.—An obstructive spirographic pattern was detected in 30 patients. The overlap group was older than the group as a whole. All patients in the overlap group were men, and almost all were smokers. In the overlap group, partial pressure of oxygen in arterial blood (PaO_2) was significantly lower and partial pressure of carbon dioxide in arterial blood ($PaCO_2$) was significantly higher. Hypoxemia and hypercapnia were more common among the patients who had overlap syndrome than in the group as a whole. The pulmonary artery mean pressure (Fig 1) was higher in the overlap group both at rest and during steady-state exercise.

Conclusions.—More than 10% of patients who have SAS have an associated obstructive airway disease. Therefore, patients who have SAS should always be examined for the presence of chronic obstructive pulmonary disease. Patients who have overlap syndrome have detectable hypoxemia, hypercapnia, and pulmonary hypertension, even in the presence of only minor bronchial obstruction. These patients are at an increased risk for respiratory insufficiency and cor pulmonale.

▶ Diagnostic findings in 1 condition may trigger clinical suspicion of associated pathology, if the clinical correlations are shown to be soundly based. In this study from France, an overlap association was found between SAS and chronic obstructive pulmonary disease, i.e., an associated airway disease was present in approximately 10% of patients who had SAS. The

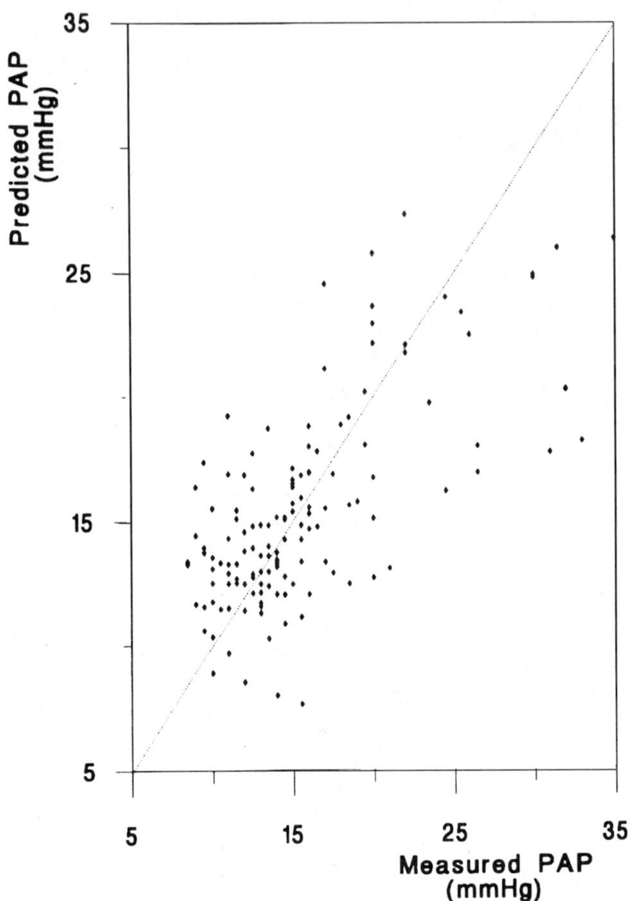

FIGURE 1.—Comparison of pulmonary artery mean pressure (*PAP*) actually measured (*x-axis*) and PAP predicted from multiple regression equation (*y-axis*). (Courtesy of Chaouat A, Weitzenblum E, Krieger J, et al: Association of chronic obstructive pulmonary disease and sleep apnea syndrome. *Am J Respir Crit Care Med* 151:82–86, 1995.)

overlap patients had higher daytime $Paco_2$ and pulmonary artery mean pressure and lower Pao_2 and higher pulmonary artery mean pressure at rest and during steady-state exercise. These patients may, as the authors suggest, be at greater risk than other patients who have SAS for respiratory insufficiency and cor pulmonale. The authors note that these findings are in French patients and, thus, in a population where many patients are likely to be heavy smokers. The authors conclude that the possibility of chronic obstructive pulmonary disease should be investigated in patients who have SAS by appropriate spirometric and air flow measurements. The overlap patients are likely to show a pattern of hypercapnia, hypoxemia, and pulmonary hypertension that is different from that of typical chronic obstructive pulmonary disease.

R.C. Bone, M.D.

21 Critical Care

Frequency and Importance of Barotrauma in 100 Patients With Acute Lung Injury

Schnapp LM, Chin DP, Szaflarski N, Matthay MA (Univ of California, San Francisco)

Crit Care Med 23:272–278, 1995 119-96-21–1

Objectives.—Barotrauma is a well-recognized complication of acute lung injury requiring mechanical ventilation. The frequency of barotrauma in patients who have acute lung injury was determined prospectively. Whether barotrauma is an independent risk factor for mortality and its contribution to mortality in these patients were also assessed.

Patients.—One hundred consecutive adult patients in the ICU at a university hospital were included. All patients met the usual criteria for diagnosis of acute lung injury requiring mechanical ventilation.

Results.—Barotrauma occurred in 13 patients (13%). The mortality rate in patients with barotrauma (76%) was not different from that of patients without barotrauma (64%). Univariate analysis showed that barotrauma was not associated with mortality. However, stepwise logistic regression analysis that accounted for other risk factors showed barotrauma as an independent risk factor for mortality (odds ratio, 6.15; confidence interval, 1.11 to 33.9) (Table 4). Nonpulmonary organ dysfunction and sepsis were also independent risk factors for mortality. If barotrauma occurred in the presence of 2 or more nonpulmonary organ dysfunctions, the mortality rate was 100% compared with 40% when barotrauma occurred with 1 dysfunction or no nonpulmonary organ failure (Table 5). Although patients who had barotrauma had a high mortality rate, only 1 death (2%) was attributed directly to barotrauma.

Conclusion.—Barotrauma occurred in 13% of patients who had acute lung injury requiring mechanical ventilation. It is an independent predictor of mortality only after accounting for other risk factors for mortality. Barotrauma directly contributes to less than 2% of all deaths, but its presence with nonpulmonary organ dysfunction is associated with a high mortality rate. Barotrauma seems to reflect the severity of underlying lung and systemic disease rather than a major cause of increased mortality.

► Limitation of barotrauma, i.e., the damage imposed by the ventilator on a seriously ill patient, is one of the major concerns associated with mechanical

TABLE 4.—Independent Predictors of Mortality Among 100 Patients With Acute Lung Injury: Multivariate Analysis

Variable	Odds Ratio (95% CI)	*P* Value
Barotrauma	11.1 (1.4–84)	0.001
Nonpulmonary organ failure	3.1 (1.9–5.0)	<0.001
Associated acute lung injury diagnosis (others)	0.1 (0.003–0.4)	<0.001

Abbreviation: CI, confidence interval.
(Courtesy of Schnapp LM, Chin DP, Szaflarski N, et al: Frequency and importance of barotrauma in 100 patients with acute lung injury. *Crit Care Med* 23:272–278, 1995.)

ventilation.[1] When the ventilated patient has acute lung injury, the injury may be exacerbated. However, the development of ventilator-induced lung injury may be difficult to observe, because its appearance may be masked by an underlying disease process that the ventilator is being used to treat.[2]

In this study, Schnapp et al. found that the mortality rate associated with barotrauma in patients with acute lung injury may reflect the severity of the underlying lung and systemic disease, rather than ventilator-induced lung injury. In their population of 100 patients with acute lung injury, the rate of occurrence of barotrauma was 13%. In univariate analysis, barotrauma was not associated with mortality; however, in a multivariate analysis that the authors used to adjust for confounding factors, barotrauma was an independent risk factor for mortality, which was one of the hypotheses stated in their study objectives. Only 1 patient's death was found to be directly attributable to barotrauma; of 10 with barotrauma who died, 8 had 2 or more nonpulmonary organ dysfunctions. Nonpulmonary organ failure was a significant predictor of mortality in this population. The authors state that different ventilator strategies probably would not have substantially changed mortality, e.g., only 1 patient died as a result of barotrauma. The authors focus our attention on underlying disease and the damage to lung epithelium found in patients with acute lung injury.

R.C. Bone, M.D.

TABLE 5.—Potential Predictor Variables of Mortality Among 13 Barotrauma Patients

	Died	Survived	*P* Value
Nonpulmonary Organ System Failure			0.035
≤ 1	2	3	
> 1	8	0	
Lowest $Pa{O_2}/F{I}{O_2}$ (mean)	78	93	0.60
No. of days intubated (mean)	38	32	0.8
Age (yr) (mean)	48	47	0.96

Abbreviations: PaO_2, partial pressure of oxygen in arterial blood; *FIO_2,* fraction of inspired oxygen.
(Courtesy of Schnapp LM, Chin DP, Szaflarski N, et al: Frequency and importance of barotrauma in 100 patients with acute lung injury. *Crit Care Med* 23:272–278, 1995.)

References

1. ACCP Consensus Conference: Mechanical ventilation. *Chest* 104:1833–1859, 1993.
2. Rouby JJ, Lherm T, Martin de Lassale E, et al: Histologic aspects of pulmonary barotrauma in critically ill patients with acute respiratory failure. *Intensive Care Med* 19:383–389, 1993.

A Look Into the Nature and Causes of Human Errors in the Intensive Care Unit

Donchin Y, Gopher D, Olin M, Badihi Y, Biesky M, Sprung CL, Pizov R, Cotev S (Hadassah-Hebrew Univ, Jerusalem; Israel Inst of Technology, Jerusalem)
Crit Care Med 23:294–300, 1995 119-96-21–2

Background.—To address the deficit of studies on the nature of human errors in critical care, human errors in the ICU were studied with the use of approaches proposed by human factors engineering. The association between human beings and their working environment, with a particular emphasis on technology, was studied.

Setting.—During a 4-month concurrent incident study in a medical-surgical ICU of a university hospital, 4 errors reported by physicians and nurses immediately after they were discovered were recorded. In addition, activity profiles on a random sample of patients were collected on the basis of 24-hour continuous bedside observations by investigators with human engineering experience. Human error was defined as a deviation from standard conduct, including addition or omission of actions relating to standard operational instructions or routines; medical decisions were ex-

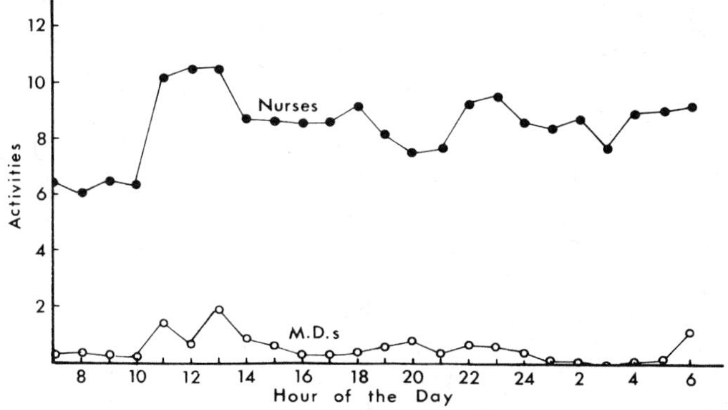

FIGURE 1.—Diurnal distribution of physician and nurse activities in the intensive care unit. Activity was measured as activity per patient per hour. Peak activity occurred during the late morning. Although the intensity of activity performed by physicians decreased sharply, nurses maintained a high rate of activity. (Courtesy of Donchin Y, Gopher D, Olin M, et al: A look into the nature and causes of human errors in the intensive care unit. *Crit Care Med* 23:294–300, 1995.)

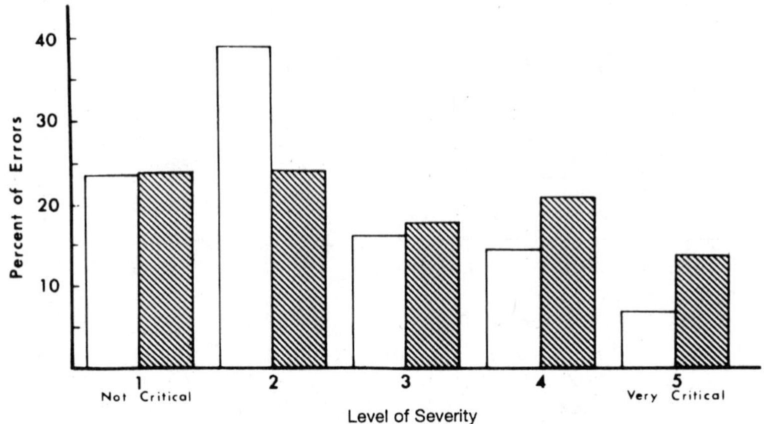

FIGURE 2.—Distribution of the severity of errors. The graph displays the joint distribution and the separate rating of errors performed by physicians (*open bars*) and nurses (*hatched bars*). (Courtesy of Donchin Y, Gopher D, Olin M, et al: A look into the nature and causes of human errors in the intensive care unit. *Crit Care Med* 23:294–300, 1995.)

cluded. Errors were rated for severity and classified on the basis of the body system and type of medical activity involved.

Findings.—Five hundred fifty-four human errors were recorded; 476 errors were by physicians and nurses, and 78 were detected by observers during an average of 178 activities per patient per day. The estimated number of errors per patient per day was 1.7. Twenty-nine percent of errors were graded as severe or potentially detrimental; such errors occurred, on average, twice a day. Errors were more likely to occur with input activities and CNS activities.

Peak activity occurred during the late morning and early afternoon hours for both physicians and nurses (Fig 1). The number of activities performed by physicians decreased sharply outside this period, whereas

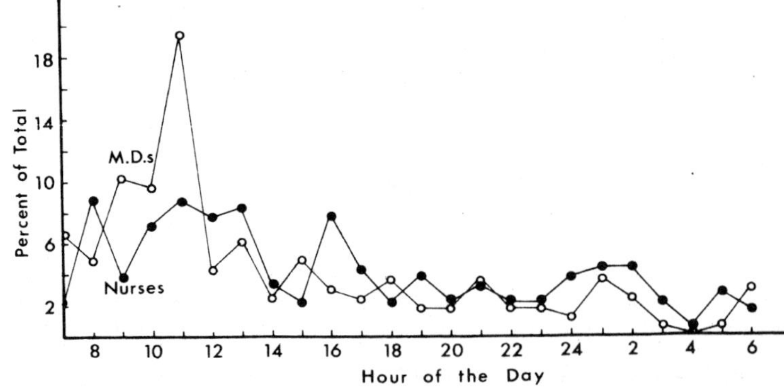

FIGURE 3.—Diurnal distribution of commitment of errors. The errors are expressed as a percentage of the total errors. (Courtesy of Donchin Y, Gopher D, Olin M, et al: A look into the nature and causes of human errors in the intensive care unit. *Crit Care Med* 23:294–300, 1995.)

nurses' activity remained high at all hours. Although nurses committed more errors than did physicians, 55% vs. 45% (Fig 2), physicians carried out only 4.7% of the daily activities compared with 84% performed by nurses. Most errors were committed in the morning, with physicians showing 1 distinct peak around the time of the physician's morning rounds. Errors committed by nurses peaked similarly, but with a 1-hour delay, and peaked as well during each shift change (Fig 3). Verbal exchanges between physicians and nurses were surprisingly high (37%) in error reports, but verbal communications constituted only 2% of the overall activity profile.

Conclusions.—A significant number of human errors occur in the ICU, and many of these errors could be attributed to problems of communication between the physicians and nurses. The tools and concepts provided by cognitive psychology and human factors engineering may be useful in the analysis of human errors in a specific ICU. The nature and causes of the errors identified in this ICU are not unique and may have general relevance for other ICUs.

► Human errors by physicians, nurses, and other health care professionals occur more frequently than they should. They also occur more frequently than most of us know, e.g., many errors are minor "slips" that are unnoticed or quickly forgotten. In this study, Donchin et al. estimated that more than 1,000 human errors were committed in a 6-bed ICU during a 4-month period, and not quite half of these were discovered and self-reported by the medical and nursing staffs. Twenty-nine percent of errors were graded as severe or potentially detrimental to the patients—a rate of approximately 2 severe errors per day in this 6-bed unit. The diurnal distribution of errors showed clustering at peak hours of physician and nurse activity. The complexity of activities also appeared to have a relationship with the probability for error occurrence. This finding is not surprising but reinforces the necessity to simplify and formalize activities that may cause confusion and/or force physicians and nurses to improvise. The study also reminds us of the absolute necessity for clear and continuous communication between physicians and nurses. The authors posit that an unusually heavy physician-nurse communication that was recorded in association with errors represented "informal" exchanges that were likely to be misunderstood or misinterpreted.

R.C. Bone, M.D.

The SUPPORT Prognostic Model: Objective Estimates of Survival for Seriously Ill Hospitalized Adults

Knaus WA, Harrell FE Jr, Lynn J, Goldman L, Phillips RS, Connors AF Jr, Dawson NV, Fulkerson WJ Jr, Califf RM, Desbiens N, Layde P, Oye RK, Bellamy PE, Hakim RB, Wagner DP (George Washington Univ, Washington, DC; Duke Univ, Durham, NC; Dartmouth Med School, Hanover, NH; et al)
Ann Intern Med 122:191–203, 1995 119-96-21-3

Background.—The Study to Understand Prognoses and Preferences for Outcomes and Risks of Treatments (SUPPORT), a multicenter trial, assessed outcomes and clinical decision-making for seriously ill hospitalized patients. A major hypothesis was that the accurate prediction of risk for death would assist physicians' clinical decision-making by reducing uncertainty and promoting communication among physicians, patients, and

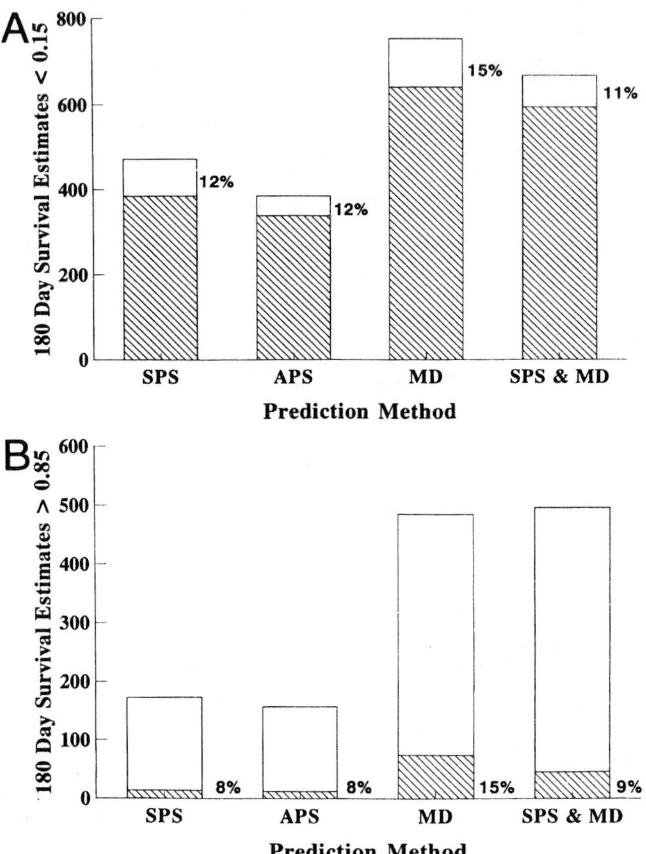

FIGURE 3.—Comparison in high and low ends of the prognostic range, of the predictive ability of 4 prognostic models. Results are based on 4,028 phase II patients who were followed for 180 days and for whom physician estimates were obtained. The *vertical axes* represent the number of patients in each sample. *Cross-hatched sections* indicate the proportion of patients who died; *open sections* indicate survivors. **A,** number of phase II patients with a 180-day survival probability of less than 0.15. Physicians predicted a survival less than 0.15 for more patients (n = 753), but within this risk group, had the highest survival rate and the lowest calibration of the 3 prognostic models. The SUPPORT physician-enhanced model had the lowest survival rate when predicting low probability of survival and the second highest number of patients (n = 668). **B,** number of phase II patients with a survival probability of greater than 0.85. The physician-enhanced prognostic model predicted the largest sample (n = 496) and had a 91% survival rate; the physician-estimated sample had an 85% mortality rate. *Abbreviations: SPS,* SUPPORT prognostic model; *APS,* SUPPORT prognostic model with the APACHE III acute physiology score; *MD,* physician's prediction; and *SPS & MD,* physician-enhanced SUPPORT model. (Courtesy of Knaus WA, Harrell FE Jr, Lynn J, et al: The SUPPORT prognostic model: Objective estimates of survival for seriously ill hospitalized adults. *Ann Intern Med* 122:191–203, 1995.)

families. The development, performance, and validation of the SUPPORT prognostic model were assessed prospectively in a cohort study.

Methods.—Five tertiary care academic centers in the United States participated. A total of 4,301 hospitalized adults were chosen for phase 1 of the study on the basis of diagnosis and severity of disease. In addition, 4,028 patients from phase 2 were included in the analysis. The survival model included the predictor variables diagnosis, age, number of days in the hospital before study entry, presence of cancer, neurologic function, and 11 physiologic measures recorded on day 3 after study entry.

Findings.—The area under the receiver-operating characteristics curve for predicting 180-day survival was 0.79 in phase 1 and 0.78 in the phase 2 independent validation. The receiver-operating characteristics curve was 0.78 when the acute physiology score from the Acute Physiology, Age, Chronic Health Evaluation III prognostic scoring system was substituted for the SUPPORT physiology score. The SUPPORT model displayed equal discrimination and slightly improved calibration compared with physicians' estimates for the patients in phase 2. Combining the SUPPORT model with physicians' estimates increased accuracy and the ability to identify patients with high probabilities of survival or death (Fig 3).

Conclusions.—With readily available clinical data, long-term survival estimates as accurate as physicians' can be determined. The best survival estimates combine an objective prognosis and the physician's clinical judgment.

► Knaus et al. make the point that clinicians, by and large, do not usually incorporate "event probabilities" into routine decision-making—even though data for such projections are increasingly available. The clinician is understandably suspicious of "probability" characteristics drawn from groups of patients; experience tells the clinician that an individual's risks may not be accurately predicted from such data. Knaus et al. state their belief, however, that within a selected group of high-mortality diagnoses, a limited amount of clinical information can produce probabilities of survival that are as accurate as those of a treating physician and may be helpful in refining decisions to limit or withdraw life support. The authors found it particularly promising that their SUPPORT model complements simultaneous prognostic estimates by physicians. The best use of the SUPPORT model would thus be to use it in complementary fashion with treating physician estimates regarding the probability of survival or death within the 180-day period covered by the study. The availability of a probabilities-for-survival-or-death model would have great potential for use by physicians in consultation with patients and families who must face wrenching decisions regarding ongoing care.

R.C. Bone, M.D.

Decisions to Limit or Continue Life-Sustaining Treatment by Critical Care Physicians in the United States: Conflicts Between Physicians' Practices and Patients' Wishes

Asch DA, Hansen-Flaschen J, Lanken PN (Univ of Pennsylvania, Philadelphia; Veterans Affairs Med Ctr, Philadelphia)

Am J Respir Crit Care Med 151:288–292, 1995 119-96-21–4

Objective.—The decision to limit or withdraw life-support by critical care physicians is generally accepted in principle. Few studies, however, have measured actual physician practice. Decisions by critical care physicians to withhold or withdraw life support on the basis of medical futility or to continue life support against the wishes of the patient or surrogate were examined.

Methods.—A survey was mailed to all 1,970 members of the Critical Care Section of the American Thoracic Society to determine their attitudes and practices with regard to withholding or withdrawing life support on the basis of medical futility or continuing life support against the wishes of the patient or surrogate.

Results.—A total of 879 surveys were included in the analysis. Self-reporting results showed that 96% of respondents had discontinued treatment with the expectation that the patient would die. In the past year, 85% had discontinued mechanical ventilation at least once, 29% had withdrawn it 3–5 times, and 26% more than 5 times. On the basis of medical futility, 83% had withheld life-sustaining treatment, and 73% had withdrawn it. Many had withdrawn or withheld treatment without the consent or knowledge of the patient or the family, and some did so over the objections of patients or family.

Conclusion.—Physicians do not automatically accept patients' or surrogates' decisions to continue or discontinue treatment. The requests are weighed along with other factors, including the possible medical futility of continuing treatment.

▶ Very few topics have been exposed to more public debate in recent years than have those of "medical futility" and the related "right to die." As a result, few people could be unaware of the issues; however, there is not yet a consensus on the ethical and legal bases for making decisions regarding limitation, continuation, or withdrawal of life-sustaining treatment. The results of the survey reported by Asch et al. indicate that critical care physicians are increasingly willing to make such decisions—even when the decisions may be less than totally acceptable to patients and their families. The ground on which they stand in making these decisions is "good faith," i.e., the best use and interpretation of medical skill, technology, and experience indicate the futility of initiating or continuing treatment. Conversely, one third of physicians who responded to the survey questionnaire reported refusal to limit treatment despite requests by a patient and/or family; in most instances, they assessed the prognosis to be good enough to indicate a reasonable chance for the patient's recovery, but they also often took legal and ethical considerations into account.

The degree to which this group of critical care physicians has incorporated medical futility decision-making into their practices is indicated by the number who reported withholding or withdrawing life-sustaining treatment without the oral or written consent of the patient or family (25%), without the knowledge or the patient or family (14%), and despite the objections of the patient or family (3%). It would be most interesting to know what led to these unilateral decisions by physicians. Questions such as these should be addressed in research directed toward learning how and why treatment vs. nontreatment decisions are made.

R.C. Bone, M.D.

Adrenal Insufficiency Occurring During Septic Shock: Incidence, Outcome, and Relationship to Peripheral Cytokine Levels

Soni A, Pepper GM, Wyrwinski PM, Ramirez NE, Simon R, Pina T, Gruenspan H, Vaca CE (Lincoln Med and Mental Health Ctr, Bronx, NY; New York Med College, Valhalla)

Am J Med 98:266–270, 1995 119-96-21–5

Background.—The serum level of cortisol usually is increased in patients who have sepsis and septic shock. Adrenal insufficiency (AI) has been described in connection with septic shock, although not consistently. Endotoxemia increases circulating levels of several cytokines that mediate septic shock and stimulate the pituitary-adrenal axis. Some immune products may inhibit adrenal function and cortisol production. Plasma levels of cortisol, tumor necrosis factor-α (TNF-α), and interleukin-6 were determined in patients who had septic shock.

Method.—Twenty-one consecutive patients who had septic shock and 11 healthy individuals were included. The determinations were repeated within 24 hours of diagnosis after the infusion of adrenocorticotropic hormone (ACTH) in doses of 1 and 250 μg. Patients who had subnormal adrenal responses to ACTH received stress doses of glucocorticoids.

Results.—The ACTH infusion test results of 5 patients who had septic shock (24%) suggested AI. One other patient had an inadequate cortisol response to low-dose ACTH but a normal response to the standard dose; the patient recovered without glucocorticoid treatment. Three patients who had AI had rapid hemodynamic improvement when given supplemental steroid treatment. Autopsies of 2 patients who had AI demonstrated intact adrenal cortices. In patients who had adequate adrenal responses to ACTH, but not in those who had AI, the level of TNF-α correlated inversely with the mean arterial pressure. Nevertheless, average levels of TNF-α were similar in the 2 groups. Levels of interleukin-6 tended to be lower in patients who had AI. Eighty percent of patients who had AI and 44% of those who had adequate ACTH responses had died after 4 weeks.

Implications.—Adrenal insufficiency should be suspected in any patient who has septic shock and does not respond to conventional measures. When the results of a brief ACTH infusion test suggest AI, stress doses of glucocorticoids should be given.

▶ This is a fascinating study. Nearly one quarter of patients with septic shock had AI. This needs to be confirmed by a larger study, but I agree with the findings. If your patient with septic shock does not respond to conventional treatment, at least consider that AI might be contributing to the impaired response.

Cortisol has a profound influence on the complex set of reactions evoked by trauma and infections. If feedback loops may influence production of cortisol in the patient who has septic shock, as Soni et al. hypothesize, an intervention with glucocorticoid therapy could be clinically rational. The authors believe that AI may be suspected in any patient with septic shock who does not respond to conventional therapy. They would rule out AI when the serum levels of cortisol are 18 µg/dL or greater. The suggested intervention is, admittedly, a measure that can improve only short-term survival, but the authors would justify it as a life-saving measure that might permit the patient to survive until more definitive therapy could prevail. The evidence from this abstracted study, however, is not optimistic regarding survival of these patients.

R.C. Bone, M.D.

Evaluation of Transesophageal Echocardiography as a Diagnostic and Therapeutic Aid in a Critical Care Setting

Poelaert JI, Trouerbach J, De Buyzere M, Everaert J, Colardyn FA (Univ Hosp, Ghent, Belgium)

Chest 107:774–779, 1995 119-96-21–6

Objective.—Transesophageal echocardiography (TEE) with the color Doppler technique is a reliable and noninvasive means of real-time imaging that may be used for bedside monitoring. Experience with TEE was reviewed in 108 consecutive critically ill patients who were evaluated during a 7-month period. Some of these patients had a pulmonary artery catheter (PAC) in place. Post–cardiac surgery patients were not included.

Indications and Methods.—Most studies were done either on specific primary indications or when transthoracic echocardiography or the PAC provided inadequate information. Sixty-three patients who had cardiac disease and 37 who had sepsis were included. Approximately half the studies were done to estimate global and regional contractility, but many patients were examined to evaluate cardiac filling or assess valvular function. The TEE probe was readily inserted in all patients, and there were no serious complications.

Results.—Transesophageal echocardiography provided information that was helpful to management in three fourths of patients. In approximately one fourth of patients, the study ruled out suspected abnormalities.

Abnormal regional wall motion was detected in many patients who had cardiac disease. In 2 instances, unexpected thrombi or intracardiac vegetations were visualized. Treatment was altered because of the TEE findings in 29 of 66 patients who had a PAC in place. In many of these patients, dobutamine was added or the dose was increased. Treatment was altered in 13 of 24 patients who had sepsis and had a PAC in place. It also was modified in 41% of patients who did not undergo PAC monitoring.

Conclusions.—Transesophageal echocardiography frequently led to modified management in these critically ill patients, regardless of whether a PAC was present. The most comprehensive approach is to combine invasive pressure monitoring with TEE estimates of intracardiac flow and volume.

► Concerns about cost-effectiveness in treating hospitalized patients (e.g., the costs associated with "overtesting" patients) must be carefully balanced against concerns about undertreating patients because of examinations not done. In this retrospective study, Poelaert et al. point out the potential value of TEE findings in ICU patients, including those who are already being monitored with a PAC. In subgroups of the patients in this study (e.g., patients with sepsis monitored by PAC), TEE provided the information to initiate or modify the dose of dobutamine and to adjust the IV fluid regimen. Overall, TEE was valuable independent of the presence of PAC monitoring, but a combination of TEE and PAC may be a superior modality in properly selected patients.

R.C. Bone, M.D.

An Outbreak of *Burkholderia* (Formerly *Pseudomonas*) *cepacia* Respiratory Tract Colonization and Infection Associated With Nebulized Albuterol Therapy

Hamill RJ, Houston ED, Georghiou PR, Wright CE, Koza MA, Cadle RM, Goepfert PA, Lewis DA, Zenon GJ, Clarridge JE (Veterans Affairs Med Ctr, Houston; Baylor College of Medicine, Houston; Texas Southern Univ, Houston)

Ann Intern Med 122:762–766, 1995 119-96-21–7

Background.—The improper use of multiple-dose medication vials and reliance on benzalkonium chloride as a medication preservative continue to result in outbreaks of nosocomial infections. An outbreak of respiratory tract colonization and infection caused by *Burkholderia cepacia* among mechanically ventilated patients who received nebulized albuterol was described.

Methods and Findings.—Forty-two mechanically ventilated patients in whom respiratory tract colonization or infection developed and 135 ventilator-dependent patients in whom such colonization and infection did not occur were included in a retrospective, case-control, bacteriologic study. Faulty infection control procedures were observed among ICU and respiratory care personnel. Case patients received 95 nebulized albuterol treatments, compared with 67.5 among control patients. Albuterol solutions in use had unstable pH values. Concentrations of benzalkonium chloride declined over time to levels that could support bacterial growth. *Burkholderia cepacia* was discovered in medication nebulizers and albuterol bottles in use. Molecular fingerprints of patient isolates and environmental *B. cepacia* isolates were identical. After appropriate infection control procedures were implemented, no further isolates of *B. cepacia* were identified.

Conclusions.—Appropriate respiratory care and infection control practices must be followed to avoid outbreaks of *B. cepacia* respiratory tract colonization and infection in mechanically ventilated patients, particularly when multiple-dose medication vials are used. Benzalkonium chloride may not be an appropriate medication preservative, as it often does not provide effective bacteriostasis.

▶ This report by Hamill et al. should encourage critical care physicians and directors of ICUs to review nosocomial infection control measures at their institutions and on their units in particular. Especially in today's environment of cost control and staff reductions, lapses may occur, as much because stretched-out staff are trying to "get the job done" as because of conscious laxness. The result in loss of infection control is the same, however.

The authors' suggestion that benzalkonium chloride may not provide effective bacteriostasis may be noted by pharmaceutical firms, but any action taken would be at some time in the future. A check of drugs from the formulary in one's own microbiology laboratory would be in order; the question regarding bacteriostatic effectiveness of benzalkonium chloride has been raised and is worth reviewing.[1]

Each institution must weigh the usefulness and cost-effectiveness of multiple-dose medication containers against potential hazard. As noted in this report, multiple-dose dispensers may be a rational choice, but the decision must be made with the full knowledge of one's own environment.

R.C. Bone, M.D.

Reference

1. Donowitz LG: Benzalkonium chloride is still in use. *Infect Control Hosp Epidemiol* 12:186–187, 1991.

Gastric Emptying in Critically Ill Patients Is Accelerated by Adding Cisapride to a Standard Enteral Feeding Protocol: Results of a Prospective, Randomized, Controlled Trial

Spapen HD, Duinslaeger L, Diloter M, Gillet R, Bossuyt A, Huyghens LP
(Vrije Universiteit Brussel, Belgium)
Crit Care Med 23:481–485, 1995 119-96-21–8

Introduction.—Critical illness imposes significant metabolic stress, which results in rapid loss of weight and muscle mass and compromises the patient's immunity. These patients, therefore, should receive early nutritional support, preferably enterally. Providing early nutrition may be complicated, however, by delayed or absent gastric motility in many critically ill patients. The effect of a new prokinetic agent, cisapride, on gastric emptying was studied prospectively in a randomized, controlled trial.

Methods.—Twenty-one critically ill, sedated, and mechanically ventilated patients were given enough enteral feeding liquid to satisfy individual protein and caloric intake requirements via a nasogastric tube. Ten patients received only the enteral nutrition; 11 patients also received cisapride. Two hours after the end of nutritional infusion each day, the gastric residues were measured. Bedside scintigraphic gastric emptying studies were performed on the fifth and seventh days after instillation of technetium 99m–labeled nutrition.

Results.—The 2 groups were comparable for age, body weight, antibiotic treatment, and patient acuity. The enteral nutrition group had a significantly higher mean gastric residue measurement than the cisapride group (94.5 vs. 17.7 mL). Scintigraphic studies revealed a significant delay in gastric emptying on days 5 and 7 in the enteral nutrition group compared with the cisapride group (78 vs. 40 minutes). The 2 groups had a comparable prevalence of loose stools and overt diarrhea. In the enteral nutrition group, 6 patients had significant vomiting and 3 had abdominal distention; these complications did not occur in the cisapride group.

Discussion.—Mean gastric emptying times were significantly faster in the cisapride group than in the enteral nutrition group. Further comparative and placebo-controlled studies are required, however, to confirm a treatment benefit before generalized use can be advocated.

► The risk associated with delayed or absent gastric motility in a critically ill patient is to be avoided if at all possible and often leads the critical care physician to consider alternatives to nasogastric feeding. Invasive techniques, such as direct enteral feeding through percutaneous jejunostomy, are associated with complications and gastrointestinal symptoms. Prokinetic drugs, such as metoclopramide and domperidone, have begun to be considered for their effect on gastric motility, but the critical care physician will note the lack of clinical trials that objectively assess these drugs in an ICU setting. This small, prospective, randomized, controlled trial of cisapride in mechanically ventilated patients offers some support for this drug as a viable modality. The authors themselves note that the generalized use of cisapride in ICU patients to "head off" gastric emptying problems would not be justified on the strength of the findings of their trial.

R.C. Bone, M.D.

Early Enteral Administration of a Formula (Impact®) Supplemented With Arginine, Nucleotides, and Fish Oil in Intensive Care Unit Patients: Results of a Multicenter, Prospective, Randomized, Clinical Trial

Bower RH, Cerra FB, Bershadsky B, Licari JJ, Hoyt DB, Jensen GL, Van Buren CT, Rothkopf MM, Daly JM, Adelsberg BR (Univ of Cincinnati, Ohio; Univ of Minnesota, Minneapolis; Research Support Inc, New Hope, Minn; et al)

Crit Care Med 23:436–449, 1995 119-96-21–9

Background.—Patients who receive early enteral nutrition after an injury may have fewer infectious complications than those given total parenteral nutrition. There have been no studies, however, comparing the effects of different enteral formulas on postinjury outcomes. Certain nutrients, such as arginine, nucleotides, and the omega-3 polyunsaturated fatty acids, may have specific effects on organ function, aside from their general nutritional effects. The effects of early enteral feeding with Impact, a formula supplemented with arginine, dietary nucleotides, and fish oil, in ICU patients were compared with those of Osmolite HN, a common-use control formula, in a prospective, randomized, double-blind, multicenter trial.

Methods.—Two hundred ninety-six patients admitted to the ICU after an event such as trauma, surgery, or sepsis were included. All had an Acute Physiology and Chronic Health Evaluation II score of 10 or greater or a Therapeutic Intervention Scoring System score of 20 or greater. Patients were randomly selected to receive either the experimental or control formula beginning within 48 hours of the study entry event. The experimental formula included additional β-carotene and higher levels of vitamin E and selenium, which have potential antioxidant and immune enhancing properties.

Results.—Early enteral feeding was well tolerated by both groups. The mortality rate was significantly less than predicted by admission severity scores, with no difference between groups. Among patients who received at least 821 mL/day of the experimental formula, the median hospital stay was reduced by 8 days. Among patients who had sepsis, use of the experimental formula reduced the median hospital stay by 10 days and dramatically reduced the frequency of acquired infections. Among patients who had sepsis and received at least 821 mL/day of the experimental formula, the median hospital stay decreased by 11.5 days, with a major reduction in acquired infections.

Conclusions.—In ICU patients, early enteral feeding with an experimental formula supplemented with arginine, dietary nucleotides, and fish oil is safe and well tolerated. Patients who receive this formula, particularly those who have sepsis at ICU admission, have significantly shorter hospital stays and lower rates of acquired infection. Studies to confirm to benefits of the experimental diet and to determine the specific components responsible for those benefits are needed.

► Arginine, nucleotides, and omega-3 polyunsaturated fatty acid are 3 of a number of so-called pharmaconutrients under evaluation for their effect on specific metabolic functions in critically ill patients. Others include the branched-chain amino acids leucine, isoleucine, and valine for their role in improving nitrogen retention with reduced ureagenesis and improved protein synthetic function; glutamine, which participates in a variety of metabolic processes, including the immune response; and nutrients with antioxidant properties (e.g., selenium, vitamins C and E, β-carotene) that may have roles in preventing or ameliorating the effect of oxygen radicals suggested in some stress models.

In addition to evaluation of individual macro- and micronutrients at pharmacologic levels (i.e., at doses exceeding those used in general nutrition therapy), combinations of these nutrients, such as the formula of arginine, fish oil, nucleic acid reported by Bower et al., are under evaluation. Most of these nutrients have no established requirement in ICU patients, but requirements may be established as well-designed clinical trials pursue the pharmaconutrient approach to intervening in the inflammatory response. The long-chain *n*-3 polyunsaturated fatty acid derived from fish oils—eicosapentanoic acid and docosahexanoic acid—enrich the plasma membrane so that eicosanoids synthesized are of the trienoic family, diminishing production of dienoic prostaglandins.[1] The relative ratio of *n*-3 to *n*-6 polyunsaturated fatty acid appears to play an important role in the regulation of synthesis of eicosanoids involved in immune function.[2] It is important to remember that administration of single or mixtures of pharmaconutrients must be carried out in a setting of balanced nutrition support.

R.C. Bone, M.D.

References

1. Katz DP, Schwartz S, Askanazi J: Therapeutic value of omega-3 fatty acids derived from fish oil: Biochemical and cellular basis. *Nutrition* 9:113–118, 1993.
2. Wan JM, Teo CT, Babayan VK, et al: Invited comment: Lipids and the development of immune dysfunction and infection. *JPEN J Parenter Enteral Nutr* 12:43S–52S, 1988.

22 Sepsis

The Natural History of the Systemic Inflammatory Response Syndrome (SIRS): A Prospective Study

Rangel-Frausto MS, Pittet D, Costigan M, Hwang T, Davis CS, Wenzel RP (Univ of Iowa, Iowa City; Univ Hosp, Geneva)

JAMA 273:117–123, 1995 119-96-22–1

Background.—Recent understandings of sepsis and septic shock have allowed for more specific definitions of aspects of "sepsis syndrome." Currently, sepsis syndrome is subdivided into systemic inflammatory response syndrome (SIRS), sepsis, severe sepsis, and septic shock. The rates and distribution of these stages of sepsis in hospitalized patients have not been studied. Epidemiology and natural history of SIRS, sepsis, severe sepsis, and septic shock were examined prospectively.

Methods.—Surveys of 2,527 hospitalized patients who had 2 or more symptoms of SIRS were performed 5 days per week for 1 year in 3 critical care units and 3 wards in a single hospital. The status of all patients was followed for 28 days or until discharge. The patients were reexamined 3 and 6 months later, and developments of criteria of the more advanced stages of sepsis or other complication were noted.

Results.—Sepsis developed in 649 patients (26%) during the 28-day follow-up. Severe sepsis developed in 467 patients (18%), and septic shock developed in 110 (4%). An additional 892 patients (35%) were thought to have had sepsis and were given antibiotics; however, no organism could be cultured. Patients in any inflammatory class who had cardiovascular disease or trauma were approximately 1.5 times more likely to have negative than positive bacterial cultures, whereas patients who had sepsis and gastrointestinal or respiratory disease were 1.4–2.3 times more likely to have negative than positive cultures. The number of symptoms of SIRS was positively associated with the likelihood of progressing to more severe inflammatory stages and negatively associated with the time required to make the transition (Fig 1). End organ dysfunction became more likely with meeting of increasing numbers of criteria of SIRS and with culture-positive vs. culture-negative sepsis. Similarly, the mortality rate increased with increasing numbers of SIRS criteria and with the progression from SIRS or sepsis to severe sepsis to septic shock (Fig 2).

Conclusions.—These data validate the hypothesis that the natural history of the inflammatory response to infection can be described as a

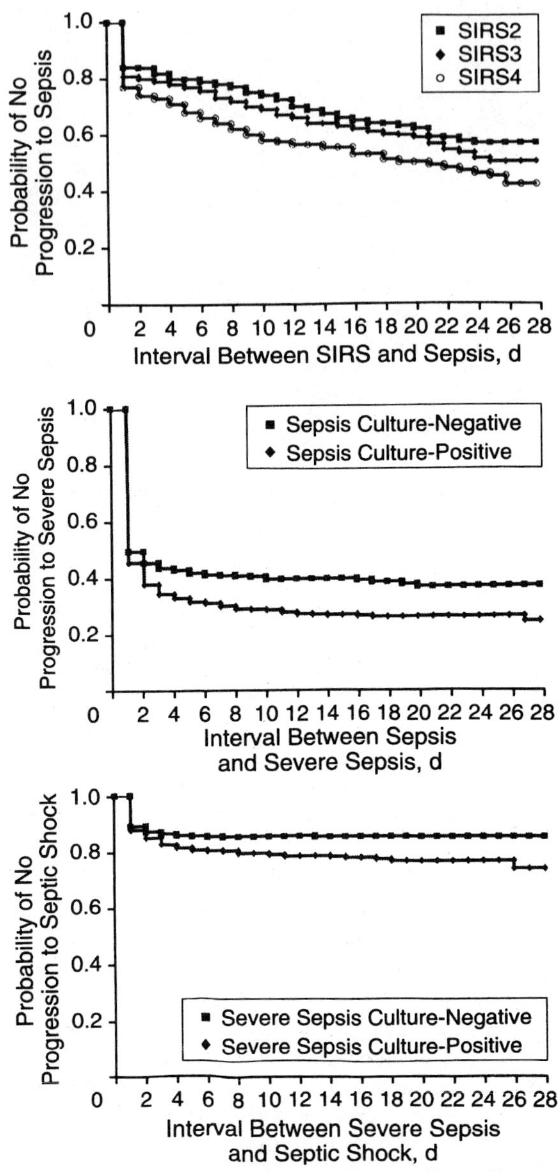

FIGURE 1.—Top, progression of patients who met the SIRS criteria for sepsis. Data include only patients with culture-proven infection meeting Consensus Conference criteria (*Crit Care Med* 20:864–875, 1992). The interval to sepsis was progressively shorter as more criteria were met. **Middle,** progression of sepsis to severe sepsis. The time to sepsis was similar among patients with culture-negative and culture-positive sepsis. **Bottom,** progression of severe sepsis to severe shock. The time to septic shock was similar among patients with culture-negative and culture-positive severe sepsis. *Abbreviations: SIRS2,* 2 of the criteria for systemic inflammatory response syndrome were met; *SIRS3,* 3 of the criteria were met; and *SIRS4,* 4 of the criteria were met. (Courtesy of Rangel-Frausto MS, Pittet D, Costigan M, et al: The natural history of the systemic inflammatory response syndrome (SIRS): A prospective study. *JAMA* 273:117–123, 1995, Copyright 1995, American Medical Association.)

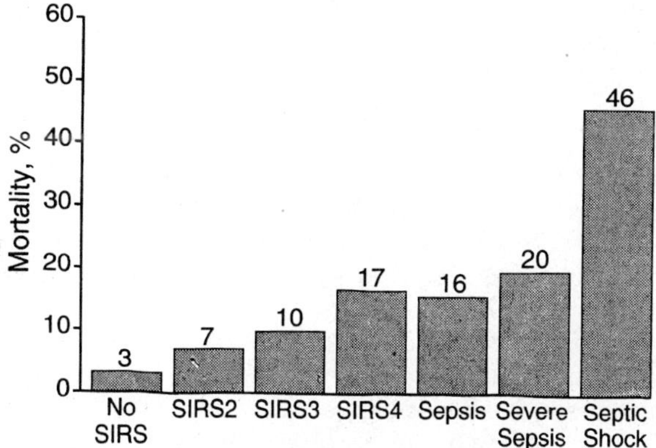

FIGURE 2.—Mortality in systemic inflammatory response syndrome (*SIRS*). A progressively higher mortality was observed as more severe inflammatory response criteria were met. Only data for patients meeting the Consensus Conference criteria (*Crit Care Med* 20:864–875, 1992) were included. The mortality rates in the group with culture-negative syndromes were similar to those with positive cultures: 10% for culture-negative sepsis, 16% for culture-negative severe sepsis, and 46% for culture-negative septic shock. *Abbreviations: SIRS2,* 2 of the criteria for SIRS were met; *SIRS3,* 3 of the criteria were met; *SIRS4,* 4 of the criteria were met. (Courtesy of Rangel-Frausto MS, Pittet D, Costigan M, et al: The natural history of the systemic inflammatory response syndrome (SIRS): A prospective study. *JAMA* 273:117–123, 1995, Copyright 1995, American Medical Association.)

continual progression from SIRS to septic shock. Although one half the patients who had sepsis did not have a documented infection, it is premature to conclude different pathogeneses for culture-negative and culture-positive syndromes. Cardiovascular disease and trauma may be participatory in patients who have culture-negative sepsis.

► Given the decades-long history of sepsis and septic shock as a clinical Gordian knot, it may seem strange that no clinical studies had systematically examined the rates and distribution of syndromes that could define sepsis in hospitalized patients. This is less puzzling when one considers that the technical and conceptual tools have only recently become available for such a study. Rangel-Frausto et al. used the recent definitions of SIRS, sepsis, severe sepsis, and septic shock[1] in designing the study described in this paper. The prospective cohort of 3,708 patients, 2,527 of whom met the criteria for SIRS, validated the authors' hypothesis that SIRS, sepsis, severe sepsis, and septic shock represent a hierarchical continuum of inflammatory response to infection. The authors noted with interest that patients who had negative cultures and met criteria for the various stages of the SIRS hierarchy equaled the number of patients who manifested positive cultures and demonstrated similar morbidity and mortality rates.

The epidemiologic evidence is convincing that SIRS represents a hierarchical continuum of an increased inflammatory response to both infectious and noninfectious stimuli. Rangel-Frausto et al. found that SIRS occurred frequently in the patients they surveyed and that outcomes can be correlated with meeting 2, 3, or 4 of the criteria that define SIRS:

1. Body temperature greater than 38°C or less than 36°C
2. Heart rate greater than 90 beats per minute
3. Tachypnea (respiratory rate > 20 breaths per minute or $Paco_2$ < 32 mm Hg)
4. Alterations in white blood cell counts (> 12 × 10^9/L, < 4.0 × 10^9/L) or the presence of > 0.1 immature neutrophils (bands)

Application of these criteria should improve detection of SIRS and allow earlier intervention. We still need, however, improved understanding of the cellular and immunologic mechanisms that cause sepsis and organ failure.[2]

In a recent editorial review,[3] Baue shared his many years of perspective and experience as a clinician and investigator of sepsis and septic shock. He defines multiple organ failure as simply the final common pathway for a large number of diseases and, thus, believes it would better serve the patient to support organ function and treat the disease than to seek a "magic bullet" to block mediators.

R.C. Bone, M.D.

References

1. American College of Chest Physicians/Society of Critical Care Medicine Consensus Conference: Definitions for sepsis and organ failure and guidelines for the use of innovative therapies in sepsis. *Crit Care Med* 20:864–875, 1992.
2. Bone RC: Sepsis, sepsis syndrome, and the systemic inflammatory response syndrome (SIRS) (editorial). *JAMA* 273:155–156, 1995.
3. Baue AE: Multiple organ failure, multiple organ dysfunction syndrome, and the systemic inflammatory response syndrome: Where do we stand? *Shock* 2:385–397, 1994.

Circulating Interleukin-1 Receptor Antagonist Concentrations Are Increased in Adult Patients With Thermal Injury

Mandrup-Poulsen T, Wogensen LD, Jensen M, Svensson P, Nilsson P, Emdal T, Mølvig J, Dinarello CA, Nerup J (Steno Diabetes Ctr, Gentofte, Denmark; Univ Hosp of Copenhagen, Hvidovre; Novo Nordisk A/S, Gentofte, Denmark; et al)

Crit Care Med 23:26–33, 1995 119-96-22–2

Introduction.—A central role in the host response to infection and injury is played by interleukin-1 (IL-1). Interleukin-1 and its natural inhibitor, IL-1 receptor antagonist (IL-1Ra), are both produced by monocytic and phagocytic cells by different processes. Most of the known actions of IL-1 are blocked by IL-1Ra. Some inflammatory conditions are reduced in the presence of IL-1Ra. The balance of the pro- and anti-inflammatory actions of these antagonists may play a significant role in the outcome of immunologic and degenerative changes. Plasma concentrations of IL-1Ra increase in surgical patients and in those who have sepsis and peak about 2 hours after IL-1. The severe acute-phase response to thermal injury of the skin is an ideal model for the study of the interaction of regulatory factors and cytokine response. The concentrations of IL-1Ra in patients who had burn injuries were assessed.

Methods.—Fifteen patients with burn injury and 15 age-matched controls were included. The patients sustained second- and third-degree burns over 7% to 78% of their body. Levels of IL-1β, tumor necrosis factor-α (TNF-α), IL-1Ra, endotoxin and albumin and rectal temperatures were determined for both groups. Three patients who had inhalation injury died.

Findings.—Among the patients, there was a marked elevation of IL-1Ra on the day of admission. Patients averaged 1,615 pg/mL, whereas the controls averaged 494 pg/mL. The concentration of IL-1Ra normalized in 12–21 days in the survivors. For the nonsurvivors, peak concentration of IL-1Ra occurred on days 1–3. When the survivors were compared with the nonsurvivors, the concentrations of IL-1Ra were 1,344 vs. 2,166 pg/mL, respectively. There was a small but significant correlation between IL-1Ra and degree of thermal injury. The concentration of IL-1Ra doubled after débridement and skin transplantation. Increases in level of IL-1Ra were related to a decrease in level of albumin and an increase in rectal temperature.

Conclusion.—Thermal injury results in a significant increase in concentration of IL-1Ra, more so in patients who have inhalation injuries. Interleukin-1 receptor antagonist may be a more sensitive marker of inflammation than either IL-1β or TNF-α.

► Assessment of inflammation by means of biochemical markers can present equivocal data. In this study of adult burn patients, plasma levels of IL-1β and TNF-α are shown to be exceeded (100-fold for IL-1β) by plasma levels of IL-1Ra, a naturally occurring inhibitor of IL-1. Therefore, IL-1Ra may be a more sensitive marker of inflammation than either IL-1β or TNF-α. Interleukin-1 receptor antagonist was present in plasma over a sustained period, and plasma concentrations were higher in burn patients who had inhalation injuries. The successful cloning of IL-1Ra was reported in 1990.[1,2] Characterization of its pathways of production in monocytic and phagocytic cells followed in 1991.[3, 4] Interleukin-1 receptor antagonist was found to block binding of IL-1 to receptors competitively, inhibiting IL-1 activity and reducing severity of sepsis and a variety of other conditions in animals. Via molecular biology, another potentially valuable clinical tool may be placed in the hands of the critical care physician.

R.C. Bone, M.D.

References

1. Eisenberg SP, Evans RJ, Arend WJ, et al: Primary structure and functional expression from complementary DNA of a human interleukin-1 receptor antagonist. *Nature* 343:341–346, 1990.
2. Carter DB, Deibel MRJ, Dunn CJ, et al: Purification, cloning, expression and biological characterization of an interleukin-1 receptor antagonist protein. *Nature* 344:633–638, 1990.

3. Arend WP, Smith MF, Janson RW, et al: IL-1 receptor antagonist and IL-1β production in human monocytes are regulated differently. *J Immunol* 147:1530–1536, 1991.
4. Poutsiaka DD, Clark BD, Vannier E, et al: Production of interleukin-1 receptor antagonist and interleukin-1β by peripheral blood mononuclear cells is differently regulated. *Blood* 78:1275–1281, 1991.

23 Acute Respiratory Distress Syndrome

Improved Survival of Patients With Acute Respiratory Distress Syndrome (ARDS): 1983–1993

Milberg JA, Davis DR, Steinberg KP, Hudson LD (Univ of Washington, Seattle)

JAMA 273:306–309, 1995 119-96-23–1

Background.—Despite advances in supportive care, the death rate among patients who have acute respiratory distress syndrome (ARDS) is widely thought to have remained high since ARDS was recognized in 1967. It is difficult to compare fatality rates in published reports, however, and no study has examined fatality rates with time. The temporal trends in ARDS fatality rates since 1983 at 1 institution were reported.

Methods.—A total of 918 consecutive adults who met ARDS criteria between 1983 and 1993 were identified through daily surveillance of ICUs. The causes of ARDS were sepsis syndrome in 37% of patients and major trauma in 25%. Thirty-seven percent of the patients had other risk factors.

Findings.—Overall fatality rates did not change between 1983 and 1987, decreased slightly in 1988 and 1989, and decreased to a low of 36% in 1993. Adjustment for age, the risk for ARDS, and sex distribution did not markedly affect the crude rates. Although patients younger than 60 years of age and those 60 years of age or older had decreases in fatality rates, a greater reduction occurred in the younger group. In patients who had sepsis, ARDS fatality rates declined steadily from 67% in 1990 to 40% in 1993. The decrease in the sepsis-related ARDS fatality rate was mainly limited to patients younger than 60 years of age. The fatality rates among trauma victims and all other patients were also reduced after 1987, although these trends were not as strong and consistent as in patients who had sepsis (Fig 1).

Conclusions.—Fatality rates were decreased significantly in this large series, mostly in patients younger than 60 years of age and in those who had sepsis syndrome. The extent to which experimental treatments or other changes in treatment contributed to the observed reduction in ARDS fatality rates could not be determined.

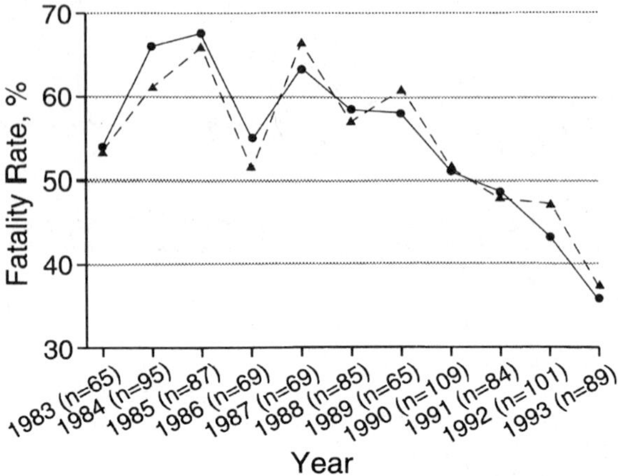

FIGURE 1.—Crude (*solid line*) and adjusted (*dashed line*) acute respiratory distress syndrome (ARDS) fatality rates, total population, Harborview Medical Center, 1983 through 1993. The rates are adjusted for ARDS risk group, age, and sex. (Courtesy of Milberg JA, Davis DR, Steinberg KP, et al: Improved survival of patients with acute respiratory distress syndrome (ARDS): 1983–1993. *JAMA* 273:306–309, 1995. Copyright 1995, American Medical Association.)

► This report by Milberg et al. immediately brings to mind an observation and a question. The observation: If improved survival of patients with ARDS is seen to occur, it is probably least surprising to see the report coming from an institution such as Harborview Medical Center, which is noted for the quality of its research as well as the quality of its patient care in pulmonary and critical care medicine. The question: Are there institution-specific elements that make it more likely to see an increased survival in patients with ARDS at 1 medical center but not at another? The authors speculate that any or all of several elements may be involved in the observed decrease in ARDS mortality seen over a decade in patients younger than 60 years of age: (1) patients in recent years are less ill or less severely injured than patients seen before 1983; (2) supportive care for critically ill patients has improved; (3) experimental drug therapies have been beneficial; or; (4) there has simply been random annual variation.

Although the study covered the period 1983–1993, the greatest decrease and downward trend in the overall ARDS mortality rate occurred in years after 1989. The most notable decrease in ARDS mortality since 1989 was in those patients younger than 60 years of age whose risk for ARDS was sepsis syndrome. Unfortunately, the authors could not determine whether experimental therapies in clinical trials may have influenced the downward trend in ARDS mortality; most of these trials were still blinded. If these therapies were an influence, the authors found it difficult to explain why the therapeutic effect was more notable in patients younger than age 60. The authors recommend that investigators planning clinical trials in ARDS pay particular attention to up-to-date, institution-specific mortality rates and take patient age and clinical risk for ARDS fully into account.

R.C. Bone, M.D.

Pressure-Controlled, Inverse Ratio Ventilation That Avoids Air Trapping in the Adult Respiratory Distress Syndrome

Armstrong BW Jr, MacIntyre NR (Scripps Clinic and Research Found, La Jolla, Calif; Duke Univ Med Ctr, Durham, NC)

Crit Care Med 23:279–285, 1995 119-96-23–2

Background.—Conventional mechanical ventilation for patients who have adult respiratory distress syndrome (ARDS) consists of volume-cycled breaths in conjunction with applied positive end-expiratory pressure (PEEP). The goal is to provide adequate ventilation and oxygenation by positive pressure that recruits and stabilizes alveoli. In recent years, the use of longer inspiration times has been proposed as an additional support technique for patients who have severe lung injury. This approach is usually reserved for patients who do not respond to aggressive conventional ventilation. The physiologic findings and outcomes of patients who had ARDS who were switched from volume-cycled conventional ratio ventilation to pressure-controlled inverse ratio ventilation that did not produce air trapping and intrinsic PEEP were assessed retrospectively in a crossover study.

Methods.—Fourteen patients who had ARDS and were in a medical ICU were included. All were receiving mechanical ventilation with volume-cycled, conventional ratio ventilation before they were switched to pressure-controlled, inverse ratio ventilation for clinical reasons. The tidal volumes and applied PEEP values of the 2 approaches were similar. The volume-cycled, conventional ratio ventilation technique used inspiratory times to increase mean airway pressure instead of additional applied PEEP as it sought to avoid air trapping, or intrinsic PEEP.

Results.—Pressure-controlled, inverse ratio ventilation reduced peak airway pressure from 53 to 40 cm H_2O as it increased mean airway pressure from 20 to 30 cm H_2O. There were no significant changes in tidal volume, mean inflation pressure, or compliance. There was an improvement in partial pressure of oxygen in arterial blood (PaO_2), from 57 to 94 mm Hg. However, there was little change in oxygenation index, which was calculated as mean airway pressure × forced inspiratory oxygen (FIO_2) × 100/PaO_2: 26 vs. 27. Minute ventilation decreased from 17.4 to 15.8 L/min, but PaO_2 and pH were not significantly changed. Other than a slight decrease in cardiac index, the hemodynamic values remained stable. Eleven patients died.

Conclusion.—In patients who have ARDS, oxygenation is mainly a function of mean airway pressure and can be increased by the use of longer inspiratory times as an alternative to applied PEEP. Lung inflation pressures and delivered volumes remain stable with increased expiratory times as long as no air trapping occurs. Because this study included only patients who were refractory to conventional ventilation, the poor outcomes were not surprising.

► Ventilation of the patient who has ARDS always presents a clinical challenge and the possibility of complications, including barotrauma. One problem that has been repeatedly noted is that ARDS causes changes in the lung as the pathologic condition moves from early to late stages.[1] The clinician therefore must deal with an evolving clinical picture and changing conditions that may pose a balancing act between low end-expiratory lung volume and overdistention.[2]

This study by Armstrong and MacIntyre sets the stage for ongoing investigations of pressure-controlled, inverse-ratio ventilation as a ventilator strategy to avoid air being trapped in the lung of a patient with ARDS. The authors base their hypothesis on the observation that pressure-controlled breaths with inspiratory times that exceed expiratory times can result in improvement in oxygenation, reduction in peak airway pressure, decreased need for PEEP, reduction in minute ventilation, decreased ratio of deadspace to tidal volume, and improvement in alveolar ventilation.[3] However, the reports on which these observations are based are case studies or are anecdotal in nature. The authors, therefore, are careful to call for randomized studies to compare pressure-controlled, inverse ratio ventilation with volume-cycles, conventional ratio ventilation.

R.C. Bone, M.D.

References

1. Gattioni L, Bombino M, Pelosi P, et al: Lung structure and function in different stages of severe adult respiratory distress syndrome. *JAMA* 271:1772–1779, 1994.
2. Dreyfuss D, Saumon G: Should the lungs be rested or recruited? The Charybdis and Scylla of ventilatory management. *Am J Respir Crit Care Med* 149:1066–1068, 1994.
3. Gurevitch MJ, Van Dyke J, Young ES, et al: Improved oxygenation and lower peak airway pressures in severe adult respiratory distress syndrome. *Chest* 89:211–213, 1986.

Persistent Elevation of Inflammatory Cytokines Predicts a Poor Outcome in ARDS: Plasma IL-1β and IL-6 Levels Are Consistent and Efficient Predictors of Outcome Over Time

Meduri GU, Headley S, Kohler G, Stentz F, Tolley E, Umberger R, Leeper K (Univ of Tennessee Med Ctr, Memphis; Regional Med Ctr, Memphis, Tenn; Veteran Affairs Med Ctr, Memphis, Tenn)
Chest 107:1062–1073, 1995 119-96-23–3

Objective.—Levels of inflammatory cytokines have been associated with the development of adult respiratory distress syndrome (ARDS) as well as shock and multiorgan dysfunction. An adverse outcome of ARDS, therefore, could correlate with persistent inflammation. Levels of cytokines were monitored prospectively in patients who had severe ARDS.

Methods.—Twenty-seven consecutive patients who had severe ARDS of medical origin were included. Plasma levels of tumor necrosis factor-α (TNF-α) and interleukin-1β (IL-1β), IL-2, Il-4, IL-6, and IL-8 were measured with the use of enzyme-linked immunosorbent assays at frequent intervals during the first 2 weeks and then every 3 days during mechanical ventilation.

Results.—Fourteen patients (52%) died. The mortality rates were 86% in patients who had sepsis and 38% in the others. Nonsurvivors had significantly higher plasma levels of TNF-α and all interleukins on the first day of ARDS. Those who had sepsis had especially higher levels of TNF-α and IL-1β, IL-6, and IL-8. Initial plasma levels of IL-1β and IL-2 reflected current values of IL-6 and IL-4, respectively, and also predicted future levels of these cytokines. Nonsurvivors had consistently increased plasma levels of IL-1β, whereas survivors had markedly lower values after the first week of illness.

Conclusion.—The intensity and duration of inflammation, as reflected by plasma levels of cytokines, may determine the ultimate outcome in patients who have ARDS.

► As much as is known about the important regulatory molecules called cytokines and their role in the inflammatory response, we may be certain that our knowledge is still a fraction of what is yet to be learned. To date, more than 100 structurally dissimilar and genetically unrelated cytokines have been identified. Each cytokine is secreted by particular cell types in response to specific stimuli and produces a characteristic constellation of effects on the growth, mobility, differentiation, or function of target cells. They may be secreted individually or as a part of a coordinated response along with other, unrelated cytokines, and their activities often overlap considerably. One cytokine may, in fact, induce or suppress the secretion of others, thereby resulting in a cascade of effects.

This study by Meduri et al. indicates that monitoring of cytokine levels involved in the inflammatory response cascade can yield data useful in predicting morbidity in ARDS. That an early, sustained increase in IL-1β is one of those predictors should not be surprising. Interleukin-1 and TNF-α are potent mediators, almost interchangeable in action at times, that induce synthesis of endothelial adhesion molecules and production of other mediators by neutrophils and monocytes. Their role in the pathogenesis of ARDS has been reported.[1, 2] Meduri et al. found that high values of IL-1β were prognostic of death independent of the presence of sepsis or shock. More studies will be needed to confirm the authors' suggestion that the evaluation of ARDS from acute to chronic inflammation, as a result of a persistent inflammatory response, may explain the histologic, laboratory, clinical, and physiologic findings in patients who have late ARDS and do not improve. Over time, additional understanding of the cytokines at both molecular and clinical levels may be necessary for better therapeutic approaches to ARDS.

R.C. Bone, M.D.

References

1. Jacobs RF, Tabor DR, Burks AW, et al: Elevated interleukin-1 release by human alveolar macrophages during the adult respiratory distress syndrome. *Am Rev Respir Dis* 145:A453, 1992.

2. Dinarello CA: The proinflammatory cytokines interleukin-1 and tumor necrosis factor and treatment of the septic shock syndrome. *J Infect Dis* 163:1177–1184, 1991.

Efficacy of Inhaled Nitric Oxide in Patients With Severe ARDS

Rossaint R, Gerlach H, Schmidt-Ruhnke H, Pappert D, Lewandowski K, Steudel W, Falke K (Freie Universität Berlin)
Chest 107:1107–1115, 1995 119-96-23–4

Background.—Selective pulmonary vasodilation can be produced by inhalation of low concentrations of nitric oxide (NO). In patients who have severe acute respiratory distress syndrome (ARDS), inhalation of NO induces vasodilation primarily in ventilated lung areas. To date, there is no information on whether NO inhalation positively affects survival in these patients. The initial and long-term effects of NO inhalation in patients who had severe ARDS were studied retrospectively.

Methods.—Eighty-seven patients who had severe ARDS were included. Thirty patients received low concentrations of inhaled NO for more than 48 hours in addition to standard treatment. The initial and long-term effects of NO inhalation were assessed in terms of hemodynamics, gas exchange, and methemoglobin formation. The survival rates of matched pairs of patients who did and did not receive NO inhalation were also compared.

Results.—Among the NO group, the ratio of arterial Po_2 to the fraction of inspired O_2 (Pao_2/FIO2) increased by at least 10 mm Hg in 83% of patients. Venous admixture (QVA/QT) decreased by at least 10% in 87% of patients, and mean pulmonary artery pressure decreased by at least 3 mm Hg in 63% of patients. The 30 patients received a mean of 17 days of NO inhalation at an average concentration of 11.5 ppm. During brief daily interruptions of NO inhalation, Pao_2/FIO2 consistently decreased by 81 mm Hg. At the same time, QVA/QT increased by 8% and pulmonary artery pressure by 5 mm Hg. Tachyphylaxis did not occur over time, nor did the effects of NO inhalation become more pronounced. There was a significant increase in level of methemoglobin, from 0.74% to 0.98%. There was no difference in survival between patients who did and those who did not receive NO.

Conclusions.—For most patients who have severe ARDS, inhalation of NO is beneficial. In some patients and for no obvious reason, however, inhalation of NO may fail to improve pulmonary gas exchange or reduce pulmonary hypertension. Large, randomized, prospective trials would be needed to show a potential increase in survival with NO inhalation therapy.

► This report by Rossaint et al. leaves open the definitive question regarding inhalation of NO by patients who have severe ARDS: Does it improve survival? Earlier work by this group indicated that inhaled NO induces vasodilation predominantly in ventilated lung areas in patients who have severe ARDS.[1] Other investigators showed that NO inhalation is not always able to reduce mean pulmonary artery pressure and increase the PaO_2.[2] This retrospective study did tend to confirm findings of the authors' previous study that continuous inhalation of low concentrations of NO remains effective for more than 2 weeks in improving pulmonary gas exchange and reducing pulmonary hypertension. However, it also confirmed the finding of a previous investigation[2] that inhalation of NO is not always effective in improving arterial oxygenation. The possibility of NO toxicity in these severely ill patients appears to have been ruled out in this retrospective analysis of patient data. A need for more data, gathered in large, controlled randomized trials, is the major finding of this study.

R.C. Bone, M.D.

References

1. Rossaint R, Falke KJ, Lopez F, et al: Inhaled nitric oxide in adult respiratory distress syndrome. *N Engl J Med* 328:399–405, 1993.
2. Ricou B, Suter PM: Variable effects of nitric oxide (NO) in ARDS patients. *Am Rev Respir Dis* 147:350A, 1993.

24 Mechanical Ventilation

Continuous Aspiration of Subglottic Secretions in Preventing Ventilator-Associated Pneumonia

Vallés J, Artigas A, Rello J, Bonsoms N, Fontanals D, Blanch L, Fernández R, Baigorri F, Mestre J (Hosp de Sabedell, Barcelona; Universitat Autónoma, Barcelona)

Ann Intern Med 122:179–186, 1995 119-96-24–1

Background.—Several strategies have been recommended to reduce the incidence of ventilator-associated pneumonia. Further study is needed to define the role of selective digestive decontamination in selected patients in ICUs. The value of continuous aspiration of subglottic secretions in preventing ventilator-associated pneumonia in a medical-surgical ICU was investigated in a randomized, controlled, blinded study.

Methods.—One hundred ninety patients admitted to an ICU over 33 months were enrolled. All patients had conditions that suggested the need for prolonged intubation. Seventy-six patients were randomly selected to receive continuous aspiration of subglottic secretions (Fig 1), and 77 received the usual care.

Findings.—The incidence rate of ventilator-associated pneumonia in patients who received continuous aspiration of subglottic secretions was 19.9 episodes per 1,000 ventilator days. The incidence in the control group was 39.6 episodes per 1,000 ventilator days. This difference resulted from a significant decrease in the number of gram-positive cocci and *Haemophilus influenzae* organisms in the patients given continuous aspiration. There were no differences in the number of *Pseudomonas aeruginosa* or *Enterobacteriaceae* organisms. Episodes of ventilator-associated pneumonia occurred at a mean of 12 days in patients who received continuous aspiration and at a mean of 5.9 days in the control group. In 85% of patients, the microorganisms isolated from protected specimen brush or bronchoalveolar lavage cultures in patients who had ventilator-associated pneumonia were the same as those previously isolated from cultures of subglottic secretions. There were no significant differences in outcomes.

Conclusions.—The use of a simple method to reduce the long-term microaspirations through the cuff of endotracheal tubes can significantly

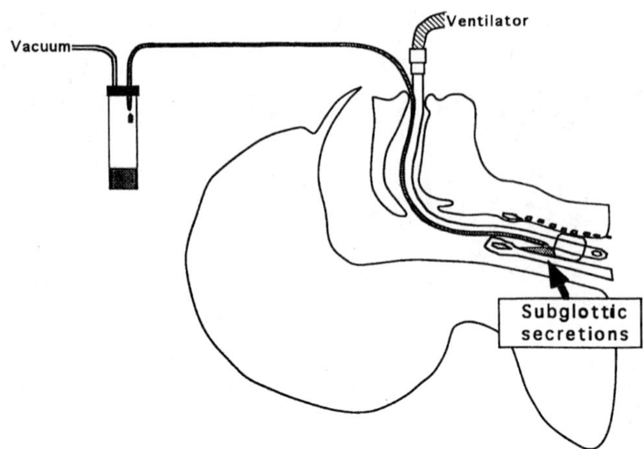

FIGURE 1.—Diagram of continuous aspiration of subglottic secretions. (Courtesy of Vallés J, Artigas A, Rello J, et al: Continuous aspiration of subglottic secretions in preventing ventilator-associated pneumonia. *Ann Intern Med* 122:179–186, 1995.)

decrease the incidence of nosocomial pneumonia in intubated patients. This method is inexpensive and does not increase the cost of treating patients with a conventional artificial airway. It also helps decrease the antibiotic dosage. Other methods of prevention may be combined with it.

▶ Two recent studies have suggested that the chronic aspiration of subglottic secretions by the ventilated patient might be prevented, either by changes in body position[1] or by manual intermittent aspiration of subglottic secretions.[2] In the study reported by Vallés et al., the continuous aspiration of subglottic secretions in ventilated patients reduced the incidence of nosocomial pneumonia by 43.4% and increased the number of days on mechanical ventilation before pneumonia developed. The overall decrease in incidence was caused by a significant reduction in the incidence of pneumonia during the first days of mechanical ventilation. That there was a direct relationship between aspiration of secretions and reduction in pneumonia incidence was indicated by the close association observed between microorganisms isolated from subglottic secretions and the pathogens commonly identified in ventilator-associated pneumonia.

The most important element in prevention of ventilator-associated pneumonia is the interruption of the pathogenetic chain. One approach has been gut decontamination with antibiotics to reduce the pathogenicity of the inoculum delivered from the digestive tract to the oropharynx and bronchial tract. The accumulated data do not show that this technique decreases mortality. Continuous aspiration of subglottic secretions decreases the volume of oropharyngeal secretions and, thus, should decrease the inoculum to the bronchial tract. With continuous aspiration of subglottic secretions, the pattern of nosocomial pneumonia was shifted in this study—a point of clinical significance. Perhaps because the size of the inoculum was altered by continuous aspiration of secretions, the authors saw a delay in the development of *P. aeruginosa* pneumonia and a decrease of *H. influenzae* pneumonia in patients who underwent aspiration. As the authors note, the study implies the potential for reducing the use of antibiotics in ventilated patients, thus reducing costs for caring for these patients and lowering the potential for development of antibiotic-resistant pathogens.

R.C. Bone, M.D.

References

1. Torres A, Serra-Batlles J, Ros E, et al: Pulmonary aspiration of gastric contents in patients receiving mechanical ventilation: The effect of body position. *Ann Intern Med* 116:540–543, 1992.
2. Mahul P, Auboyer C, Jospe R, et al: Prevention of nosocomial pneumonia in intubated patients: Respective role of mechanical subglottic secretions drainage and stress ulcer prophylaxis. *Intensive Care Med* 18:20–25, 1992.

Incidence of Tricuspid Regurgitation and Vena Caval Backward Flow in Mechanically Ventilated Patients: A Color Doppler and Contrast Echocardiographic Study

Jullien T, Valtier B, Hongnat J-M, Dubourg O, Bourdarias J-P, Jardin F (Hôpital Ambroise Paré, Boulogne, France)

Chest 107:488–493, 1995 119-96-24–2

Objective.—Ventricular dimensions and oxygen consumption in patients receiving mechanical ventilation are usually measured by thermodilution. Tricuspid regurgitation (TR) and vena cava backflow (VCBF), however, can alter the thermodilution curve. The relationship between TR and VCBF and the cyclic effect of mechanical ventilation on TR were studied.

Methods.—Respiratory mechanics were measured, and color Doppler, continuous-wave Doppler, and contrast echocardiography were performed in 40 patients receiving mechanical ventilation.

Results.—All 40 patients had TR; it was mild in 21 patients, moderate in 9, and severe in 10. Tricuspid regurgitation increased significantly during mechanical ventilation. Systolic or pancardiac regurgitation was seen with contrast echocardiography in 22 patients, with systolic regurgitation apparent during the entire respiratory cycle in 7 patients, and during the expiratory phase in 9 patients. Six patients who had mild TR had isolated pancardiac regurgitation during lung inflation. Pancardiac VCBF was detected in 15 patients.

Conclusions.—The incidences of TR and VCBF were high. Severe TR occurred in 25% of patients. The incidence of TR in patients receiving mechanical ventilation compares with that of patients not receiving mechanical ventilation. Because of inaccuracies in the measurement of TR and the lack of relationship between VCBF and the severity of TR, the thermodilution method is not a reliable way of measuring cardiac output in patients receiving mechanical ventilation.

▶ Tricuspid regurgitation during mechanical ventilation has been noted in the literature for many years, but its incidence and severity have not been studied to any large extent. A study of TR with regard to the measurement of cardiac output by thermodilution, as reported by Jullien et al., is relevant in regard to the clinical importance one should assign to the thermodilution curve.[1] This abstracted study allows the authors to question the adequacy of the thermodilution technique for measuring cardiac output or right ventricular ejection fraction in ventilated patients. The contrast echocardiographic studies done in these patients indicated that lung inflation might induce VCBF, thus producing regurgitation of microcavitations into the inferior vena cava and hepatic veins. The authors therefore suggest that VCBF is not necessarily reflective of TR; indeed, the studies showed that VCBF always started at systole, which has been considered to be reflective of TR. Tricuspid regurgitation was found by color Doppler and contrast echocardiographic study to be more marked during mechanical ventilation than during brief periods of spontaneous breathing.

R.C. Bone, M.D.

Reference

1. Cigarroa R, Lange R, Williams R, et al: Underestimation of cardiac output by thermodilution in patients with tricuspid regurgitation. *Am J Med* 86:417–420, 1989.

A Comparison of Four Methods of Weaning Patients From Mechanical Ventilation

Esteban A, for the Spanish Lung Failure Collaborative Group (Hosp Universitario de Getafe, Madrid)

N Engl J Med 332:345–350, 1995 119-96-24-3

Background.—Weaning patients in the ICU from mechanical ventilation is challenging. It is usually done in an empirical manner, as no standardized approach has been developed. Patients ready to be weaned were assessed prospectively in a randomized, multicenter trial.

Methods.—Five hundred forty-six patients who were mechanically ventilated for a mean of 7.5 days were enrolled. All were judged ready for weaning by their physicians. One hundred thirty patients who had had respiratory distress during a 2-hour trial of spontaneous breathing were randomly assigned to 1 of 4 weaning methods. Twenty-nine patients received intermittent mandatory ventilation, in which the ventilator rate was initially set at a mean of 10 breaths per minute and then reduced, if possible, at least twice a day, usually by 2–4 breaths per minute. Thirty-seven patients received pressure-support ventilation, in which support was set initially at 18 cm of water then reduced, if possible, by 2–4 cm of water

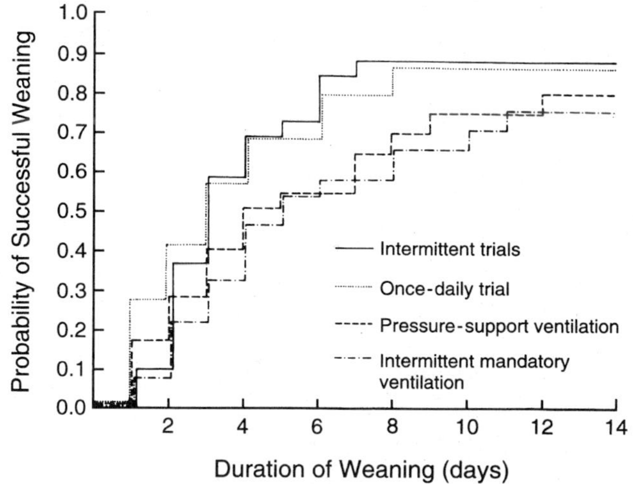

FIGURE 1.—Kaplan-Meier curves of the probability of successful weaning. After adjustment for baseline characteristics in a Cox proportional-hazards model, the rate of successful weaning with a once-daily trial of spontaneous breathing was 2.83 times higher than that with intermittent mandatory ventilation ($P < 0.006$) and 2.05 times higher than that with pressure-support ventilation ($P < 0.04$). (Reprinted by permission of *The New England Journal of Medicine*. Esteban A, for the Spanish Lung Failure Collaborative Group: A comparison of four methods of weaning patients from mechanical ventilation. *N Engl J Med* 332:345–350, 1995. Copyright 1995, Massachusetts Medical Society.)

at least twice daily. Thirty-three patients received intermittent trials of spontaneous breathing, done 2 or 4 times a day if possible. Thirty-one patients received a once-daily trial of spontaneous breathing.

Findings.—The median durations of weaning for the 4 groups were 5 days, 4 days, 3 days, and 3 days, respectively (Fig 1). After adjustment for other covariates, the rate of successful weaning was greater with a once-daily trial of spontaneous breathing than with pressure-support ventilation or intermittent mandatory ventilation. No significant differences were found in the rate of success between once-daily trials and multiple trials of spontaneous breathing (Tables 3 and 4).

Conclusions.—Extubation with a once-daily trial of spontaneous breathing was achieved approximately 3 times faster than with intermittent mandatory ventilation and approximately 2 times faster than with pressure-support ventilation. Multiple daily spontaneous breathing trials were just as successful.

► Weaning from mechanical ventilation has been, and continues to be, a topic that (1) will stimulate heated debate at any gathering of physicians who consider themselves experts on the subject and (2) will, at a medical meeting on the topic, fill a large seminar room with practicing physicians who struggle each day with the difficulties and uncertainties of weaning ventilated patients. In an earlier paper, Esteban et al. observed that more than 40% of the time a patient receives mechanical ventilation is devoted to attempts to wean.[1]

TABLE 3.—Rate of Successful Weaning With the Various Techniques and According to Baseline Characteristics

Variable	Relative Rate of Successful Weaning (95% Confidence Interval)	*P* Value
Weaning technique		
Once-daily trial of spontaneous breathing vs. intermittent mandatory ventilation	2.83 (1.36–5.89)	<0.006
Once-daily trial of spontaneous breathing vs. pressure-support ventilation	2.05 (1.04–4.04)	<0.04
Once-daily trial of spontaneous breathing vs. intermittent trials of spontaneous breathing	1.24 (0.64–2.41)	<0.54
Duration of ventilator support before weaning begun (1-day increments)	0.94 (0.90–0.98)	<0.005
Time to failure of first trial of spontaneous breathing (10-min increments)	1.15 (1.07–1.24)	<0.001
Age (10-yr increments)	0.83 (0.71–0.96)	<0.02

Note: Proportional hazards regression analysis was used to estimate the 95% confidence interval of the relative rate of successful weaning.

(Reprinted by permission of *The New England Journal of Medicine*. Esteban A, for the Spanish Lung Failure Collaborative Group: A comparison of four methods of weaning patients from mechanical ventilation. *N Engl J Med* 332:345–350, 1995. Copyright 1995, Massachusetts Medical Society.)

Each currently available method of weaning has its proponents, but there have been few well-designed comparative studies. A study from France[2] compared traditional T-tube weaning, intermittent mandatory ventilation, and pressure-support ventilation; it was found that pressure-support ventilation was associated with shorter duration of weaning and lower failure rate than the other methods. Esteban et al. found that a once-daily trial or intermittent trials of spontaneous breathing led to extubation more quickly than did intermittent mandatory ventilation or pressure-support ventilation. Approximately 15% of patients who successfully underwent a 2-hour trial of spontaneous breathing required reintubation within 48 hours, but 22.6% eventually were reintubated. The authors observe that a once-daily trial of spontaneous breathing and a prolonged period of rest may be more effective than other weaning methods in assisting the patient to adapt to nonassisted breathing. In addition, the authors note that a once-daily spontaneous breathing trial does not require the changes in ventilator settings and subsequent arterial blood-gas measurements needed for weaning via pressure-support ventilation—a potentially serious consideration in our era of cost consciousness.

Is the study by Esteban et al. a final or semi-final evaluation of weaning methods? It is not likely to be accepted as such, although it will gain recognition as a carefully performed study with potentially important clinical

TABLE 4.—Outcomes in Patients Who Were Difficult to Wean From Mechanical Ventilation

Weaning Technique	Successful Weaning and Extubation	Reintubation	Continued Mechanical Ventilation After 14 Days
		no. of patients (%)	
Intermittent mandatory ventilation	20 (69.0)	4 (13.8)	5 (17.2)
Pressure-support ventilation	23 (62.2)	7 (18.9)	4 (10.8)
Intermittent trials of spontaneous breathing	27 (81.8)	5 (15.2)	1 (3.0)
Once-daily trial of spontaneous breathing	22 (71.0)	7 (22.6)	1 (3.2)

Note: The percentages do not total 100% in the groups that received pressure-support ventilation and a once-daily trial of spontaneous breathing because 1 patient died in each group and weaning was interrupted because of an intercurrent illness in 2 patients in the pressure-support group.

(Reprinted by permission of *The New England Journal of Medicine.* Esteban A, for the Spanish Lung Failure Collaborative Group: A comparison of four methods of weaning patients from mechanical ventilation. *N Engl J Med* 332:345–350 1995. Copyright 1995, Massachusetts Medical Society.)

implications. The number of patients in each weaning-trial group was not large enough to avoid skewing of comparisons by patients who were extraordinarily difficult to wean. Also, the percentage of patients (22.6%) who required reintubation after a once-daily trial of spontaneous breathing is not a particularly impressive indicator of success by some standards. The potential for cost savings should not be interpreted as an indication to decrease the overall monitoring of the patient during once-daily trials of spontaneous breathing; any weaning method can result in electrolyte disorders, infection, anemia, heart failure, or other factors that are reversible if promptly observed and treated.

R.C. Bone, M.D.

References

1. Esteban A, and the Spanish Lung Failure Collaborative Group: Modes of mechanical ventilation and weaning: A national survey of Spanish hospitals. *Chest* 106:1188–1193, 1994.
2. Brochard L, Rauss A, Benito S, et al: Comparison of three methods of gradual withdrawal from ventilatory support during weaning from mechanical ventilation. *Am Rev Respir Crit Care Med* 150:896–903, 1994.

Work of Breathing After Extubation

Ishaaya AM, Nathan SD, Belman MJ (Cedars Sinai Med Ctr, Los Angeles; Univ of California, Los Angeles)
Chest 107:204–209, 1995 119-96-24–4

Background.—Work of breathing is higher in the period immediately after extubation in comparison with spontaneous breathing through an endotracheal tube. The glottis and trachea were studied as possible sites of increased airway resistance after extubation.

Patients and Methods.—Eight patients (mean age, 71 years) were included. The mean duration of intubation was 5.5 days. Breathing pattern, work of breathing, and pressure time product were assessed during weaning from mechanical ventilation. The trachea was examined, and the cross-sectional area of the glottis was measured during bronchoscopy at extubation.

Results.—Significantly lower work of breathing and pressure time product were observed during pressure support ventilation, at 0.43 J/L and 101 cm H_2O·sec/min, compared with 1.49 J/L and 299 cm H_2O·sec/min during spontaneous breathing after extubation. Both indices, however, were significantly higher after extubation, at 1.49 J/L and 299 cm H_2O·sec/min, compared with 0.95 J/L and 196 cm H_2O·sec/min when breathing through the endotracheal tube (Fig 4). None of the patients had tracheal or glottic narrowing during bronchoscopy. Successful measurements of the glottic cross-sectional area were obtained in 4 patients at the onset of inspiration; the mean measurement was 140 mm^2.

Conclusions.—Increased work of breathing after extubation does not result from tracheal or laryngeal disease. Rather, upper airway narrowing at a more proximal site, (e.g., the oropharynx or velopharynx) may be the cause of increased respiratory work.

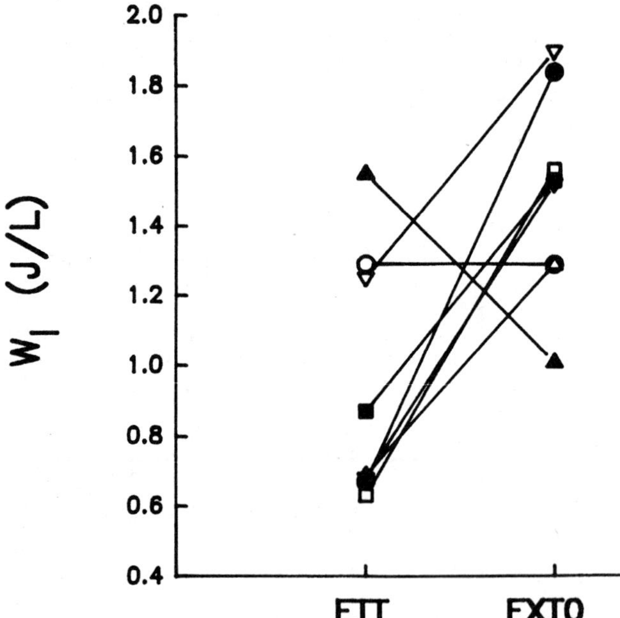

FIGURE 4.—The individual values for work of breathing (W_I) during endotracheal tube (*ETT*) and postextubation (*EXTO*). All patients apart from 1 showed an increase in W_I. (Courtesy of Ishaaya AM, Nathan SD, Belman MJ: Work of breathing after extubation. *Chest* 107:204–209, 1995.)

► The pulmonary group at Cedars Sinai Medical Center and the University of California, Los Angeles, have been working to define the anatomical and physiologic events associated with extubation and weaning in the ventilated patient. In a 1993 paper, they reported the unexpected finding that the work of breathing was significantly increased in the immediate postextubation period as compared with the work of breathing spontaneously through an endotracheal tube.[1] The study abstracted here was designed to determine whether the increased work of breathing in the postextubation period could be caused by changes in the trachea and glottis as a result of damage caused by intubation. Using bronchoscopy to examine the trachea and glottis at the time of extubation, the investigators could not confirm that hypothesis; rather, no tracheal or glottal narrowing was detected. Future studies will now be undertaken to determine whether the increase in work of breathing after extubation may be caused by upper airway narrowing at the oropharynx or velopharynx. Of more immediate clinical interest, the investigators suggest that tolerance of low levels of pressure support may not be a reliable predictor of successful extubation.

R.C. Bone, M.D.

Reference

1. Nathan SN, Ishaaya AM, Koerner SK, et al: Prediction of pressure support during weaning from mechanical ventilation. *Chest* 103:1215–1219, 1993.

Medical Effectiveness of Esophageal Balloon Pressure Manometry in Weaning Patients From Mechanical Ventilation

Gluck EH, Barkoviak MJ, Balk RA, Casey LC, Silver MR, Bone RC (North Chicago VA Med Ctr, Ill; Rush-Presbyterian-St Luke's Med Ctr, Chicago; Med College of Toledo, Ohio)

Crit Care Med 23:504–509, 1995 119-96-24–5

Objective.—The cost of mechanical ventilation of a patient in the ICU can be as high as $3,500 a day. The cost-effectiveness and predictive value of an esophageal balloon pressure monitor, which uses a weaning algorithm, was compared prospectively with the conventional clinical weaning.

Methods.—The results of attempts to wean 23 patients from mechanical ventilation with the use of 2 scoring systems, 1 based on clinical weaning parameters and 1 based on esophageal balloon data, were examined. Protocols were evaluated on aggressiveness of weaning and patient tolerance of the process. Criteria for failure of the weaning process were established.

Results.—One hundred thirty-eight weaning decisions were made. In 40.5% of decisions, the esophageal weaning protocol was more aggressive and was correct. Clinical weaning and esophageal protocol decisions predicted the same number of weaning steps in 39.8% of decisions. In 11.6%

of decisions, the clinical weaning protocol was more aggressive and was correct. Overall, the esophageal protocol was significantly more aggressive than was the clinical protocol. The mean duration of mechanical ventilation was 5.33 days. Had the patient been weaned by the clinical protocol, the average would have been 7.81 days.

Conclusion.—When the rigid esophageal protocol was used, patients were weaned from mechanical ventilation an average of 1.7 days faster than when the clinical protocol was used, without an increase in patient intolerance.

▶ The amount of time that a ventilated patient spends in weaning can be a substantial portion of the entire time spent on the ventilator.[1] Therefore, weaning can account for a large part of the costs associated with mechanical ventilation and will likely attract more and more attention as an area in which costs can be reduced if success in weaning can be improved and time to weaning shortened. However, the determinants of the outcome of weaning are a complex of physiologic and psychological factors that pose difficulty for the physician who must make a clinical decision regarding weaning strategy. The new respiratory monitor described by Gluck et al., which uses esophageal balloon pressure manometry to provide physiologic data, permitted the investigators to formulate a rigorous weaning protocol that reduced reliance on subjective clinical judgment. Their statistical analysis demonstrated to their satisfaction that the esophageal weaning protocol resulted in more aggressive weaning than a clinical protocol. Confirmation of these promising results awaits the outcome of a planned multicenter trial.

R.C. Bone, M.D.

Reference

1. Esteban A, Alia I, Ibanez J, et al: Modes of mechanical ventilation and weaning: A national survey of Spanish hospitals. *Chest* 106:1188–1193, 1994.

25 Transplantation

Bronchiolitis Obliterans in Single-Lung Transplant Recipients

Nathan SD, Ross DJ, Belman MJ, Shain S, Elashoff JD, Kass RM, Koerner SK
(Cedars Sinai Med Ctr, Los Angeles; Univ of California, Los Angeles)

Chest 107:967–972, 1995 119-96-25–1

Introduction.—The chief event compromising long-term survival in lung transplant recipients is bronchiolitis obliterans (BO), a disorder of presumed immunologic origin that accompanies chronic pathologic rejection of the transplant. Reported incidence rates range from 10% to 50%. The course of BO in individual recipients is not clear. Serial spirometric readings of single lung transplant recipients were reviewed.

Patients.—Fifteen patients in whom BO developed were included. Bronchiolitis obliterans was defined by a lasting reduction of at least 20% in forced expiratory volume in 1 second. These patients were among 26 single lung recipients who lived longer than 6 months. Twelve patients underwent transplantation for pulmonary fibrosis or chronic obstructive lung disease. Bronchiolitis obliterans was confirmed histologically in 11 patients.

Outcome.—Six patients (group 1) had a rapid onset of functional decline and a relentlessly progressive course. Four others (group 2) also had a rapid onset and decrease in function but subsequently stabilized. Five patients (group 3) had an insidious onset and course of functional compromise. Five patients in group 1 died of progressive respiratory failure a mean of 6.5 months after the onset of BO. Two of these patients had evidence of pulmonary embolism at autopsy. One patient in group 2 died of complications from cytomegalovirus colitis. One patient in group 3 died of post-transplant lymphoproliferative disease and aminoglycoside-related renal failure. Thirteen patients received at least 1 course of pulsed solumedrol therapy for BO. Four of 21 pulses appeared to improve lung function transiently, but only 1 of these patients responded for longer than 1 month.

Conclusion.—Monitoring the forced expiratory volume in 1 second will help predict the outcome in single lung transplant recipients in whom BO develops.

► Nathan et al. point out that development of BO during the postoperative course of single lung transplantation can be difficult to identify histologically via a transbronchial biopsy specimen. Clinical diagnosis using forced expiratory volume in 1 second is gaining acceptance.[1] This work builds on that hypothesis and offers the finding that persistent reduction in forced expiratory flow 25% to 75% may be the earliest indicator of BO in recipients of single lung transplants.

Not to be left out of postoperative complication monitoring in recipients of single lung transplants is the remaining native lung. This lung can be a source of significant pathology, resulting in increased morbidity, prolonged hospitalization, and the potential for increased mortality. Transplant complications arising from the native lung include ventilation flow mismatch, pulmonary infarction, and infection.[2]

R.C. Bone, M.D.

References

1. International Society for Heart and Lung Transplantation: A working formulation for the standardization of nomenclature and for clinical staging of chronic dysfunction in lung allografts. *J Heart Lung Transplant* 12:713–716, 1993.
2. Frost AE, Keller CA, Noon GP, et al: Outcome of the native lung after single lung transplant. *Chest* 107:981–984, 1995.

PART THREE

HEMATOLOGY AND ONCOLOGY

MARTIN J. CLINE, M.D.

Introduction

This year I have given more than usual emphasis to the section on "classical hematology," and I have included articles on the treatment of pruritus in polycythemia rubra vera, on the management of essential thrombocytosis, and on the optimization and problems of anticoagulant therapy. In 1995, we included information on "a newly defined genetic hypercoagulable syndrome leading to thrombosis at a young age," i.e., hereditary resistance to activated protein C caused by a mutation in the gene for factor V. As noted, "this abnormality may be 10 times more common in thrombosis-prone young individuals than any other known deficiency of anticoagulant proteins." This year, several articles that put this new syndrome into perspective are included in this section. Surprisingly, carrying the mutant gene may not increase the risk of heart attacks in men.

Leukemias

We continued to make steady progress in the treatment of acute myeloid leukemia, and several articles on this subject are included in this YEAR BOOK. We are not so fortunate with regard to the treatment of acute lymphoid leukemia in adults, and I have little news to report. However, in the rare disorder known as adult T-cell leukemia/lymphoma, the cause of which is a retrovirus, a combination of interferon and a drug used to treat AIDS apparently works miracles.

Lymphomas

As noted in the previous 2 YEAR BOOKS, in the treatment of high-grade lymphomas, we seem to be returning to the original recipe of cyclophosphamide, doxorubicin, vincristine, and prednisone (CHOP). In the past few years, we have acquired a host of new drugs for indolent B-cell tumors, including deoxycoformycin, fludarabine, and 2-chlorodeoxadenosine. These agents often work in treating disease that is resistant to alkylating agents, but it is still not clear whether they have a role in first-line therapy.

Perhaps the most interesting observation in this section of the YEAR BOOK is that an AIDS-associated lymphoma called "body-cavity lymphoma" is linked to the same herpesvirus that may cause Kaposi's sarcoma.

Bone Marrow Transplantation and Gene Therapy

In bone marrow transplantation, the emphasis continues to be on determining the usefulness of autologous transplantation in leukemias and advanced lymphomas. We did not hear much this year about the usefulness of autologous bone marrow transplantation in diverse malignancies such as advanced breast and ovarian cancers, so we still do not know whether it is useful.

There have been no "breakthroughs" in gene therapy, but a few reported disappointments appeared in the pages of *The New England Journal of Medicine*. Nevertheless, steady progress is being made. Look for routine use in the clinic for some diseases by the beginning of the next century.

Oncology

As observed in previous YEAR BOOKS, basic molecular biology continues to make enormous contributions to our understanding of the mechanisms of malignant diseases. Two genes for familial forms of breast cancer have been identified: the *BRCA1* gene, located on the long arm of chromosome 17, and the *BRCA2* gene, found on the long arm of chromosome 13. We are also getting a clearer picture of the molecular mechanisms of colon cancer.

Prostate cancer is emerging as a very important disease in a progressively aging population. The efficacy and usefulness of screening for prostate cancer are analyzed in important articles, and we continue to examine the roles of limited and aggressive therapy of this cancer.

Martin J. Cline, M.D.

26 Red Cells, White Cells, and Hemostasis

Long-Term Treatment With Interferon-α2b for Severe Pruritus in Patients With Polycythaemia Vera

Muller EW, De Wolf JTM, Egger R, Wijermans PW, Huijgens PC, Halie MR, Vellenga E (Univ Hosp Groningen, The Netherlands; Leyenburg Hosp, The Hague, The Netherlands; Free Univ, Amsterdam, The Netherlands)

Br J Haematol 89:313–318, 1995 119-96-26–1

Background.—Local or generalized pruritus can be particularly problematic in patients who have polycythemia vera (PV). Standard antipruritic treatment, such as antihistamines, H2-receptor antagonists, aspirin, and cholestyramine, is generally ineffective in the majority of patients. In contrast, a favorable treatment effect has recently been noted with interferon-α therapy. This agent has the added benefit of antiproliferative action, resulting in a decreased need for phlebotomy and chemotherapy. However, the number of patients receiving interferon-α treatment and the duration of follow-up have thus far been limited. The efficacy and safety of long-term interferon-α treatment were therefore investigated.

Patients and Methods.—Fifteen patients (mean age, 68 years) who had PV and severe pruritus were included. All patients were treated with subcutaneous recombinant human interferon-α2b at a starting dose of 3 MU given 3 times weekly. Doses were increased when pruritus symptoms failed to decrease after 3 months and when the drug was well tolerated. Laboratory, histologic, and clinical evaluations were conducted throughout the study. The median follow-up was 13 months.

Results.—Pruritus symptoms were significantly improved with interferon-α treatment in 12 of the 15 patients. Long-term relief of symptoms was maintained during treatment, and patients also experienced improvements in general well-being, sleep, and physical and social activities. The mean number of phlebotomies decreased from 4.3 in the year preceding the study to 1.8 in patients undergoing interferon-α treatment. Significant decreases in leukocyte and platelet numbers also were observed. Erythropoietin-independent erythroid colony formation was found to persist during treatment; the effects of interferon-α therefore could not be attributed to the disappearance of the abnormal erythroid progenitor clone or to an inhibitive effect on histamine production. All but 1 patient experienced initial adverse treatment-related effects, including flulike symptoms, myalgia, bone pain, and low-grade fever. Five patients were subsequently withdrawn from the study because of drug intolerability.

Conclusions.—Long-term treatment with interferon-α is both feasible and effective, although side effects are a significant concern. Additional studies are needed to identify an optimal dose that will be tolerated by patients, provide relief from pruritus symptoms, and offer adequate hematologic control.

► Intractable pruritus is a frequent problem in patients who have polycythemia vera. The mechanism is unknown, and the pruritus cannot simply be ascribed to the increased levels of blood histamine associated with increased numbers of basophils because basophilia but not pruritus is more prominent in chronic myelocytic leukemia.

The pruritus of polycythemia vera is often exacerbated by contact with water, and some patients avoid baths and showers. Most conventional antipruritic measures are not effective against the pruritus that accompanies polycythemia vera. This article suggests that interferon-α may provide relief from pruritus in those patients who can tolerate the flulike side effects.

Interferon relieved pruritus in 12 of 15 patients, but an additional 5 patients subsequently refused to take interferon because its side effects were worse than the itching. Overall, 7 of the 15 patients experienced long-term relief.

M.J. Cline, M.D.

Hydroxyurea for Patients With Essential Thrombocythemia and a High Risk of Thrombosis

Cortelazzo S, Finazzi G, Ruggeri M, Vestri O, Galli M, Rodeghiero F, Barbui T (Ospedali Riuniti di Bergamo, Italy; Ospedale Civile S Bortolo di Vicenza, Italy)

N Engl J Med 332:1132–1136, 1995 119-96-26–2

Introduction.—Patients with essential thrombocythemia who are older than 60 years and those who have already had a thrombolic event have been shown to have a high vascular complication rate. These patients could be candidates for platelet count reduction. Hydroxyurea reduces platelet count, but there is no evidence that it decreases thrombotic episodes in patients with essential thrombocythemia. In a prospective, randomized trial, it was determined whether keeping the platelet count below 600,000 mm^3 would reduce the incidence of thrombosis in high-risk patients.

Methods.—A total of 114 patients who had essential thrombocythemia were 60 or more years of age and had a platelet count of $1,500,000/mm^3$ or less. Hemostatic and coagulation studies were done at baseline and at appropriate intervals throughout the trial. Fifty-six patients were randomly assigned to receive hydroxyurea treatment and 58 patients to have no hydroxyurea treatment.

Results.—The patients were followed for a median of 27 months. All patients randomized to receive hydroxyurea had a decrease in platelet count to below 600,000/mm^3 (median count, 459,000 mm^3) within 2–8 weeks. This level was maintained throughout long-term treatment. This is in agreement with an earlier finding of a reduced rate of thrombosis in patients with platelet counts below 600,000/mm^3. Fourteen of 58 untreated controls and 2 of 56 patients treated with hydroxyurea had vascular occlusive events. Hemorrhagic complications occurred in 5 patients, all of whom were taking aspirin or ticlopidine prophylactically. Cigarette smoking was significantly associated with thrombosis, as confirmed by an earlier study.

Conclusion.—Unlike busulfan, hydroxyurea is not an alkylating agent. Concern about its leukemogenic effects, prolonged myelosuppression, and pulmonary and gonadal toxicity eliminates busulfan as a first-line therapy for essential thrombocythemia. Hydroxyurea used in the treatment of essential thrombocythemia was effective in reducing platelet count and preventing thrombosis. However, it must be taken continuously. If inadvertently stopped, an excessive rebound increase in the platelet count could occur.

► Essential thrombocytosis is one of the myeloproliferative disorders characterized by increased numbers of megakaryocytes in the bone marrow and increased numbers of circulating platelets. It is an uncommon disorder that must be distinguished from other conditions with increased numbers of platelets, e.g., chronic blood loss, polycythemia vera, and chronic myelocytic leukemia. Occasionally, essential thrombocytosis makes a transition to another myeloproliferative disorder.

Patients with essential thrombocytosis are at risk of both thromboses and bleeding. There have been arguments as to whether observation alone or maneuvers (such as hydroxyurea treatment) to reduce the platelet count is the best management strategy. In the absence of clear-cut guidelines, I have usually begun treatment with hydroxyurea when the platelet count approaches 1 million per cubic millimeter. This article now provides clear guidelines: *treat with hydroxyurea.*

M.J. Cline, M.D.

Quality of Hematologic Recovery in Patients With Aplastic Anemia Following Cyclosporine Therapy

Yamaguchi M, Nakao S, Takamatsu H, Chuhjo T, Shiobara S, Matsuda T (Kanazawa Univ, Japan)

Exp Hematol 23:341–346, 1995 119-96-26–3

Background.—Antilymphocyte globulin (ALG) and antithymocyte globulin (ATG) have been used to treat patients with aplastic anemia (AA). Although hematologic remission and long-term survival are realized by more than 50% of these patients, treatment with ALG/ATG is associated with a high risk of late clonal complications, including paroxysmal nocturnal hemoglobinuria and myelodysplastic syndrome. Cyclosporine (CyA) also has been used to treat AA, with successful results reported. Unlike ALG and/or prednisolone therapy, CyA does not directly affect hematopoietic progenitor cells, and therefore may differ from other agents in terms of quality of hematologic recovery. Therefore, the effects of CyA therapy on quality of hematologic recovery in patients with AA were retrospectively examined.

Patients and Methods.—Twenty-five patients with AA (13 females and 12 males) who had been treated with oral CyA, 5 or 6 mg/kg, each day for at least 1 month were included. None of the patients had previously received ATG or ALG therapy. Polymorphonuclear leukocytes (PMNCL) were evaluated for clonality using 3 different X-linked gene probes and for glycosyl-phosphatidylinositol (GPI)-anchored membrane protein expression by flow cytometric analysis.

Results.—Clonal hematopoiesis was not detected in 7 of the CyA-responsive female patients. Two of the 6 female patients who failed to respond to CyA treatment showed evidence of clonal hematopoiesis, although 1 of the 2 women had demonstrated monoclonality before therapy. With the exception of 1 patient, the GPI-linked membrane proteins CD55, CD59, and CD16 were expressed normally on PMN in all patients treated with CyA, despite response. In the former patient, a small proportion of GPI-anchored membrane protein-negative cells had been noted before therapy. At 41 months after therapy induction, the proportion of the paroxysmal nocturnal hemoglobinuria cell population had remained unchanged.

Conclusions.—Patients with AA who are successfully treated with CyA do not appear to be at high risk for clonal complications, such as paroxysmal nocturnal hemoglobinuria and myelodysplastic syndrome. The follow-up period of this series of patients was, however, relatively short (median, 30 months) in comparison with studies evaluating patients treated with ALG. The probability of late clonal complications occurring among CyA-treated patients therefore remains to be determined.

▶ The prognosis for patients with untreated severe aplastic anemia is poor, and median survival is less than 18 months. Younger patients with an HLA-matched sibling are generally treated by bone marrow transplantation. Older patients and those without a donor have generally been treated with ALG or ATG. Approximately 50% of patients respond with long-term improvement in their hematologic status. However, it has recently been recognized that treated patients may have clonal hematologic disorders, such as paroxysmal nocturnal hemoglobinuria or one of the myelodysplastic syndromes. In my view, this monoclonal hematopoiesis is more likely to be a component of the defect underlying the aplastic anemia than a consequence of the therapy, but this is not known for certain.

Recently another immunosuppressive, CyA, has also been shown to be effective therapy for some patients with severe aplastic anemia. The long-term consequences of CyA therapy are not known. This study examines 25

Japanese patients with severe aplastic anemia who were treated with CyA. The authors noted no clonal hematopoiesis 15 months to 13 years after CyA therapy for severe aplastic anemia.

M.J. Cline, M.D.

Life Expectancy in Primary Myelodysplastic Syndromes: A Prognostic Score Based Upon Histopathology From Bone Marrow Biopsies of 569 Patients

Maschek H, Gutzmer R, Choritz H, Georgii A (Pathologisches Institut, Medizinische Hochschule Hannover, Germany)

Eur J Haematol 53:280–287, 1994 119-96-26–4

Introduction.—The French-American-British Cooperative Study group (FAB) classification of primary myelodysplastic syndromes (MDS) is based on blast counts in bone marrow aspirates. Considerable prognostic importance is placed on these reports even though there is substantial variation within FAB classifications. Approaches have been modified and scoring systems developed, but the impact of histopathologic features has not been thoroughly examined.

Methods.—Core bone marrow biopsy specimens were obtained from 569 patients who were evaluated for primary MDS. These patients had been registered between 1982 and 1992. Patients whose MDS was secondary or therapy related were not included. Demographics and laboratory data were obtained from medical records. Serial semi-thin sections were stained with Wright-Giemsa, trichrome Masson-Goldner, Gomori's silver staining, and the Prussian Blue reaction. The tissue was classified using the FAB criteria. Fiber increases were graded as 1 (slight increase) to 3 (severe increase). The onset of MDS was the time of the diagnostic biopsy. The survival time was the time to death or last contact.

Results.—Refractory anemias were determined in 45% of the patients and refractory anemias with excess of blasts were found in 24% of the patients. The remaining 3 classes had 9% each. A sixth group, MDS not otherwise specified, included 4% of the patients. The average survival time was 16 months. The shortest period was for patients who had acute leukemia; their median survival was 12.2 months. The best prognosis, 41.9 months, was in patients with refractory anemia with ringed sideroblasts. The best predictor of short survival was dysgranulopoiesis with increased quantity. An increase in mast cells suggested a longer survival. Siderin storage was inversely proportional to survival time. There was still a wide variation in survival time within each FAB group. The most important histopathologic parameters were quantity of myeloblasts, myelofibrosis, and abnormal localization of immature precursors. The scoring system based on histopathology stratified 3 risk groups with different survival times.

Conclusion.—The scoring system gave prognostic information predicting the survival time in patients with MDS. Histopathologic scoring based on current methods should be used for objective predictions independently of hematologic, cytologic, or laboratory data.

► The myelodysplastic syndromes are a heterogeneous collection of disorders, which, almost certainly, have different pathogenetic mechanisms. Six categories of myelodysplastic syndromes are recognized; they vary in clinical aggressiveness from a simple anemia refractory to conventional therapy to a clear-cut leukemia. There are transitions among the various categories, and it is not always easy to predict which cases will evolve into a leukemia. In general, those cases with excessive numbers of blast cells in the bone marrow and those with chromosomal abnormalities are more likely to develop a leukemic picture. The leukemia is usually an acute myeloid leukemia and is usually poorly responsive to conventional therapy.

This study of more than 500 patients with the myelodysplastic syndromes attempts to identify additional features of disease that predict behavior. The large number of patients is one of the impressive aspects of this report, because the myelodysplastic syndromes are relatively uncommon.

As in previous smaller studies, refractory anemia with ringed sideroblasts (RARS) is the most "benign" of these disorders, and in this series, the median survival from diagnosis was 42 months. Refractory anemia with excess blasts in transition (RAEB-t) was the most aggressive of the 6 categories and median survival was only 4 months. An adverse prognostic sign was morphologic abnormalities of granulopoiesis with increased numbers of granulocyte precursors. Prediction of disease behavior is increasingly important in the myelodysplastic syndromes because some patients are now being treated by allogeneic bone marrow transplantation.

M.J. Cline, M.D.

Cisplatin-Associated Anemia: An Erythropoietin Deficiency Syndrome

Wood PA, Hrushesky WJM (Stratton Veterans Affairs Med Ctr, Albany, NY; Albany Med College, NY)

J Clin Invest 95:1650–1659, 1995 119-96-26–5

Objective.—Patients receiving cisplatin-based chemotherapy may demonstrate a cumulative anemia that is out of proportion to the effects on other blood cells. A deficiency in erythrocyte production predominates, suggesting that the anemia may arise partly from deficient renal production of erythropoietin (EPO) caused by cisplatin-induced renal toxicity. Cisplatin-induced renal toxicity and anemia were studied in human beings and in rats.

Clinical Study.—In a study of 47 patients with cancer, the severity of treatment-induced anemia and the associated transfusion requirements were correlated with cisplatin-induced renal tubular dysfunction. The ratio of observed to expected serum levels of EPO decreased as cisplatin therapy continued, in proportion to the severity of patients' renal dysfunction. When cisplatin therapy was halted, the anemia, observed/expected serum EPO ratios, and renal tubular dysfunction resolved. There were permanent decreases in creatinine clearance, however.

Rat Study.—Progressive renal dysfunction developed in rats treated with cisplatin. The anemia persisted for many weeks and did not affect the animals' white blood cell counts. The expected EPO and reticulocyte responses did not occur. Cisplatin-treated rats given EPO showed a greater reticulocyte response and hematocrit increase than did non–cisplatin-treated rats given EPO. This finding suggested that cisplatin caused minimal erythroid precursor cell damage.

Conclusions.—A transient but persistent erythropoietin deficiency syndrome—caused by cisplatin-induced renal tubular damage—appears to be the primary cause of cisplatin-associated anemia. Giving EPO replacement therapy can prevent or treat the renal tubular damage.

► Nephrotoxicity is a well-recognized complication of cisplatin administration, and the serum level of creatinine or the creatinine clearance is monitored during drug administration. If an excessive drug amount is given, renal damage with creatinine elevation can be permanent.

The kidneys are the principal source of erythropoietin production. This article points out that the synthesis of erythropoietin may be affected by cisplatin administration. The effect is reversible with cessation of cisplatin therapy.

Anemia secondary to decreased erythropoietin production is a well-recognized complication of chronic renal failure and is generally treated by transfusion or exogenous erythropoietin administration. That nephrotoxic drugs might also impair erythropoietin production seems obvious, yet I am unaware of studies on this point with drugs such as cyclosporine or amphotericin. Most of these drugs are given in clinical settings in which multiple factors influence the development of anemia and we do not usually single out the effect of a drug on erythropoietin production.

M.J. Cline, M.D.

Differences in Intravenous and Subcutaneous Application of Recombinant Human Erythropoietin: A Multicenter Trial

Schaller R, Sperschneider H, Thieler H, Dutz W, Hans S, Voigt D, Marx M, Engelmann J, Schöter K-H, Scigalla P, Stein G (Friedrich Schiller Universität, Jena, Germany; Medizinische Hochschule Erfurt, Germany; Bezirkskrankenhaus Potsdam, Germany; et al)

Artif Organs 18:552–558, 1995 119-96-26-6

Purpose.—Recombinant human erythropoietin (rhEPO) is used to manage anemia among patients undergoing routine hemodialysis. A randomized, multicenter parallel group comparison study was performed to determine the maintenance doses for IV and subcutaneous (SC) delivery of rhEPO and to evaluate any differences in efficacy, tolerability, and weekly increases of packed cellular volume (PCV) with IV and SC delivery of rhEPO from different production sites.

Patients and Methods.—Ninety patients with end-stage renal failure who were undergoing routine hemodialysis for at least 6 months were included. Patient age ranged from 19 to 77 years. Recombinant human erythropoietin used in the study was produced by the Genetics Institute, Cambridge, Massachusetts, and by Boehringer Mannheim, Penzberg, Germany. The study consisted of a 1-week pretreatment phase, an 8-week double-blind phase, and a final open phase, which included both a correction and a maintenance period. During the double-blind phase, patients were randomly assigned to IV or SC administration of Penzberg-EPO or IV or SC administration of Cambridge-EPO and were treated 3 times per week with a single dose of 40 units/kg. After the first 8 weeks, all patients were treated with either IV or SC Penzberg-EPO. The doses were increased every 4 weeks as needed until the target hematocrit was achieved (correction phase). After the target hematocrit was reached, patients were treated with a maintenance dose.

Results.—The rhEPO production site had no effect on drug efficacy, tolerability, or weekly PCV increases. To maintain a target PVC of 30–35 volume %, the median dose of rhEPO needed with IV administration was 33 units per kg body weight 3 times per week, compared with 22 units per kg when administered subcutaneously. The occurrence or exacerbation of hypertension was noted with rhEPO therapy. This was particularly evident during the correction phase and was seen more commonly in the SC group. No critical differences were observed between the SC and IV groups during the maintenance phase.

Conclusions.—The efficacy and tolerability of rhEPO is not influenced by production site. Weekly increases in PVC also were not affected by production site. On average, the rhEPO dosage required to maintain the target hematocrit was 30% lower with SC administration. Patients receiving rhEPO should undergo frequent blood pressure checks, as this agent is associated with the occurrence or aggravation of hypertension. Individuals with established hypertension also should not receive rhEPO unless their blood pressure is well controlled.

► This is a careful study that provides practical information:

1. It takes about one third more rhEPO to maintain the hematocrit in patients undergoing chronic dialysis when the rhEPO is given by the IV route rather than the SC route.

2. Monitor blood pressure carefully when administering rhEPO to patients. Severe hypertension may develop in some patients.

M.J. Cline, M.D.

Effect of Hydroxyurea on the Frequency of Painful Crises in Sickle Cell Anemia

Charache S, Terrin ML, Moore RD, Dover GJ, Barton FB, Eckert SV, McMahon RP, Bonds DR, and the Investigators of the Multicenter Study of Hydroxyurea in Sickle Cell Anemia (Johns Hopkins Univ, Baltimore, Md; Maryland Med Research Inst, Baltimore, Md; Natl Heart, Lung, and Blood Inst, Bethesda, Md)

N Engl J Med 332:1317–1322, 1995 119-96-26–7

Introduction.—A previous trial using hydroxyurea in patients with sickle-cell anemia showed that fetal hemoglobin increased, with only mild myelotoxicity. In a randomized, double-blind, placebo-controlled trial, it was determined whether hydroxyurea could reduce the frequency of painful crisis in 279 patients with sickle-cell anemia.

Methods.—Eligible patients were enrolled from 21 sites in the United States and Canada. Patients needed to be at least 18 years of age, have known sickle-cell anemia, and have reported at least 3 crises in the previous year. Those randomly assigned to a treatment group received an initial hydroxyurea dose of 15 mg/kg/day, which was increased by 5 mg/kg/day every 12 weeks, unless marrow depression occurred. Treatment was discontinued in the event of marrow depression but was restarted when blood counts recovered. The resumed dose was lower by 2.5 mg/kg/day than the dose associated with marrow depression. A painful crisis was defined as one requiring a visit to a medical facility that lasted more than 4 hours.

Results.—The median rate of crisis per year was 2.5 in the treatment group and 4.5 in the placebo group. These rates were 1.0 and 2.4, respectively, when crises were severe enough to cause hospitalization. No significant differences were noted in the 2 groups in the incidence of death, stroke, and hepatic sequestration. The treatment group had significantly less development of chest syndrome, fewer blood transfusions, and longer median time to first and second vaso-occlusive crisis than did the placebo group.

Conclusion.—There was a 44% reduction in the median annual rate of painful crisis in patients receiving hydroxyurea. Although this result is statistically and clinically meaningful, questions remain regarding: the mechanism by which hydroxyurea reduced the frequency of painful crisis, optimal dose schedule, safety of long-term therapy (in respect to leukemogenesis), and long-term effects on growth, development progression of organ damage, and mortality. A 44% reduction in disease manifestations in adults may not be enough to encourage physicians to prescribe this potent drug for long-term treatment. Continued study is needed.

► In 1982 it was reported that the chemotherapeutic agent 5-azacytidine increased the amount of fetal hemoglobin in baboons. It was subsequently observed that several cytotoxic agents had this effect. Because increased levels of fetal hemoglobin ameliorate the effects of hemoglobin S on cell sickling, cytotoxic drugs were considered as possible therapeutic agents in patients with sickle-cell anemia who had severe complications and frequent painful crises. Hydroxyurea was chosen for clinical trials because it has relatively few side effects and because its myelosuppression is readily reversible when administration of the drug is stopped.

The authors of this multi-institution, randomized, double-blind study evaluated the effectiveness of hydroxyurea in preventing severe painful crises in sickle-cell anemia. The results suggest that hydroxyurea can ameliorate the course of disease in some adults with 3 or more painful crises per year. It generally takes many weeks or months for the fetal hemoglobin levels to increase with treatment, and the beneficial results require prolonged and careful observation. In clinical practice, hydroxyurea therapy should probably be reserved for those patients who have the most severe disease, because the long-term complications of treatment are still unknown. In particular, one worries about the possible development of leukemia.

M.J. Cline, M.D.

Mutation in the Gene Coding for Coagulation Factor V and the Risk of Myocardial Infarction, Stroke, and Venous Thrombosis in Apparently Healthy Men

Ridker PM, Hennekens CH, Lindpaintner K, Stampfer MJ, Eisenberg PR, Miletich JP (Harvard Med School, Boston; Children's Hosp, Boston; Harvard School of Public Health, Boston, et al)

N Engl J Med 332:912–917, 1995 119-96-26–8

Background.—A point mutation in the gene coding for coagulation factor V has been associated with a form of activated protein C that resists degradation, and which, therefore, may increase the risk of venous thrombosis. It is not clear, however, whether healthy individuals are at increased risk. The mutation involves a substitution for guanine at nucleotide 1691.

Objective.—The G1691A mutation was in 374 initially healthy male physicians enrolled in the Physicians' Health Study who subsequently had myocardial infarction, 209 with stroke, and 121 with deep venous thrombosis and/or pulmonary embolism. The same number of enrollees who remained healthy served as a control group.

Findings.—The prevalence of the factor V mutation was 6.1% in men who subsequently had myocardial infarction and 4.3% in those with stroke, which is not significantly different from the 6.0% rate in those who remained free of cardiovascular disease. The mutation was, however, found in 11.6% of men who had venous thrombosis or pulmonary embolism during follow-up. The adjusted relative risk of thrombosis/embolism in heterozygous subjects was 2.7, and the risk of primary venous thrombosis was 3.5. The increased relative risk was apparently found chiefly in older men. One fourth of the men older than 60 years of age who had primary venous thrombosis exhibited the mutation.

Conclusion.—The G1691A mutation of the factor V gene is the most common inherited factor known to predispose to venous thrombosis.

► Protein C and its co-factor, protein S, are part of a naturally occurring, physiologically important system that is a negative regulator of blood clotting. When activated, protein C inactivates blood clotting factors V and VIII.

The observation that resistance to activated protein C is one of the most common genetic abnormalities associated with an increased risk of thromboembolic disease was reported in 1993, and it was one of the most important discoveries in clinical coagulation to be made in the past decade. It is now known that this resistance is usually the result of a single mutation in the factor V gene that makes the factor V protein resistant to degradation by activated protein C. The abnormal gene is apparently quite common and appears to be worldwide in its distribution. Between 3% and 7% of northern Europeans may harbor the mutation.

In this study of a large cohort of apparently healthy men, the presence of the abnormal gene increased the risk of venous thrombosis but was not associated with an increased risk of myocardial infarction or stroke. It is important to note that men with this gene defect may not have their first episode of venous thrombosis until after the age of 60 years.

M.J. Cline, M.D.

Protein C Deficiency in a Controlled Series of Unselected Outpatients: An Infrequent But Clear Risk Factor for Venous Thrombosis (Leiden Thrombophilia Study)

Koster T, Rosendaal FR, Briët E, van der Meer FJM, Colly LP, Trienekens PH, Poort SR, Reitsma PH, Vandenbroucke JP (Univ Hosp Leiden, The Netherlands; Anticoagulation Clinics of Leiden, Amsterdam, and Rotterdam, The Netherlands)

Blood 85:2756–2761, 1995 119-96-26–9

Background.—Along with protein S and antithrombin, protein C is a physiologic component of anticoagulation, and a deficiency may impede inhibitory processes and promote thrombosis. Heterozygosity for protein C deficiency has been related to a predisposition to venous thrombosis. Such defects may be present in 3% to 8% of patients with thrombosis. Their frequency in the general population remains uncertain.

Objective.—Plasma levels of protein C, protein S, and antithrombin were estimated in 474 consecutive, unselected patients younger than 70 years of age who were seen with a first episode of deep venous thrombosis. Thrombosis was confirmed objectively in all cases, and malignant disease was excluded. The same number of matched healthy control subjects were studied. Ten percent of the patients were receiving long-term coumarin treatment.

Findings.—The relative risk of thrombosis in patients with low levels of protein C was 3.1, and it was nearly 4 for those with persistently low values. The protein C gene was mutated in 13 patients whose initial levels were less than 0.67 units/mL, as well as in 2 controls. Slightly more controls than patients had initially and persistently low levels of total protein S. When low levels of both total and free protein S were taken as criteria for the deficient state, the relative risk of thrombosis was 1.7. Two consecutive low antithrombin values conferred a relative risk of 5.0. Spontaneous thrombosis was by no means limited to protein-deficient patients.

Conclusions.—Hereditary protein C deficiency and below-normal plasma levels of protein S and antithrombin are not very frequent in the general population. Nevertheless, protein C deficiency clearly increases the risk of venous thrombosis.

► As noted in the preceding abstract, proteins C and S are part of a physiologically important system that negatively regulates blood coagulation. As detailed in this article, deficiency of protein C carries approximately the same risk of venous thrombosis as does the common mutation in factor V that confers resistance to protein C. Both men and women may be affected by these disorders of "hypercoagulability."

M.J. Cline, M.D.

Brief Report: Variability of Thrombosis Among Homozygous Siblings With Resistance to Activated Protein C Due to an Arg→Gln Mutation in the Gene for Factor V

Greengard JS, Eichinger S, Griffin JH, Bauer KA (Scripps Research Inst, LaJolla, Calif; Brockton West Roxbury Veterans Affairs Med Ctr, Boston; Harvard Med School, Boston)

N Engl J Med 331:1559–1562, 1994 119-96-26–10

Introduction.—Patients with idiopathic deep-vein thrombosis frequently have resistance to activated protein C. This resistance is commonly attributable to a mutation in the factor V gene that replaces the arginine in residue 506 with glutamine (Arg→Gln mutation). Resistance to activated protein C was reported in a white family with familial thrombosis in which 4 of 5 children were homozygous for the Arg→Gln mutation in the factor V gene.

Methods.—Blood samples were collected in all but one family member (who was receiving long-term warfarin therapy) for: activated protein C, total and free protein S, antithrombin III activity, prothrombin fragment F_{1+2}, genomic DNA, and factor V complementary DNA sequence.

Results.—Two homozygous sons with the Arg→Gln mutation and 1 heterozygous son experienced severe and recurrent thromboembolic episodes, with an onset ranging from 16 to 33 years. Two homozygous daughters (28 and 33 years of age) have had no thromboembolic episodes. Neither daughter has experienced major surgical procedures, taken oral contraceptives, or been pregnant. However, they are considered to be at high risk for thromboembolic events. The heterozygous father has had no thromboembolic episodes, but the heterozygous mother had an episode of venous thrombosis during pregnancy. Three of 4 children who were homozygous for the Arg→Gln mutation and their heterozygous mother had markedly elevated levels (more than 2 SD) of prothrombin fragment F_{1+2}, and 1 homozygous son and his father were within 1 SD above the mean for normal. All other coagulation studies were within normal limits.

Conclusion.—The severity of resistance to activated protein C correlated with the heterozygous and homozygous genotypes in a kindred with familial thrombosis. It is possible that other defects influence thrombosis.

► We are still learning about the consequences and natural history of homozygous and heterozygous mutations in the factor V gene. In the previous articles, we have seen that the mutation carries a moderate rather than a dramatic risk of venous thromboembolism when large populations are analyzed. This article examines the heterogeneity of expression of the mutation within a single family. The observations suggest that there is an increased risk of venous thromboembolism in some heterozygous individuals. It also suggests that factors in addition to resistance to activated protein C may influence the development of venous thromboses in affected individuals.

M.J. Cline, M.D.

Risk Factors for Intracranial Hemorrhage in Outpatients Taking Warfarin

Hylek EM, Singer DE (Massachusetts Gen Hosp, Boston)

Ann Intern Med 120:897–902, 1994 119-96-26–11

Objective.—To use anticoagulant therapy rationally, particularly in the elderly population, it is necessary to balance its antithrombotic efficacy with the risk of bleeding. A case-control study was planned at a large general hospital to estimate the risk of intracranial hemorrhage in adult outpatients who were given warfarin therapy.

Study Population.—A review of 1,881 patients admitted to the hospital with intracranial hemorrhage in 1981–1991 revealed that 121 were taking warfarin at the time. Each of these patients was matched with 3 control outpatients who also received anticoagulant therapy. Seventy-seven of the study patients had intracerebral bleeding and 44 had subdural hemorrhage. The respective mortality rates were 46% and 20%.

Observations.—The prothrombin time ratio (PTR) was the predominant risk factor for both types of hemorrhage. The risk was markedly increased for PTR values greater than 2.0. Age also was a risk factor, especially for subdural bleeding. The PTR also was the most prominent risk factor for both intracerebral and subdural bleeding on multiple logistic analysis. A history of cerebrovascular disease, the presence of a prosthetic heart valve, and age also were risk factors.

Conclusion.—These findings emphasize the need to closely control anticoagulant therapy at the lowest level that is effective, particularly in older patients. The PTR should be kept below 2.0.

► More than 6% of the patients admitted to this large hospital for intracranial hemorrhage were taking warfarin at the time of the bleeding. This is consistent with other data indicating that more than 10% of patients receiving chronic anticoagulant therapy may experience a serious bleeding episode. The seriousness of this complication is emphasized by the associated mortality being between 20% and 46%.

Although age is one factor in predicting a warfarin-associated intracranial bleed, the most important factor is the prothrombin time ratio. The risks of bleeding increase significantly when the ratio rises above 2.0.

There is an expanding use of long-term anticoagulation with the report that anticoagulants reduced the risk of stroke in patients with atrial fibrillation. In the use of such anticoagulation, one must always balance the potential risks against the potential benefits. In my experience, young physicians who are in training often do not appreciate the very high risks of long-term anticoagulation. I usually stress that the risks are greater than the rewards unless (1) the patient has a good level of understanding of the process of anticoagulation; (2) the patient is compliant; (3) the treating physician is knowledgeable about the drug interactions that can affect warfarin therapy; and (4) there are financial and social resources available for meticulously monitoring the prothrombin time ratio. In general, for most purposes (except an actively propagating thrombus), the prothrombin time ratio can be kept near 1.7.

M.J. Cline, M.D.

A Distinct Coagulopathy Associated With Interleukin-2 Therapy

Oleksowicz L, Strack M, Dutcher JP, Sussman I, Caliendo G, Sparano J, Wiernik PH (Albert Einstein Cancer Ctr, Bronx, NY; Montefiore Med Ctr, Bronx, NY)

Br J Haematol 88:892–894, 1994 119-96-26–12

Background.—Although high doses of interleukin-2 (IL-2) have been shown to have significant antineoplastic activity in patients with melanomas and renal cell carcinoma, such therapy is associated with considerable toxicity, including coagulopathy. Coagulation factor assays were performed on blood samples obtained from patients before and after IL-2 treatment to help further characterize this coagulopathy.

Patients and Methods.—Fourteen patients with advanced metastatic cancer were included. Peripheral venous blood specimens were obtained before the initiation of IL-2 treatment, 6 hours after the last dose of IL-2 was administered, and 2–3 days after IL-2 was discontinued. Pretreatment coagulation profiles were analyzed and compared with values obtained after treatment.

Results.—A significant 43% increase in mean partial thromboplastin time (PTT) was noted 6 hours after administration of IL-2 treatment, as were significant decreases in functional levels of factors II, IX, X, XI, and XII. No significant changes in mean prothrombin time (PT) or in the functional activity of factors V, VII, and VIII were observed with IL-2 treatment. Coagulation profiles returned to normal 2–3 days after IL-2 was discontinued. No evident bleeding was observed during IL-2 administration, and there were no associations between the degree of coagulopathy and clinical response or severity of coagulopathy and dose of IL-2 or interferon.

Conclusions.—Patients undergoing treatment with IL-2 show a distinct transient and mild coagulopathy, which is not associated with bleeding. Despite the fact that reduced activities of the intrinsic coagulation proteins IX, X, XI, and XII and PTT characterize this coagulopathy, it is not entirely explained by DIC or fibrinolysis.

► Interleukin-2 (IL-2) occupies a minor place in the therapeutic armamentarium and is sometimes used in the treatment of renal cancer and melanoma. Treatment with IL-2 is associated with multiple side effects, some of which can be life-threatening. These include hypotension, hepatic dysfunction, oliguria, and edema resulting from capillary leak. The authors of this article observed abnormalities of the activated PTT or PT in 75 of 100 patients treated with IL-2. Although the coagulopathy with IL-2 is relatively mild and resolves within a few days of stopping treatment, one should be aware of this phenomenon if one uses this cytokine to treat patients.

M.J. Cline, M.D.

A Comparison of Six Weeks With Six Months of Oral Anticoagulant Therapy After a First Episode of Venous Thromboembolism

Schulman S, Rhedin A-S, Lindmarker P, Carlsson A, Lärfars G, Nicol P, Loogna E, Svensson E, Ljungberg B, Walter H, Viering S, Nordlander S, Leijd B, Jönsson K-Å, Hjorth M, Linder O, Boberg J, and the Duration of Anticoagulation Trial Study Group (Karolinska Hosp, Stockholm; Huddinge Hosp, Sweden; Danderyd Hosp, Sweden; et al)

N Engl J Med 332:1661–1665, 1995 119-96-26–13

Background.—Prophylactic oral anticoagulants are given routinely to patients with deep-vein thrombosis or pulmonary embolism to prevent recurrence. However, the optimal duration of anticoagulant therapy has been debated. The efficacy of 6 weeks of therapy was compared with that of 6 months of therapy in preventing recurrence, hemorrhagic complications, and death in patients after a first episode of deep-vein thrombosis or pulmonary embolism.

Methods.—Consecutive patients who were at least 15 years old, with a diagnosed first episode of either pulmonary embolism or deep-vein thrombosis, were randomly assigned to receive oral anticoagulation therapy for either 6 weeks or 6 months after prothrombin times were stable within the target range (international normalized ratio of 2.0 to 2.85). The patients were followed for 2 years to determine the incidence of recurrent venous thromboembolism, major hemorrhage, and death in each treatment group.

Results.—Of the 897 patients enrolled, 443 were assigned to receive 6 weeks of therapy, and 454 were assigned to receive 6 months of therapy. There were major hemorrhages in 1 patient in the 6-week group and in 5 patients in the 6-month group; none were fatal. Three of these patients were receiving anticoagulant doses exceeding the target range. Twenty-two patients in the 6-week group and 17 patients in the 6-month group died during the 2-year study period. There were 123 episodes of recurrent venous thromboembolism, with a significantly higher incidence in the 6-week than in the 6-month group (18.1% vs. 9.5%). The incidence of recurrence was sharply increased immediately after anticoagulant therapy was discontinued in the 6-week group.

Conclusions.—The risk of recurrent thromboembolism was reduced significantly by increasing the duration of oral anticoagulant therapy from 6 weeks to 6 months, which supports the use of at least 6 months of anticoagulant therapy after an initial thromboembolic episode. However, the monthly incidence of recurrent thromboembolism was comparable in the 2 groups after 6 months, suggesting that venous thromboembolism is an ongoing condition with a persistent risk of recurrence.

▶ This important study of more than 900 patients with venous thromboembolism addresses the question of the optimal duration of oral anticoagulant therapy. The results are clear-cut and provide a useful guideline for physicians treating this common disorder: *6 months is better than 6 weeks.*

M.J. Cline, M.D.

27 Leukemia

Treatment of Adult T-Cell Leukemia-Lymphoma With a Combination of Interferon Alfa and Zidovudine

Gill PS, Harrington W Jr, Kaplan MH, Ribeiro RC, Bennett JM, Liebman HA, Bernstein-Singer M, Espina BM, Cabral L, Allen S, Kornblau S, Pike MC, Levine AM (Univ of Southern California, Los Angeles; Univ of Miami, Fla; North Shore Univ Hosp, Manhasset, NY; et al)

N Engl J Med 332:1744–1748, 1995 119-96-27–1

Introduction.—Adult T-cell leukemia-lymphoma is a heterogeneous disease; in the acute and lymphomatous forms, it resists cytotoxic chemotherapy, and it has a survival rate of 3.7–6 months. New treatments are needed for this disease. In 1 patient who was co-infected with HIV type 1, human T-cell lymphotropic virus type I (HTLV-1), and adult T-cell leukemia-lymphoma, the combination of zidovudine and interferon-α induced a rapid and durable response. The efficacy of zidovudine and interferon-α was evaluated in adult T-cell leukemia-lymphoma.

Methods.—Oral zidovudine (200 mg given 5 times daily) and interferon-α (Intron A, 5 million to 10 million units given subcutaneously each day) were administered to 19 patients (12 female and 7 male patients; median age, 48 years) with acute or lymphomatous forms of adult T-cell leukemia-lymphoma, 7 of whom had a relapse after multiagent cytotoxic chemotherapy or failed to respond to cytotoxic chemotherapy. Resolution of all malignant disease for 4 weeks or more was considered a complete response.

Results.—In 58% of patients (11 of 19), major responses were achieved; 26% had complete remission (5 of 19). In the group of 7 patients who had failed cytotoxic therapy, 4 had major responses, 2 of which were complete remissions. Two of 5 patients with complete responses had HIV-1 infection. Six patients with complete or partial response survived more than 1 year. Since the discontinuation of treatment, the longest remission has lasted more than 59 months. Toxic effects included grade 4 neutropenia in 5 patients, low-grade fever in 8, fatigue in 7, diarrhea in 2, and nausea in 3 patients.

Conclusion.—Even in patients in whom prior cytotoxic therapy has failed, the combination of zidovudine and interferon alfa has activity against adult T-cell leukemia-lymphoma. For its role in the treatment of adult T-cell lymphoma, this regimen should be further evaluated to determine optimum uses for the combination and their precise mechanism.

▶ Adult T-cell leukemia-lymphoma is the only human leukemia that is known to be consistently associated with a retroviral infection. Human T-cell lymphotropic virus type I is the etiologic agent. Infection is endemic in parts of Japan and the Caribbean basin, and cases have been described in other parts of the world, including the United States. The disease is known to be transmissible by infected blood products and may be transmitted by mother's milk.

Adult T-cell leukemia-lymphoma is an interesting disease with a long natural history. It may remain asymptomatic or display only a blood lymphocytosis for many years. Infection with virus may occur in infancy, but clinical manifestations may not occur for 30 or more years. The HTLV-I can also cause a multiple sclerosis–like picture, usually after a shorter latent period than that of the leukemia.

Cellular immunodeficiency may lead to opportunistic infections. Leukemia/lymphoma develops in less than 5% of individuals infected with HTLV-I. It is often a chronic indolent disease, but an acute phase may develop with skin, visceral, and bone involvement and hypercalcemia. The acute phase generally has a poor response to the multiagent chemotherapy programs used in other leukemias, and survival in this phase is often 6 months or less.

A few years ago, some of the authors treated a patient with adult T-cell leukemia-lymphoma who was co-infected with HTLV-I and HIV. They used a combination of interferon-α and zidovudine and observed a good response. They then extended their trial to 19 other patients with adult T-cell leukemia-lymphoma and observed that 5 achieved a complete remission of disease, which was, in some cases, prolonged. This is a gratifying, if surprising, result.

M.J. Cline, M.D.

2-Chlorodeoxyadenosine Activity in Patients With Untreated Chronic Lymphocytic Leukemia

Saven A, Lemon RH, Kosty M, Beutler E, Piro LD (Ida M and Cecil H Green Cancer Ctr, Scripps Clinic and Research Found, La Jolla, Calif)
J Clin Oncol 13:570–574, 1995 119-96-27-2

Introduction.—Chronic lymphocytic leukemia (CLL) is caused by clonal proliferation of B lymphocytes. The purine analogue 2-chlorodeoxyadenosine (2-CdA) has activity in patients with CLL who do not respond to alkylator therapy. A phase II trial of 2-CdA was conducted in 20 patients with previously untreated CLL.

Methods.—All patients received 2-CdA, 0.1 mg/kg/day, in a 7-day continuous IV infusion every 4–5 weeks. Treatment continued until the maximum response was achieved or until prohibitive toxicity occurred.

Results.—The median number of courses administered was 4. The complete response rate was 25% and the partial response rate was 60%, for an overall response rate of 85%. The responses lasted for a median of more than 8 months. The main form of toxicity was myelosuppression. Grade III or IV thrombocytopenia occurred in 20% of patients. Opportunistic infections developed a median of 19 months after cessation of 2-CdA therapy in 3 patients, all of whom received corticosteroids.

Conclusions.—Major activity of 2-CdA occurs in patients with previously untreated CLL. Response rates are lower in previously treated patients, perhaps partly because of poor marrow reserve related to prior therapy. Randomized studies are needed to compare the efficacy of 2-CdA, fludarabine, and chlorambucil in the treatment of CLL.

► For many years, an alkylating agent such as chlorambucil combined with intermittent prednisone was the standard treatment for CLL. This therapy frequently causes some regression of disease but rarely produces a complete hematologic remission. This treatment controls disease manifestations in most patients for a certain period and probably, but not certainly, contributes to longer survival.

In the past few years, other agents have appeared that are cytotoxic for the mature B cells that constitute the malignant population in CLL, notably, the nucleotide analogues, 2-CdA and fludarabine. It has previously been demonstrated that CLL that is resistant to alkylating agents will often respond to treatment with 2-CdA. Now, this study examines 2-CdA used as first-line therapy in previously untreated patients with CLL. The complete response rate was 25%, and the partial response rate was 60%, which is quite satisfactory. However, the myelosuppression was greater than that usually encountered with conventional alkylating agent therapy. There is no evidence yet that 2-CdA constitutes superior treatment and randomized studies are needed to decide which is the best therapy.

M.J. Cline, M.D.

The Immunological Profile of B-Cell Disorders and Proposal of a Scoring System for the Diagnosis of CLL

Matutes E, Owusu-Ankomah K, Morilla R, Marco JG, Houlihan A, Que TH, Catovsky D (Royal Marsden Hosp, London; Inst of Cancer Research, London)

Leukemia 8:1640–1645, 1994 119-96-27-3

Introduction.—Cell morphologic features and immunologic markers are the basis for the characterization of the chronic lymphoid leukemias. Some overlap in marker expression has been found among the various B-cell diseases and disorders other than chronic lymphocytic leukemia (CLL), such as mantle-cell non-Hodgkin's lymphoma. By examining circulating cells from a large group of patients, the ability of immunologic markers to distinguish among the various B-cell lymphoproliferative disorders involved with leukemia was examined.

Methods.—Flow cytometry was used to analyze circulating cells from 666 patients with a panel of markers. Chronic lymphocytic leukemia was found in 400 patients; 100 had splenic lymphoma with villous lymphocytes; 40 had hairy-cell leukemia; 26 had follicular lymphoma; 25 had lymphoplasmacytic lymphoma; 22 had prolymphocytic leukemia; 20 had mantle-cell lymphoma; 18 had large-cell lymphoma; and 15 had a hairy-cell leukemia variant. A scoring system was based on the reactivity of the monoclonal antibodies CD5, CD23, and FMC7 and the intensity of expression of CD22 and membrane immunoglobulins to provide evidence that this scoring system can clearly distinguish between CLL and other B-cell diseases. These 5 markers were given a value of 1 or 0 according to whether they are typical or atypical for CLL. Scores range from 0 (atypical for CLL) to 5 (typical for CLL).

Results.—After the scoring system was applied to all of the cases, 87% of markers for CLL scored 5 and 4, whereas 0.4% of markers scored 0 or 1; 89% of markers for other B-cell leukemias scored 0 or 1 and 72% of markers for lymphomas scored 0 or 1. In the B-cell leukemia group, there was 1 score of 4 but no scores of 5.

Conclusion.—No differences were seen between CLL with high and low scores; however, higher scores were seen in patients with more typical morphologic features. No single marker distinguished CLL from other diseases, but the most reliable were FMC7 and surface immunoglobulin intensity. Application of a combination of membrane markers can help distinguish CLL from other B-cell malignancies. The classification and diagnosis of B-cell lymphoproliferative disorders can be facilitated by the proposed score.

► This is a valiant effort to categorize the chronic B-cell lymphoproliferative disorders on a rational basis using B-cell markers as the discriminating parameters. More than 600 patients with various disorders and 5 markers were studied. Unfortunately, lymphocyte biology is quite complex, and there was considerable overlap between CLL and other lymphoproliferative disorders, such as the leukemic phase of some B-cell lymphomas. Apparently, one must still review the clinical picture and look at the blood smear under the microscope in assessing B-cell malignancies.

Sometimes a marker profile is useful in distinguishing atypical CLL. The common markers for CLL are CD5+, CD23+, and low-density surface immunoglobulin. However, no single marker can distinguish CLL from other B-cell lymphoproliferative diseases.

M.J. Cline, M.D.

Improved Survival for Patients With Acute Myelogenous Leukemia

Mitus AJ, Miller KB, Schenkein DP, Ryan HF, Parsons SK, Wheeler C, Antin JH (Brigham and Women's Hosp, Boston; Beth Israel Hosp, Boston; Children's Hosp, Boston)

J Clin Oncol 13:560–569, 1995 119-96-27-4

Objective.—Despite advances in chemotherapy and supportive care, overall survival for patients with acute myelogenous leukemia (AML) is still poor. Cure rates are no higher than 25% to 30%. A multicenter trial designed to improve survival in patients with AML by improving the induction and consolidation phases of therapy was initiated in 1987. The results in 94 patients were evaluated.

Methods.—In an attempt to increase remission rate, the standard 3+7 days chemotherapy protocol of daunorubicin and cytarabine was modified with the addition of high-dose cytarabine on days 8 through 10 to create a 3+7+3 regimen. Toward decreasing the rate of leukemic relapse, all patients who entered complete remission were offered allogeneic or autologous bone marrow transplantation (BMT). Ninety-four patients were enrolled from 1987 to 1993; the results were analyzed by intention to treat.

Results.—The complete response rate was 89%. The remission rate was so high that previously identified outcome predictors—including cytogenetic findings, white blood cell count, French-American-British classification, age, and sex—were not prognostically useful. Five-year survival was 55% overall. Bone marrow transplantation was performed in 60% of all patients who had complete remission. Five-year event-free survival was 56% in patients receiving allogeneic BMT and 45% in those receiving autologous BMT, a nonsignificant difference.

Conclusions.—This new approach to therapy for AML—using a 3+7+3 chemotherapy regimen to increase remission rate and BMT to decrease the rate of leukemic relapse—yields excellent long-term disease-free survival. The improvement over historical data probably results from the very high rate of induced remission and the effectiveness of consolidation therapy. This new approach offers the possibility of cure to many patients with AML.

▶ This paper describes an apparently minor modification of the standard treatment program for adults with AML, which may result in improved survival. Three days of high doses of cytarabine were added to the standard induction program. The complete remission rate was 89% in a patient population that does not seem to be unusual. This is considerably higher than the rate of approximately 70% observed in most series. The patients were then treated with between 1 and 3 cycles of "consolidation" chemotherapy, followed by either allogeneic or autologous bone marrow transplantation. The results are a very impressive 55% 5-year survival of the entire cohort of 94 patients. As I review 15 years of YEAR BOOKS, it seems clear that we make slow but steady progress against AML.

M.J. Cline, M.D.

Timed Sequential Chemotherapy for Previously Treated Patients With Acute Myeloid Leukemia: Long-Term Follow-Up of the Etoposide, Mitoxantrone, and Cytarabine–86 Trial

Archimbaud E, Thomas X, Leblond V, Michallet M, Fenaux P, Cordonnier C, Dreyfus F, Troussard X, Jaubert J, Travade P, Troncy J, Assouline D, Fiere D (Hôpital Edouard Herriot, Lyon, France; Hôpital André Michallon, Grenoble, France; Hôpital Claude Huriez, Lille, France; et al)

J Clin Oncol 13:11–18, 1995 119-96-27–5

Background.—Timed sequential chemotherapy is intended to maximize the number of leukemic cells killed by cytotoxic drugs by recruiting cells initially and administering a second sequence of cycle-active drugs when cell numbers peak. This has proved to be effective as first-line treatment of acute myeloid leukemia (AML) and, also, in patients who have a relapse after conventional chemotherapy.

Objective.—A timed sequential chemotherapy regimen of mitoxantrone, etoposide, and cytarabine was evaluated in 133 patients with AML, 111 in relapse and 22 who had failed to respond to previous chemotherapy. All but 2 patients had a World Health Organization performance status of 2 or less at the outset.

Management.—Mitoxantrone was given on days 1–3, etoposide on days 8–10, and cytarabine at both intervals. A second course of induction therapy was allowed if there was no complete remission. Some patients received maintenance treatment with reduced drug doses for 6 months. The median follow-up was 40 months.

Results.—Complete remission was achieved in 60% of patients and in 76% of those who were in first relapse of AML. Twenty-nine percent of patients failed to respond to treatment. The projected 5-year disease-free survival rates for patients younger than 60 years of age who achieved a complete response ranged from 20% to 46%. Previous resistance to treatment was the most prominent adverse prognostic factor for both complete response and survival. Eleven percent of the patients died of toxic drug effects. More than half the patients became septic.

Conclusion.—Approximately 1 in 5 patients with treatment-resistant or relapsed AML can expect prolonged disease-free survival after receiving timed sequential chemotherapy.

► The management of patients with AML whose disease relapses or fails to respond to initial therapy has always been extremely difficult. If an HLA-matched sibling is available, bone marrow transplantation has usually been considered a reasonable option in patients younger than 60 years of age. However, because most patients do not have such a sibling, there has been a steady search since the early 1970s for effective second-line chemotherapy programs that will induce remissions and prolong disease-free survival.

The 3-drug combination reported in this article appears to be an unusually effective "salvage" program, although its effectiveness extracts a high price in toxicity, with 11% of patients dying of drug-related side effects. If one pays this price, it is reported that a remarkable 60% of patients achieve a complete hematologic remission. Most of these remissions are of relatively short duration, but about 1 in 10 patients who has a remission is still alive at 5 years. In other words, of every 100 patients with refractory disease, 6 will have prolonged survival with this program without bone marrow transplantation.

M.J. Cline, M.D.

Autologous or Allogeneic Bone Marrow Transplantation Compared With Intensive Chemotherapy in Acute Myelogenous Leukemia

Zittoun RA, for the European Organization for Research and Treatment of Cancer (EORTC) and the Gruppo Italiano Malattie Ematologiche Maligne Dell'Adulto (GIMEMA) Leukemia Cooperative Groups (Hôtel-Dieu, Paris)

N Engl J Med 332:217–223, 1995 119-96-27-6

Background.—The majority of patients with primary acute myelogenous leukemia who enter complete remission after induction therapy relapse in spite of various types of maintenance chemotherapy. In adult patients younger than 60 years, treatment after initial induction of remission has been intensified. More and more patients in complete remission are treated with allogeneic or autologous bone marrow transplantation. Results of bone marrow transplantation are often from single institutions or registries and may carry a selection bias. In a prospective trial, disease-free survival and overall survival were examined after 3 postremission treatments.

Methods.—Patients with untreated acute myelogenous leukemia underwent induction treatment with daunorubicin (45 mg/m^2 of body surface area) and cytarabine (200 mg/m^2). Those in a complete remission received intensive consolidation chemotherapy of intermediate-dose cytarabine (1,000 mg/m^2) and amsacrine (120 mg/m^2). Patients with an HLA-identical sibling underwent allogeneic bone marrow transplantation; the others randomly underwent autologous bone marrow transplantation with unpurged bone marrow, or a second course of intensive chemotherapy of high-dose cytarabine (2 g/m^2) and daunorubicin (45 mg/m^2). Comparisons were made on the basis of intention to treat.

Results.—The median follow-up was 3.3 years. A complete remission was achieved in 623 patients; 576 of these had received the first course of intensive consolidation chemotherapy. Of the 623 in a complete remission, 168 were assigned to allogeneic bone marrow transplantation, and 254 were randomly assigned to the other 2 groups. Of the 623 patients, 343 completed the treatment assignment. The relapse rate was the highest in the group receiving intensive chemotherapy; it was the lowest in the group receiving allogeneic transplantation. The mortality rate was the highest in the group receiving allogeneic transplantation and the lowest in the group receiving intensive chemotherapy. Adverse prognostic factors were: French-American-British class other than M2 or M3, longer interval from diagnosis to complete remission, need for more than 1 course of induction chemotherapy to achieve a complete remission, poor or intermediate prognosis according to cytogenetic classification of Keating et al., a high white blood cell count, and increased serum lactate dehydrogenase concentration. The projected rates of disease-free survival at 4 years were 55% for allogeneic transplantation, 48% for autologous transplantation, and 30% for intensive chemotherapy (Fig 2). After complete remission, overall survival was similar for the 3 groups because more patients who had relapse after a second course of intensive chemotherapy responded to subsequent autologous bone marrow transplantation. Hematopoietic recovery occurred later after autologous transplantation, and the duration of hospitalization was longer with bone marrow transplantation.

Conclusions.—Autologous and allogeneic bone marrow transplantation result in better disease-free survival than does intensive consolidation chemotherapy with cytarabine and daunorubicin during a first complete remission in acute myelogenous leukemia. Transplantation immediately after a relapse or during a second complete remission might also yield good results. Other prospective studies have reported different regimens of intensive consolidation chemotherapy to be superior to conventional regimens or equivalent to bone marrow transplantation.

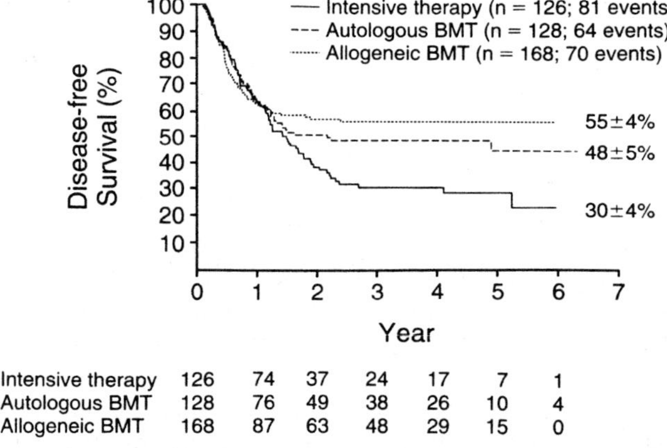

Intensive therapy	126	74	37	24	17	7	1
Autologous BMT	128	76	49	38	26	10	4
Allogeneic BMT	168	87	63	48	29	15	0

FIGURE 2.—Kaplan-Meier plots of disease-free survival, according to whether patients were assigned to autologous or allogeneic bone marrow transplantation (*BMT*) or a second course of intensive consolidation therapy. The number of patients at risk is shown below each time point. Plus-minus values are the projected disease-free survival rates (± standard error) at 4 years. The events considered were relapse or death during a first complete remission. (Reprinted by permission of *The New England Journal of Medicine,* Zittoun RA, for the European Organization for Research and Treatment of Cancer (EORTC) and the Gruppo Italiano Malattie Ematologiche Maligne Dell'Adulto (GIMEMA) Leukemia Cooperative Groups: Autologous or allogeneic bone marrow transplantation compared with intensive chemotherapy in acute myelogenous leukemia. *N Engl J Med* 332:217–223, Copyright 1995, Massachusetts Medical Society.)

► Whether bone marrow transplantation, either allogeneic or autologous, is superior to chemotherapy alone in the treatment of leukemia is of perennial interest to hematologists and others who treat patients with leukemia. This is a well-organized study comparing the rates of survival and leukemia-free survival in 3 treatment groups of patients with acute myeloid leukemia. Only patients younger than 60 years of age were included.

As anticipated, the results were better for allogeneic bone marrow transplantation than for conventional intensive chemotherapy: 55% vs. 30% disease-free survival at 4 years. The results for autologous bone marrow transplantation were also surprisingly good: 48% at 4 years. In view of these and related data reviewed in previous YEAR BOOKS, how should one manage the patient younger than 60 years who has acute myeloid leukemia? My suggestion is as follows: after remission induction and consolidation, use allogeneic bone marrow transplantation if an HLA-matched sibling is available. If no sibling is available, the patient's bone marrow or peripheral blood stem cells should be cryopreserved and stored against future need. The patient can then be carefully followed. Should disease recur, then autologous bone marrow transplantation can be undertaken.

M.J. Cline, M.D.

Acute Lymphocytic Leukemia in Adults: A Retrospective Study and Analysis of Current Management Options

Ho TC, Tefferi A, Su JQ, Litzow MR, Hoagland HC, Noël P (Mayo Clinic Rochester, Minn; Mayo Clinic Scottsdale, Ariz)

Mayo Clin Proc 69:937–948, 1994 119-96-27-7

Introduction.—Advances in chemotherapy for acute lymphocytic leukemia (ALL) have improved long-term disease-free survival in children to greater than 70%, whereas in adults this figure is less than 40%. Reproducible prognostic factors have been identified to allow appropriate risk stratification and risk-adjusted management in children; it remains to be seen whether a similar approach will improve outcome in adults. There is currently no standard treatment for adult ALL. A treatment experience with 90 adult patients with ALL was reviewed to assess the current therapeutic options, analyze the prognostic variables, and make treatment recommendations.

Patients and Outcomes.—Ninety of 384 patients with ALL treated from 1982 to 1992 were older than 15 years of age. Induction chemotherapy was used in 80 patients, most with Adriamycin or daunorubicin in combination with vincristine and prednisone. Long-term survival was 25% overall. There were 10 patients younger than 18 years of age, none of whom underwent bone marrow transplantation (BMT); long-term survival in this group was 80%. A complete remission (CR) was achieved with induction chemothcrapy in 42 of the 70 patients aged 18 years or older. Thirty-one of those 42 did not receive BMT, and their long-term survival was less than 13%. Survival was 100% when BMT was performed during a first CR, 50% when BMT was done during a later CR, and 17% when BMT was done in patients not in CR. Patients undergoing chemotherapy were older than those undergoing BMT, 50 vs. 34 years; age was the only significant prognostic factor overall.

Conclusions.—With current chemotherapeutic regimens, the outcome of ALL in adult patients remains dismal. The results improve significantly for patients younger than 18 years and for those who receive BMT after CR. Current issues regarding management for adult ALL cannot be resolved by any available information. The only way to determine the best therapy for these patients is to enter them in comparative trials.

► Although this paper presents little new data, it does provide a good discussion of the options for treatment of adults with ALL.

The effect of age on prognosis in this disease is well known. Response to treatment and survival is much better in children than in those older than 18 years.

The options for treating adult ALL are: (1) multiagent chemotherapy; (2) allogeneic bone marrow transplantation if an HLA-matched sibling donor is available; and (3) intensive chemotherapy followed by autologous bone marrow transplantation.

As the authors of this article point out, long-term survival with chemotherapy alone is approximately 10% in this series and approximately 25% in other series. The results are somewhat better with allogeneic bone marrow transplantation, with survival data varying between 40% and 60%. As noted, if allogeneic bone marrow transplantation is to be undertaken, it is best done early in disease—preferably in the first complete remission of disease.

The usefulness of autologous bone marrow transplantation in this disease is still unknown and is being investigated in many studies. For the moment, this approach is best reserved for patients willing to participate in protocol studies.

It should be noted that this analysis applies to adults in the age range of 18–60 years. Older patients do not do as well with intensive chemotherapy or allogeneic bone marrow transplantation. They have a higher incidence of serious graft-vs.-host disease and complications of therapy. More conservative therapeutic approaches are often used in the elderly.

M.J. Cline, M.D.

Low Doses of Interferon-α Are as Effective as Higher Doses in Inducing Remissions and Prolonging Survival in Chronic Myeloid Leukemia

Schofield JR, Robinson WA, Murphy JR, Rovira DK (Univ of Colorado, Denver)

Ann Intern Med 121:736–744, 1994 119-96-27-8

Background.—Recombinant human interferon-α is the treatment of choice for most patients with chronic myeloid leukemia. Although high doses of this agent are generally used, these are associated with significant toxicity. Low-dose interferon-α was thus investigated in patients with chronic myeloid leukemia to determine its effect on remission status, prolonged survival, and toxicity.

Patients and Methods.—Forty-one patients with newly diagnosed or previously treated chronic-phase, Philadelphia chromosome-positive chronic myeloid leukemia were included. Therapy consisted of daily interferon-α at a dose of 2×10^6 units/m^2 of body surface area for 28 days and then 3 times per week. Hematologic remission and toxicity were evaluated monthly via complete blood counts and physical examination. Bone marrow cytogenetic analyses were undertaken every 6 months to assess karyotypic response in patients with complete hematologic remission. The survival curves and median survival values were also determined. Results were compared with those of historical controls and other series in which higher doses of interferon-α were used.

Results.—Within 12 months of diagnosis, 70% of the patients had achieved a complete hematologic response, with 22% of those showing a major or complete karyotypic response. The Kaplan-Meier estimated 5-year survival rate was 73%. The approximate annual cost of low-dose interferon-α was $5,953, compared with a median of $24,375 for higher doses used by other investigators. Less toxicity was also noted with low-dose treatment.

Conclusions.—Similar patient populations receiving higher doses of interferon-α have reportedly achieved complete hematologic remission rates of 50% to 70%, major and complete karyotypic response rates of 16% to 29%, and survival rates comparable to those obtained in this study. Low-dose treatment is thus as effective as higher-dose interferon-α in inducing remissions and prolonging survival in patients with chronic myeloid leukemia and is also associated with less expense and toxicity.

► This study compares low-dose and high-dose interferon-α in patients with chronic myeloid leukemia (CML). By using historical controls the authors conclude that low-dose therapy is just as effective, has less toxicity, and costs less (approximately $6,000 vs. $24,000 for a year of treatment).

Although the authors state that "for now recombinant human interferon-α remains the treatment of choice for most patients [with CML]," I am not certain that their data support this contention. The presumed advantage of interferon therapy of CML over treatment with busulfan or hydroxyurea is that interferon can induce complete remissions with return of the marrow karyotype to normal. Such a reversion is usually associated with prolonged remission of disease. However, in this series of 41 patients treated with interferon, 70% achieved a hematologic remission—a result no better than that achieved with chemotherapy—and only 3 of the 41 achieved a complete karyotypic remission (7% of the series). The authors suggest that patients started on interferon early in the disease do better.

In view of the greater cost and toxicity of interferon relative to treatment with hydroxyurea therapy, we clearly need a side-by-side comparison of the 2 therapies in CML to reach a conclusion about best therapy. For the moment, allogeneic bone marrow transplantation remains the treatment of choice in patients younger than 60 years who have an HLA-matched sibling donor.

M.J. Cline, M.D.

Prolonged Administration of Interferon-α in Patients With Chronic-Phase Philadelphia Chromosome-Positive Chronic Myelogenous Leukemia Before Allogeneic Bone Marrow Transplantation

Beelen DW, Graeven U, Elmaagacli AH, Niederle N, Kloke O, Opalka B, Schaefer UW (Univ Hosp of Essen, Germany)

Blood 85:2981–2990, 1995 119-96-27–9

Introduction.—In the treatment of chronic myelogenous leukemia, recombinant or partially pure human leukocyte interferon-α has shown promising activity. The only established treatment with a high potential of eradicating the disease is allogeneic bone marrow transplantation in patients with suitable family marrow donors. A variety of prognostic factors have influenced the outcome of allogeneic bone marrow transplantation in patients with chronic myelogenous leukemia, including administration of interferon-α, which may inhibit hematopoietic cell and marrow fibroblast growth, enhance expression of major histocompatibility antigens, and increase the activity of lymphocytes mediating antigen-specific and nonspecific cytotoxicity. The influence of pretransplant cytoreductive agents, particularly interferon-α, was evaluated to determine the outcome of allogeneic bone marrow transplant in patients with chronic phase Ph^1-chromosome-positive chronic myelogenous leukemia.

Methods.—The influence of interferon-α was studied in 133 patients with chronic myelogenous leukemia: 103 received marrow grafts from HLA-identical family donors and 30 received marrow grafts from alternative donors. Interferon-α was previously administered to 50 (39%) patients for a median duration of 14 months, or a range of 1 to 61 months. Hydroxyurea and/or busulfan therapy was previously given to 83 patients (62%) for a median of 15 months before the transplant.

Results.—Administration of interferon-α for longer than 12 months was identified as the only significant pretransplant therapy-related predictor of transplant outcome using proportional hazards regression analysis. Compared with other pretransplant therapy, the adjusted risk ratio of transplant-related mortality was 2.5 times higher with interferon-α, which was attributed to a 3.1-fold higher risk ratio of fatal posttransplant infections after treatment with interferon-α for longer than 12 months before the transplant. Patients with alternative donors had marrow graft failure (7 of 30, or 23%), and this was further restricted to those patients who had been previously administered interferon-α. In the alternate donor group, the probability of graft failure was 49% ± 28% in 17 patients given interferon-α compared with 0% for the other 13 patients. In the alternate donor group with previous interferon-α treatment, a significant delay was seen in neutrophil and platelet count reconstitution.

Conclusion.—In patients with chronic-phase Philadelphia chromosome-positive chronic myelogenous leukemia, prolonged treatment with interferon-α before bone marrow transplant is strongly associated with an increased risk of fatal transplant-related complications and an inferior outcome. The impact of treatment duration of cumulative doses of interferon-α or other cytoreductive agents given to patients with chronic-phase chronic myelogenous leukemia before transplant should be analyzed in the future.

► The previous study (Abstract 119-96-27–8) examined low- vs. high-dose recombinant interferon-α in patients with chronic myelocytic leukemia. In my comments on that article, I expressed the reservation that it was not yet proven that interferon was necessarily superior to conventional single-agent chemotherapy in this disease. In this article, the authors examined the effects of prior prolonged interferon treatment on the subsequent outcome with bone marrow transplantation in chronic myelocytic leukemia. Remember, bone marrow transplantation is the treatment of choice in patients younger than 60 years of age with an HLA-matched sibling donor.

The authors report an effect of interferon on the outcome of bone marrow transplantation that is considerably more dramatic than I might have anticipated. Interferon had a significant adverse effect with a 2.5 times higher mortality. This was ascribed to the effects of myelosuppression and of graft failure.

One should be wary of using interferon therapy in chronic myelocytic leukemia if one anticipates the possible use of subsequent bone marrow transplantation.

M.J. Cline, M.D.

28 Lymphoma and Myeloma

Comparison of CHOP Chemotherapy With Autologous Bone Marrow Transplantation for Slowly Responding Patients With Aggressive Non-Hodgkin's Lymphoma

Verdonck LF, van Putten WLJ, Hagenbeek A, Schouten HC, Sonneveld P, Van Imhoff GW, Kluin-Nelemans HC, Raemaekers JMM, van Oers RHJ, Haak HL, Schots R, Dekker AW, deGast GC, Löwenberg B (Univ Hosp, Utrecht, The Netherlands; Dr Daniel denHoed Cancer Ctr, Rotterdam; Univ Hosp, Maastricht, The Netherlands; et al)

N Engl J Med 332:1045–1051, 1995 119-96-28–1

Background.—It has been suggested that patients with disseminated, aggressive non-Hodgkin's lymphoma who have complete remission after first-line chemotherapy are more likely to be cured than patients who respond more slowly. The efficacy of high-dose marrow-ablative therapy with autologous bone marrow transplantation in patients with disseminated, aggressive non-Hodgkin's lymphoma who respond slowly to chemotherapy has been assessed since 1987. In patients with slow responses to chemotherapy, the benefits of continued chemotherapy, or high-dose chemoradiotherapy and autologous bone marrow transplantation, were compared prospectively in a multicenter study.

Methods.—Patients who had a slow response to 3 courses of cyclophosphamide, doxorubicin, vincristine, and prednisone (CHOP) were randomly assigned to undergo either another 5 courses of CHOP or high-dose chemoradiotherapy and autologous bone marrow transplantation.

Results.—Of 286 patients who received 3 courses of CHOP, 38% had fast responses and 47% had slow responses: there was no response in 15%. A total of 69 patients with slow responses to 3 courses of CHOP and lymphoma-negative marrow were randomly assigned to either continued therapy with CHOP or transplantation. Complete remission was achieved in 74% of patients who continued therapy with CHOP and 68% of those who underwent transplantation. In patients who continued therapy with CHOP, overall survival was 85%, disease-free survival was 72%, and event-free survival was 53% at 4 years. In patients who underwent transplantation, overall survival was 56%, disease-free survival was 60%, and event-free survival was 41% at 4 years. The disease-free survival rate of patients with fast responses to CHOP who were not randomized was 54% at 4 years.

Conclusions.—There was no significant benefit from early marrow-ablative chemoradiotherapy with autologous bone marrow transplantation in patients with disseminated, aggressive non-Hodgkin's lymphoma with slow responses to first-line chemotherapy. There appears to be no prognostic value to the rate at which complete remission occurs.

▶ This is an important article in that it provides some clear guidelines for the management of "aggressive" non-Hodgkin's lymphoma. In general, these high-grade lymphomas have a more aggressive natural history than low-grade lymphomas, but they are more apt to remit and be cured by modern therapy programs.

Several points may be taken from this study: First, the disease-free survival rate (which is a reasonable approximation of the cure rate in this disease) with conventional chemotherapy at 4 years was about 50%. Second, there was no benefit from early autologous bone marrow transplantation in patients who had a slow response to chemotherapy. Third, unlike in acute leukemia, there appears to be no prognostic value in the rate at which the disease responds to therapy. Finally, the results with CHOP chemotherapy are generally as good as those achieved with much more aggressive programs—a point that has previously been made in the 1994 and 1995 editions of the YEAR BOOK OF MEDICINE.

M.J. Cline, M.D.

AIDS-Related Burkitt's Lymphoma: Morphologic and Immunophenotypic Study of Biopsy Specimens

Carbone A, Gloghini A, Gaidano G, Cilia AM, Bassi P, Polito P, Vaccher E, Saglio G, Tirelli U (Istituto Nazionale di Ricovero e Cura a Carattere Scientifico, Aviano, Italy; Università di Torino, Italy; Centro Regionale di Riferimento Oncologico, Aviano, Italy)

Am J Clin Pathol 103:561–567, 1995 119-96-28–2

Introduction.—A special committee of the World Health Organization determined that Burkitt's tumor was a distinct pathologic entity different from other poorly differentiated lymphomas. The tumor was to be called "malignant lymphoma, undifferentiated, Burkitt's type." This lymphoma was first identified in a male homosexual in 1982. Subsequent reports suggested that Burkitt's lymphoma (BL) is associated with AIDS whether the AIDS is of East African (endemic) form, from outside Africa (sporadic form), or from an HIV infection. The classic small noncleaved-cell (SNCC) lymphoma included both Burkitt's and non-Burkitt's subtypes, both of which have been seen in European and American patients with BL. The morphologic features of the lymphoma do not differ between the endemic or sporadic forms. The boundaries between morphologic variants are very vague and may bias the appropriate discrimination of SNCC from such lymphomas as BL. A recent categorization of HIV-related non-Hodgkin's lymphoma (NHL) offers guidelines for classification of tumors.

Methods.—During a 10-year period, 114 patients with HIV were treated. The HIV lymphomas were classified as SNCC, large-cell immunoblastic, diffuse large-cell, and a few cases were intermediate between SNCC and plasmablastic differentiation and plasmacytoid immunoblasts. The presence of the HIV antibody was confirmed and CD4+ counts were performed using flow cytometry. This study focused on 69 cases of NHL. Biopsy results were classified according to the Working Formulation. The following were determined on frozen tissues: surface immunoglobulins, common acute lymphoblastic leukemia antigen, as well as B- and T-cell differentiating antigens. Overexpression of p53 was tested on lymphoma samples.

Findings.—The CD4+ counts were lowest among patients with immunoblastic lymphomas (IBL). Both subunits of SNCC tumors were evident. Overexpression of p53 and Epstein-Barr virus were found in half of the BL and one quarter of the subtypes of SNCC and all but 1 of the intermediate lymphomas. Immunoblastic lymphoma tissues were consistently negative for p53 overexpression while having a high association with the Epstein-Barr virus.

Conclusion.—Pathologic classification of HIV-related lymphomas is normally based on the recognition of Burkitt's and non-Burkitt's subtypes. However, an intermediate class deserves recognition. Lymphomas that show intermediate features are a unique subgroup distinct from SNCC and IBL. The intermediate tissues bear a closer resemblance to SNCC.

▶ In patients with AIDS there is a high incidence of NHL and, to a lesser extent, of Hodgkin's lymphomas. The non-Hodgkin's lymphomas are almost all of an aggressive B-cell phenotype, and, unlike sporadically occurring non-Hodgkin's lymphomas, they often show a predilection for involvement of the brain.

Although the sporadic form of Burkitt's lymphoma is encountered worldwide, it is a relatively rare lymphoma. It is more common in equatorial Africa, where it is endemic. Burkitt's lymphoma is readily recognized by a typical "starry sky" appearance caused by infiltrating macrophages in a sea of dark-staining lymphoblasts. Burkitt's lymphoma is one of the common types of non-Hodgkin's lymphomas that occur in individuals infected with HIV. As discussed in this and the preceding article, it should be regarded as part of a morphologic spectrum of aggressive B-cell lymphomas. Once any of the NHLs become manifest in an individual with AIDS, the outlook for survival is poor.

M.J. Cline, M.D.

High-Dose Therapy and Autologous Bone Marrow Transplantation for Intermediate and High Grade Non-Hodgkin's Lymphoma in Patients Aged 55 Years and Over: Results From the European Group for Bone Marrow Transplantation

Sweetenham JW, Pearce R, Philip T, Proctor SJ, Mandelli F, Colombat P, Goldstone AH, on behalf of the EBMT Lymphoma Working Party (Univ College Hosps, London)

Bone Marrow Transplant 14:981–987, 1994 119-96-28–3

Background.—High-dose therapy with autologous stem-cell transplantation is being increasingly used as initial therapy for some patients with intermediate- or high-grade non-Hodgkin's lymphoma (NHL). Often, patients older than 59 years of age are not treated with high-dose therapy because of anticipated poor tolerance. A retrospective analysis of patients 55 years of age and older who had NHL and underwent high-dose therapy and autologous bone marrow transplantation was performed.

Methods.—During a 13-year period, 901 adult patients with intermediate- or high-grade NHL who underwent high-dose therapy with autologous bone marrow transplantation were reported to the Lymphoma Registry of the European Group for Bone Marrow Transplantation. After an initial comparison (Fig 1), each of the 82 patients who were 55 years or older at the time of transplantation was matched with a patient younger than 55 years of age for the following criteria: disease status and presence of bone marrow or CNS involvement at the time of transplantation. The median age for the group 55 years of age and older was 57 years and for the younger group was 37 years.

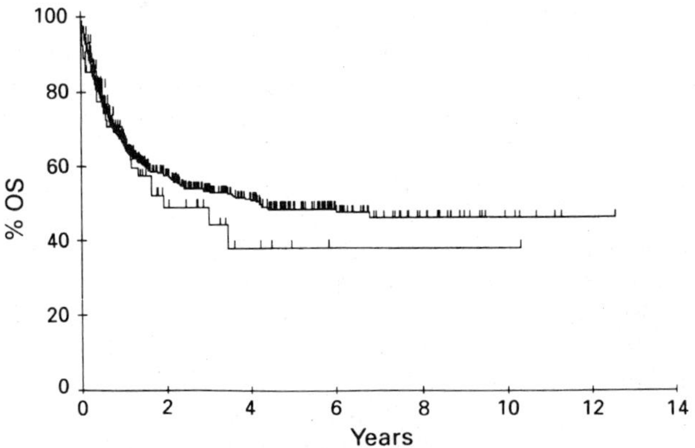

FIGURE 1.—Actuarial overall survival (*OS*) for 82 patients aged ≥ 55 years (**upper curve**) compared with 819 patients aged < 55 years (**lower curve**). Upper curve: OS at 5 years = 48%, $n = 849$. Lower curve: OS at 5 years = 38%, $n = 82$. $P = 0.383$. (Courtesy of Sweetenham JW, Pearce R, Philip T, et al: High-dose therapy and autologous bone marrow transplantation for intermediate and high grade non-Hodgkin's lymphoma in patients aged 55 years and over: Results from the European Group for Bone Marrow Transplantation. *Bone Marrow Transplant* 14:981–987, 1994.)

Results.—The 5-year actuarial progression-free survival for patients aged 55 years or older was 37%, and for patients younger than 55 years, it was 33%. The overall survival was 38% for the younger and 39% for the older group. Histologic subtype did not affect outcomes. The toxic death rate was higher in the older patients who received total body irradiation.

Conclusions.—Patients aged 55 years and older with NHL treated with high-dose therapy with autologous bone marrow transplantation do not have a lower progression-free or overall survival than younger patients. Because total body irradiation is associated with a higher toxic death rate in these older patients, they should probably receive chemotherapy only high-dose treatment regimens. It appears likely that peripheral blood progenitor cell transplantation will allow the use of high-dose therapy in selected patients up to age 70 years. Because the basis on which these patients were selected for autologous bone marrow transplantation is not clear and the study is retrospective, these findings must be cautiously interpreted.

▶ The subject of autologous bone marrow transplantation in non-Hodgkin's lymphoma was reviewed in the 1994 and the 1995 YEAR BOOKS OF MEDICINE. The 1995 study examined high-dose chemotherapy combined with either autologous bone marrow transplant or peripheral stem-cell transplantation in 158 patients with refractory NHL of intermediate histologic grade. Approximately one third of the patients were alive and in remission at 21 months after treatment. A subgroup of patients with a good prognosis for response to this therapy was identified. Interestingly, in this group, the rate of disease-free survival at 3 years was twice as high when peripheral stem-cell transplantation rather than autologous bone marrow transplantation was used.

Until recently, high-dose therapy with autologous stem-cell transplantation in patients with intermediate- and high-grade NHL has been restricted to those with relapsed or refractory disease. Now, a few studies are addressing the question of whether this intensive therapy should be applied early in the course of disease in patients who have poor prognostic factors. The previous study addressed this question in one type of disease. In any event, NHL is common in older populations, and patients older than 60 years of age constitute a large proportion of those seeking treatment. One has generally hesitated to use very aggressive treatment programs in older patients.

This study compares high-dose therapy with autologous stem-cell transplantation in patients younger than 55 years and those older than 55 years of age. The results are comparable in the 2 groups, although the authors warn against the inclusion of whole body irradiation in the older patients.

The take-away message is the following: It is still uncertain that high-dose therapy with autologous stem-cell transplantation provides real benefit to patients with NHL. For the moment, it should be reserved for patients with NHL that has relapsed or is refractory to treatment. The age of the patient (within reasonable limits) should not be a major factor in deciding whether to use high-dose therapy with autologous stem-cell transplantation.

M.J. Cline, M.D.

Value of Lymphangiography in the Staging of Hodgkin Lymphoma

Libson E, Polliack A, Bloom RA (Hadassah Univ Hosp, Ein Kerem, Jerusalem, Israel)

Radiology 193:757–759, 1994 119-96-28–4

Objective.—The value of lymphangiography was examined in 39 adult patients with Hodgkin's disease in whom CT scanning had failed to demonstrate abnormal abdominal lymph nodes or disease in parenchymal organs. All patients were previously untreated and had supradiaphragmatic disease.

Results.—None of the 29 patients with normal lymphangiograms had abnormal nodes on exploration, but 1 had disease in the spleen. Of 10 patients whose lymphangiograms demonstrated architecturally abnormal but normal-sized lymph nodes, only 2 had involved nodes. Nodes in the other patients exhibited merely reactive hyperplasia. One patient with and 1 without node involvement had splenic Hodgkin's disease.

Conclusion.—Lymphangiography has no value in staging Hodgkin's disease.

► This nice, succinct article informs us that with the advent of CT scans of the abdomen, lymphangiography no longer has a place in the staging of Hodgkin's disease. Although this may have seemed obvious, one wonders whether lymphangiography would have picked up normal-sized but architecturally abnormal nodes involved by disease. The answer is apparently "no."

M.J. Cline, M.D.

Treatment of Waldenstrom's Macroglobulinemia Resistant to Standard Therapy With 2-Chlorodeoxyadenosine: Identification of Prognostic Factors

Dimopoulos MA, Weber D, Delasalle KB, Keating M, Alexanian R (Univ of Texas, Houston)

Ann Oncol 6:49–52, 1995 119-96-28–5

Background.—Approximately one half of the patients with Waldenstrom's macroglobulinemia respond to standard treatment with alkylating agents and steroids. 2-Chlorodeoxyadenosine (2-CdA) has been effective for about 40% of patients who are resistant to treatment or experience relapse. A series of patients with resistant macroglobulinemia were followed to identify those most likely to benefit from 2-CdA.

Methods.—The study included 46 consecutive patients with Waldenstrom's macroglobulinemia that had failed to respond to standard therapy.

There were 25 women and 21 men (median age, 60 years). Most patients were treated because of progressive anemia, lymphadenopathy or organomegaly, or hyperviscosity syndrome. Twenty patients had primary resistance, 17 had refractory relapse, and 9 had a relapse while not receiving treatment. All received 2 courses of 2-CdA on an outpatient basis. The dosage was 0.1 mg/kg/day, given by 7-day continuous infusion with a portable pump via a central venous catheter.

Results.—A response to 2-CdA was achieved in 43% of patients. The response rate was 78% in patients who had a relapse while not receiving treatment and 57% in those with primary resistance within the first year compared with 22% for those in later stages of disease. Response was unrelated to patient age or sex, presence of lymphadenopathy or splenomegaly, pretreatment hemoglobin, severity of blood or marrow lymphocytosis, serum level of abnormal protein or β_2-microglobulin, or pretreatment CD4+ or CD8+ lymphocyte count. For responders, median survival after treatment was 28 months and median progression-free survival was 12 months. Patients with primary refractory disease had a projected median survival of 36 months compared with a median survival of 13 months for patients with refractory relapse.

Conclusions.—For patients with macroglobulinemic lymphoma that is resistant to standard therapy, 2-CdA is a potentially beneficial treatment. The response rates are best for patients who experience relapse while not receiving treatment or during their first year of primary refractory disease. For patients in later phases of resistant disease, 2-CdA appears to be of little help; alternative treatments should be given in this situation.

► This study examines the role of 2-CdA in Waldenstrom's macroglobulinemia resistant to standard treatment. Standard treatment in this disorder consists of plasmapheresis for acute manifestations of hyperviscosity and then alkylating agents, usually given over several months.

Forty-six patients with resistant disease were examined in this study. This is a remarkably large number, considering that most patients respond to conventional therapy provided it is given over sufficient time. One must therefore question the authors' criteria for "resistant" disease. Nevertheless, 43% of the patients were said to respond to 2-CdA therapy. The response was even higher (78%) in those whose disease relapsed while treatment was discontinued, but it was much lower in those with advanced disease.

Despite my misgivings about the validity of the authors' definition of "refractory" macroglobulinemia, I shall tuck away the fact that 2-CdA may be effective in this disease. This is not too surprising in view of the fact that it works in most indolent B-cell neoplasms if one is willing to pay the price of myelosuppression.

M.J. Cline, M.D.

Treatment of Multiple Myeloma According to the Extension of the Disease: A Prospective, Randomised Study Comparing a Less With a More Aggressive Cytostatic Policy

Riccardi A, for the Cooperative Group of Study and Treatment of Multiple Myeloma (Università and Istituto di Ricovero e Cura a Carattere Scientifico Policlinico S Matteo, Pavia, Italy)

Br J Cancer 70:1203–1210, 1994 119-96-28–6

Background.—The focus of attempts to improve survival of patients with multiple myeloma has mainly been on the development of more aggressive chemotherapies with little attention paid to the tailoring of treatment according to the stage of the disease. Whether the prognostic significance of staging in multiple myeloma is influenced by the aggressiveness of effective induction treatment and/or by maintenance chemotherapy was investigated.

Methods.—After receiving a diagnosis of multiple myeloma, patients were staged using standard criteria. They were then randomly assigned to either less or more aggressive induction cytostatic protocols for stage I and II disease using melphalan and prednisone for 6 courses or for stage III disease, Peptichemio, vincristine, and prednisone for 4 courses. Upon completion of induction, patients from all 3 stage groups were randomly assigned to the discontinuation of chemotherapy after maximal tumor reduction was reached or the continuation of chemotherapy indefinitely until relapse.

Results.—Three hundred forty-one patients entered the study, 301 receiving induction therapy and 40 patients with stage I disease who received no cytostatics until progression. The response rate to induction chemotherapy was, overall, 43.8%, with no significant difference between groups. Those left initially untreated had progression of the disease that was not significantly different from those treated. The median duration of the first response to induction chemotherapy was not different among those with continuation of chemotherapy and those in whom it was discontinued. The median survival was independent of receiving or not receiving maintenance for all responsive patients. Independent of protocol, median survival was more than 78 months in the stage I group, 46.3 months in the stage II group, and 24.3 months in the stage III group.

Conclusions.—Treatment in patients with early-stage multiple myeloma may be delayed. Independent of stage, the overwhelming majority of patients can be managed with melphalan and prednisone as initial treatment.

► Multiple myeloma is typically a disease of middle or old age. The well-known clinical manifestations of multiple myeloma are produced by replacement of normal hematopoietic cells from the bone marrow, osteolysis, and the effects of high concentrations of paraprotein. Lytic lesions of bone may be the result of production of osteoclast activating factor by plasma cells. The lesions may be localized, widespread, or may manifest as generalized osteoporosis.

The paraprotein produced by the myeloma cells is excreted by the kidneys and may cause damage to the tubules. This may be exacerbated by nephrocalcinosis produced by high concentrations of calcium mobilized from bone and by pyelonephritis. Some cases of multiple myeloma also have amyloid deposition in the tissues with resultant hepatospenomegaly, macroglossia, and cardiac and renal damage.

Death in patients with multiple myeloma usually occurs as a result of renal failure or infection, usually within 3–5 years of diagnosis. One gauges the results of therapy in this disease by following the level of paraprotein in the blood and urine and by performing repeated aspirations of bone marrow for the evaluation of the number of plasma cells. For decades, the standard treatment of multiple myeloma has been a combination of an alkylating agent such as melphalan or cyclophosphamide with corticosteroid. The combination often reduces the body burden of plasma cells and occasionally improves azotemia but rarely produces complete remission of disease.

This study addresses questions that are frequently asked in multiple myeloma. Should minimal disease be treated or merely observed until evidence of progression? Is more aggressive treatment superior to conventional melphalan-prednisone therapy? Is maintenance therapy of benefit once disease has responded to treatment?

A number of studies done during the course of more than 1 decade indicate that in early multiple myeloma, there is no benefit from aggressive chemotherapy. This study confirms that there is little difference between observation and early treatment for minimal disease.

A number of studies have compared standard with aggressive chemotherapy, but there has not been strong evidence favoring one approach over another. This study also failed to find benefit from aggressive treatment, which carried a higher price in toxicity than did standard therapy. Finally, maintenance therapy did not alter the median duration of the initial response. Although the current management of multiple myeloma is not very satisfactory, it appears that, for the present, *less* is *better.*

M.J. Cline, M.D.

Impact of Response to Treatment on Survival in Multiple Myeloma: Results in a Series of 243 Patients

Bladé J, López-Guillermo A, Bosch F, Cervantes F, Reverter J-C, Montserrat E, Rozman C (Univ of Barcelona)

Br J Haematol 88:117–121, 1994 119-96-28–7

Background.—Before alkylating agents were introduced, patients with multiple myeloma often survived less than 1 year. With standard chemotherapy, median survival is between 2 and 3 years. A higher response rate

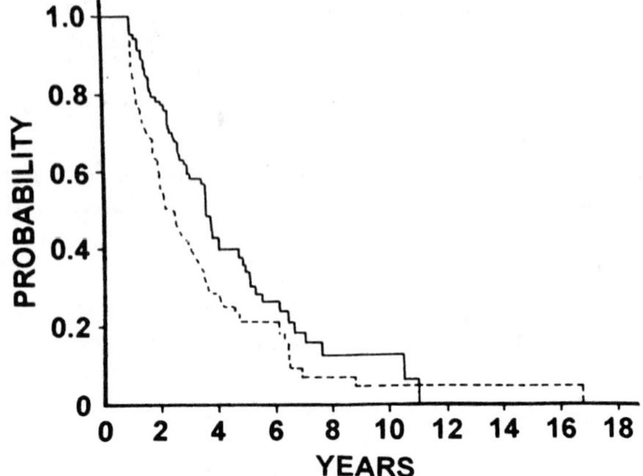

FIGURE 1.—Survival of responders (*thick line*) vs. nonresponders (*thin line*) by the landmark method with the landmark at 12 months after starting chemotherapy (χ^2 = 5.7058; P = 0.0169). (Courtesy of Bladé J, López-Guillermo A, Bosch F, et al: Impact of response to treatment on survival in multiple myeloma: Results in a series of 243 patients. *Br J Haematol* 88:117–121, 1994. Reprinted with permission from Blackwell Science Ltd.)

to combination chemotherapy has not always resulted in significantly longer survival. Therefore, it is unclear whether response to treatment has an effect on survival.

Methods and Objective.—The cases of 243 patients with multiple myeloma treated with standard chemotherapy during a 22-year period were assessed. The patient response to treatment and the impact of this response on patient survival were determined.

Results.—Data were available for 229 patients. The overall response rate was 50.1%. The median survival of patients with an objective response to treatment was 43.4 months, and the median survival of patients with a partial response was 42.8 months. For patients who did not respond to treatment, the median survival was 19 months. Complete remission was seen in 14 patients; their median survival was 42 months. Rapid response to treatment was seen in 21 patients; median survival was 43.3 months. With the landmark method (Fig 1) and the Mantel and Byar and Cox regression methods, there was a significant correlation between response and survival.

Conclusions.—Degree of response and response kinetics do not have a significant effect on survival of patients with multiple myeloma who respond to treatment. Response to therapy, however, is associated with significantly longer survival in these patients.

► The authors of the preceding article (Abstract 119-96-28–6) reviewed the effects of different therapeutic strategies in a large group of patients with multiple myeloma and concluded that aggressive therapy had no advantage over standard treatment with melphalan and prednisone. This study examines whether standard therapy has any impact on survival.

The results of treatment of 243 patients with multiple myeloma were examined. The authors of this study, like those of many previous studies, conclude that those patients who have multiple myeloma and show response to treatment live longer than do those whose disease does not respond: a median survival of approximately 3½ years vs. approximately 19 months.

M.J. Cline, M.D.

Double High-Dose Chemoradiotherapy With Autologous Stem Cell Transplantation Can Induce Molecular Remissions in Multiple Myeloma

Björkstrand B, Ljungman P, Bird JM, Samson D, Gahrton G (Karolinska Inst, Sweden; Charing Cross Hosp, London)

Bone Marrow Transplant 15:367–371, 1995 119-96-28–8

Background.—Although autotransplant regimens are associated with substantially increased complete remission rates among patients with multiple myeloma, most patients will have relapse after a median response duration of 24–30 months. For this reason, more effective treatment regimens are needed. The practicality and efficacy of repeated cycles of myeloablative cytotoxic therapy with autologous stem-cell support were therefore investigated in a group of patients with early, chemotherapy-responsive multiple myeloma.

Patients and Methods.—Fifteen patients with stage II–III multiple myeloma (median age, 48 years) were included. The patients were scheduled for 2 consecutive cycles of myeloablative chemoradiotherapy with autologous bone marrow or blood stem-cell transplantation after responding to primary induction chemotherapy. Bone marrow grafts were used in 3 of the 15 first transplants and peripheral blood stem cells in 2 of the first and all of the second transplants. The pretransplant preparative regimen consisted of melphalan (200 mg/m^2) for the first transplant and melphalan (140 mg/m^2) plus total body irradiation (10 Gy) for the second transplant.

Results.—Twelve patients were in partial and 3 in complete remission before the first transplant. After the first procedure, 7 were in partial and 7 in complete remission. Three patients with incomplete hematopoietic reconstitution after transplantation and 1 patient who experienced early death underwent only 1 cycle of myeloablative therapy. Second transplants were performed in the remaining 11 patients, 6 of whom were then in complete and 5 in partial remission. An additional 2 patients experienced complete remission after the second procedure, and 3 remained in partial remission. At a mean of 20 months after first transplants, 8 patients remained in continuous complete remission and 3 in partial remission. Polymerase chain reaction (PCR) analysis of the clone-specific immunoglobulin gene rearrangement was performed in 5 patients with complete remission to determine minimal residual disease. Of these 5 individuals, 4 remained PCR negative for up to 33 months after the first transplant. There was 1 transplant-related death, and another patient died of progressive disease.

Conclusions.—Application of repeated cycles of myeloablative treatment with hematopoietic stem-cell rescue is both practical and effective, with long-term complete remissions achieved in a large percentage of patients with multiple myeloma. Larger groups of patients with longer follow-up need to be evaluated to help clarify the therapeutic role of this superintensive regimen.

► This is the third of the 4 articles on multiple myeloma to be found in the 1996 YEAR BOOK OF MEDICINE. Its authors clearly take a more aggressive view than the minimal standard therapy approach presented by the authors of the first article selected. Fifteen relatively young patients who had multiple myeloma responsive to chemotherapy were subjected to 2 cycles of intensive chemotherapy and whole body irradiation plus rescue with autologous marrow or peripheral blood stem cells. This group of selected patients did remarkably well, and 8 of the 15 patients remained in remission at a median of 20 months after initiating treatment. More remarkably still, 4 of the patients had no evidence of disease by a highly sensitive PCR analysis at 17–33 months' post transplant. This is a promising technique in selected patients with multiple myeloma.

M.J. Cline, M.D.

Treatment of Myeloma Using Intensive Therapy and Allogeneic Bone Marrow Transplantation

Reece DE, Shepherd JD, Klingemann H-G, Sutherland HJ, Nantel SH, Barnett MJ, Spinelli JJ, Phillips GL (Leukemia/Bone Marrow Transplantation Program of British Columbia, Canada; Vancouver Hosp, BC, Canada)
Bone Marrow Transplant 15:117–123, 1995 119-96-28–9

Objective.—A few case reports have suggested that more intensive chemotherapy regimens, including myeloablative therapy given before bone marrow transplantation (BMT), could be an effective treatment for patients with myeloma. It may even be possible to produce a "graft-vs.-myeloma" effect in patients receiving allogeneic marrow support. An experience with allogeneic BMT in 26 patients with multiple myeloma was evaluated.

Patients.—Intensive therapy and allogeneic BMT were considered for 65 patients aged 55 years or less with myeloma during a 5-year period. Allogeneic BMT was performed in 26. The patients had had myeloma for a median of 4 months, and they had received a median of 1 previous regimen. The myeloma was chemosensitive in all patients but 5. Conditioning therapy varied, including busulfan, cyclophosphamide (CY), and melphalan (MEL) in 14 patients; BUCY2 in 8; and CY and total body irradiation in 4. Nineteen patients received marrow from HLA-matched siblings, 3 from 1-antigen-mismatched siblings, and 4 from unrelated donors. Cyclosporine was given to all patients: additionally, 5 received methylprednisolone and 19 received methotrexate with or without other agents.

Results.—Only 3 patients had grade III or IV regimen-related toxicity, including none of those who received the new 3-drug conditioning regimen. Twenty patients had grade II–IV acute graft-vs.-host disease (GVHD), and 3 died of it. Another 3 patients died of chronic GVHD. There were 21 assessable patients. Thirteen attained complete remission, for a rate of 62%, and 6 had partial remission. At a median follow-up of 14 months, actuarial progression-free survival (PFS) was 52%. This figure was 52% in chemoresponsive patients vs. 0% in chemoresistant patients.

Conclusions.—With intensive therapy and allogeneic BMT, it is possible to achieve long-term progression-free survival in some patients with myeloma. This treatment would be more effective if ways could be found to reduce GVHD and optimize the use of alternative donors. The authors consider transplantation for all patients with myeloma who are medically fit, have an identified matched related donor, and have chemosensitive disease.

▶ This is the last of this year's selection of articles on multiple myeloma. It, too, takes an aggressive approach to the treatment of this disease using allogeneic BMT with either a family member or matched unrelated individual as bone marrow donor. The authors were quite aggressive in their approach; in some cases, they used family members who had a single mismatch as donors. This situation is known to be associated with a high incidence of graft-vs.-host disease.

To summarize the study, allogeneic BMT was performed in 26 patients younger than 55 years of age who had multiple myeloma. Seven of the 26 patients had a less-than-ideal bone marrow donor. To prepare the patients for BMT, 3 different intensive "conditioning" programs were used. The results were as follows:

1. Twenty of the 26 patients had severe GVHD—a very high incidence by any standard—and 6 died of its complications.
2. Thirteen of the 26 patients (50%) achieved a complete remission.
3. Five patients were in remission more than 18 months after treatment; one of these received a less-than-ideal marrow.

The authors are encouraged by these results and want to use transplantation for more patients with multiple myeloma.

M.J. Cline, M.D.

29 Bone Marrow Transplantation and Gene Therapy

Bone Marrow Transplant-Associated Thrombotic Microangiopathy: A Case Series

Zeigler ZR, Shadduck RK, Nemunaitis J, Andrews DF, Rosenfeld CS (Western Pennsylvania Cancer Inst, Pittsburgh)

Bone Marrow Transplant 15:247–253, 1995 119-96-29–1

Introduction.—Bone marrow transplant (BMT) can be a curative treatment for patients with benign and malignant diseases. However, several complications can develop, including thrombotic microangiopathy (TM). Reported mortality rates associated with thrombotic microangiopathy have ranged from 0% to 100%. The experience in 1 regional institution with BMT-TM was evaluated.

Methods.—During a 7-month period, 52 allogeneic and 65 autologous BMTs were performed. All patients who subsequently had elevated lactate dehydrogenase levels had blood smears examined for fragmented erythrocytes. Data collected in these patients included the time to development of BMT-TM, the treatment and treatment response, other complications, and the clinical outcome. Clinical parameters were also measured in 17 control patients who received allogeneic BMT and had no clinical evidence of BMT-TM. A grading system, ranging from grade 0 to grade 4, was used to classify the lactate dehydrogenase level and the percentage of fragmented cells, which were used to interpret BMT-TM severity.

Results.—Of the 17 controls, 10 had grade 0 BMT-TM and 7 had grade 1 BMT-TM, which was found at a median of 61 days after the patient underwent allogeneic BMT. Bone marrow transplantation–associated thrombotic microangiography of grade 2 or higher developed in 22 patients, with higher grades associated significantly with male sex and with the cyclophosphamide/total body irradiation preparative regimen. Patients with BMT-TM of grades higher than 1 were seen at a median of 36 days after BMT. Among the clinical parameters measured, the lactate dehydrogenase platelet count ratio increased in association with the grade

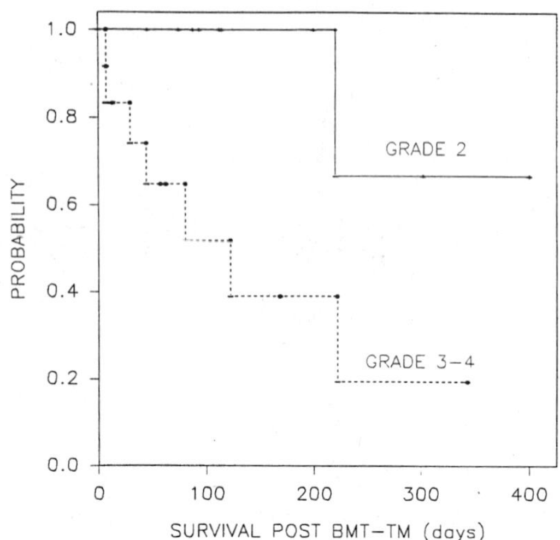

FIGURE 1.—Kaplan-Meier plot of survival from day of diagnosis of bone marrow transplantation–associated thrombotic microangiograph (*BMT-TM*). Patients with grade 2 BMT-TM (*solid line*) $n = 10$; patients with grades 3–4 BMT-TM (*dotted line*) $n = 12$. $P = 0.018$ by log rank test. (Courtesy of Zeigler ZR, Shadduck RK, Nemunaitis J, et al: Bone marrow transplant-associated thrombotic microangiography: A case series. *Bone Marrow Transplant* 15:247–253, 1995.)

of BMT-TM and serum creatinine values increased significantly only in patients with grade 4 severity. The severity of BMT-TM generally correlated positively with the severity of acute graft-vs.-host disease and negatively with survival (Fig 1). The BMT-TM was manifested clinically in various symptoms, including hypertension, edema, neurologic symptoms, hemorrhagic cystitis, fever, and diarrhea. Complete resolution was seen in 7 patients with grade 2 BMT-TM (spontaneous in 5 and after discontinuation of cyclosporine in 2) but in none of the patients with grade 3 or 4 BMT-TM. Exchange with cryosupernatant produced a greater (though partial) response in patients with grade 4 BMT-TM than did exchange with fresh frozen plasma.

Conclusions.—Thrombotic microangiopathy is a common complication of BMT, particularly in patients who receive allogeneic BMT with cyclosporine prophylaxis. The grading of the disorder varies considerably and correlates with survival and response rate, suggesting that the percentage of fragmented cells is a significant prognostic indicator. Patients with grade 3–4 BMT-TM may improve with exchange using cryosupernatant and/or protein A immunoadsorption.

► A microangiopathic hemolytic anemia with fragmented red cells on the blood smear and release of lactic acid dehydrogenase from lysing red cells is an occasional complication of allogeneic bone marrow transplantation. Its pathogenesis is not clear, although there may be correlation with graft-vs.-host disease and with intensive chemotherapy-irradiation regimens.

These authors have developed a grading system for this thrombotic microangiopathy based on the level of lactate dehydrogenase and the number of fragmented erythrocytes. High-grade microangiopathy and thrombotic disease is associated with a high mortality. The treatment procedures such as plasmapheresis used in other microangiopathic disorders, such as thrombotic thrombocytopenic purpura, are not obviously effective in this situation.

M.J. Cline, M.D.

Desferrioxamine Therapy Accelerates Clearance of Iron Deposits After Bone Marrow Transplantation for Thalassaemia

Giardini C, Galimberti M, Lucarelli G, Polchi P, Angelucci E, Baronciani D, Gaziev D, Erer B, La Nasa G, Barbanti I, Muretto P (Ospedale di Pesaro, Italy; Università di Cagliari, Pesaro, Italy)

Br J Haematol 89:868–873, 1995 119-96-29–2

Introduction.—The definitive cure for homozygous β-thalassemia is allogeneic bone marrow transplantation (BMT). The current medical treatment centers around red blood cell transfusion and iron chelation. The iron chelation is related to survival and reduced iron-induced complications. The quality of iron chelation therapy, age, and the number of transfusions influences the tissue iron overload from BMT. Only a small portion of the iron accumulated is a result of steady-state erythropoiesis that follows BMT restoration of hematopoiesis. Whether from transfusional iron overload or hereditary hemochromatosis, the degree of increase in tissue iron can depend on the time in which the liver, pituitary, and heart are exposed to iron. Therefore, prompt reduction of tissue iron is essential. Unfortunately, a method of rapid removal of iron stores for the ex-thalassemic patient has not been described. Phlebotomy is a viable, if limited, method. Hepatic iron, in the presence of continuous iron accumulation, can be reduced with nightly subcutaneous deferoxamine. The ex-thalassemic patient should be able to reduce iron in the absence of iron accumulation. The response of these patients to this therapy is unknown.

Methods.—Eighteen ex-thalassemic patients, following BMT, were selected for deferoxamine therapy. Serum ferritin levels exceeded 2,000 μg/L for a minimum of 1 year. Transferrin saturation exceeded 90%. Deferoxamine, 40 mg/kg, was infused 6 nights per week, over a 12-hour period, for 9 months. Once the serum ferritin levels had reduced below 1,000 μg/L, the deferoxamine was reduced to every other day. Diet was controlled and routine laboratory tests were performed monthly. Liver biopsy specimens were obtained before BMT, before the start of deferoxamine, and between 6 and 20 months later. The histologic sections were graded as 0 (no stainable iron) to 3 (highest degree of siderosis).

Results.—The median ferritin levels were significantly lowered from 3,607 to 1,188 μg/L. In addition, serum iron and serum alanine aminotransferase were significantly reduced. Before therapy, stainable iron was moderate to severe in the liver parenchyma in 15 of the 18 patients and moderate to severe at the level of the mesenchyme in all 18. This was reduced to changes in the liver parenchyma in 5 patients and at the level of mesenchyme in 10 patients after deferoxamine therapy.

Conclusion.—Iron deposits can be safely reduced with chelation therapy. Thus, an alternative to phlebotomy is now available.

► The thalassemias arise from genetic abnormalities in the synthesis of the α- or β-globin chains. Unbalanced globin chain production leads to unstable hemoglobin molecules and premature destruction of the developing red blood cell with ineffective erythropoiesis in the bone marrow and hemolytic anemia.

The clinical manifestations of the thalassemias vary from none to a severe fatal anemia with intrauterine death. In thalassemia major, all the characteristics of a chronic severe hemolytic anemia are present. Because the disorder begins early in life, bony abnormalities occur from the intense erythropoietic activity unless transfusion therapy is given to maintain the blood count. Bone fractures and a characteristic facial appearance are frequent. With the passage of time, iron overload is inevitable, and if untreated, it leads to some of the principal complications of thalassemia major: skin pigmentation, endocrine gland dysfunction, delayed puberty, diabetes mellitus and, eventually, cardiomyopathy.

With supportive treatment by transfusion and iron chelation, many patients are now living into adult life, whereas previously they often died in childhood or adolescence. The only curative treatment at present is allogeneic BMT. The mortality associated with the procedure depends on several factors, of which an important one is the presence or absence of iron-related tissue damage at the time of the transplant. In good-risk patients, cure by BMT is greater than 70%.

Because tissue damage by iron is a function of the iron concentration in tissues as well as the duration of exposure to high levels of iron, it seems reasonable to bring the iron concentration down toward normal levels as quickly as possible. This article examines the use of desferoxamine in thalassemic patients after bone marrow transplantation. The authors conclude that it is a valid treatment for iron reduction if used over 5–20 months. I am not certain that they have demonstrated that it is better than phlebotomy. It takes 10–25 days of deferoxamine treatment to remove the iron that is taken off in a single unit of blood. My own view is that deferoxamine should be reserved for those patients who cannot tolerate phlebotomy.

M.J. Cline, M.D.

Successful Bone Marrow Transplantation for Idiopathic Hypereosinophilic Syndrome

Fukushima TR, Kuriyama K, Ito H, Miyazaki Y, Arimura K, Hata T, Saitoh M, Tomonaga M (Nagasaki Univ, Japan)

Br J Haematol 90:213–215, 1995 119-96-29-3

Background.—The rare disorder that causes multiple organ failure from the infiltration of eosinophils is termed idiopathic hypereosinophilic syndrome (HES). The patient will respond to corticosteroids, indicating an immunologic mechanism, or not, in the case of myeloproliferative disorder (MPD). A patient with HES/MPD was successfully treated with allogeneic bone marrow transplantation.

Case Report.—Man, 21, was admitted because of a heart abnormality that was diagnosed as Epstein's anomaly. He improved when treated with diuretics, but was also found to have eosinophilia. Eosinophilic infiltration was proved on a skin biopsy from the upper chest. The spleen and liver were both extended beyond their respective costal margins. The white blood cell count, 60×10^9/L, was 65% eosinophils. His hemoglobin was 121 g/L. Bone marrow smears showed 19.8% eosinophils that were uneven with no excess blasts. The leukocyte alkaline phosphatase score was 41. There was moderate fibrosis in the bone marrow and eosinophilic infiltration in the heart tissue.

He was initially treated with methylprednisolone, which was unsuccessful at controlling the eosinophilia and skin rash. Eosinophils decreased to $2.5–3.5 \times 10^9$/L after the administration of hydroxyurea, 500 mg every other day. This response was transient. Because he had an HLA-identical, MLC-negative sister, an allogeneic bone marrow transplantation was performed. After a reconditioning program, the bone marrow cells were harvested and injected into the patient. Morbidity included ascites and hepatomegaly that appeared on day 2 after the transplant. By day 30, eosinophils constituted 35% of the peripheral blood leukocytes. The eosinophils continued to decrease without treatment. Abnormal taste sensation, nausea, and elevated hepatobiliary enzymes were eventually tolerated. The patient continued to survive more than 1 year without a relapse.

Conclusion.—Allogeneic bone marrow transplantation appears to be a potential treatment for patients with HES/MPD.

▶ When there are increased numbers of eosinophils in the blood, one commonly thinks of parasitic diseases, allergic conditions, some dermatopathies or, more rarely, neoplastic diseases. Idiopathic HES is a fascinating disorder or group of disorders characterized by high levels of blood eosinophils without obviously detectable cause accompanied by organ dysfunction. A few cases ultimately prove to be variants of MPD, as evidenced by chromosomal abnormalities; however, in most cases, the etiology is never determined.

Many organ systems may be affected in this condition, but involvements of the heart and lungs are particularly prominent. The cardiomyopathy accompanying this disorder is characterized by fibrosis and infiltration of the myocardium with eosinophils.

Because organ damage is associated with infiltration with high numbers of eosinophils, those patients who fail to respond to corticosteroids are often treated with a cytotoxic agent such as hydroxyurea. However, because idiopathic HES is relatively rare, there have been no controlled trials of the benefits of such treatment.

Because disease that is responsive to conventional therapy has a high mortality, the patient described in this report from Japan underwent bone marrow transplantation from an HLA-matched sibling. After a relatively arduous course, he apparently recovered and is free of disease. One wonders, however, whether the conditions that provoked the idiopathic HES in the first place will cause problems for the grafted marrow. Reviews of the idiopathic HES can be found in 1982 and 1994 publications.[1, 2]

M.J. Cline, M.D.

References

1. Fauci AS, Herley JB, Roberts WC, et al: The idiopathic hypereosinophilic syndrome: Clinical, pathophysiological, and therapeutic considerations. *Ann Intern Med* 97:78–82, 1982.
2. Weller PF, Bubley GJ: The idiopathic hypereosinophilic syndrome. *Blood* 83:2759–2779, 1994.

Regulated High-Level Human β-Globin Gene Expression in Erythroid Cells Following Recombinant Adeno-Associated Virus-Mediated Gene Transfer

Einerhand MPW, Antoniou M, Zolotukhin S, Muzyczka N, Berns KI, Grosveld F, Valerio D (Univ of Leiden, The Netherlands; Natl Inst for Med Research, London; State Univ of New York, Stony Brook; et al)

Gene Therapy 2:336–343, 1995 119-96-29–4

Introduction.—Erythrocyte function is severely compromised in β^0-thalassemia and sickle-cell anemia. In the former, the β-globin is insufficient, and in the latter, the β-globin chain has mutated. Patients or carriers with persistent fetal hemoglobin have either no disease or a milder form of the disease, which suggests that an intact β- or γ-globin chain can ameliorate the phenotype. Because of this, gene therapy focuses on integrating a human β-globin gene into the patient's stem cells. There are a variety of methods for locating and obtaining β-globin expression. An adenoassociated virus in which human β-globin gene is controlled by the β–locus control region (β-LCR) at elements HS 4, 3, and 2 was designed. Expression of β-globin is observed in murine erythroleukemia (MEL) cells.

Major Finding and Comment.—In transduced and G418 MEL cell clones, the gene expression of human β-globin was controlled and increased to levels that were comparable with endogenous β^{maj}. This indicates that adeno-associated virus vectors are promising methods for gene therapy in patients with hemoglobinopathies.

► For gene therapy to work, the following conditions must be met: (1) there has to be an effective vector for inserting the new genes; (2) the introduced gene must be in a form in which it will be expressed at levels sufficient to have a therapeutic effect; (3) the target cells must be accessible; and (4) the target cells should be stem cells, which are capable of proliferation and dissemination of the new gene among the affected cell population.

The authors of this article are experimenting with a system that tries to meet these requirements. They use adenovirus as the vector and the naturally occurring promoter of the β-globin gene to control gene expression. For the present, they are using a tissue culture model system rather than the ultimate targets—human hematopoietic stem cells. The results are encouraging.

M.J. Cline, M.D.

Gene Transfer to Primary Chronic Granulomatous Disease Monocytes

Thrasher AJ, Casimir CM, Kinnon C, Morgan G, Segal AW, Levinsky RJ (Inst of Child Health, London; Univ College London)

Lancet 346:92–93, 1995 119-96-29–5

Introduction.—Lesions of the gene that encodes NADPH oxidase are a class of primary immunodeficiencies including chronic granulomatous disease (CGD). A membrane-bound flavocytochrome b_{558} translocates to the membrane once a cell is activated. All subunits of the b_{558} are affected in CGD except p21*rac*. In 60% of the cases, the lesion is found in the X-linked gene encoded gp91*phox*. Lesions on the other subunits have an autosomal recessive pattern.

Methods.—A complementary DNA–encoded p47*phox* was cloned to rescue the recombinant virus p47AD2. Monocytes from 3 patients with CGD were stimulated with myristate acetate to reduce nitroblue-tetrazolium to dark-blue-staining formazan within 24 hours after infection. Cells from patients with CGD cannot perform this reaction.

Patients.—Patient 1, a boy, had known p47*phox* deficiency. Two girls (patients 2 and 3) had newly diagnosed CGD, but the site of the molecular lesion was not known. Transduction by p47AD2 caused a proportion of monocytes from the first 2 patients to reduce nitroblue-tetrazolium. The cells from the third patient could not perform the reaction. In patient 2, NADPH oxidase activity was significant only when exposed to p47AD2, whereas patient 3 had no activity under any condition. Western blot analysis showed that patient 2 had no immunoreactive p47*phox*. Patient 3 had normal levels of p67*phox* but lacked the similar cytosolic factor.

Comment.—The transduction of monocytes by adenoviral vectors can aid in the identification of defects of NADPH oxidase components. Restoration of function can also be documented by nitroblue-tetrazolium staining. The method is simple, does not require a large number of cells, and may have therapeutic potential.

► In the next few years, we are going to see an increasing number of reports of attempts at gene therapy, both in inherited diseases and in cancer. Chronic granulomatous disease is a good candidate for a gene therapy trial. It is a severe disease, often resulting in the early death of those affected; it involves hematopoietic cells, which are easily accessible for insertion of new genes; and the success or failure of the experiment is easily tested by a simple histochemical reaction.

This study uses an adenovirus as vector to insert the defective gene into CGD monocytes rather than the more popular retroviral vectors. The experiment apparently worked, at least transiently. This is encouraging for the future of such novel therapy.

M.J. Cline, M.D.

30 Basic Oncology

Localization of a Breast Cancer Susceptibility Gene, *BRCA2*, to Chromosome 13q 12-13

Wooster R, Neuhausen SL, Mangion J, Quirk Y, Ford D, Collins N, Nguyen K, Seal S, Tran T, Averill D, Fields P, Marshall G, Narod S, Lenoir GM, Lynch H, Feunteun J, Devilee P, Cornelisse CJ, Menko FH, Daly PA, Ormiston W, McManus R, Pye C, Lewis CM, Cannon-Albright LA, Peto J, Ponder BAJ, Skolnick MH, Easton DF, Goldgar DE, Stratton MR (Inst of Cancer Research, Surrey, England; Univ of Utah, Salt Lake City; McGill Univ, Montreal, Canada; et al)

Science 265:2088–2090, 1994 119-96-30–1

Background.—Recent studies have indicated that the breast cancer susceptibility gene, *BRCA1*, may be largely responsible for a subset of familial breast cancers. To identify other genes that might confer a high risk to breast cancer, a linkage study was performed in patients with a family history of early-onset breast cancer who had a negative lod score for markers surrounding the *BRCA1* gene.

Patients and Methods.—A genomic linkage search was performed in 15 families who had multiple cases of early onset breast cancer that were not linked to *BRCA1*. Lod scores were computed with FASTLINK, using a familial breast cancer model based on the Cancer and Steroid Hormone Study.

Results.—Genotyping with polymorphic microsatellite repeats indicated the presence of a susceptibility gene on chromosome 13. Two-point lod scores obtained from markers on chromosome 13q were used to further refine the position. An admixture test indicated that rather than a single location, there was a significant degree of heterogeneity. Flanking markers indicated that the location of the identified *BRCA2* gene was at 13q12–13. This newly identified gene also confers a high risk of early-onset breast cancer. In contrast to *BRCA1*, however, the *BRCA2* phenotype confers a lower risk of ovarian cancer but an apparently increased risk for male breast cancer.

Conclusions.—Genes *BRCA1* and *BRCA2* probably account for most, but not all, of those cases of early-onset breast cancer occurring in families with multiple reported cases.

► In 1990, a breast cancer susceptibility gene designated *BRCA1* on the long arm of chromosome 17 was identified. The *BRCA1* gene accounts for most families in which there is early onset of both breast and ovarian cancers but does not account for all breast cancer–prone families. Now these investigators have defined another breast cancer susceptibility gene on chromosome 13, which they have called *BRCA2*. Mutations in this gene confer a high risk of breast cancer but not ovarian cancer.

Other familial gene abnormalities that involve a high risk of breast and other cancers include the *p53* gene on the short arm of chromosome 17 and the ataxia telangiectasia gene on chromosome 11.

In family members who have abnormalities of either *BRCA1* or *BRCA2*, the risk of breast cancer developing by 80 years of age is almost 90%. These 2 genes appear to account for the vast majority of familial breast cancers. Their recognition opens the way to new screening tests for individuals at risk for breast cancer.

M.J. Cline, M.D.

Mutation of a *mutL* Homolog in Hereditary Colon Cancer

Papadopoulos N, Nicolaides NC, Wei Y-F, Ruben SM, Carter KC, Rosen CA, Haseltine WA, Fleischmann RD, Fraser CM, Adams MD, Venter JC, Hamilton SR, Petersen GM, Watson P, Lynch HT, Peltomäki P, Mecklin J-P, de la Chapelle A, Kinzler KW, Vogelstein B (Johns Hopkins Oncology Ctr, Baltimore, Md; Human Genome Sciences Inc, Rockville, Md; Inst for Genomic Research, Gaithersburg, Md; et al)

Science 263:1625–1629, 1994 119-96-30–2

Background.—Hereditary nonpolyposis colorectal cancer (HNPCC) is one of the most prevalent genetic disorders; as many as 1 in 200 individuals are affected. Mendelian inheritance was inferred from the finding that markers on chromosome 2p segregated with disease in large kindreds with HNPCC. Some cases of HNPCC have been related to alterations in a *mutS*-related mismatch repair gene.

Objective.—To learn whether mutations of other mismatch repair genes might cause HNPCC, a large database of expressed sequence tags derived from random complementary DNA (cDNA) clones was searched.

Findings.—Three genes not previously described were found to bear significant resemblance to the bacterial *mutL* at their 5' ends. The gene most similar to the yeast *mutL* gene *MLH1*, termed h*MLH1*, was found to reside on chromosome 3p21 within 1 centimorgan of markers that have been linked with susceptibility to cancer in HNPCC kindreds. Affected individuals from 7 Finnish kindreds all had a heterozygous deletion of codons 578 to 632 of h*MLH1*, and 5 of the 7 kindreds could be traced to a common ancestor. When HNPCC kindreds not suitable for linkage studies were evaluated by a random cDNA sequencing approach, a complex 371-nt deletion was found, starting at the first position of codon 347. This alteration was present in heterozygous form.

Implications.—It seems very likely that HNPCC is associated with heritable defects in any of several mismatch repair genes. Studies using the H6 tumor-cell line are consistent with a model of HNPCC in which a second mutation is required for tumorigenesis.

► The genetic basis of inherited familial cancers is being elucidated for a number of common as well as rare malignancies. The preceding article (Abstract 119-96-30–1) discussed 2 genes that are implicated in the great majority of familial breast cancers. This article describes another gene that is frequently altered in the type of familial colon cancer that is not associated with hereditary polyposis—a disease sometimes designated hereditary non-polyposis colorectal cancer, or HNPCC. This disorder, one of the most common inherited cancers of man, may affect 1 in 200 individuals. One of the defective genes in this disorder is found on the short arm of chromosome 2. It is a gene that is involved in the repair of mistakes that occur in DNA replication or with DNA damage and is similar in structure to more primitive genes found in unicellular organisms. It is likely that other so-called "mismatch repair" genes are involved in this type of colon cancer.

The authors hypothesize that affected individuals are born with one abnormal gene. When a mutation occurs in the corresponding normal allele, mutations rapidly accumulate and cancer develops. Why the cancers should be specifically colon cancer is not clear at this time. Knowledge of these genetic abnormalities that predispose to familial cancers will eventually lead to strategies for early detection of disease.

M.J. Cline, M.D.

Inhibition of Angiogenesis In Vivo by Interleukin 12

Voest EE, Kenyon BM, O'Reilly MS, Truitt G, D'Amato RJ, Folkman J (Harvard Med School, Boston; Hoffmann-La Roche Inc, Nutley, NJ)

J Natl Cancer Inst 87:581–586, 1995 119-96-30–3

Introduction.—Potent antitumor and antimetastatic activities have been demonstrated in several murine tumor models by interleukin-12 (IL-12), formerly called natural killer cell–stimulatory factor or cytotoxic lymphocyte maturation factor. Interleukin-12 has been effective in in vivo studies but had little effect in in vitro studies, suggesting that IL-12 may have antiangiogenic properties to account for its tumor-inhibitory effects. For tumors to enlarge, angiogenesis is fundamental, and growth of tumors has been suppressed by preventing the development of new blood vessels in tumors. Interleukin-12 was evaluated in mice to determine whether it has antiangiogenic properties.

Methods.—To evaluate the effects of IL-12 and interferon-γ on angiogenesis in vivo, basic fibroblast growth factor–induced corneal neovascularization was used in mice. For 5 consecutive days, IL-12 (1 μg/day) was given to different strains of male mice: immunocompetent C57BL mice; severe combined immunodeficient mice; natural killer cell–deficient beige mice; and T-cell–deficient nude mice. The maximal vessel length and the corneal circumference involved in new formation of blood vessels were measured to assess the extent of neovascularization in response to a basic fibroblast growth factor pellet and the inhibition of neovascularization by IL-12 or interferon-γ. In Lewis lung carcinoma–bearing mice, the antitumor activities of IL-12 and of the angiogenesis inhibitor AGM-1470 were evaluated.

Results.—Corneal neovascularization was almost completely inhibited in C57BL/6, severe combined immunodeficient mice, and natural killer cell–deficient beige mice with IL-12 treatment. Suppression was mediated through interferon-γ, as the administration of interferon-γ–neutralizing antibodies prevented the suppression of angiogenesis. During treatment with IL-12, the administration of interferon-γ reproduced the antiangiogenic effects. In Lewis lung carcinoma–bearing mice, combined treatment with AGM-1470 and IL-12 did not increase toxicity and enhanced antitumor effects.

Conclusion.—Neovascularization is strongly inhibited by IL-12. A specific cell type of the immune system does not mediate this effect. Rather, interferon-γ is induced by IL-12, showing that interferon-γ plays a critical role in mediating the antiangiogenic effects of IL-12. Further studies are needed to recognize the mechanisms of the antiangiogenic properties of IL-12 so that its clinical applications with other neovascularization inhibitors may be planned.

► I included this article in the 1996 YEAR BOOK OF MEDICINE because it describes a potentially novel approach to the treatment of human cancers—an approach based on the interruption of the new vascular supply that supports tumor growth. In this study, the authors used one of the lymphokines designated as IL-12 to interfere with neovascularization of tumors and demonstrated that its mechanism of action is probably mediated via production of interferon-γ.

In the past 2 years, several studies have shown that interruption of neovascularization inhibits growth of tumors in model systems in mice. We await transfer of these observations to human cancers.

M.J. Cline, M.D.

31 Clinical Oncology

Age and Clinical Decision Making in Oncology Patients

Yellen SB, Cella DF, Leslie WT (Rush-Presbyterian-St Luke's Med Ctr, Chicago)

J Natl Cancer Inst 86:1766–1770, 1994 119-96-31–1

Background.—It has been reported that older adults who have cancer are less likely to receive aggressive treatment, to be presented with alternative treatments, and to receive adjuvant therapy. There is little or no information about the treatment preferences of older adults with cancer, although many clinicians assume that these patients do not prefer aggressive cancer treatment. The treatment preferences of older adults with cancer were investigated.

Methods.—In an interview, 244 patients, aged 23–83 years, who had cancer were presented with 2 sets of hypothetical situations describing a person of the same sex with the same type of cancer as the patient. The patients were asked to make hypothetical treatment decisions on the basis of the details given. In the first set of situations, patients had to decide whether to accept treatment. The second set of situations presumed acceptance of cancer treatment.

Results.—In the first set of situations, acceptance of treatment was unaffected by the age or stage of cancer of the actual patient. Older adults and younger adults made similar decisions about chemotherapy for curative and palliative purposes. In the second set describing hypothetical early disease, younger adults changed their preference to a more toxic treatment to increase survival at an earlier point than did older adults. In the second set describing hypothetical advanced disease, treatment decisions were unaffected by the stage of cancer of the actual patient, and there was no interaction between age and stage of disease.

Discussion.—Older and younger patients with cancer may make similar decisions about aggressive therapy for curative or palliative purposes. Older patients may be less willing to trade quality of life for longer survival, i.e., they may prefer less aggressive therapy once they have decided to accept treatment. The choices made by these patients seemed to be affected by their prior experience with chemotherapy. The hypothetical treatment situations are described in detail.

▶ This fascinating study examines the relationship between the age of patients with cancer and how they feel about different treatment programs.

In general, older patients opt for the same choices as younger patients, except they are less apt to want more aggressive therapy, even if it increases the chances for long-term survival.

I suspect that making decisions about the therapeutic options for cancer is as much influenced by the age of the treating physician as it is by the age of the patient. This might be the subject of the next study by these authors.

M.J. Cline, M.D.

A Prospective Evaluation of Plasma Prostate-Specific Antigen for Detection of Prostatic Cancer

Gann PH, Hennekens CH, Stampfer MJ (Harvard Med School, Boston; Harvard School of Public Health, Boston)

JAMA 273:289–294, 1995 119-96-31–2

Objective.—Prostate cancer, the second leading cause of cancer death among men in the United States, can be detected by measuring the level of prostate-specific antigen (PSA) in the serum. Because levels of PSA are directly proportional to tumor volume and because testing is relatively inexpensive, some advocate routine screening of men for prostate cancer. Others argue that because PSA does not measure severity of the disease, routine screening is not cost-effective. The results of a prospective evaluation of the specificity and sensitivity of the test, as well as the lead time, cutoff levels, and relative risks associated with levels of PSA, were reported.

Methods.—A total of 366 men with prostate cancer and 1,098 randomly selected controls participated in the 10-year study. Prostate-specific antigen titers were compared, and sensitivity and specificity were determined for each year of follow-up. There were 183 aggressive (stage C or D) tumors, 160 nonaggressive (stage A or B) tumors, and 23 intermediately aggressive tumors.

Results.—Overall sensitivity at the standard cutoff of 4.0 ng/mL was 46%, but it decreased significantly with time since last blood collection, particularly for younger men. Sensitivity was 87% for aggressive tumors and 53% for nonaggressive tumors. The overall specificity was 91% and changed little from year to year. Maximum validity was achieved at a cutoff of 3.3 ng/mL. The diagnostic lead time was estimated at 5.5 years. Only 40% of cancers detected after 5 years were nonaggressive. Men with levels of PSA between 2.0 and 3.0 ng/mL had a relative risk of 5.5 compared with men whose PSA values were less than 1.0 ng/mL.

Conclusion.—One PSA test had a high specificity and sensitivity for detecting prostate cancer within 4 years. Prostate-specific antigen values below the standard cutoff were associated with a significantly increased risk of prostate cancer. The value of routine screening must be assessed in terms of cost and prognosis for patients with prostate cancer.

► This article reviews the sensitivity and specificity of PSA as a screening test for prostate cancer. The population examined included 366 men with known prostate cancer and 1,098 randomly selected controls. The study covered a 10-year period.

At a cutoff point of 4.0 ng/mL, PSA had a surprisingly low overall sensitivity of 46%. This sensitivity decreased with time after the last blood collection, especially in younger men. Sensitivity was higher for aggressive tumors than for nonaggressive prostatic cancer. The overall specificity was good—91%.

Men with an increased level of PSA (2.0–3.0 ng/mL), which was below the cutoff point of 4.0, had a 5.5-fold risk of prostatic cancer relative to those with a value of less than 1.0 ng/mL.

From this report one concludes that prostatic acid phosphatase is a pretty good but not perfect screening test for prostatic cancer, but is it worth the effort and cost? Read the next article and see.

M.J. Cline, M.D.

Screening for Prostate Cancer: A Decision Analytic View

Krahn MD, Mahoney JE, Eckman MH, Trachtenberg J, Pauker SG, Detsky AS (Univ of Toronto; Toronto Hosp; Wellesley Hosp, Toronto; et al)

JAMA 272:773–780, 1994 119-96-31–3

Background.—Digital rectal examination (DRE) and measurement of serum prostate-specific antigen (PSA) are widely used in screening for prostatic cancer in men older than 50 years. Transrectal ultrasound (TRUS) is also used in the attempt to detect prostatic cancer at an early stage. However, the benefits of early detection remain unproven, taking into consideration the indolent nature of many prostatic cancers, the advanced age of the patients, the invasiveness and complications of treatment, and the high cost of screening. In a decision analytic cost-utility analysis, the clinical and economic effects of screening for prostate cancer with PSA, TRUS, and DRE were determined.

Methods.—Four potential screening programs involving various combinations of DRE, TRUS, and PSA were considered, each starting with a single episode of screening. The 4 policies were compared with a conservative policy of treatment only when symptoms developed. Each combination of tests was assumed to predict the rate of cancer detection and stage distribution. Radical prostatectomy was the assumed treatment for localized cancer. The 5 strategies were compared for calculated life expectancy, quality-adjusted life expectancy (QALE), and cost-utility ratios for unselected and high-prevalence populations.

Results.—For unselected men between 50 and 70 years of age, PSA or TRUS screening resulted in prolongation of unadjusted life expectancy. On its own, because it detects only more advanced tumors, DRE yielded no increases in life expectancy at any age. Assuming that perioperative mortality increased along with age-related comorbidity, a net loss in life expectancy was estimated to occur with screening in men older than 70 years. For older men with more advanced cancer at the time of detection, the life expectancy gains decreased or disappeared. Screening was predicted to produce a net loss in QALE of 3–13 days. Calculated cost-effectiveness ratios for the various screening programs ranged from $113,000 to $729,000 per incremental life-year saved. Although screening with PSA alone was the most attractive screening policy at all ages, its cost-effectiveness ratio remained high. A similar pattern was observed in high-prevalence populations.

Conclusions.—Prostate cancer screening does not appear to be justifiable as a rational health policy. Although screening programs may marginally reduce mortality from prostatic cancer, this benefit is more than outweighed by the morbidity of treatment. Contrary to some recommendations and to current practice trends, these authors do not advocate PSA or TRUS screening for asymptomatic men. An editorial comment on this study suggests that physicians should counsel their patients about the potential trade-offs associated with screening and treatment, providing them with the accurate information needed to make a decision regarding testing.

▶ Prostate cancer is gaining in importance as a medical problem. It is now the second leading cause of cancer deaths among men. As a result of both an aging population and increased application of screening procedures, the rates for radical prostatectomy have risen sixfold between 1984 and 1990.

Radical surgery for prostate cancer is associated with high morbidity and a high rate of permanent unpleasant complications such as incontinence. Intensive radiotherapy also often exacts a high price in terms of complications such as cystitis and proctitis. Because patients who have prostate cancer are often elderly and because the disease is often indolent, the value of screening is uncertain.

The authors of this study estimate that it costs between $113,000 and $729,000 for each incremental year of life, and they conclude that screening for prostate cancer is probably not worthwhile when both cost and quality of life are considered in the equation. In the words of the authors, "screening will result in net harm rather than net health benefit." Although others may disagree with this conclusion, I can find no flaw in their analysis.

M.J. Cline, M.D.

Kaposi's Sarcoma–Associated Herpesvirus-Like DNA Sequences in AIDS-Related Body-Cavity–Based Lymphomas

Cesarman E, Chang Y, Moore PS, Said JW, Knowles DM (New York Hosp-Cornell Med Ctr, NY; Columbia Univ, New York; Cedars-Sinai Med Ctr, Los Angeles)

N Engl J Med 332:1186–1191, 1995 119-96-31–4

Background.—In patients who have AIDS, there is a 40% chance that cancer, especially Kaposi's sarcoma or non-Hodgkin's lymphoma, will develop. Two novel DNA fragments were recently found in 90% of Kaposi's sarcoma lesions from patients with AIDS. In patients with AIDS who did not have Kaposi's sarcoma, these DNA fragments were also found in 6 of 39 tissue samples. These DNA fragments were not found in patients who did not have AIDS. The DNA fragments resembled DNA from 2 herpesviruses. In patients without AIDS, an association between Kaposi's sarcoma and lymphoid cancer has been reported, and in patients with AIDS-related Kaposi's sarcoma, a high-risk of malignant lymphoma has been reported. The etiologic relation between these neoplasms is unclear. Tissue samples of AIDS-related and non–AIDS-related lymphoid neoplasms were examined for Kaposi's sarcoma–associated herpesvirus sequences.

Methods.—The DNA of 193 lymphoid neoplasms from 42 patients with AIDS and 151 patients without AIDS was analyzed. Southern blot hybridization and the polymerase chain reaction were used to identify sequences of Kaposi's sarcoma–associated herpesvirus. Polymerase chain reaction products in positive samples were compared with Kaposi's sarcoma–associated herpesvirus sequences in Kaposi's sarcoma tissue from patients with AIDS.

Results.—In 8 lymphomas in patients with AIDS, Kaposi's sarcoma–associated herpesvirus sequences were identified (Fig 2). These 8 were body-cavity–based lymphomas and contained the Epstein-Barr viral genome. In the other 185 lymphomas, no Kaposi's sarcoma–associated herpesvirus sequences were found. In the body-cavity–based lymphomas,

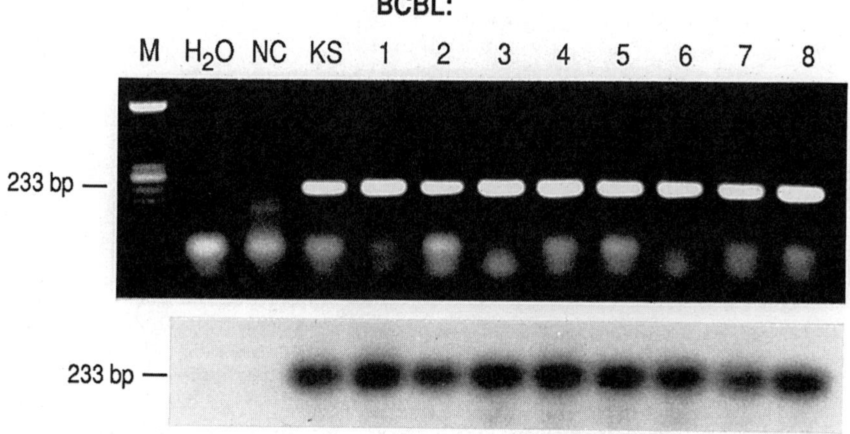

FIGURE 2.—Polymerase chain reaction (*PCR*) amplification of DNA from AIDS-related body-cavity–based lymphomas, using the $KS330_{233}$ primers. The **upper panel** shows the ethidium bromide–stained agarose gel of the amplification products of DNA from a molecular-weight marker (*M; Hind*III-digested lambda and *Hae*III-digested Phi-X DNA), water (*H_2O*), and DNA from a negative control (*NC*; HL-60 cell line), a positive control (*KS*), and lymphomas 1 through 8. The **lower panel** shows specific hybridization of the PCR products to an internal oligonucleotide probe end-labeled with phosphorus-32, after transfer to nitrocellulose filters. (Reprinted by permission of *The New England Journal of Medicine.* Cesarman E, Chang Y, Moore PS, et al: Kaposi's sarcoma–associated herpesvirus-like DNA sequences in AIDS-related body-cavity–based lymphomas. *N Engl J Med* 332:1186–1191, Copyright 1995, Massachusetts Medical Society.)

there were 40–80 times more Kaposi's sarcoma–associated herpesvirus sequences than in Kaposi's sarcoma lesions.

Conclusions.—These 8 lymphomas are distinct clinicopathologic entities. Kaposi's sarcoma–associated herpesvirus is associated with Kaposi's sarcomas; the neoplastic nature of Kaposi's sarcoma is unclear. Body-cavity–based lymphomas are malignant, however. The presence of Kaposi's sarcoma–associated herpesvirus sequences in these lymphomas indicates that a novel herpesvirus has a role in their development.

► In 1994, DNA sequences of a previously unidentified human herpesvirus were found to be frequently associated with Kaposi's sarcoma in patients who had AIDS.[1] The virus, which has come to be known as Kaposi's sarcoma–associated herpesvirus (KSHV), is also sometimes found in patients with AIDS who do not have Kaposi's sarcoma. It is still not proven with certainty that Kaposi's sarcoma is a monoclonal malignancy. Nevertheless, a causative role for KSHV in the development of the lesions of Kaposi's sarcoma seems likely. Epstein-Barr virus, another herpesvirus, has been implicated in the development of nasopharyngeal carcinoma and Burkitt's lymphoma.

The lymphomas that develop in patients with AIDS are usually of B-cell origin. They are about equally divided between 3 types of lymphoma: small noncleaved-cell, large-cell, and large-cell immunoblastic plasmacytoid. A rare type of lymphoma in patients who have AIDS is so-called body-cavity lymphoma in which the malignant cells grow as an effusion rather than as a solid mass in pleural, pericardial, or peritoneal spaces.

The authors of this study found that there is a frequent association between these body-cavity lymphomas and KSHV, an association not found in other types of lymphoma. This association strongly suggests that the virus is the causative agent of this unusual lymphoma, and it strengthens the concept that some herpesviruses are the pathogenetic agents in some human cancers.

M.J. Cline, M.D.

Reference

1. Chang Y, Cesarman E, Pessin MS, et al: Identification of herpesvirus-like DNA sequences in AIDS-associated Kaposi's sarcoma. *Science* 266:1865–1869, 1994.

Quality of Life After Palliative Radiotherapy in Patients With Hormone-Resistant Prostate Cancer: Single Institution Experience

Fosså SD (Norwegian Radium Hosp, Oslo, Norway)

Br J Urol 74:345–351, 1994 119-96-31–5

Background.—The goal of treatment of patients with hormone-resistant prostate cancer is to improve their quality of life. It is difficult to determine whether this goal is being met because there are few methods of assessing quality of life. A self-administered questionnaire addressing the quality of life of these patients was developed in 1986 and later improved. The efficacy of radiotherapy in relieving pain and improving the quality of life of patients with hormone-resistant prostate cancer was assessed.

Methods.—The questionnaire was completed by 137 patients aged 48–87 years who had hormone-resistant prostate cancer. Patients received either strontium-89 (150 MBq) or external beam radiotherapy. Quality of life was assessed before treatment and at 3 months in surviving patients.

Results.—The validity and reliability of the questionnaire were acceptable. Physicians' assessment and patients' perception of physical function correlated significantly. The median scale scores of physical function, pain, and overall quality of life as assessed by the patient distinguished significantly those with a poor life expectancy from those with a more favorable life expectancy. Alkaline phosphatase, performance status, and physical function were significant independent prognostic factors. At 3 months, patients who received palliative radiotherapy reported some pain relief; 35% of patients who were assessable had reduced the amount of analgesic they took; and overall quality of life was unchanged.

Conclusions.—It is possible to assess the quality of life of patients with hormone-resistant prostate cancer, and this assessment can offer valuable information. Palliative radiotherapy was less effective in patients with very advanced disease than is suggested in the literature and should be started at an earlier stage of disease. Questionnaires addressing quality of life continue to be improved.

► In the 1993 YEAR BOOK OF MEDICINE, we abstracted articles that examined whether aggressive treatment was indicated in advanced prostate cancer. The general conclusion at that time was that aggressive therapy was, in general, not indicated. This article continues the analysis of the management of prostate cancer. It addresses the issue of whether palliative radiotherapy provides benefit with regard to quality of life in patients with advanced hormone-resistant prostate cancer. The answer: *not much.*

M.J. Cline, M.D.

Long-Term Follow-Up of the First Randomized Study of Cisplatin Versus Carboplatin for Advanced Epithelial Ovarian Cancer

Taylor AE, Wiltshaw E, Gore ME, Fryatt I, Fisher C (Royal Marsden Hosp, London)

J Clin Oncol 12:2066–2070, 1994 119-96-31–6

Introduction.—In women with ovarian cancer, cisplatin has had a response rate as high as 65% in untreated patients and 27% in previously treated patients, but its side effects include neurotoxicity, nephrotoxicity, ototoxicity, and a high incidence of severe emesis. A less toxic analogue, carboplatin, has had a response rate of 25% in women with relapsed carcinoma, but with no evidence of neurotoxicity, nephrotoxicity, or ototoxicity, and considerably less vomiting. The efficacy of single-agent cisplatin and single-agent carboplatin was compared in untreated women with stage III or IV ovarian cancer in an 8-year study.

Methods.—Carboplatin was given to 67 women, and cisplatin was administered to 64 women. Every 4 weeks for 10 courses, cisplatin was administered, with courses 1–5 given at a dosage of 100 mg/m^2 and courses 6–10 given at a dosage of 30 mg/m^2. Carboplatin was also given every 4 weeks for 10 courses with a dosage of 400 mg/m^2. After 5 courses of chemotherapy, women who had clinical or radiologic evidence of responses had second-look surgery. In this crossover study, women were crossed over to the other drug because of nonresponse, progressive disease, or toxicity.

Results.—Cisplatin had an overall response rate of 53.8% and carboplatin had an overall response rate of 38.4%. With cisplatin, there were 16 (30.8%) complete remissions, and with carboplatin, there were 14 (26.9%) complete remissions. There was no statistical significance in the responses between the 2 drugs. With the cisplatin, the median duration of response was 21 months and the 5-year relapse-free survival rate was 22%. With the carboplatin, the median duration of response was 17 months, and the 5-year relapse-free survival rate was 25%. The median duration of survival for the cisplatin was 19.5 months, and its 5-year survival rate was 15%. For the carboplatin, median duration of survival was 13 months, and its 5-year survival rate was 19%. The median follow-up of patients was 9 years. Cisplatin caused more crossover because of toxicity than carboplatin, with 50% of women crossing over from cisplatin and 3.3% of women crossing over from carboplatin.

Conclusion.—Similar long-term survival results were found with cisplatin and carboplatin in women with advanced ovarian cancer. Carboplatin is equally as effective as cisplatin, yet with fewer side effects, in short-term and in long-term survival.

▶ In 1973, cisplatin was first described as an effective chemotherapeutic agent for ovarian cancer. It soon became a standard component of multiagent chemotherapy programs in this and other epithelial cancers. It is, however, a relatively difficult agent to use and has a number of significant toxicities including nephrotoxicity, neurotoxicity, and ototoxicity. It also causes severe nausea and vomiting. As a result of a search for a less toxic analogue, carboplatin was developed and entered into clinical trials in the early 1980s. Carboplatin is myelosuppressive but lacks the other toxicities of cisplatin.

A number of previous reports have suggested that carboplatin is about as effective as cisplatin in treating ovarian cancer. This study did a direct long-term comparison between the 2 agents in 131 patients with stages III and IV ovarian cancer. The results show that cisplatin and carboplatin have similar long-term effects on survival and disease-free survival. This is an important observation because it means that the less toxic drug can be used.

M.J. Cline, M.D.

Ten-Year Results of a Randomized Trial Evaluating Prolonged Low-Dose Adjuvant Chemotherapy in Node-Positive Breast Cancer: A Joint European Organization for Research and Treatment of Cancer: Dutch Breast Cancer Working Party Study

Clahsen PC, van de Velde CJH, Welvaart K, van Driel OJR, Sylvester RJ, and Cooperating Investigators (European Organization for Research and Treatment of Cancer Data Ctr, Brussels, Belgium; Univ Hosp Leiden, The Netherlands)

J Clin Oncol 13:33–41, 1995 119-96-31–7

Background.—Although preliminary results of adjuvant chemotherapy in axillary node-positive breast cancer have been promising, questions concerning both the effects of such treatment on overall survival and the disadvantages of short- or long-term side effects have remained. The effects of prolonged low-dose adjuvant chemotherapy on survival and toxicity in patients with axillary node-positive breast cancer were thus investigated.

Patients and Methods.—Four hundred fifty-two patients who received postoperative irradiation were included. Patients were prospectively randomized in a trial (European Organization for Research and Treatment of Cancer 09771) comparing surgery and prolonged low-dose chemotherapy vs. surgery alone. Chemotherapy was administered for 24 months and included monthly courses of cyclophosphamide, 50 mg/m^2 orally on days 1–14; methotrexate, 15 mg/m^2 IV on days 1 and 8; and fluorouracil, 350 mg/m^2 IV on days 1 and 8 (CMF).

Results.—A trend for treatment effect in favor of chemotherapy was observed for disease-free survival, with a 10-year disease-free survival rate of 43% for the chemotherapy group and a rate of 36% noted for the controls. Overall survival time was significantly increased in the patients who received chemotherapy. A 10-year overall survival rate of 59% was observed for the chemotherapy arm, compared with 50% for the control arm. Time to local relapse was also significantly prolonged in the chemotherapy group (hazards ratio, 0.63). A particular benefit of chemotherapy was observed in patients with 1–3 positive axillary nodes and those with estrogen receptor–negative tumors. Toxicity was observed in 93% of the patients, although no toxic deaths occurred.

Conclusions.—Prolonged low-dose adjuvant CMF can significantly increase overall survival in women with node-positive axillary breast cancer. Toxicity, however, is considerable, despite reduction of the dose of chemotherapy by 50%. Thus, conventional dose short-term regimens may be preferable in the treatment of node-positive breast cancer.

► The first trial of using adjuvant chemotherapy to treat patients with breast cancer who were undergoing surgery was initiated in 1958. Combination chemotherapy for breast cancer was introduced in the early 1960s, and the first study of the use of CMF as adjuvant chemotherapy for poor-risk breast cancer was initiated in 1973. Today, 6 months of treatment with CMF is generally considered the standard adjuvant treatment for patients younger than 50 years of age who have breast cancer and risk factors for recurrence of disease.

Because in 1973–1976 the long-term effects of adjuvant therapy were unknown, this study was started to examine prolonged (2-year) adjuvant therapy with low doses of CMF. The results indicate that such a program provides a benefit over and above that of no adjuvant therapy, but toxicity is substantial. Therefore, *there appears to be no advantage of prolonged treatment over a conventional 6-month program of treatment with CMF.*

M.J. Cline, M.D.

First Isolated Locoregional Recurrence Following Mastectomy for Breast Cancer: Results of a Phase III Multicenter Study Comparing Systemic Treatment With Observation After Excision and Radiation

Borner M, for the Swiss Group for Clinical Cancer Research (Inst of Med Oncology, Inselspital, Bern, Switzerland)

J Clin Oncol 12:2071–2077, 1994 119-96-31–8

Background.—Because effective local therapy does not prevent the development of distant metastases, micrometastases are generally thought to develop long before locoregional recurrence is detected and, in many patients, before the primary tumor is found. To date, there have been no prospective randomized clinical trials of the effect of systemic therapy on the outcomes of patients with isolated locoregional recurrence after local therapy.

Methods.—The study subjects were 167 low-risk patients with estrogen receptor–positive (ER+) recurrence or, when receptor status was unknown, a disease-free interval (DFI) of more than 12 months and no more than 3 recurrent tumor nodules. Seventy-nine percent were postmenopausal. By random assignment, the patients were treated with observation after local therapy or tamoxifen (TAM) until disease progression.

Findings.—Overall, the median observation was 6.3 years. The median duration of disease-free survival (DFS) was 26 months in the patients under observation and 82 months for those receiving TAM. This was primarily the result of a reduction in further local recurrences. The occurrence of early distant metastases was delayed. In a multivariate analysis, DFI and TM therapy were identified as significant prognostic factors for DFS. The respective overall survival rates at 5 years were 76% and 74%. Also, DFI was a prognostic indicator for overall survival.

Conclusions.—Compared with observation alone, systemic treatment with TAM after isolated locoregional breast cancer recurrence significantly increased 5-year DFS rates from 36% to 59% and prolonged median DFS by more than 4.5 years in patients with ER+ tumors or with a DFI of longer than 12 months with minimal tumor burden. Currently, TAM has no significant effect on overall survival, but the median survival duration of the population studies has not been reached.

▶ When breast cancer recurs locally without evidence of distant metastases, one must institute local therapy such as irradiation to control local disease. Should one, in addition, give systemic treatment at this point in the natural history of the disease? This study compares doing nothing (observation) with tamoxifen administration in 167 patients. By every parameter one can think of, tamoxifen wins. Note that most of the patients were postmenopausal and had favorable prognosis, estrogen receptor–positive disease. Nevertheless, the message is clear: *Tamoxifen is worth trying along with measures to control the local recurrence of breast cancer.*

M.J. Cline, M.D.

PART FOUR

THE HEART AND CARDIOVASCULAR DISEASE

ROBERT A. O'ROURKE, M.D.

Introduction

During the past year, many important basic and clinical research studies have been published that likely will modify preventive measures, diagnostic assessment, and treatment for many patients with suspected or definite clinical cardiovascular disease. Many of these reports are detailed and discussed in the Heart and Cardiovascular Disease section of the 1996 YEAR BOOK OF MEDICINE.

This section of the 1996 YEAR BOOK OF MEDICINE includes 9 chapters and a total of 55 abstracted publications plus editorial comments based on these and many additional references. The contents of Chapter 32, Risk Factors for Coronary Artery Disease, provide further support for the protective role of high-density lipoprotein cholesterol (HDL-C) in the clinical manifestations of atherosclerosis. The combination of low HDL-C and high triglyceride levels particularly appears to be associated with an increased risk of atherosclerotic disease among individuals with a borderline high or high total cholesterol level. Two reports indicating reductions in the risk of cardiovascular death and other coronary events in patients treated with the hepatic hydroxymethylglutaryl coenzyme A (HMG-CoA) reductase inhibitors simvastatin or pravastatin are highlighted. Also included in this chapter are discussions concerning the effects of estrogen and estrogen/progestin regimens on coronary disease risk factors in postmenopausal women and the improvement in myocardial perfusion abnormalities as determined by positron emission tomography after long-term intense risk factor modification. A report from the Cardiovascular Health Study details the usefulness of subclinical disease criteria for identifying high-risk older individuals who may be candidates for more acute intervention.

Chapter 33, Acute Coronary Syndromes, forms the largest component of this section of the YEAR BOOK. Information concerning the incremental value of the leukocyte differential and the rapid creatinine kinase–MB isoenzyme for the early diagnosis of myocardial infarction is presented. There is a discussion concerning the greater benefit of low–molecular weight heparin as compared with heparin or heparin plus aspirin in patients with acute coronary syndromes. This benefit appears to be attributable to the high and sustained plasma antithrombin activity that is achieved with the administration of low–molecular weight heparin. Chapter 33 also contains information concerning the relative cost-effectiveness of thrombolytic therapy with tissue plasminogen activator as compared with streptokinase for acute myocardial infarction, and it emphasizes the lower rate of recurrent ischemia after primary coronary angioplasty as compared with reperfusion therapy with thrombolytic agents. Evidence is presented for a favorable effect of infarct coronary artery patency on prognosis after acute myocardial infarction; however, the problem of reocclusion of an initially patent infarct-related artery persists. Data concerning the results of coronary artery bypass graft surgery after thrombolytic therapy in patients with acute myocardial infarction are also discussed. Additional information indicates that the resting left ventricular ejection fraction before discharge provides prognostic information for patients receiving thrombolytic therapy for myocardial infarction as it does in patients who are not treated with thrombolytic agents. However, the increased mortality rate at any reduced level of left ventricular ejection fraction is far less than in those patients who did not receive thrombolytic therapy. The Fourth International Study of Infarct Survival (ISIS-4) clinical trial using early administration of oral captopril, oral mononitrate, and IV magnesium sulfate in a large number of patients with acute myocardial infarction is discussed in detail.

In this chapter on Acute Coronary Syndromes, the usefulness of β-blocker treatment in older postinfarction patients is discussed, as is the ongoing debate as to how often β-blocking drugs are underused in the secondary prevention treatment of patients who have recovered from an acute myocardial infarction. Data from Europe concerning a role of the concentration of fibrinogen, tissue plasminogen activator antigen, and von Willebrand factor in the risk for acute coronary artery syndromes are also presented.

The magnitude of left ventricular dysfunction in patients with painful as compared with asymptomatic episodes of myocardial ischemia, as determined by exercise echocardiography, is the subject of a report in Chapter 34, Chronic Coronary Heart Disease. Chapter 34 contains an extensive discussion of the medical and revascularization therapies available for patients with silent myocardial ischemia. Several recent reports from the Asymptomatic Cardiac Ischemia Pilot (ACIP) study are emphasized. The benign prognosis of patients with syndrome X and the results of diagnostic testing and treatment of patients with this syndrome are considered, as is an intravascular ultrasound study that showed an abnormal vasomotor response in patients who had atheroma or intimal thickening by ultrasound despite having had relatively normal coronary arteriograms. There also is considerable discussion concerning the selection of medical treatment for stable angina pectoris as well as the recent controversy concerning the usefulness and possible adverse effects of calcium antagonists in patients with coronary heart disease. Comparison of quality-of-life scores in patients with angina pectoris after single-vessel coronary angioplasty and in patients with medical therapy (ACME Trial) is detailed, as is the role of coronary arteriography and myocardial revascularization before noncardiac vascular surgery.

In Chapter 35, Coronary Interventional Procedures, the selection of coronary angioplasty as compared with coronary artery bypass surgery for patients with symptomatic three-vessel coronary artery disease is addressed. There is a discussion of the usefulness of directional atherectomy vs. balloon angioplasty for coronary ostial and nonostial left anterior descending coronary artery lesions, and a multicenter randomized trial of coronary angioplasty vs. directional atherectomy for patients with saphenous vein bypass graft lesions is also presented. Data indicating that stent implantation in aorta ostial saphenous vein graft lesions has a high probability of procedural success, a relatively low morbidity, and uncommon adverse clinical events are provided. New information is given concerning the in-hospital costs of percutaneous coronary revascularization. Also, the 3-year costs of myocardial revascularization in the Emory Angioplasty vs. Surgery Trial (EAST) are mentioned.

Chapter 36 concerns cardiomyopathy heart failure. In this chapter, an important study concerning the usefulness of immunosuppressant drugs in patients with myocarditis presents results that are largely negative. Information concerning the variability and phenotype expression of β-myosin heavy chain mutations and the potential relationship to sudden cardiac death in patients with hypertrophic cardiomyopathy is discussed. The dissociation between exertional symptoms and circulatory function in patients with heart failure is emphasized, and data are provided concerning the potential mechanisms of hemodynamic improvement by dual-chamber pacing for patients who have severe left ventricular dysfunction.

In Chapter 36, information is provided concerning (1) the predictors of systolic and diastolic improvement in patients who have dilated cardiomyopathy treated with metoprolol, and (2) the hemodynamic and clinical improvement in such patients treated with the vasodilating β-blocker, carvedilol. Several papers pertain to patients with cardiac transplantation, with one delineating the characteristics of patients surviving more than 10 years after cardiac transplantation, another indicating the high incidence of transplant coronary artery disease detected by intravascular ultrasound, and a third suggesting that the HMG-CoA reductase inhibitors slow the progression of coronary arteriopathy in patients after transplant by more than just their effect on cholesterol reduction.

Valvular heart disease is the subject of Chapter 37. In this chapter, a long-term prospective follow-up study indicates a favorable outcome for most patients with severe asymptomatic chronic aortic regurgitation. An important study indicates that left ventricular contractile impairment is not irreversible in all patients who have long-term severe mitral regurgitation. Significant mitral regurgitation in patients with rheumatic mitral disease who are receiving anticoagulants is described as being associated with a marked decrease in the relative risk of thrombus formation as determined by transesophageal echocardiography. Also presented is a report detailing the correlation of high levels of serotonin with valvular abnormalities in patients with the carcinoid syndrome, as are data concerning the optimal oral anticoagulation therapy for patients with various types of mechanical heart valves.

Chapter 38 concerns noninvasive testing. In this chapter, data are provided indicating that both silent and symptomatic ischemia during exercise ECG testing have an adverse effect on the 12-year survival rate in women and in men with known coronary heart disease. Also discussed is the role of adenosine thallium-201 tomography in defining the long-term risk in patients after acute myocardial infarction; the absolute extent of scintigraphic myocardial ischemia is a strong predictor of overall cardiac risk, particularly when combined with a low ejection fraction, in patients who do or do not receive thrombolytic therapy. In Chapter 38, low-dose dobutamine echocardiography compared favorably with thallium single-photon emission computed tomography (SPECT) in predicting improvement in regional left ventricular function after surgical myocardial revascularization. Several references are discussed that compare different types of stress testing using myocardial perfusion imaging or echo wall motion assessment in the detection of reversible myocardial ischemia. Specific information is provided concerning the biphasic response of echocardiographic wall thickening during low- and high-dose dobutamine infusion for determining areas of ischemic but viable myocardium. The usefulness of MRI in assessing the severity of mitral regurgitation and its comparison with invasive techniques is the subject of an important clinical research report.

Arrhythmia is the subject of Chapter 39. A large patient study concerning the natural history of atrial fibrillation documents the association of atrial fibrillation with subsequent congestive heart failure, independent of the effect of ischemic heart disease or hypertension. A serial transesophageal echocardiographic evaluation of patients with nonrheumatic atrial fibrillation shows that reduced thromboembolic complications with 4 weeks of precardioversion anticoagulation are related to atrial thrombus resolution. Another report contained in this chapter defines the best predictive criteria of the signal-averaged ECG for predicting serious arrhythmic events in patients who have had myocardial infarction.

Chapter 39 includes a study of the mechanisms responsible for spontaneous sustained ventricular tachycardia in the Electrophysiologic Study vs. Electrocardiographic Monitoring (ESVM) Trial, and a report from the Cardiac Arrhythmia Suppression Trial (CAST) indicates that almost 50% of the patients with both congestive heart failure syndrome and an ejection fraction less than 30% did not achieve arrhythmia suppression. Preliminary data suggesting that increased QT dispersion interval may be a marker of increased risk for life-threatening arrhythmias after a previous myocardial infarction are also included.

An important study concerning the efficacy of amiodarone in patients with congestive heart failure and asymptomatic ventricular arrhythmia is detailed. In this large multicenter trial, amiodarone was effective in suppressing arrhythmias and in improving ventricular function, but it did not reduce the frequency of sudden death or prolong survival. Another abstract in this chapter confirms that the internal cardioverter defibrillator (ICD) is an extremely effective device that accurately detects and successfully terminates ventricular tachyarrhythmias.

"Other topics" comprise Chapter 40. Evidence is presented that cocaine affects left ventricular function primarily by increasing left ventricular afterload and not by a persistent reduction in myocardial contractility. The management of cocaine-associated myocardial ischemia in patients with chest pain resulting from the use of this illicit drug is also discussed. The relationship of the third heart sound on cardiac auscultation to deceleration of transmitral valve flow velocity is reviewed, and the differences in the rate of deceleration in elderly and young patients with third heart sounds are elucidated. The efficacies of different treatment strategies for neurocardiogenic syncope are discussed in detail. The recur rence rate of symptoms in severely symptomatic patients treated with head-up tilt-guided pharmacologic therapy is lower than in those receiving empiric therapy or given no medication.

Also discussed in the Other Topics chapter is single-lung transplantation for pulmonary hypertension. In one institution's experience, optimal survival for the entire group of 34 patients was reasonable, with 91% surviving and being discharged from the hospital after transplantation. The early post-transplant normalization of pulmonary vascular resistance and right ventricular ejection fraction appears to persist during follow-up in survivors, at least up to 3 years.

Robert A. O'Rourke, M.D.

32 Risk Factors for Coronary Artery Disease

Combined Effects of HDL Cholesterol, Triglyceride, and Total Cholesterol Concentrations on 18-Year Risk of Atherosclerotic Disease

Burchfiel CM, Laws A, Benfante R, Goldberg RJ, Hwang L-J, Chiu D, Rodriguez BL, Curb JD, Sharp DS (Natl Heart, Lung, and Blood Inst, Honolulu, Hawaii; Stanford Univ, Palo Alto, Calif; Kuakini Med Ctr, Honolulu, Hawaii; et al)

Circulation 92:1430–1436, 1995 119-96-32–1

Background.—Although individual lipids and lipoproteins are known to play an important role in the development of atherosclerotic disease, the combined effects of high-density lipoprotein cholesterol (HDL-C), triglyceride (TG), and total cholesterol (TC) levels on the risk of coronary heart disease (CHD) have not been well established. Data on Japanese-American men enrolled in the Honolulu Heart Program were analyzed prospectively to determine the combined effects of HDL-C, TG, and TC on the incidence of atherosclerotic disease.

Methods.—A total of 1,646 men aged 51–72 years were included in the analysis. All were free of CHD, stroke, and cancer, and none were taking lipid-reducing medication at the time of enrollment. These men had been assessed periodically since 1965–1968. The mean follow-up was 15.9 years.

Findings.—Atherosclerotic events developed in 318 men during follow-up. These included angina, coronary insufficiency, aortic aneurysm, definite CHD, or thromboembolic stroke. Definite CHD developed in 170 men between 1970 and 1988 (Fig 2). A Cox regression analysis was performed after the subjects were stratified according to levels of TC, HDL-C, and TG. With high levels of HDL-C and low TG as the reference, age-adjusted relative risks (RR) of atherosclerotic events were significantly

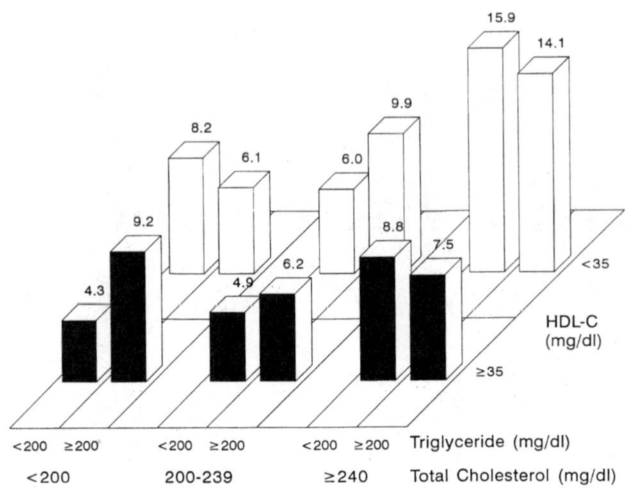

FIGURE 2.—Age-adjusted incidence of coronary heart disease per 1,000 person-years by high-density lipoprotein cholesterol (*HDL-C*), triglyceride, and total cholesterol levels for the Honolulu Heart Program, 1970–1988. (Reproduced with permission [*Circulation*]. Copyright [1995] American Heart Association.)

increased in men with low HDL-C and high TG at borderline-high and high levels of TC but not in those with desirable TC levels. The increased risks were unaffected by blood pressure, obesity, fat distribution, diabetes, smoking status, and alcohol intake.

Conclusions.—Men with low HDL-C and high TG levels apparently have an increased risk of atherosclerotic disease when their TC is borderline-high or high. This increased risk is independent of other cardiovascular risk factors. Thus, the combined effects of HDL-C and TG may be important to consider in screening efforts.

► This study was conducted in men of Japanese-American ancestry, who have been characterized as having a somewhat lower incidence of coronary heart disease relative to other Caucasian populations. The results from this study provide support for a protective role of HDL-C in the clinical manifestations of atherosclerosis. The protective effect of HDL-C, apparent when evaluating HDL-C without taking triglycerides into account, was more evident at higher levels of *total cholesterol* and may be attributable to the role of HDL-C in reversing cholesterol transport or in impeding oxidative modification of low-density lipoprotein cholesterol. The combination of low HDL-C and high TG levels appears to be associated with an increased risk of atherosclerotic disease among individuals with a borderline-high or high *total cholesterol* level. At desirable levels of *total cholesterol,* the risks of atherosclerotic disease and coronary heart disease were not increased in subjects with the combination of low HDL-C and high TG levels.

In a report from the Program on the Surgical Control of the Hyperlipidemias (POSCH), Buchwald and associates[1] analyzed the disease-free intervals and calculated the freedom from atherosclerotic events. An overall mortality rate of 10% occurred at 6.7 years in the control group and at 9.4 years in the group undergoing partial ileal bypass, both of whom had coronary heart disease and hypercholesterolemia. The 2.7-year gain in the disease-free interval in the intervention group was statistically significant. The marked lipid modification achieved by partial ileal bypass in the POSCH trial led to demonstrable increases in the disease-free intervals for overall coronary heart disease mortality, confirmed nonfatal myocardial infarction, and coronary intervention procedures.

R.A. O'Rourke, M.D.

Reference

1. Buchwald H, Campos CT, Boen JR, et al: Disease-free intervals after partial ileal bypass in patients with coronary heart disease and hypercholesterolemia: Report from the program on the surgical control of the hyperlipidemias (POSCH). *J Am Coll Cardiol* 26:351–357, 1995.

Baseline Serum Cholesterol and Treatment Effect in the Scandinavian Simvastatin Survival Study (4S)

Scandinavian Simvastatin Survival Study Group (Aker Hosp, Oslo, Norway)

Lancet 345:1274–1275, 1995 119-96-32-2

Background.—In the Scandinavian Simvastatin Survival Study (4S), the administration of simvastatin to patients with previous myocardial infarction or stable angina pectoris reduced the risk of death by 30%, as a result of a 42% reduction in the risk of death from coronary heart disease, and reduced the risk of major coronary events (coronary death and nonfatal myocardial infarction) by 34%. Data from the 4S were used to determine whether lipid levels were relevant to the prognosis in these patients.

Methods.—The risk of major coronary events (coronary death and nonfatal myocardial infarction) in relation to baseline levels of cholesterol was studied in 4,444 men and women aged 35–70 years with coronary heart disease randomized to placebo or simvastatin, 20–40 mg daily. The patients' serum level of total cholesterol ranged from 5.5 to 8.0 mmol/L, and the level of triglyceride was 2.5 mmol/L or less in those following a lipid-lowering diet.

Results.—Simvastatin significantly reduced the risk of major coronary events in all quartiles of baseline total, high-density lipoprotein (HDL) and low-density lipoprotein (LDL) cholesterol. The risk reductions produced by simvastatin compared with placebo were similar in each quartile of baseline lipid concentration and did not differ significantly between quartiles for any lipid variable. The relative risk reduction in the simvastatin group was 35% in the lowest quartile and 36% in the highest quartile of baseline LDL cholesterol. There was no significant treatment by baseline-value interaction for any lipid.

Conclusion.—The reduction in the relative risk of major coronary events produced by simvastatin is independent of baseline concentration of lipids. This observation is only valid for patients with coronary heart disease with serum total cholesterol ranging from 5.5 to 8.0 mmol/L and other characteristics similar to the patients included in the 4S.

▶ This short report is an important follow-up of the 4S trial reported in September 1994.[1] It is of great interest that simvastatin significantly reduced the risk of major coronary events in all quartiles of baseline total, HDL, and LDL cholesterol, and by a similar amount in each quartile of baseline lipid concentration.

Recently, Shepherd and colleagues, of the West of Scotland Coronary Prevention Study Group, reported their findings on preventing coronary heart disease by using pravastatin in men with hypercholesterolemia.[2] They randomly assigned 6,595 men who were 45–64 years of age and had a mean plasma cholesterol level of 272 ± 23 mg/dL to receive either pravastatin or placebo. The average follow-up was 4.9 years. Pravastatin lowered plasma cholesterol levels by 20% and LDL cholesterol levels by 26%, whereas there was no change with placebo. There was a relative reduction in the risk of nonfatal myocardial infarction or death from coronary heart disease of 31% ($P < 0.001$) in the pravastatin group. There were similar reductions in the risk of definite nonfatal myocardial infarction, death from coronary heart disease, and death from all cardiovascular causes. This study reported a 22% reduction in the risk of death from any cause in the pravastatin group. These results with pravastatin are comparable to those previously reported with simvastatin, with pravastatin reducing the incidence of myocardial infarction and death from cardiovascular causes without adversely affecting the risk of death from noncardiovascular causes in men with moderate hypercholesterolemia and no history of myocardial infarction.

R.A. O'Rourke, M.D.

References

1. Scandinavian Simvastatin Survival Group: Randomised trial of cholesterol lowering in 4444 patients with coronary heart disease: The Scandinavian Simvastatin Survival Study (4S) *Lancet* 344:1383–1389, 1994.
2. Shepherd J, Cobbe SM, Ford I, et al: Prevention of coronary heart disease with pravastatin in men with hypercholesterolemia. *N Engl J Med* 333:1301–1307, 1995.

Effects of Estrogen or Estrogen/Progestin Regimens on Heart Disease Risk Factors in Postmenopausal Women: The Postmenopausal Estrogen/Progestin Interventions (PEPI) Trial

The Writing Group for the PEPI Trial (Nat Insts of Health, Bethesda, Md)
JAMA 273:199–208, 1995 119-96-32–3

Background.—Previous studies have shown that unopposed oral estrogens can increase high-density lipoprotein cholesterol (HDL-C), decrease low-density lipoprotein cholesterol (LDL-C), and reduce the risk of heart disease in postmenopausal women. Conversely, progestins have been shown to act as an estrogen antagonist on lipoprotein levels. The effects of unopposed estrogen and estrogen/progestin regimens on specific heart disease risk factors were examined.

Participants and Methods.—A randomized, double-blind study segregated 875 menopausal women into 1 of 5 treatment groups. Patients were treated with either placebo, conjugated equine estrogen (CEE), 0.625 mg/day; CEE, 0.625 mg/day, and cyclic medroxyprogesterone acetate (MPA, 10 mg/day) for 12 days per month; CEE, 0.625 mg/day, and consecutive MPA at 2.5 mg/day; or CEE, 0.625 mg/day, plus cyclic micronized progesterone (MP) at 200 mg/day for 12 days per month. Follow-up was conducted at 3, 6, and 12 months, and every 6 months thereafter for 3 years.

Results.—All active treatment regimens resulted in a significantly increased level of HDL-C compared with placebo (Fig 1). Administration of unopposed CEE and CEE with MP had significantly greater effects than other treatments. All active treatments also resulted in a similar decrease in LDL-C levels over time, which stabilized at their lowest levels after 6–12 months of treatment. Triglyceride levels were significantly increased in all active treatment regimens when compared with placebo. Neither systolic nor diastolic blood pressure was affected by these treatment regimens. Although mean changes in 2-hour insulin did not differ among treatment assignments, 2-hour glucose levels increased significantly among those assigned to active treatment compared with placebo recipients. Pairwise comparisons indicated that women receiving placebo had increased fibrinogen compared with those on active regimens. All women gained weight during the study; however, those receiving placebo gained the most weight, whereas those receiving unopposed CEE gained significantly less. Women receiving unopposed CEE had significantly more adenomatous (27 patients) and atypical hyperplasia (14 patients) and were more likely to have a hysterectomy (7 patients) than any other women. Additionally, breast cancer developed in 8 patients during the 3-year follow-up.

Conclusions.—Although the addition of MPA to CEE therapy involves significant decreases in HDL-C, lipoprotein profiles are still improved and fibrinogen levels lowered when compared with placebo. Furthermore, the high rate of adenomatous or atypical endometrial hyperplasia found in women receiving unopposed CEE therapy argues strongly for joint CEE and MP therapy in menopausal women with a uterus.

► This is an extremely important study relative to the reduction of risk for coronary artery disease in postmenopausal women. The PEPI study confirms that oral estrogen taken either alone or with progestin is associated with improved lipoprotein and lower fibrinogen levels compared with placebo and shows that the magnitude of these differences is likely to be clinically significant. The PEPI trial also resulted in significant increases from baseline in HDL-C, the most important readily measured determinant of cardioprotection in women, even when progestin was added to estrogen therapy. However, the 10% annual rate of adenomatous or atypical endometrial hyperplasia observed in women assigned to receive estrogen only makes

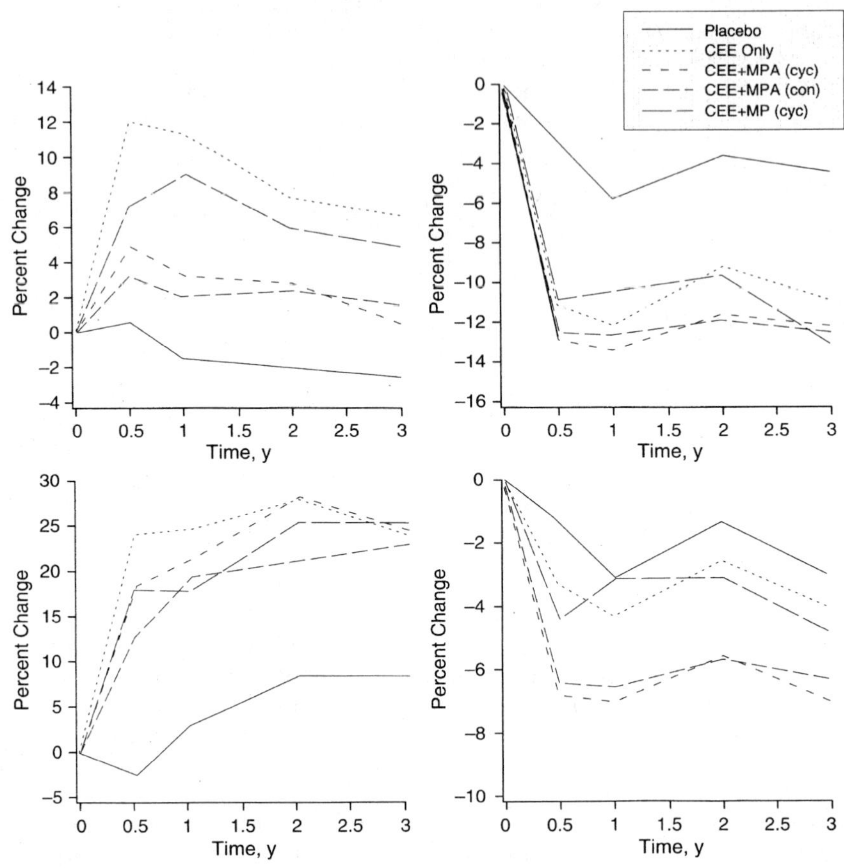

FIGURE 1.—Mean percent change from baseline by treatment arm for high-density lipoprotein cholesterol (**top left**), low-density lipoprotein cholesterol (**top right**), triglycerides (**bottom left**), and total cholesterol (**bottom right**). *Abbreviations: CEE,* conjugated equine estrogen; *MPA,* medroxyprogesterone acetate; *MP,* micronized progesterone. (Courtesy of The Writing Group for the PEPI Trial: Effects of estrogen or estrogen/progestin regimens on heart disease risk factors in postmenopausal women: The Postmenopausal Estrogen/Progestin Interventions (PEPI) Trial. *JAMA* 273:199–208, Copyright 1995, American Medical Association.)

combination hormone therapy the treatment of choice for women with a uterus. For women without a uterus, there is no need for the addition of the progestin. For these women with a uterus, estrogen plus progestin appears to spare the endometrium and preserve the bulk of estrogen's favorable effect on risk factors, including HDL-C. Large clinical trials are currently under way in the United States to determine whether and how much hormone therapy will reduce the risk of heart disease in healthy women (Women's Health Initiative) or the risk of new cardiovascular events in women who already have heart disease (Hormone Estrogen/Progestin Replacement Study). These studies will also assess the incidence of breast cancer in postmenopausal women receiving long-term estrogen therapy.

Proudler et al.[1] studied the effect of estrogen/progestin on serum angiotensin-converting enzyme (ACE) activity in postmenopausal women. After 6 months, ACE activity was reduced by 20% ($P < 0.001$) in 28 treated women but remained unchanged in 16 controls. Such changes in serum ACE levels may represent a novel mechanism by which hormone replacement therapy reduces coronary heart disease risk in women in addition to its effect on hyperlipidemia and HDL-C.

In another report relative to the risk of coronary heart disease in women, Fuchs and associates[2] assessed the risk for coronary heart disease in relation to the amount and type of alcoholic beverages consumed in 85,709 female nurses who were followed every 2 years from 1980 to 1992. The data, similar to that previously reported in men, indicate that light-to-moderate intake of alcohol is associated with a significantly lower risk of death than occurs in nondrinkers or heavy drinkers, primarily because of a lower risk of cardiovascular disease. This apparent survival benefit with light-to-moderate alcohol consumption appeared largely confined to women at greater risk for coronary heart disease.

R.A. O'Rourke, M.D.

References

1. Proudler AJ, Ahmed AI, Crook D, et al: Hormone replacement therapy and serum angiotensin-converting-enzyme activity in postmenopausal women. *Lancet* 346:89–90, 1995.
2. Fuchs CS, Stampfer MJ, Colditz GA, et al: Alcohol consumption and mortality among women. *N Engl J Med* 332:1245–1250, 1995.

Changes in Myocardial Perfusion Abnormalities by Positron Emission Tomography After Long-Term, Intense Risk Factor Modification

Gould KL, Ornish D, Scherwitz L, Brown S, Edens RP, Hess MJ, Mullani N, Bolomey L, Dobbs F, Armstrong WT, Merritt T, Ports T, Sparler S, Billings J
(Univ of Texas, Houston; Univ of California, San Francisco)
JAMA 274:894–901, 1995 119-96-32–4

Objective.—A randomized study was undertaken to monitor myocardial perfusion abnormalities in patients with coronary artery disease who either received conventional care by their own physicians or participated in a strict program of risk factor modification.

Study Plan.—Thirty-five patients 41–70 years of age were entered into the study after angiography had documented the presence of coronary artery disease. None were taking lipid-lowering drugs or had recently had myocardial infarction. The left ventricular ejection fraction exceeded 25%. Fifteen patients were randomly assigned to receive usual care, which primarily consisted of antianginal treatment. Twenty patients were assigned to a program that included a very low fat vegetarian diet, mild-to-moderate aerobic exercise 3 times per week, stress management, and group support. The fat content of the diet was less than 10% of total energy intake.

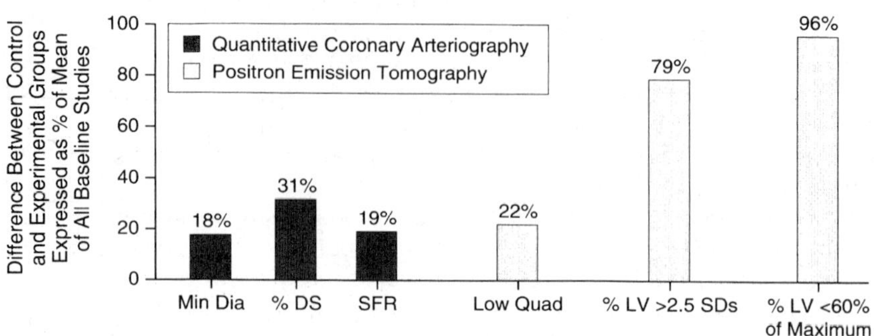

FIGURE 6.—Comparison of changes by positron emission tomography (*PET*) and quantitative coronary arteriography (*QCA*). The PET measures were myocardial quadrant with the lowest average activity (*Low Quad*), percentage of left ventricle (*LV*) outside 2 SDs of normals, and percentage of LV activity less than 60% of maximal activity. Measurements by QCA were minimum absolute lumen diameter (*Min Dia*), percent diameter stenosis (*%DS*) and stenosis flow reserve (*SFR*) derived from the integrated effects of absolute lumen diameter, %DS, and cumulative length effects based on fluid dynamic equations, all as previously validated and reported. The absolute difference in changes between the control and experimental groups (without the minus or plus sign for direction of change) was expressed as a percentage of the mean of each measurement at baseline for all patients. (Courtesy of Gould KL, Ornish D, Scherwitz L, et al: Changes in myocardial perfusion abnormalities by positron emission tomography after long-term, intense risk factor modification. *JAMA* 274:894–901, Copyright 1995, American Medical Association.)

Assessment.—Quantitative coronary angiography and dipyridamole positron emission tomography (PET) were done at baseline and 5 years after randomization.

Results.—Perfusion abnormalities on dipyridamole PET images improved after 5 years of risk factor modification but became worse in control patients. The percent of the left ventricle with activity that was less than 60% of peak activity on the PET image of normalized counts increased by 13.5% in controls and decreased by 4.2% in the experimental group. Both the extent and intensity of perfusion abnormalities on resting PET images were lessened significantly in the experimental group. Improvement in myocardial perfusion was at least as great as, or greater than, the change in angiographic coronary stenosis (Fig 6).

Conclusion.—In patients with coronary artery disease who undergo intensive risk factor modification, a modest regression of coronary stenosis is accompanied by significant improvement in myocardial perfusion.

▶ This interesting study indicates that the size and severity of myocardial perfusion abnormalities documented by PET at rest and after dipyridamole stress decrease or improve in patients undergoing intense risk factor modification in comparison with an increase or worsening in perfusion abnormalities in patients treated with standard therapy.

The authors of this study suggest that the modest regression of coronary artery stenosis after intense risk factor modification in patients with coronary atherosclerosis is associated with significantly decreased size and severity of perfusion abnormalities by rest-dipyridamole (PET) perfusion imaging as compared with a worsening of myocardial perfusion in control patients treated with standard antianginal therapy at 5 years of follow-up. Although the results of this study are encouraging and are consistent with those of recent studies on the decreased morbidity and mortality in patients undergoing intensive risk factor reduction, additional confirmatory studies in larger numbers of patients will be of great interest.

Recently, the American Heart Association published a "Guide to Comprehensive Risk Reduction for Patients with Coronary and Other Vascular Disease."[1] In this guide, risk interventions include cessation of smoking, management of lipids, physical activity, and weight management, as well as the use of estrogens in postmenopausal women. For lipid management, the primary goal is to reduce serum low-density lipoprotein cholesterol to less than 100 mg/dL, whereas the secondary goal is to increase the serum level high-density lipoprotein cholesterol above 35 mg/dL while reducing serum triglycerides below 200 mg/dL. Specific recommendations related to weight management and physical activity, cessation of smoking, and the use of antilipid drugs are given in these guidelines.

In a report from the Health Professionals Follow-Up Study of 44,895 males 40–75 years of age,[2] no significant association between dietary intake of *n*-3 fatty acids or fish intake and the risk of coronary heart disease could be shown. For men in the top one fifth of the group in terms of intake of *n*-3 fatty acids, the relative risk of coronary heart disease was 1.12 as compared with the men in the bottom one fifth. For men who consumed 6 or more servings of fish per week as compared with those who consumed 1 serving per month or less, the relative risk of coronary disease was only 1.14. These data suggest that increasing fish intake from 1–2 servings per week to 5–6 servings per week does not substantially reduce the risk of coronary heart disease among men who are initially free of cardiovascular disease.

Another report[3] concerns a nested case-control study that was conducted among the 14,916 participants in the Physicians' Health Study with a sample of plasma obtained before randomization. Each participant with a myocardial infarction occurring during the first 5 years of follow-up was matched by smoking status and age with a randomly chosen control participant who had not had coronary heart disease. The mean levels of plasma fish oils in case and control participants, expressed as percent of total fatty acids, were not statistically significantly different. Results adjusted for major cardiovascular risk factors showed no association between the initial fish oil levels and the incidence of myocardial infarction.

R.A. O'Rourke, M.D.

References

1. Smith SC Jr, and the Secondary Prevention Panel: Preventing heart attack and death in patients with coronary disease. *Circulation* 92:2–4, 1995.
2. Ascherio A, Rimm EB, Stampfer MJ, et al: Dietary intake of marine n-3 fatty acids, fish intake, and the risk of coronary disease among men. *N Engl J Med* 332:977–982, 1995.
3. Guallar E, Hennekens CH, Sacks FM, et al: A prospective study of plasma fish oil levels and incidence of myocardial infarction in U.S. male physicians. *J Am Coll Cardiol* 25:387–394, 1995.

Subclinical Disease as an Independent Risk Factor for Cardiovascular Disease

Kuller LH, Shemanski L, Patsy BM, Borhani NO, Gardin J, Haan MN, O'Leary DH, Savage PJ, Tell GS, Tracy R (Univ of Pittsburgh, Pa; Univ of Washington, Seattle; Univ of California-Irvine, Davis; et al)
Circulation 92:720–726, 1995 119-96-32-5

Objective.—Individuals who have subclinical cardiovascular disease (CVD) are at higher risk of having atherosclerotic disease at another site. In the longitudinal observational Cardiovascular Health Study, individuals with a history of clinical CVD were evaluated, as were the high- and low-risk groups without a history of clinical CVD among adults 65 years and older.

Methods.—Ankle-brachial blood pressure, carotid artery stenosis, and wall thickness were measured; echocardiography and ECG responses were evaluated; and responses to the Rose Angina and Claudication questionnaire were tallied for 2,239 men and 2,962 women aged 65 years or older. The patients were followed twice a year for an average of 2.39 years. The incidence of fatal and nonfatal events was recorded.

Results.—On the basis of clinical disease criteria, 3 groups were established: 1,617 patients had clinical disease, 1,942 had subclinical CVD, and 1,642 had clinical CVD (Table 1). Patients with clinical disease had the highest mortality rate. Both men and women with subclinical disease had a significantly higher incidence of coronary heart disease (CHD), nonfatal myocardial infarction (MI), and angina pectoris. Women had a higher incidence of MI, and men had a higher incidence of CHD events. The

TABLE 1.—Criteria for Clinical and Subclinical Disease in the Cardiovascular Health Study

Clinical Disease Criteria	Subclinical Disease Criteria
Atrial fibrillation or pacemaker	Ankle-arm index ∞ 0.9 mm Hg
History of intermittent claudication or peripheral vascular surgery	Internal carotid wall thickness > 80th percentile
	Common carotid wall thickness > 80th percentile
History of congestive heart failure	Carotid stenosis > 25%
History of stroke, transient ischemic attack, or carotid surgery	Major ECG abnormalities*
	Abnormal ejection fraction on echocardiogram
History of coronary artery bypass graft surgery or percutaneous transluminal coronary angioplasty	Abnormal wall motion on echocardiogram
	Rose questionnaire claudication positive
History of angina or use of nitroglycerin	Rose questionnaire angina positive
History of myocardial infarction	

* According to Minnesota Code, ventricular conduction defects (7-1, 7-2, 7-4); major Q/QS-wave abnormalities (1-1, 1-2); left ventricular hypertrophy (high-amplitude R waves with major or minor ST-T abnormalities (3-1, 3-3, and 4-1–4-3 or 5-1–5-3); isolated major ST/T-wave abnormalities (4-1, 4-2, 5-1, 5-2).

(Courtesy of Kuller L, Borhani N, Furberg C, et al: Prevalence of subclinical atherosclerosis and cardiovascular disease and association with risk factors in the Cardiovascular Health Study. *Am J Epidemiol* 139:1164–1179, 1994.)

increased risk of CHD for men with subclinical disease was 2.0, and for women it was 2.5. The increased risk of death was 2.9 for men and 1.7 for women. Subclinical and clinical disease were independent predictors of death. Men had significantly higher mortality rates than women. Lipoprotein levels, blood pressure, smoking history, and diabetes had little effect on the significant association between subclinical disease and risk of CVD.

Conclusion.—Subclinical disease is an independent risk factor for cardiovascular disease and may be useful in identifying older individuals at high risk for clinical disease.

► This report from the Cardiovascular Health Study (CHS) is interesting. The use of the subclinical disease criteria indicated in Table 1 may become an appropriate approach for identifying high-risk older individuals who may be candidates for more active intervention to prevent the onset of clinical disease and its complications. The measurement of subclinical disease used in the CHS can be done primarily by technicians. These tests could be used to identify high-risk individuals, especially older individuals. The costs of the various measures of subclinical disease are important in determining their usefulness for identifying certain older individuals who are at high risk of clinical disease. The follow-up of the CHS cohort will provide the opportunity to determine the best combination of measures of subclinical disease for the prediction of incident clinical disease and the relative costs.

In a study of 1,809 consecutive black patients who underwent both coronary arteriography and M-mode echocardiography as part of a diagnostic evaluation, the effect of echocardiographically determined left ventricular hypertrophy (LVH) on survival was compared with the number of stenosed coronary vessels and left ventricular systolic dysfunction.[1] When left ventricular hypertrophy, number of diseased coronary vessels, and left ventricular dysfunction (ejection fraction < 45%) were subjected to multivariant analysis, hypertrophy conferred a relative risk of 2.4 (95% confidence interval, 1.7–3.2). By comparison, the presence of a single stenosed vessel did not increase the risk of death, and multivessel disease and ejection fraction of < 45% were associated with a relative risk of 1.6 and 2.0, respectively. Therefore, LVH was associated with greater relative risk for mortality than were other traditional measures of coronary disease severity. The high prevalence and powerful risk of left ventricular hypertrophy likely make an important contribution to the adverse survival rates among black patients with heart disease and may account partially for the black/white differential.

Another interesting report concerns the prognosis of left ventricular geometric patterns in the Framingham Heart Study.[2] The goal of this study was to determine the incremental prognostic value of left ventricular geometric patterns (consisting of normal geometry, concentric hypertrophy, eccentric hypertrophy, and concentric remodeling) beyond that provided by risk factors for CVD, including left ventricular mass. Framingham Heart Study subjects, who were free of CVD, had a prevalence of abnormal left ventricular geometry of approximately 24% in men and approximately 28% in women. The use of echocardiography to classify left ventricular geometry provided little incremental prognostic information beyond left ventricular mass and other cardiovascular risk factors. Although abnormal left ventricular geometry was associated with cardiovascular events and all-cause mortality, it was also associated with differences in left ventricular mass. Adjustment for cardiovascular risk factors and left ventricular mass attenuated the strength of the association of geometric patterns with outcomes.

It has been hypothesized that occupations that have both high psychological demands and low decision latitude (job strain) can lead to coronary artery disease. Recently, Hlatky and his associates[3] assessed the job duties and work environment of 1,489 patients undergoing diagnostic coronary arteriography. Seventy-six percent of the patients were male and 80% were white. By design, all patients were employed, 60% in white-collar jobs and only 16% in jobs requiring heavy labor. Traditional cardiac risk factors were more prevalent in the 922 patients with significant coronary artery disease. In a multivariate analysis, job strain did not correlate significantly with the presence of coronary disease, nor did it correlate with angina frequency at the time of arteriography. Job strain did not predict cardiac events during follow-up.

R.A. O'Rourke, M.D.

References

1. Liao Y, Cooper RS, McGee DL, et al: The relative effects of left ventricular hypertrophy, coronary artery disease, and ventricular dysfunction on survival among black adults. *JAMA* 273:1592–1597, 1995.
2. Krumholz HM, Larson M, Levy D: Prognosis of left ventricular geometric patterns in the Framingham Heart Study. *J Am Coll Cardiol* 25:879–884, 1995.
3. Hlatky MA, Lam LC, Lee KL, et al: Job strain and the prevalence and outcome of coronary artery disease. *Circulation* 92:327–333, 1995.

33 Acute Coronary Syndromes

Incremental Value of the Leukocyte Differential and the Rapid Creatine Kinase–MB Isoenzyme for the Early Diagnosis of Myocardial Infarction
Thomson SP, Gibbons RJ, Smars PA, Suman VJ, Pierre RV, Santrach PJ, Jiang N-S (Mayo Clinic and Found, Rochester, Minn)
Ann Intern Med 122:335–341, 1995 119-96-33–1

Objective.—The potential value of leukocyte differential for the diagnosis of myocardial infarction has been limited by the great variations in the traditional manual leukocyte differential. Using the more accurate automated hematology analyzers, the potential incremental value of the leukocyte differential as an early marker of myocardial infarction was studied, particularly when combined with the rapid creatine kinase–MB isoenzyme.

Study Design.—In a prospective, blinded study, 511 consecutive adult patients seen in the emergency department with chest pain were studied. Automated leukocyte differentials, rapid creatine kinase–MB levels, cortisol levels, and routine clinical measurements were obtained at the time of initial assessment.

Results.—Sixty-nine patients had myocardial infarction. These patients had higher total creatine kinase and creatine kinase–MB levels, lower relative lymphocyte count, higher total and relative granulocyte counts, and higher cortisol levels than patients without infarction. Among patients with myocardial infarction, the sensitivity of a diagnostic ST-segment elevation was 39%, specificity was 99%, and positive predictive value was 93%. Although cortisol was the most sensitive marker (68%), it was also the least specific (86%), with a positive predictive value of only 52%. The sensitivity of relative lymphocytopenia (lymphocyte decrease < 20.3%) was 58%, and that of an increased rapid creatine kinase–MB level was 56%; specificities were 91% and 93%, respectively; and positive predictive values were 58% and 66%, respectively. The combination of relative lymphocytopenia and increased rapid creatine kinase–MB level had a sensitivity of 44%, but increased specificity to 99.7% and positive predictive value to 97% (Fig 4). Multivariate logistic regression analysis showed that both relative lymphocytopenia and increased rapid creatine kinase–MB level were significant independent predictors of infarction in patients

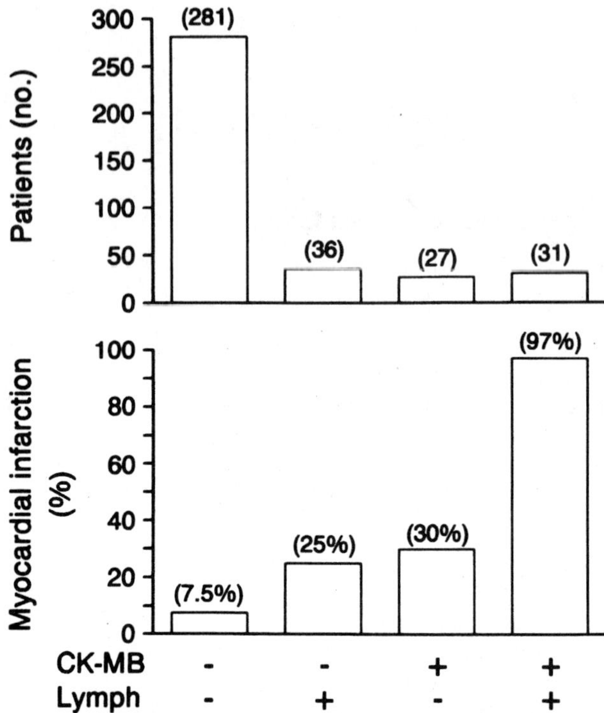

FIGURE 4.—Combinations of results for relative lymphocyte percentages and rapid creatine kinase–MB levels. Patient subgroups were determined by relative lymphocyte percentages (*lymph*) and rapid creatine kinase–MB (*CK-MB*) levels; *plus* indicates abnormal results; *minus* indicates normal results. The number of patients with each combination of relative lymphocyte percentages and CK-MB levels (**top**) and the prevalence of acute myocardial infarction (**bottom**) are shown. (Courtesy of Thomson SP, Gibbons RJ, Smars PA, et al: Incremental value of the leukocyte differential and the rapid creatine kinase–MB isoenzyme for the early diagnosis of myocardial infarction. *Ann Intern Med* 122:335–341, 1995.)

without ST-segment elevation. If the criterion for the diagnosis of myocardial infarction was the presence of both relative lymphocytopenia and increased rapid creatine kinase–MB level or ST-segment elevation, then the sensitivity for the diagnosis of infarction increased from 39% (with ST-segment elevation alone) to 65%, and both specificity (99%) and positive predictive value (94%) remained high.

Conclusion.—The combination of a relative lymphocytopenia and increased rapid creatine kinase–MB level is an accurate early marker of myocardial infarction, even in some patients without ST-segment elevation. This combination improves the sensitivity of early diagnosis when compared with that of ST-segment elevation alone.

► The differentiation of patients seen in the emergency room with myocardial infarction but no ECG ST-segment elevation from patients with unstable angina and other acute chest-pain syndromes is difficult. Markers reported for the early identification of acute myocardial infarction in such patients include initial clinical variables and initial and, often, serial measurements of creatinine kinase–MB, creatine kinase–MB isoforms, myoglobin, troponin T, and cortisol. The noninvasive technique results used to rule out myocardial infarction include no echocardiographic evidence of abnormal wall motion and the presence of no myocardial infarction perfusion abnormalities with technetium sestamibi radionuclide imaging.

In this particular study, relative lymphocytopenia obtained by automated leukocyte differential plus increased rapid creatine kinase–MB measurements were useful for the early diagnosis of acute myocardial infarction. Because of the low prevalence of infarction in patients with chest pain, any current individual marker, with the exception of ECG ST-segment elevation, is not specific enough to ensure a high positive predictive value. However, the presence of both a relative lymphocytopenia and an elevated rapid creatine kinase–MB level had a greater positive predictive value than either individual marker alone and may lead to the identification of patients with impending myocardial infarction.

In recent years, there has been considerable enthusiasm for the use of cardiac troponin T blood levels for the detection of myocardial necrosis. The marker cardiac troponin T has several potential advantages over creatine kinase–MB because it persists longer in the circulation than creatine kinase–MB, has a higher proportional increase in the blood above the discriminator value, and is a cardiac-specific molecule that can be differentiated from skeletal muscle isoforms by monoclonal antibodies. Its clinical value has been limited by the rather long turnaround time of 90 minutes for the usual enzyme immunoassay. Recently, Müller-Bardorff and colleagues[1] developed a whole-blood rapid assay device for cardiac troponin T, using gold-labeled and biotin-labeled monoclonal antibodies that give a positive or negative result in less than 20 minutes. A clinical analysis showed the same high sensitivity and specificity in the diagnostic time window for this rapid assay than did the less rapid conventional enzyme-linked immunoassay measurement of troponin T as an indicator for myocardial cell damage.

R.A. O'Rourke, M.D.

Reference

1. Müller-Bardorff M, Freitag H, Scheffold T, et al: Development and characterization of a rapid assay for bedside determinations of cardiac troponin T. *Circulation* 92:2869–2875, 1995.

Thrombin Generation and Activity During Thrombolysis and Concomitant Heparin Therapy in Patients With Acute Myocardial Infarction

Merlini PA, Bauer KA, Oltrona L, Ardissino D, Spinola A, Cattaneo M, Broccolino M, Mannucci PM, Rosenberg RD (Ca' Granda Niguarda Hosp, Milan, Italy; Harvard Med School, Boston; IRCCS Policlinico San Matteo, Pavia, Italy; et al)

J Am Coll Cardiol 25:203–209, 1995 119-96-33–2

Purpose.—Patients undergoing thrombolytic therapy show increased thrombin generation and activity. Although concomitant IV heparin is known to suppress increased thrombin activity, its effects on thrombin generation are unknown. Thrombin generation and activity were prospectively studied during thrombolysis and concomitant administration of heparin.

Methods.—Serial blood samples were obtained from 15 patients receiving streptokinase, 15 receiving recombinant tissue-type plasminogen activator, and 13 receiving anistreplase. These specimens were taken before the thrombolytics were administered as well as 90 minutes and 24 and 48 hours afterward. Before therapy began, the patients received a 5,000-IU IV bolus of heparin, followed by an infusion of 1,000 units/hr to maintain an activated partial thromboplastin time greater than 1.5 times baseline. Prothrombin fragment 1+2 was measured to assess thrombin generation, and plasma levels of fibrinopeptide A were measured to evaluate plasma levels of thrombin–antithrombin complex and thrombin activity.

Results.—Plasma levels of prothrombin fragment 1+2 increased during thrombolytic and concomitant heparin therapy, from 1.08 nmol/L at baseline to 2.73 nmol/L at 90 minutes. At the same time, thrombin–antithrombin complex increased from 6.5 to 17.1 μg/mL. No significant change occurred in fibrinopeptide A.

Conclusions.—Thrombolytic therapy is accompanied by increased thrombin generation, even if IV heparin is given at the same time. This is true whether fibrin-specific or non–fibrin-specific thrombolytic drugs are used.

▶ The finding of increased thrombin generation during thrombolysis despite the concomitant administration of heparin raises a number of questions. In addition to catalyzing the conversion of fibrinogen to fibrin, thrombin is a potent activator of a variety of cell events, including platelet aggregation, secretion and formation of thromboxane A_2, contraction of smooth muscle cells, and expression of tissue factor on endothelial cells, all of which may have a detrimental effect at the site of highly unstable postthrombolysis residual lesions. In the setting of coronary thrombolysis, thrombin is the main factor responsible for platelet activation. Accordingly, the beneficial results obtained with aspirin, which only inhibits the thromboxane induced by platelet aggregation, probably will be enhanced by direct thrombin inhibition.

There is increasing evidence from clinical trials that low–molecular weight heparin is effective in the treatment of venous and arterial thrombosis.

Low–molecular weight heparin appears to have a more favorable effect than heparin or heparin plus aspirin in patients who have acute coronary syndromes. Recently, Agnelli and associates[1] performed a pharmacokinetic study to compare the relative half-lives of prophylactic and therapeutic doses of low–molecular weight heparins by assessing antithrombin activity. High and sustained plasma antithrombin activity was achieved when low–molecular weight heparin was administered in therapeutic doses used in contemporary clinical trials with only a moderate prolongation of the activated partial thromboplastin time. Therefore, low–molecular weight heparin may be better than regular heparin for preventing recurrent coronary artery thrombosis in patients undergoing thrombolytic therapy.

Gurfinkel and associates[2] compared low–molecular weight heparin plus aspirin, regular heparin plus aspirin, and aspirin alone in the treatment of unstable angina and silent ischemia. In this study, aspirin plus low–molecular weight heparin given twice daily subcutaneously was superior to administration of aspirin plus regular IV heparin or aspirin alone in preventing episodes of recurring angina, nonfatal myocardial infarction, and the need for urgent revascularization. The incidence of silent myocardial ischemia by ECG monitoring also was significantly lower in those receiving low–molecular weight heparin plus aspirin.

R.A. O'Rourke, M.D.

References

1. Agnelli G, Iorio A, Renga C, et al: Prolonged antithrombin activity of low-molecular-weight heparins: Clinical implications for the treatment of thromboembolic diseases. *Circulation* 92:2819–2824, 1995.
2. Gurfinkel EP, Manos EJ, Mejaíl RI, et al: Low molecular weight heparin versus regular heparin or aspirin in the treatment of unstable angina and silent ischemia. *J Am Coll Cardiol* 26:313–318, 1995.

Cost Effectiveness of Thrombolytic Therapy With Tissue Plasminogen Activator as Compared With Streptokinase for Acute Myocardial Infarction

Mark DB, Hlatky MA, Califf RM, Naylor CD, Lee KL, Armstrong PW, Barbash G, White H, Simoons ML, Nelson CL, Clapp-Channing N, Knight JD, Harrell FE Jr, Simes J, Topol EJ (Duke Univ, Durham, NC; Stanford Univ, Palo Alto, Calif; Univ of Toronto; et al)

N Engl J Med 332:1418–1424, 1995 119-96-33–3

Background.—In the recent Global Utilization of Streptokinase and Tissue Plasminogen Activator for Occluded Coronary Arteries (GUSTO) trial, patients with acute myocardial infarction who received tissue plasminogen activator (t-PA) over 1½ rather than 3 hours, with two thirds of the dose given in the first 30 minutes, had a 30-day mortality that was 15% lower than that in streptokinase-treated patients.

Objective and Methods.—Based on data from the GUSTO study, the cost-effectiveness of t-PA treatment was compared with that of streptokinase. Life expectancy was projected from data on survivors of myocardial infarction in the Duke Cardiovascular Disease Database. The primary analysis assumed that no added treatment costs accrued because of the use of t-PA after the first year and that the survival benefit of using t-PA remained evident 1 year after enrollment.

Findings.—The consumption of resources in the first year was generally similar for the t-PA and streptokinase groups, although there was a trend toward more angioplasties and more readmissions in the former group. Survival at 1 year was slightly greater in the t-PA group (91% vs. 89.9%). The comparative primary cost-effectiveness ratio for using t-PA rather than streptokinase was approximately $33,000 per year of life saved. Variations in the higher costs of t-PA therapy influenced the cost-effectiveness ratio (Fig 3). A value of $50,000 was reached when the added cost of t-PA, including that of thrombolytic agents, exceeded $4,350 per patient. The cost-effectiveness ratio was reduced to $42,400 when the higher risk of disabling stroke attending t-PA treatment was taken into account.

Projection.—If accelerated t-PA therapy were to routinely replace streptokinase for patients with acute myocardial infarction, the cost would amount to about $500 million each year, but patients would gain 3.5 million additional years of life.

▶ The substitution of accelerated t-PA streptokinase in the treatment of acute myocardial infarction increased health benefits at a cost comparable to those of other expensive therapies routinely considered worthwhile. It should be emphasized that the cost-effectiveness ratios were less favorable

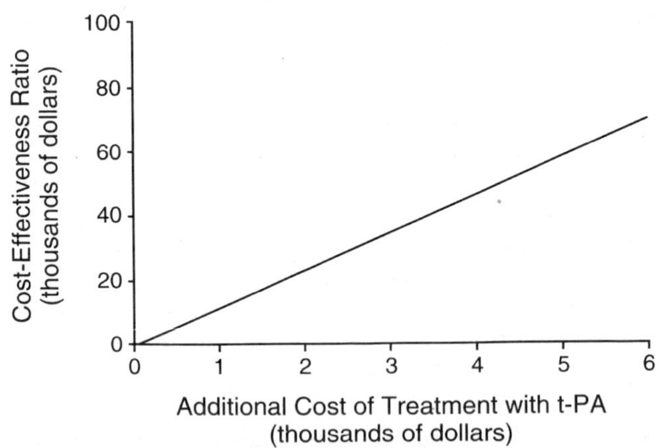

FIGURE 3.—Sensitivity analysis of the cost difference between treatment with tissue plasminogen activator (*t-PA*) and treatment with streptokinase, assuming no cost differences beyond the first year after treatment. The *y* axis shows cost-effectiveness ratios expressed as dollars per additional year of life saved. The *x* axis shows the increased cost per patient associated with treatment with t-PA. In the primary analysis, the increased cost per patient was $2,845. (Reprinted by permission of *The New England Journal of Medicine*. Mark DB, Hlatky MA, Califf RM, et al: Cost effectiveness of thrombolytic therapy with tissue plasminogen activator as compared with streptokinase for acute myocardial infarction. *N Engl J Med* 332:1418–1424, Copyright 1995, Massachusetts Medical Society.)

for all patients 40 years of age or younger and for patients 60 years of age or younger who had inferior wall myocardial infarctions. These groups had the lowest 1-year mortality rates and the smallest increase in survival attributable to treatment with t-PA. It is possible that careful subgroup analysis might indicate certain patients at low risk for subsequent cardiac events and mortality for whom streptokinase is the more cost-effective method of thrombolytic therapy.

In another report from the GUSTO-I trial, Gore and associates[1] analyzed the stroke incidence and outcomes in this international study of 4 thrombolytic therapies. The GUSTO-I trial demonstrated significant increases in total stroke and primary intracranial hemorrhage as a function of thrombolytic assignment, particularly in the combination treatment (streptokinase plus t-PA). This excess incidence of stroke with more aggressive thrombolytic therapy added 7 deaths per 1,000 patients treated to the mortality rate with accelerated t-PA compared with 5 deaths per 100 patients treated with streptokinase. However, because of the high mortality rate associated with stroke in this setting, there were similar proportions of disabled stroke survivors in the accelerated t-PA group, the streptokinase and subcutaneous heparin group, and the streptokinase and IV heparin group. Stroke remains a rare but often catastrophic complication of thrombolysis. Additional studies should assess the net clinical benefit of thrombolysis in high-risk subgroups, particularly in the elderly and in patients with hypertension or prior cerebrovascular events.

R.A. O'Rourke, M.D.

Reference

1. Gore JM, Granger CB, Simoons ML, et al: Stroke after thrombolysis: Mortality and functional outcomes in the GUSTO-I trial. *Circulation* 92:2811–2818, 1995.

Implications of Recurrent Ischemia After Reperfusion Therapy in Acute Myocardial Infarction: A Comparison of Thrombolytic Therapy and Primary Angioplasty

Stone GW, Grines CL, Browne KF, Marco J, Rothbaum D, O'Keefe J, Hartzler GO, Overlie P, Donohue B, Chelliah N, Timmis GC, Vlietstra R, Puchrowicz-Ochocki S, O'Neil WW (Cardiovascular Inst, El Camino Hosp, Mountain View, Calif; William Beaumont Hosp, Royal Oak Mich; Lakeland Regional Med Ctr, Lakeland, Fla; et al)

J Am Coll Cardiol 26:66–72, 1995 119-96-33–4

Background.—Early reperfusion during acute myocardial infarction has been shown to reduce mortality. Although thrombolytic therapy can be easily administered to these patients, it is associated with a high incidence of reocclusion. Primary percutaneous transluminal coronary angioplasty is an alternative therapy that may reduce the risk of reocclusion in these patients. The incidence of recurrent ischemia after different reperfusion strategies was investigated in a large group of patients with acute myocardial infarction.

Methods.—Patients admitted to any of 12 centers within 12 hours of the onset of acute myocardial infarction were prospectively randomized to receive either recombinant tissue-type plasminogen activator (rt-PA) or primary coronary angioplasty. Sixteen clinical variables were examined in 395 patients to identify predictors of recurrent ischemia.

Results.—Ischemia reccurred in 76 patients during their hospital stay, resulting in reinfarction in 18 patients and in death in 5 patients. Ischemia reccurred in 28% of patients after rt-PA, but in only 10% after coronary angioplasty. This significant difference contributed to a higher rate of reinfarction and death, catheterization and revascularization procedures, and prolonged hospital stay after thrombolysis (Fig 1). Multivariate analysis indicated that treatment with rt-PA, as opposed to coronary angioplasty, was the strongest predictor of recurrent ischemia, especially after the second day of hospitalization.

Conclusions.—Compared with thrombolytic therapy, primary coronary angioplasty, although invasive, significantly reduces the recurrence of ischemia and contributes to improved patient outcome. The low incidence of recurrent ischemia after day 2 of hospitalization in patients with successful angioplasty could facilitate safe early discharge and reduce costs.

▶ The role of acute primary coronary angioplasty vs. acute thrombolytic therapy in various groups of patients who have acute myocardial infarction remains controversial; in many geographic sites, the facilities are not readily available for direct coronary angioplasty, even though the amount of myocardial revascularization and the residual coronary artery stenosis of the infarct-related vessel are reduced to a greater extent by primary angioplasty. In this prospective randomized study, the incidence of recurrent ischemia

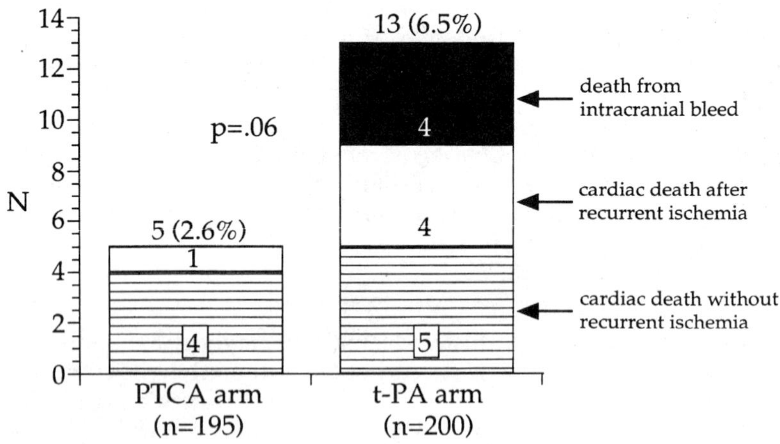

FIGURE 1.—Cause of death in 395 patients. *Abbreviations: n,* number of patients; *PTCA,* percutaneous transluminal coronary angioplasty; *t-Pa,* recombinant tissue-type plasminogen activator. (Reprinted with permission from the American College of Cardiology [*Journal of the American College of Cardiology,* 1995, 26:66–72.])

after angioplasty and after rt-PA therapy was similar within the first 2 days of admission; however, after hospital day 2, recurrent ischemia occurred in only 2 patients who received primary angioplasty compared with 27 patients who received rt-PA. Because the development of recurrent ischemia adversely affects patient outcome and increases resource utilization, the much lower rate of recurrent ischemia after primary coronary angioplasty is an important consideration in selecting reperfusion therapy when both are feasible.

In an assessment of patients with and without postinfarction angina 2 weeks after a myocardial infarction, Tabata et al.[1] performed coronary arteriography and angioscopy in 51 consecutive patients with a diagnosis of acute myocardial infarction. Coronary arteriography followed immediately by coronary angioscopy was performed in 17 patients with and 34 without postinfarction angina during the same period. The frequency of thrombus as observed by angioscopy was significantly higher in patients with than without postinfarction angina (17 of 17 vs. 5 of 34, respectively, $P < 0.01$). Therefore, infarct-related coronary artery thrombus is often present in early postinfarction angina and may be the primary pathogenic factor. Angioscopy was much more sensitive than coronary arteriography for the detection of coronary thrombus, as has been shown in other studies.

R.A. O'Rourke, M.D.

Reference

1. Tabata H, Mizuno K, Arakawa K, et al: Angioscopic identification of coronary thrombus in patients with postinfarction angina. *J Am Coll Cardiol* 25:1282–1285, 1995.

Effect of Infarct Artery Patency on Prognosis After Acute Myocardial Infarction

Lamas GA, for the Survival and Ventricular Enlargement Investigators (Mount Sinai Med Ctr, Miami Beach, Fla)

Circulation 92:1101–1109, 1995 119-96-33–5

Background.—Early restoration of infarct-related artery (IRA) patency results in the preservation of left ventricular function and improved outcomes in patients with acute myocardial infarction (AMI). However, the benefits of a patent IRA may be out of proportion to the amount of improvement in ventricular function. Also, such benefits may result not only from salvage of ischemic myocardium but also from the opening of the IRA beyond a narrow postinfarct time window. The effects of IRA patency on patient outcomes after acute MI with left ventricular ejection fraction and the extent of coronary disease were assessed, and the influence of angiotensin-converting enzyme (ACE) inhibitor therapy on patients with patent and occluded infarct arteries was determined.

Methods.—A total of 2,231 patients with documented MI and a left ventricular ejection fraction of 40% or less were enrolled in the Survival and Ventricular Enlargement (SAVE) study. By random assignment, the ACE inhibitor captopril, 50 mg 3 times/day, or placebo was given 3–16 days after MI. Mean follow-up was 3.5 years. Data on the 946 patients in whom IRA patency was established before randomization were included in the current analysis.

Findings.—Cardiac catheterization performed a mean 4.2 days after infarction demonstrated initial IRA occlusion in 30.7% of the patients. Seventeen percent of the patients had an occluded IRA after revascularization at the time of randomization. Clinical baseline characteristics were similar in those with persistently occluded IRAs and those with patent IRAs. However, patients with occluded arteries had a slightly lower ejection fraction than those with patent IRAs. In a Cox proportional-hazards analysis, the independent predictors of all-cause mortality were hypertension, number of diseased coronary arteries, occluded IRA, ejection fraction, age, and use of β-adrenergic receptor blockers. Occluded IRA, hypertension, number of diseased vessels, ejection fraction, use of β-adrenergic receptor blockers, and captopril treatment were independent predictors of a composite end point including cardiovascular mortality, morbidity, or a decrease in ejection fraction of 9 units or more.

Conclusions.—Patency of IRA within 16 days of MI predicts a favorable clinical outcome independent of the number of obstructed coronary arteries or left ventricular function. The benefits of ACE inhibition do not depend on whether the IRA is patent.

▶ The "time-independent" beneficial effect of a patent infarct-related coronary artery has been the topic of considerable discussion. In this report from the Survival and Ventricular Enlargement (SAVE) study concerning patients with a documented myocardial infarction and a left ventricular ejection fraction of 40% or less, an occluded infarct-related artery was a predictor of a composite end point consisting of cardiovascular mortality, morbidity, or reduction of ejection fraction of 9 units or more. It also is important that the use of β-blockade, although clinically determined rather than randomized, was beneficial independent of infarct-related artery patency and captopril therapy. The importance of a patent infarct-related artery may vary depending on the extent of myocardial infarction and its effect on left ventricular function, because all the patients included in the SAVE study had ejection fractions of 40% or less.

The frequent reocclusion of patent infarct-related arteries between 4 weeks and 1 year after myocardial infarction following initially successful thrombolytic therapy is well documented. White and associates[1] assessed the effect of combined aspirin and dipyridamole on long-term patency of the infarct-related artery. They studied 215 patients who had a patent infarct-related artery 4 weeks after myocardial infarction and randomized them to receive either a combination of 25 mg of aspirin and 200 mg of dipyridamole twice daily or placebo. At 1-year follow-up, 25% of 154 patients had reocclusion of the infarct-related artery; 23% of those receiving aspirin and dipyridamole had late reocclusion not different than 27% of those receiving placebo. There were no differences for the end points of cardiac death, myocardial infarction, or revascularization between those receiving antiplatelet drugs and those receiving placebo. As indicated in several studies, late reocclusion of a patent infarct-related artery is a frequent event, occurring in 25% to 30% of patients, and is not altered by antiplatelet therapy.

R.A. O'Rourke, M.D.

Reference

1. White HD, French JK, Hamer AW, et al: Frequent reocclusion of patent infarct-related arteries between 4 weeks and 1 year: Effects of antiplatelet therapy. *J Am Coll Cardiol* 25:218–223, 1995.

Coronary Artery Bypass Graft Surgery After Thrombolytic Therapy in the Thrombolysis in Myocardial Infarction Trial, Phase II (TIMI II)

Gersh BJ, Chesebro JH, Braunwald E, Lambrew C, Passamani E, Solomon RE, Ross AM, Ross R, Terrin ML, Knatterud GL, and the TIMI II Investigators (Mayo Clinic and Found, Rochester, Minn; Brigham and Women's Hosp, Boston; Maine Med Ctr, Portland; et al)

J Am Coll Cardiol 25:395–402, 1995 119-96-33–6

Background.—Thrombolytic therapy has been shown to decrease early mortality after acute myocardial infarction. Many patients undergo coronary bypass after thrombolytic therapy, but there are few data on the early and late outcomes in these patients. Data from the Thrombolysis in Myocardial Infarction trial, phase II (TIMI II) were analyzed to determine the results of coronary artery bypass grafting after thrombolytic therapy.

Methods.—Of 3,339 patients enrolled in the TIMI II trial, 390 underwent bypass surgery, a rate of about 12%. Fourteen percent of these patients had surgery within 24 hours after entry into the trial or within 24 hours of coronary angioplasty. The remaining 86% of patients had bypass surgery between 24 hours and 42 days after study entry. The results of surgery in these patients were evaluated, focusing on patient characteristics, the effects of previous percutaneous transluminal coronary angioplasty, and morbidity and mortality by patient subgroups.

Results.—Perioperative mortality was 16.7% for patients undergoing surgery within 24 hours of study entry or coronary angioplasty, compared with 3.9% for those with later surgery. The rate of perioperative myocardial infarction was about 6% in both groups; the rate of major hemorrhagic events was 74.1% in the early surgery group and 50.9% in the later surgery group. Early surgery was the only independent predictor of perioperative mortality on multivariate analysis. Multivessel disease and use of the internal thoracic artery were less frequent in the patients undergoing early bypass surgery. Among patients who survived the postoperative period, 1-year mortality rate after discharge was about 2% in both groups. There was just 1 documented case of recurrent myocardial infarction during this period.

Conclusions.—Bypass surgery after thrombolytic therapy carries an increased mortality rate, particularly for patients who have surgery within 24 hours of coronary angioplasty or during the evolving phase of acute myocardial infarction. On the other hand, the 1-year prognosis is excellent for perioperative survivors, who are generally regarded as being at elevated risk for death or recurrent infarction. This study will provide a useful baseline of information for comparison with future studies.

► In considering this study, it should be emphasized that of the 54 patients who underwent operation within 24 hours after entry into the study or after coronary angioplasty, only 1 was characterized as having an elective operation. The remainder had either persistent angina or complications after angioplasty. By contrast, in patients undergoing operation within 24 hours to 42 days from entry, approximately 65% of the patients were categorized as elective. The higher mortality rate in patients undergoing bypass surgery within 24 hours after study entry or after coronary angioplasty is consistent with other reports of mortality after emergency coronary surgical procedures and with the greater prevalence of hypotension and cardiogenic shock among these patients.

R.A. O'Rourke, M.D.

Value of Radionuclide Rest and Exercise Left Ventricular Ejection Fraction in Assessing Survival of Patients After Thrombolytic Therapy for Acute Myocardial Infarction: Results of Thrombolysis in Myocardial Infarction (TIMI) Phase II Study

Zaret BL, for the TIMI Study Group (Yale Univ, New Haven, Conn)

J Am Coll Cardiol 26:73–79, 1995 119-96-33-7

Background.—Before the introduction of thrombolytic therapy, left ventricular ejection fraction at rest and during exercise, and the difference between these 2 parameters, were important prognostic factors for patients with coronary disease. It has been suggested that these factors may have lost their prognostic importance with the advent of thrombolytic therapy.

Purpose.—The prognostic value of rest and exercise left ventricular ejection fraction was determined in coronary patients treated with thrombolytic therapy as part of the Thrombolysis in Myocardial Infarction (TIMI) trial.

Methods.—Radionuclide left ventricular ejection fraction was obtained at rest and during symptom-limited submaximal supine exercise. These measurements were compared with both cardiac and all-cause mortality. These results also were compared with those from the earlier Multicenter Postinfarction Research Group (MPRG) study.

Results.—The prognostic study cohort consisted of 3,197 patients from the TIMI II study population. There were 97 deaths during the 1-year follow-up; 75 deaths were attributable to cardiovascular factors. Radionuclide ventriculographic data were available for 2,567 patients. There was a relationship in this patient population between left ventricular rest ejection fraction and all-cause mortality. The highest mortality rate was found in patients with an ejection fraction of less than 30% (Fig 1). No

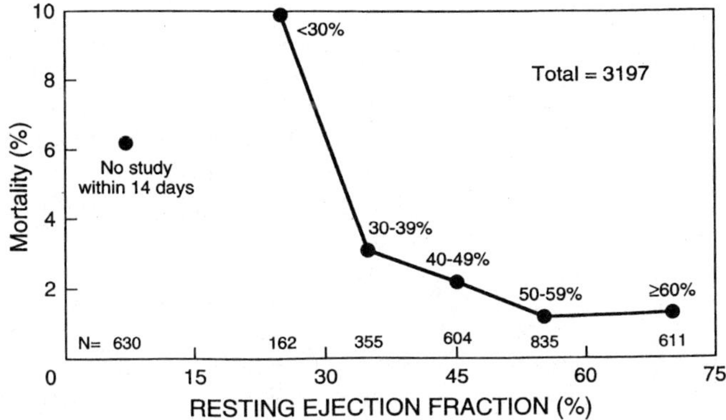

FIGURE 1.—Relation of rest ejection fraction to all-cause mortality in the Thrombolysis in Myocardial Infarction II study. Note the hyperbolic shape of the curve and the mortality rate for patients who did not undergo radionuclide ventriculography within 14 days. (Reprinted with permission from the American College of Cardiology [*Journal of the American College of Cardiology*, 1995, 26:73–79.])

additional information was provided by exercise ejection fraction data. The inability to exercise was associated with poor prognosis.

Conclusions.—Rest left ventricular ejection fraction remains an important prognostic indicator in coronary patients receiving thrombolytic therapy. Exercise ejection fraction does not provide additional prognostic information, although the inability to exercise is associated with a poor prognosis. When survival data were compared with those of the prethrombolytic therapy MPRG study (Fig 5), mortality was determined to be lower at any level of ejection fraction in the TIMI II study.

► These results indicate a prognostic value of resting left ventricular ejection fraction measurements before discharge in patients receiving throm-

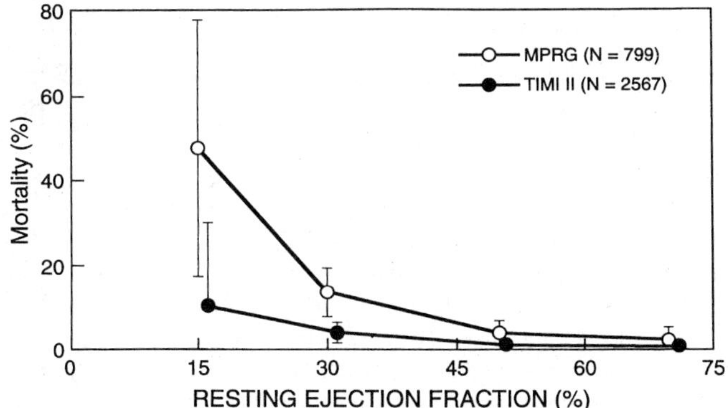

FIGURE 5.—Comparison of cardiovascular mortality rate curves in relation to rest ejection fraction. Note the increased mortality in the Multicenter Postinfarction Research Group (*MPRG*) studies at the lower levels of ejection fraction. The data from the Thrombolysis in Myocardial Infarction (*TIMI*) II trial have been regrouped according to specifications outlined in the MPRG study. *Vertical bars* represent confidence intervals. (Reprinted with permission from the American College of Cardiology [*Journal of the American College of Cardiology*, 1995, 26:73–79.])

bolytic therapy as in patients who are not treated with thrombolytic agents. The data also suggest that in addition to preserving ventricular myocardium, thrombolytic and associated therapies may enhance survival at any particular level of left ventricular function by other mechanisms. The reason for this is not readily apparent. This observation has been used to provide additional support for the "open-artery hypothesis" discussed above.

In another report relating to left ventricular systolic dysfunction after myocardial infarction, Giannuzzi and associates[1] demonstrated the presence or absence of exertional ischemia by exercise scintigraphy in patients with a left ventricular ejection fraction less than 40%. At 6-month follow-up, left ventricular dimensions did not change in the 20 patients with a left ventricular ejection fraction of less than 40% who had no evidence of exertional ischemia. However, left ventricular enlargement over time occurred in 45 patients with mild-to-moderate ischemia at 5 weeks after myocardial infarction by exercise scintigraphy and in 26 patients with severe exertional ischemia. Therefore, exercise-induced myocardial ischemia may contribute to progressive ventricular enlargement in patients with depressed left ventricular function after large anterior myocardial infarction.

R.A. O'Rourke, M.D.

Reference

1. Giannuzzi P, Marcassa C, Temporelli PL, et al: Residual exertional ischemia and unfavorable left ventricular remodeling in patients with systolic dysfunction after anterior myocardial infarction. *J Am Coll Cardiol* 25:1539–1546, 1995.

ISIS-4: A Randomised Factorial Trial Assessing Early Oral Captopril, Oral Mononitrate, and Intravenous Magnesium Sulphate in 58 050 Patients With Suspected Acute Myocardial Infarction

ISIS-4 (Fourth International Study of Infarct Survival) Collaborative Group (Radcliffe Infirmary, Oxford, England)

Lancet 345:669–685, 1995 119-96-33–8

Background.—The Fourth International Study of Infarct Survival (ISIS-4), a randomized factorial trial, was designed to determine the effects of oral captopril, oral mononitrate, and IV magnesium sulfate on mortality and major morbidity in a large series of patients with suspected acute myocardial infarction (MI). The study findings were reviewed.

Patients and Methods.—A total of 58,050 patients who were evaluated in 1,086 hospitals up to 24 hours after the onset of suspected acute MI was enrolled in the study. None of the patients showed evidence of cardiogenic shock, persistent severe hypotension, or other contraindications that would preclude participation. Approximately 29,000 patients were randomized to treatment groups, and the remainder served as controls. The treatment groups included the oral captopril group, which received an initial dose of 6.25 mg, titrated up to 50 mg twice daily for 1 month, and was compared with a matched placebo group; the oral controlled-release mononitrate group, which received an initial dose of 30 mg, titrated up to

60 mg once daily for 1 month, and was compared with a matched placebo group; and the IV magnesium sulfate group, which received an initial bolus of 8 mmol, followed by 72 mmol over 24 hours, and was compared with an open control group.

Results.—No strong interactions were observed among the effects of the 3 treatments. Treatment with captopril led to a significant 7% proportional reduction in 5-week mortality (Fig 1), corresponding to roughly 5 fewer deaths per 1,000 patients treated for 1 month, a finding consistent with that reported in other trials. Slightly higher benefits were noted in higher risk patients, such as those with a history of previous MI or with heart failure. The benefit from 1 month of early captopril treatment also appeared to persist for the first 12 months. Treatment with IV magnesium was ineffective, with no significant reductions in 5-week mortality. Additional follow-up did not show any later survival benefit. Oral mononitrate appeared to be safe, but it did not provide any significant reduction in 5-week mortality.

Conclusion.—Early initiation of converting enzyme inhibitor therapy should be considered in patients with suspected acute MI and no evident contraindications to such treatment.

► In this mega clinical trial, nitrate therapy started early in the course of acute infarction was safe and well tolerated but demonstrated no clear survival advantage. Concerning the use of IV magnesium in acute myocardial

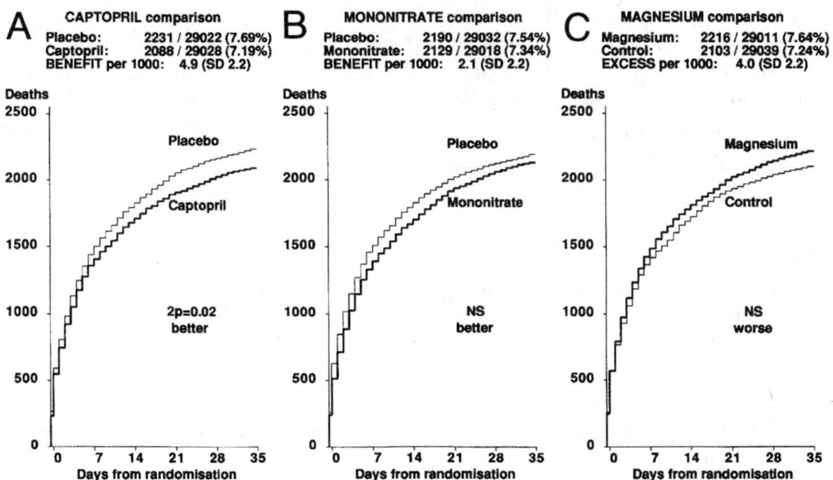

FIGURE 1.—Cumulative mortality reported on days 0–35. **A,** all patients allocated to 1 month of oral captopril (*heavy line*) vs. those allocated to a matching placebo; **B,** all patients allocated to 1 month of oral controlled-release mononitrate (*heavy line*) vs. those allocated to a matching placebo; **C,** all patients allocated to 24 hours of IV magnesium sulfate (*heavy line*) vs. those allocated to open control. (Courtesy of ISIS-4 [Fourth International Study of Infarct Survival] Collaborative Group: ISIS-4: A randomised factorial trial assessing early oral captopril, oral mononitrate, and intravenous magnesium sulphate in 58,050 patients with suspected acute myocardial infarction. *Lancet* 345:669–685, Copyright by The Lancet Ltd., 1995.)

infarction, there was no evidence of efficacy overall or in any subgroup examined. Of interest, the ISIS-4 results show no benefit for magnesium, even among the 23,000 patients randomized within 6 hours of the onset of symptoms or whether the patients also received fibrinolytic or antiplatelet therapies. A high-risk subset of patients in whom magnesium was beneficial could not be identified in ISIS-4. Consistent with other trials, the use of angiotensin-converting enzyme inhibitors (ACEI) early in acute myocardial infarction resulted in about 5 lives saved per 1,000 patients treated for 1 month. The ISIS-4 data complement the results of the SOLVD, SAVE, and AIRE trials and demonstrate that continuing ACEI therapy after the first few weeks or months in those who had evidence of left ventricular dysfunction will produce a further mortality reduction of about 2 per 1,000 patients per additional month of treatment after the first month.

Thus, one could consider starting ACE inhibitor therapy early in a wide range of patients with acute myocardial infarction, provided there is no clear contraindication (such as cardiogenic shock or persistent severe hypotension). Subsequently, after a few weeks, patients could be reviewed and treatment continued for those with clinical heart failure, low ejection fraction, or other evidence of a large infarct who are at high risk of death or severe heart failure during the next few years.

In an interesting animal study, Jugdutt and associates[1] sought to compare the effects of captopril plus isosorbide dinitrate vs. monotherapy on infarct collagen content and left ventricular remodeling and function during healing after myocardial infarction. Compared with placebo therapy, captopril, isosorbide dinitrate, or captopril plus isosorbide dinitrate improved all remodeling variables, but isosorbide dinitrate improved ventricular function more than captopril or captopril plus isosorbide dinitrate. The reduction of infarct collagen content by captopril demonstrated in this dog infarct model suggests that the well-documented benefits with captopril may represent a balance between positive and negative effects; its combination with isosorbide dinitrate might be advantageous.

R.A. O'Rourke, M.D.

Reference

1. Jugdutt BI, Khan MI, Jugdutt SJ, et al: Combined captopril and isosorbide dinitrate during healing after myocardial infarction: Effect on ventricular remodeling, function, mass and collagen. *J Am Coll Cardiol* 25:1089–1096, 1995.

Utility of Beta-Blockade Treatment for Older Postinfarction Patients

Park KC, Forman DE, Wei JY (Harvard Med School, Boston)
J Am Geriatr Soc 43:751–755, 1995 119-96-33-9

Background.—Although more than 50% of myocardial infarctions (MIs) occur in patients 65 years of age and older, most studies of the treatment of coronary artery disease (CAD) have included younger patients. It is uncertain whether the benefits of β-blocker therapy are the same for very old adults as for those younger than 65 years. In a retrospective cohort study, the hypothesis that use of a β-blocker after MI would improve clinical outcomes in older patients was evaluated.

Methods.—A total of 1,011 patients with MI between the ages of 60 and 90 years were admitted to the study institution between January 1988 and September 1989. Review of patient medical records yielded 118 patients who met eligibility requirements, including 76 treated with the β-1 selective blocking agent metoprolol and 42 controls who did not receive β-blockers. All metoprolol recipients and control patients or their families were contacted after 2 years to determine the incidence of nonfatal reinfarction, post-MI hospital admissions, and all-cause, 2-year post-MI mortality. Data from patients aged 70–89 years were also analyzed separately.

Results.—Patients in the metoprolol group received the agent at a total dosage of at least 25 mg/day for at least 5 days post-MI. Controls were significantly older than those treated with metoprolol and were less likely to have received a β-blocker in the past; the metoprolol group had a significantly higher incidence of hypertension, hypercholesterolemia, and prior percutaneous transluminal coronary angioplasty. Rates of subsequent reinfarction were similar in study and control groups, but the rate of subsequent readmission was significantly increased with use of metoprolol. Those treated with metoprolol had an age-adjusted mortality reduction of 76% compared with controls, a reduction that persisted in patients aged 70–79 years and 80–89 years. When potential confounders were excluded, the mortality reduction with metoprolol was 12%.

Conclusion.—Older patients treated with metoprolol after MI had significantly reduced mortality compared with those not given β-blocker therapy, confirming the value of β-blockade in the very old. Methodological limitations of the study may explain the lack of effect on reinfarction and readmission.

► This retrospective cohort study showed an age-adjusted mortality reduction of 76% in post–myocardial infarction patients aged 60–89 years who were treated with metoprolol. Multivariate logistic regression analysis showed a 12% reduction in mortality among older patients as a result of metoprolol therapy.

There is some debate as to how underused β-blocking drugs are in secondary prevention for patients who have recovered from an acute myocardial infarction. In a recent report, Viskin and associates[1] found that only 58% of infarct survivors with no contraindications to β-blockers received these drugs at the time of hospital discharge, and only 11% received doses equivalent to more than 50% of the dosages shown to be effective in improving long-term survival in clinical trials. The independent predictors of failure to prescribe β-blockers for infarct survivors without contraindications to these drugs were the use of diuretic agents, transient heart failure, impaired left ventricular function, and increased patient age. Failure to prescribe β-blockers after myocardial infarction was common, but in most cases it was not attributable to clear contraindications. Many patients not receiving β-blockers belong to subgroups that would derive the greatest benefit from such treatment. Finally, even when β-blockers are prescribed, the dosages used are considerably lower than those proven to be effective in preventing death after myocardial infarction.

It probably is not necessary to prescribe long-term daily β-blocker therapy for low-risk patients who have recovered from an uncomplicated myocardial infarction.[2] However, long-term β-blocker therapy definitely should be given to high-risk postinfarction patients without contraindications. This applies to high-risk patients that do not undergo myocardial revascularization as part of their initial therapy and to many patients at high risk after successful myocardial revascularization. Beta-blockers should be used as needed to manage angina, evidence of myocardial ischemia, or high blood pressure in appropriate patients after myocardial infarction. Beta-blockers are underused by physicians in secondary prevention efforts for high-risk post–infarction patients, especially when one considers the doses used in comparison to those proven to be efficacious in long-term follow-up.

R.A. O'Rourke, M.D.

References

1. Viskin S, Kitzis I, Lev E, et al: Treatment with beta-adrenergic blocking agents after myocardial infarction: From randomized trials to clinical practice. *J Am Coll Cardiol* 25:1327–1332, 1995.
2. O'Rourke RA: Are beta-blockers really underutilized in postinfarction patients? *J Am Coll Cardiol* 26:1437–1439, 1995.

Hemostatic Factors and the Risk of Myocardial Infarction or Sudden Death in Patients With Angina Pectoris

van de Loo LCW, for the European Concerted Action on Thrombosis and Disabilities Angina Pectoris Study Group (Univ of Münster, Germany)

N Engl J Med 332:635–641, 1995 119-96-33–10

Purpose.—A number of systemic thrombogenic factors may contribute to the occurrence, extent, and persistence of coronary thrombosis, which is generally recognized as the precipitating event in the transition from stable to acute ischemic heart disease. Certain laboratory tests may make it possible to detect a thrombogenic state and thereby identify patients at increased risk for cardiovascular disease. However, most studies of this issue have been conducted in healthy patients; there are few data on patients with known coronary artery disease. The link between baseline measurements of hemostatic factors and the occurrence of coronary events during follow-up was evaluated in patients with angina pectoris.

Methods.—A prospective, multicenter study included 3,043 patients with angina pectoris. All underwent coronary angiography because of suspected coronary artery disease. At baseline, selected hemostatic factors indicating a thrombophilic state or an alteration in the vascular epithelium were measured. The patients were followed for 2 years, and the hemostatic factors were analyzed in relation to the incidence of myocardial infarction or sudden coronary death.

Results.—Coronary events were more likely in patients with higher baseline concentrations of hemostatic factors, after adjustment for extent of coronary artery disease and other risk factors (Fig 1). The mean fibrinogen concentration was 3.29 g/L in patients with myocardial infarction or sudden coronary death during follow-up vs. 3 g/L in those without such events. Concentrations of von Willebrand factor antigen were 138% vs. 125%, and concentrations of tissue plasminogen activator (t-PA) antigen were 11.9 ng/mL vs. 10 ng/mL. Concentration of C-reactive protein was directly correlated with the incidence of coronary events except when the analysis was adjusted for fibrinogen concentration. Patients with high serum cholesterol levels had an increased risk of coronary events with increasing levels of fibrinogen and C-reactive protein. However, those with low fibrinogen concentrations were at low risk of coronary events even if they had high serum levels of cholesterol. Severity of coronary artery disease was still the best predictor of coronary events.

Conclusions.—Baseline concentrations of the hemostatic factors fibrinogen, von Willebrand factor antigen, and t-PA antigen are independent predictors of subsequent coronary events in patients with angina pectoris. Fibrinogen concentration is a strong predictor even within the range of normal. High fibrinogen and C-reactive protein concentrations may be useful in identifying patients with hypercholesterolemia who are at particularly high risk for coronary events. If concentrations of fibrinogen are low, even patients with increased serum levels of cholesterol are at low risk for coronary events. The findings add to the evidence that impaired fibrinolysis, endothelial-cell injury, and inflammatory activity play a pathogenetic role in the progression of coronary artery disease.

► These results indicate a role of the concentration of fibrinogen, t-PA antigen, and von Willebrand factor in the risk for acute coronary syndromes. The associatin of higher concentrations of both fibrinogen and C-reactive protein with increased coronary risk suggests that the fibrinogen concentration becomes elevated at least in part as a consequence of inflammatory reactions that occur in progressive atherosclerosis. The positive association of the risk of coronary events with the concentrations of t-PA antigen and the von Willebrand antigen, both of which are released by endothelial cells, indicates a possible role for endothelial perturbation in treating patients prone to acute coronary syndromes.

Recently, Borghi and the SMILE Study Investigators[1] assessed the effect of the angiotensin-converting enzyme (ACE) inhibitor zofenopril on mortality and morbidity after acute anterior myocardial infarction. A total of 1,556 patients were studied and randomized to receive either placebo or zofenopril for 6 weeks. The incidence of death or severe congestive heart failure at 6 weeks was significantly reduced in the zofenopril group as compared with the placebo group. The cumulative reduction in the risk of death or severe congestive heart failure was 34% and the reduction in risk of death was 25% in the group receiving the ACE inhibitor. After 1 year of observation, the mortality rate was still significantly lower (by 29%) in the

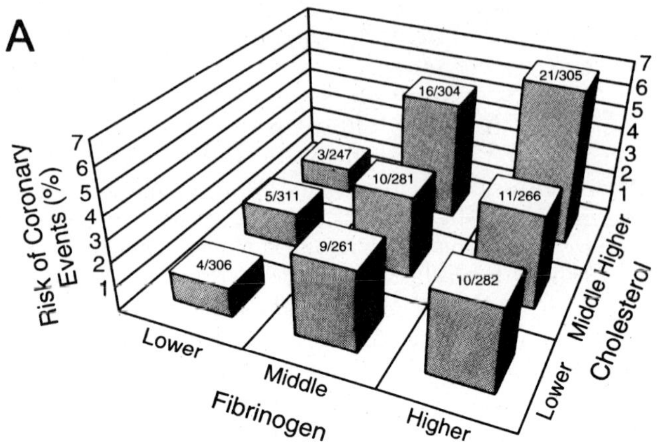

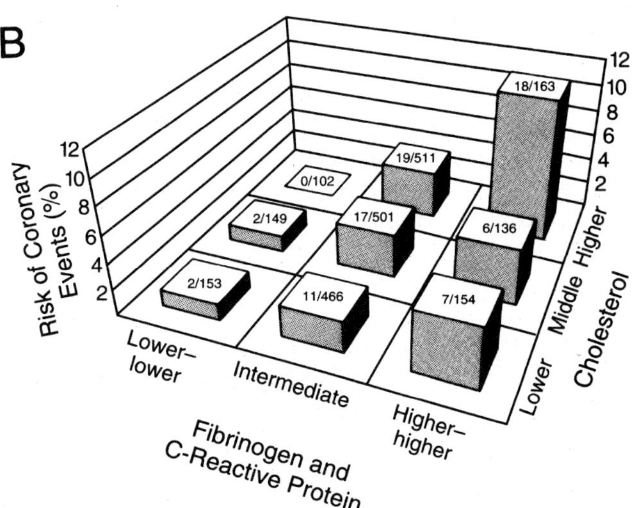

FIGURE 1.—Incidence of coronary events during 2-year follow-up, according to concentrations of fibrinogen, C-reactive protein, and total cholesterol. The risk of coronary events according to fibrinogen and total cholesterol concentrations is shown in (**A**) and the risk according to fibrinogen and C-reactive protein concentrations combined, as compared with total cholesterol concentrations, is shown in (**B**). The concentrations of these variables are divided into 3 categories (lower, middle, and higher), each containing one third of the sample, according to their respective distributions. In (**B**), "intermediate" refers to all combinations of fibrinogen and C-reactive protein concentrations other than lower–lower or higher–higher. Values used to divide the sample into thirds were 2.71 and 3.31 g/L for fibrinogen, 5.79 and 6.80 mmol/L (224 and 263 mg/dL) for cholesterol, and 0.88 and 2.17 mg/L for C-reactive protein. The number of coronary events and the number of patients at risk are shown for each group. Only patients for whom data on both fibrinogen and total cholesterol concentrations were available are included in the analysis. (Courtesy of van de Loo JCW, for the European Concerted Action on Thrombosis and Disabilities Angina Pectoris Study Group: Hemostatic factors and the risk of myocardial infarction or sudden death in patients with angina pectoris. *N Engl J Med* 332:635–641, Copyright 1995, Massachusetts Medical Society.)

zofenopril group. Therefore, the salutary effects of ACE inhibitors in such patients are again demonstrated and appear to be a "drug group" beneficial result.

R.A. O'Rourke, M.D.

Reference

1. Borghi C, for the Survival of Myocardial Infarction Long-Term Evaluation (SMILE) Study Investigators: The effect of the angiotensin-converting–enzyme inhibitor zofenopril on mortality and morbidity after anterior myocardial infarction. *N Engl J Med* 332:80–85, 1995.

34 Chronic Coronary Heart Disease

Magnitude of Myocardial Dysfunction Is Greater in Painful Than in Painless Myocardial Ischemia: An Exercise Echocardiographic Study
Nihoyannopoulos P, Marsonis A, Joshi J, Athanassopoulos G, Oakley CM (Hammersmith Hosp, London)
J Am Coll Cardiol 25:1507–1512, 1995 119-96-34–1

Introduction.—Some studies have suggested that painless episodes of myocardial ischemia are generally shorter, with less marked abnormalities of left ventricular function, than painful episodes. In other reports, however, abnormalities in left ventricular function induced by exercise were similar during painful and painless ischemia. Exercise echocardiography was used to assess the magnitude of myocardial dysfunction in 89 patients, 58 with painful and 31 with painless myocardial ischemia.

Patients and Methods.—All patients had significant coronary artery disease and positive exercise stress test results. None had previous coronary artery bypass grafting, associated valvular heart disease, or myocardial infarction. The group of 67 men and 22 women had a mean age of 59 years. Classification into painful and painless cohorts was based upon outcome of a symptom-limited treadmill exercise test, performed at least 24 hours after discontinuation of antianginal therapy. Echocardiographic images were acquired in digital format before and immediately after treadmill exercise testing.

Results.—The painful and painless ischemia groups were comparable in age, sex, risk factors, and extent of coronary artery disease. There was a higher incidence of 3-vessel disease in the painful ischemia group and of single-vessel disease in the painless ischemia group. Compared with patients with painful ischemia, those with painless ischemia had a significantly longer mean exercise duration and attained a greater maximal workload and a higher rate–blood pressure product. Nearly all patients (93%) in the group with painful myocardial ischemia had at least 1 hypokinetic or akinetic segment detected immediately after exercise; in contrast, 55% of patients with painless ischemia had at least 1 new wall motion abnormality detected. Both the total ischemic score (15.9 vs. 12) and the number of ischemic myocardial segments (16% vs. 6%) were greater in the painful myocardial ischemia group.

Conclusion.—Among patients with no previous myocardial infarction, echocardiography demonstrated that exercise-induced angina was associated with a greater magnitude of myocardial dysfunction in painful vs. painless ischemic episodes. The severity of myocardial ischemia appears to be greater in patients with painful ischemia.

▶ This study in patients with documented coronary artery disease compared patients with symptomatic myocardial ischemia during positive treadmill exercise tests with those having asymptomatic episodes of myocardial ischemia during positive exercise ECG testing. Patients with symptomatic ischemia during exercise testing had more severe regional ventricular dysfunction when documented by exercise echocardiography than those with silent ischemia. This particular study supports the hypothesis that differences in the amount of myocardium in jeopardy during painful and painless ischemia often account for the presence or absence of symptoms during an ischemic episode. However, among different patient populations, it is likely that individual variation in ischemic pain threshold and perception may be explained by visceral neuropathy (diabetes mellitus), presence of myocardial infarction, previous coronary bypass surgery, or simply by reduced perception of painful stimuli (e.g., increased beta endorphins). There are data to support each of these mechanisms for asymptomatic myocardial ischemia. Also, many episodes of silent ischemia as documented by ambulatory ECG recordings in patients with chronic stable angina may result from coronary vasoconstriction (supply ischemia) rather than from demand-driven ischemia, such as that which occurs during treadmill testing. Thus, there are likely several mechanisms for episodes of asymptomatic myocardial ischemia that are operative uniformly or variably in different subsets of patients.

R.A. O'Rourke, M.D.

Effect of Amlodipine, Atenolol and Their Combination on Myocardial Ischemia During Treadmill Exercise and Ambulatory Monitoring

Davies RF, for the Canadian Amlodipine/Atenolol in Silent Ischemia Study (CASIS) Investigators (Univ of Ottawa Heart Inst, Ont, Canada)

J Am Coll Cardiol 25:619–625, 1995 119-96-34–2

Objective.—It is not clear whether ischemia during treadmill testing and 48-hour ambulatory monitoring responds to anti-ischemic drugs in the same manner. The Canadian Amlodipine/Atenolol in Silent Ischemia Study compared the anti-ischemic efficacy of amlodipine, atenolol, and their combination during treadmill testing and 48-hour ambulatory monitoring.

Study Design.—Patients with stable coronary artery disease and ischemia during treadmill testing and ambulatory monitoring were randomly assigned to receive amlodipine (n = 51) or atenolol (n = 49) in a counterbalanced, crossover evaluation of placebo and active drug, followed by evaluation of the combination of amlodipine and atenolol. Therapy was continued for at least 2 weeks.

Results.—During treadmill testing, the onset of ischemia was significantly prolonged by 29% with amlodipine and by 34% with the combination, but not with atenolol. During ambulatory monitoring, atenolol significantly reduced the frequency of ischemia by 57% and the combination reduced it by 72%, whereas the smaller 28% reduction by amlodipine was not significant. Exercise time to angina significantly increased by 29% with amlodipine, 16% with atenolol, and 39% with the combination therapy. Amlodipine and combination therapy, but not atenolol, significantly improved exercise time only in patients with angina during treadmill testing. Despite the increase in exercise time, amlodipine did not affect the double product at onset of ischemia, suggesting that reduction of ischemia is mediated predominantly by a decrease in cardiac workload at a given level of exercise. On the other hand, atenolol reduced both the double product at onset of ischemia during treadmill testing and heart rate at onset of ischemia during ambulatory monitoring, suggesting that β-blockade reduces absolute myocardial blood supply that partially offsets the beneficial effect of lower cardiac demand.

Summary.—The relative anti-ischemic effects of amlodipine and atenolol differ during treadmill testing and ambulatory monitoring. Amlodipine is more effective in suppressing ischemia during treadmill testing, whereas atenolol is more effective during ambulatory monitoring, but the combination of both drugs is more effective than either single drug in both settings. The combination of a β-blocker with a long-acting dihydropyridine, such as amlodipine, is an effective pharmacologic strategy for suppressing both silent and symptomatic ischemia.

► In this study, the calcium blocker amlodipine appeared to be more effective in suppressing or delaying myocardial ischemia during treadmill exercise testing, and the long-acting β-blocker atenolol was more effective in suppressing episodes of myocardial ischemia during ambulatory ECG recordings. Importantly, the combination was significantly better than either single drug in both testing situations. These results are consistent with previous studies indicating that the combination of a β-blocker with a long-acting β-blocker is an effective pharmacologic strategy for suppressing both silent and symptomatic ischemia.

In a report from the Asymptomatic Cardiac Ischemia Pilot (ACIP) Study, Rogers and associates[1] detailed the outcome at 1 year for patients with asymptomatic cardiac ischemia randomized to medical therapy or revascularization. A group of 558 patients with coronary anatomy amenable to revascularization, at least 1 episode of asymptomatic ischemia on the 48-hour ambulatory ECG, and ischemia on treadmill exercise testing were randomized to 1 of 3 treatment strategies: (1) medication to suppress angina (angina-guided strategy); (2) medication to suppress both angina and ambulatory ECG ischemia (ischemia-guided strategy); or (3) revascularization strategy (angioplasty or bypass surgery). Medication was titrated atenolol-nifedipine or diltiazem-isosorbide dinitrate.

The revascularization group received less medication and had less ischemia on serial ambulatory ECG recordings and exercise testing than did those assigned to the medical strategies. The ischemia-guided group received more medication but, surprisingly, had no greater suppression of ischemia than did the angina-guided group. At 1 year, the mortality rate was 4.4% in the angina-guided group, 1.6% in the ischemic-guided group, and 0% in the revascularization group, the difference between angina-guided therapy and revascularization being statistically significant. The frequency of myocardial infarction, unstable angina, stroke, and congestive heart failure was not significantly different among the 3 strategies. Interestingly, at the 1-year visit the proportion of patients without ischemia was 42% in the angina-guided strategy group, 50% in the ischemia-guided strategy group, and 60% in the revascularization strategy group, the difference between angina-guided therapy and revascularization being statistically significant.

In another report from the ACIP study, Chaitman and associates[2] compared the results of the 3 treatment strategies on ECG exercise test parameters 12 weeks after the institution of therapy. The results indicate that myocardial revascularization significantly reduced the extent and frequency of exercise-induced myocardial ischemia compared with either medical strategy.

In a third report from the same ACIP study, Bourassa et al.[3] compared the relative efficacy of coronary angioplasty or coronary artery bypass graft surgery in suppressing ambulatory ECG and treadmill exercise myocardial ischemia between 2 and 3 months after revascularization. Even though patients assigned to bypass surgery had more severe coronary disease and more ischemic episodes at baseline than those assigned to angioplasty, ambulatory ECG ischemia was no longer present at 8 weeks after revascularization in 70% of the bypass surgery group vs. 46% of the angioplasty group ($P = 0.002$). Total exercise time in minutes on the treadmill test also increased to a significantly greater extent after bypass surgery. Although angina and ambulatory ischemia are relieved in a high proportion of patients early after revascularization, ischemia can still be induced on exercise testing, albeit at higher levels of exercise.

R.A. O'Rourke, M.D.

References

1. Rogers WJ, Bourassa MG, Andrews TC, et al: Asymptomatic cardiac ischemia pilot (ACIP) study: Outcome at 1 year for patients with asymptomatic cardiac ischemia randomized to medical therapy or revascularization. *J Am Coll Cardiol* 26:594–605, 1995.
2. Chaitman BR, Stone PH, Knatterud GL: Asymptomatic cardiac ischemia pilot (ACIP) study: Impact of anti-ischemia therapy on 12-week rest electrocardiogram and exercise test outcomes. *J Am Coll Cardiol* 26:585–593, 1995.
3. Bourassa MG, Pepine CJ, Forman SA: Asymptomatic cardiac ischemia pilot (ACIP) study: Effects of coronary angioplasty and coronary artery bypass graft surgery on recurrent angina and ischemia. *J Am Coll Cardiol* 26:606–614, 1995.

Cardiac Syndrome X: Clinical Characteristics and Left Ventricular Function: Long-Term Follow-Up Study

Kaski JC, Rosano GMC, Collins P, Nihoyannopoulos P, Maseri A, Poole-Wilson PA (St George's Hosp, London; Royal Brompton Natl Heart and Lung Hosp, London; Hammersmith Hosp, London)

J Am Coll Cardiol 25:807–814, 1995 119-96-34–3

Purpose.—The diagnostic label "syndrome X" refers to patients with exertional angina and a positive response to exercise testing but angiographically normal coronary arteries. It is a heterogeneous syndrome that includes various pathogenetic entities. The clinical characteristics and evolution of symptoms and left ventricular function were studied in a clinically homogeneous sample of 99 patients with syndrome X.

Methods.—The patients were 78 women and 21 men (mean age, 48.5 years). The patients were followed for a mean of 7 years, during which time they had cardiac catheterization, ambulatory ECG monitoring, and echocardiography of left ventricular function.

Findings.—Significantly more women than men were affected, and 61.5% of the women in the sample had passed menopause before their chest pain started. In addition to exertional angina, 41 patients also had rest angina. For most patients, the episodes of chest pain lasted more than 10 minutes on the average. For 42%, sublingual nitrate offered effective pain relief. Ambulatory ECG monitoring showed transient ST-segment depression in 64 patients and myocardial perfusion abnormalities in 22. Thirty-two patients had a 20 mm Hg or greater increase in systolic blood pressure during the first stage of exercise testing. These patients had a quicker onset of ST depression and shorter exercise times than did those whose blood pressure increased by 20% or less.

There were no deaths or myocardial infarctions during follow-up. The mean ventricular function remained stable, with a shortening fraction of approximately 35%. There was 1 case of heart failure, 8 of systemic hypertension, and 4 of conduction disturbances. The symptoms improved in 11 patients, varied or did not change in 64, and worsened in 24.

Conclusions.—Syndrome X appears to be most common in postmenopausal women. Although typical angina-like chest pain is most often present, conventional antianginal treatments often fail. A few patients will have myocardial perfusion abnormalities. Long-term survival is not negatively affected, although chest pain may interfere with the patient's lifestyle; deterioration of cardiac function is rare.

► In this study, the presence of a positive response to ECG exercise testing was necessary for the diagnosis of syndrome X in an attempt to reduce clinical heterogeneity and to identify patients whose chest pain was likely to have a cardiac origin. The results confirm previous observations of a female prevalence among patients with syndrome X. Syndrome X was associated with a benign prognosis during an average of 7 years of follow-up, in relation to cardiac mortality, the development of serious coronary events, and heart failure. However, in this study as in others, lifestyle was often impaired by prolonged recurrent chest discomfort. Diagnostic testing and treatment of patients with this syndrome are costly and therapy with conventional anti-anginal agents is rarely successful.

R.A. O'Rourke, M.D.

Anatomic and Physiologic Heterogeneity in Patients With Syndrome X: An Intravascular Ultrasound Study

Wiedermann JG, Schwartz A, Apfelbaum M (Columbia Presbyterian Med Ctr, New York; Columbia Univ, New York)

J Am Coll Cardiol 25:1310–1317, 1995 119-96-34-4

Background.—As many as 1 in 5 patients with angina who are referred for cardiac catheterization are found to have normal coronary arteries. Myocardial ischemia has been demonstrated in these patients, who are said to have "syndrome X." The mortality is quite low, but symptoms frequently persist and prevent patients from resuming their work. Evidence of impaired coronary flow reserve suggests a "microvascular" cause of angina in these patients. Reactivity of the coronary vessels may be a critical factor.

Objective.—Intravascular ultrasound imaging was used to directly clarify the morphologic features of the 3 major epicardial vessels and to document the vasomotor response to exercise and the effects of β-blockade with propranolol.

Methods.—Ultrasound studies were done using a 4.3F, 30-MHz catheter in 30 patients having a diagnosis of syndrome X, 19 women and 11 men whose average age was 50.4 years. All of them had abnormal exercise stress test results. Imaging was repeated as the patients performed supine arm exercise until the heart rate increased by at least 50%. Exercise imaging was repeated after the IV injection of propranolol, 0.1 mg/kg of body weight.

Findings.—Twelve patients had normal coronary arteries; 10 had atheromatous plaque; and 8 exhibited marked intimal thickening but no evidence of plaque. Risk factors were somewhat less in patients with normal morphologic findings, but not significantly so. Only 2 of the 12 patients with normal-appearing vessels had abnormal exercise test findings, compared with all but 1 of the 18 patients with abnormal morphologic findings by intravascular ultrasound. Those with morphologically normal vessels had an average vasodilatory response of +16.9% at peak exercise. Luminal area decreased by 17.4% and 17.6% in both groups with morphologically abnormal vessels. Propranolol blunted both the vasodilatory response to exercise in patients with normal vessels and the vasoconstrictive response in those with abnormal vessels.

Conclusions.—Most patients with syndrome X have morphologically abnormal coronary arteries, which tend to constrict, rather than dilate, on exercise. Propranolol attenuates this response and therefore may prove beneficial to patients with abnormal vessels.

► In this study, intravascular ultrasound was used to assess epicardial coronary artery morphologic features and the presence or absence of coronary artery disease. The coronary vasomotor response to exercise was also assessed by intracoronary ultrasound imaging. In this group of 30 patients studied, 18 had abnormal epicardial coronary arteries. The vasomotor response to exercise was normal in patients with syndrome X who had normal coronary arteries by intravascular ultrasound and abnormal in patients with atheroma or intimal thickening by ultrasound. Propranolol loading attenuated both the normal vasodilatory and abnormal vasoconstrictive response to exercise in patients with syndrome X. Thus, therapy with β-blockers might be of greater benefit in patients with syndrome X and abnormal coronary arteries by ultrasound.

R.A. O'Rourke, M.D.

Selection of Medical Treatment in Stable Angina Pectoris: Results of the International Multicenter Angina Exercise (IMAGE) Study

Ardissino D, Savonitto S, Egstrup K Rasmussen K, Bae EA, Omland T, Schjelderup-Mathiesen PM, Marraccini P, Merlini PA, Wahlqvist I, Rehnqvist N, on behalf of the IMAGE Study Group (IRCCS, Policlinico S Matteo, Pavia, Italy)

J Am Coll Cardiol 25:1516–1521, 1995 119-96-34–5

Objective.—A multicenter trial enrolled 290 patients with stable angina pectoris and randomly assigned them to treatment with either metoprolol, a β-adrenergic blocking agent, or nifedipine, a calcium antagonist. Investigators sought to determine which characteristics of anginal symptoms or exercise test results might predict the type of agent that would be more effective in an individual patient.

Methods.—The patients were enrolled at 25 European centers. All had typical anginal symptoms and had been stable for at least 6 months. Exclusion criteria included age older than 75 years, myocardial infarction in the 6 months before study entry, and serious concomitant diseases. After a 2-week placebo run-in period, patients completed a questionnaire on anginal symptoms and an exercise stress test. The 6-week double-blind treatment was completed by 264 of the patients, 138 in the metoprolol (200 mg once daily) group and 126 in the nifedipine (20 mg twice daily) group. Exercise tests were repeated at the end of the study, 1–4 hours after drug intake. The patients also used diary cards to record the occurrence of angina attacks throughout the study.

Results.—Although both agents prolonged exercise tolerance over baseline levels, the improvement was greater in the metoprolol group than in the nifedipine group. The 2 drugs increased time to angina and decreased the mean weekly number of anginal attacks to the same extent. In stepwise regression analysis, only lower exercise tolerance at baseline was independently related to a better response within each treatment group. Metoprolol was more effective than nifedipine at increasing exercise tolerance in 2 patient subgroups: those in the low tertiles of total exercise time and time to 1-mm ST-segment depression and those in the high tertiles of rate-pressure product at rest and at ischemic threshold.

Conclusion.—Beta-adrenergic blocking agents reduce oxygen consumption, whereas calcium antagonists increase coronary blood flow. Knowledge of the prevailing cause of ischemic episodes would allow selection of the optimal treatment for an individual patient with stable angina pectoris. The findings of this trial suggest that results of a baseline exercise test may be useful in selecting medical treatment.

▶ In this multicenter study, patients with chronic stable angina pectoris were randomly allocated to a double-blind treatment for 6 weeks with either metoprolol or nifedipine according to a parallel drug design. At the end of this period, exercise tests were repeated 1–4 hours after drug intake. Although both metoprolol and nifedipine prolonged exercise tolerance over baseline levels, the improvement was greater in the patients receiving metoprolol ($P < 0.05$). Metoprolol was more effective than nifedipine in patients with a lower exercise tolerance or with a higher rate-pressure product at rest and at the ischemic threshold. None of the characteristics of angina symptoms or exercise test results predicted a greater efficacy of nifedipine over metoprolol. Therefore, in certain patients, the baseline exercise test result may predict the likelihood of successful therapy with metoprolol, but not necessarily with nifedipine.

Patients with chronic stable angina are often treated with nitrates in addition to calcium antagonists and β-blockers. To determine whether rebound ischemia occurs during nitrate-free periods with intermittent cutaneous nitroglycerin therapy in patients with angina pectoris who are receiving background antianginal therapy, Freedman and associates[1] entered 52 patients who had stable-effort angina and were taking either a β-blocking drug or diltiazem, or their combination, into a randomized double-blind placebo-controlled crossover study of cutaneous nitroglycerin patches. Active or placebo patches were worn for 1 week, applied at 8 AM and removed at 10 PM to provide a 10-hour daily nitrate-free (or placebo-free) period. During the last 48 hours of each phase, ambulatory ECG recordings were used to detect ischemia. Most patients taking background antianginal therapy experienced no ischemia during the patch-off period. In the 44% of patients who had ischemia during this period, there was a nonsignificant increase in the duration of ischemia with active therapy. The change in the distribution of diurnal ischemia suggests that rebound ischemia may occur with intermittent cutaneous nitroglycerin, despite other background antianginal therapy.

In a very controversial communication, Furberg and associates[2] assessed the effect of the dose of dihydropyridine calcium antagonist, nifedipine, on the increased risk of mortality observed in randomized secondary-prevention trials using short-acting forms of this drug, and they reviewed the mechanisms by which this adverse effect might occur. They restricted their dose-response meta-analysis to the 16 randomized secondary-prevention trials of nifedipine for which mortality data were available. Overall, the use of nifedipine was associated with a significant adverse effect on total mortality (risk ratio, 1.16; 95% confidence interval, 1.01–1.33). In addition, their meta-analysis indicated that high doses of nifedipine were significantly associated with increased mortality.

Three editorials[3–5] appeared in the same publication as the Furberg meta-analysis. The first editorial emphasizes that the indicted agent was short-acting nifedipine and that there is no evidence that other calcium antagonists increase cardiac mortality. Many studies using nifedipine, other dihydropyridines, and nondihydropyridine calcium blockers without an increase in patient mortality are cited. The authors of the second editorial,[4] which suggests that there are several areas where additional research is desperately needed to better guide the use of calcium antagonists, strongly agree with the co-authors of the meta-analysis on this issue. This editorial states that long-term prospective randomized outcome studies are needed to assess the effects of the newer calcium-channel blockers in patients with chronic stable angina, variant angina, syndrome X, and hypertension.

The third editorial[5] recommends the use of nitrates and β-blockers as the initial treatment for relieving angina and the use of calcium antagonists only if symptoms persist, if nitrates or β-blockers are contraindicated or not tolerated, or if revascularization is inappropriate. If a calcium antagonist is used, it would be prudent to use a nondihydropyridine agent such as diltiazem or verapamil.

In my opinion, the long-acting dihydropyridine calcium blockers and other calcium blockers not of the dihydropyridine class are efficacious for clinical use in treating patients with chronic stable angina, unstable angina, and variant angina. They are useful in the treatment of many patients with hypertension, particularly when there is coincident ischemic heart disease. However, they are not agents that should be used in the secondary prevention for patients with a previous Q-wave myocardial infarction. Their use in patients with congestive heart failure should be cautious and only when the heart failure relates to left ventricular dysfunction resulting from reversible myocardial ischemia and other anti-ischemia agents are not efficacious.

Recently, Ezekowitz and associates[6] reported the results of a multicenter, double-blind crossover trial of amlodipine in chronic stable angina. Amlodipine produced a significantly greater increase in symptom-limited exercise duration and total work, and a decrease in angina-attack frequency and nitroglycerin consumption compared with placebo. Ambulatory ECG recordings revealed a significant reduction in numbers, absolute total area, and duration of ST-segment depression after treatment with amlodipine as compared with placebo. Amlodipine therapy was well tolerated, and it demonstrated anti-ischemic and antianginal efficacy in the management of stable angina.

R.A. O'Rourke, M.D.

References

1. Freedman SB, Daxini BV, Noyce D, et al: Intermittent transdermal nitrates do not improve ischemia in patients taking beta-blockers or calcium antagonists: Potential

role of rebound ischemia during nitrate-free-period. *J Am Coll Cardiol* 25:349–355, 1995.
2. Furberg CD, Psaty BM, Meyer JV: Nifedipine: Dose-related increase in mortality in patients with coronary heart disease. *Circulation* 92:1326–1331, 1995.
3. Opie LH, Messerli FH: Nifedipine and mortality: Grave defects in the dossier (editorial). *Circulation* 92:1068–1073, 1995.
4. Kloner RA: Nifedipine in ischemic heart disease (editorial). *Circulation* 92:1074–1078, 1995.
5. Yusuf S: Calcium antagonists in coronary artery disease and hypertension: Time for reevaluation (editorial)? *Circulation* 92:1079–1082, 1995.
6. Ezekowitz MD, Hossack K, Mehta JL, et al: Amlodipine in chronic stable angina: Results of a multicenter double-blind crossover trial. *Am Heart J* 129:527–535, 1995.

A Comparison of Quality of Life Scores in Patients With Angina Pectoris After Angioplasty Compared With After Medical Therapy: Outcomes of a Randomized Clinical Trial

Strauss WE, Fortin T, Hartigan P, Folland ED, Parisi AF, and the Veterans Affairs Study of Angioplasty Compared to Medical Therapy Investigators (Veterans Affairs Med Ctr, West Roxbury, Mass)
Circulation 92:1710–1719, 1995 119-96-34–6

Rationale.—Traditionally, antianginal treatments have been evaluated using objective measures such as exercise tolerance in conjunction with such subjective measures as the attack rate. Today, increasing importance is attached to how patients feel about their quality of life (QOL). Measures of QOL have been used to assess the effects of coronary angioplasty but not to compare the overall impact of angioplasty with that of medical care in patients with angina.

Study Plan.—A self-administered QOL instrument was used along with conventional measures to compare the results of percutaneous transluminal coronary angioplasty with those of medical management in patients having stable angina and positive exercise tolerance test results. All participants had 70% or greater narrowing in the proximal two thirds of a major coronary vessel. Exercise testing and coronary angiography were repeated 6 months after randomization. A total of 182 patients with single-vessel coronary disease completed the study. Physical functioning was assessed using the McMaster Health Index Questionnaire.

Results.—Baseline QOL scores were nearly identical in the 2 treatment groups. At 6 months, overall psychological well-being and combined physical and psychological functioning were significantly improved in the patients who underwent angioplasty. Overall, QOL improved only in patients whose duration of treadmill exercise increased. Improvement was most evident in angioplasty-treated patients, whose exercise duration increased by more than 2 minutes. At follow-up, both exercise duration and the number of anginal episodes in the past month were most closely correlated with the physical subscale of the QOL questionnaire. Only patients who underwent angioplasty whose coronary angiograms showed substantial improvement had significant improvement in overall QOL.

Conclusion.—This randomized trial demonstrated greater improvement in quality of life after coronary angioplasty than with conventional medical management in patients with angina.

▶ In the Angioplasty Compared to Medicine (ACME) study of patients with single-vessel coronary disease reported previously in the 1993 YEAR BOOK OF MEDICINE,[1] anginal attack rate and nitroglycerin consumption were found to be significantly less with percutaneous transluminal coronary angioplasty (PTCA) than with medical therapy. In addition, the extent of angina-free time during treadmill testing improved to a greater degree in PTCA-assigned patients. However, there were many repeat procedures in those who had coronary artery restenosis during the 6-month follow-up. In addition to the primary end points of exercise performance and rate of angina attack, patients participating in the ACME completed a standardized questionnaire assessing the psychological and physiologic parameters that indicate self-perceived quality of life. At the end of the 6-month evaluation, patients who were randomized to PTCA had a significantly greater improvement in overall quality-of-life scores. This improvement in quality of life was only noted in PTCA-assigned patients demonstrating an increase in exercise performance, and it only occurred in patients whose angiogram demonstrated at least 18.8% improvement in index lesion severity. However, among patients with mild-to-moderate myocardial ischemia and single-vessel disease, medical therapy will improve exercise performance and quality of life in some without the necessity of the higher costs of initial coronary angioplasty followed by repeat angioplasty or by coronary artery bypass graft surgery when coronary restenosis occurs.

R.A. O'Rourke, M.D.

Reference

1. 1993 YEAR BOOK OF MEDICINE, pp 339–341.

The Role of Coronary Angiography and Coronary Revascularization Before Noncardiac Vascular Surgery

Mason JJ, Owens DK, Harris RA, Cooke JP, Hlatky MA (Stanford Univ, Calif; Veterans Affairs Med Ctr, Palo Alto, Calif)

JAMA 273:1919–1925, 1995 119-96-34-7

Introduction.—Perioperative cardiac complications are an important cause of morbidity and mortality after noncardiac surgery, and the risk is particularly high for patients undergoing vascular surgery. The identification of patients at increased risk poses a dilemma for the clinician. Decision analysis was used to determine whether preoperative coronary angiography and revascularization improve the short-term outcome after elective vascular surgery.

Methods.—The decision model considered 2 basic choices: to proceed directly to vascular surgery with close monitoring of the cardiac status and aggressive treatment of myocardial ischemia or to obtain a coronary angiogram, and, depending on the coronary anatomy, proceed to vascular surgery, perform coronary revascularization, or cancel the vascular surgery. Several outcomes are possible if vascular surgery is chosen: a technically successful and uncomplicated operation, death of the patient, a technically successful operation and a nonfatal myocardial infarction, or a technically successful operation and a nonfatal stroke. The main outcome measures, mortality, nonfatal myocardial infarction, nonfatal stroke, uncorrected vascular disease, and cost, were assessed within 3 months for patients who had either no angina or mild angina before operation and a positive result on a dipyridamole-thallium scan.

Results.—In the base case analysis, proceeding directly to vascular surgery led to both lower morbidity and reduced costs. Preoperative coronary angiography led to higher mortality if vascular surgery were to proceed in patients with inoperable coronary artery disease (CAD), but it led to slightly lower mortality if vascular surgery were canceled in patients with inoperable CAD. The use of coronary angiography also led to lower mortality in patients at particularly high risk for complications during vascular surgery.

Conclusions.—This decision model indicates that the best strategy for a patient at increased risk for perioperative cardiac complications is to proceed with the planned elective vascular surgery. The coronary angiography strategy commits the patient to 3 procedures, thus 3 encounters with the risk of death, myocardial infarction, and stroke. Overall, coronary angiography before vascular surgery leads to worse outcomes, and the procedure should be reserved for patients with a substantially higher-than-average risk of mortality.

▶ The data from this study suggest that the routine use of coronary angiography before vascular surgery leads to worse outcomes even among patients with a higher-than-average risk. Coronary angiography should be reserved for those patients at risk for very high operative mortality with vascular surgery and for whom it can be reasonably anticipated that mortality of coronary revascularization would be relatively low.

A recent report from the American Heart Association/American College of Cardiology Clinical Practice Guidelines Committee concerning the Perioperative Assessment of the Cardiac Patient for Noncardiac Surgery provides guidelines as to which patients might benefit from coronary arteriography before noncardiac surgery.[1] The patient's clinical characteristics, the functional activity capacity, the severity of the necessary surgery, and the results of imaging techniques (when needed) for assessing myocardial ischemia and left ventricular function are used to reach decisions concerning the advisability of preoperative coronary arteriography.

R.A. O'Rourke, M.D.

Reference

1. Eagle KA, Brundage BH, Chaitman BR, et al: Guidelines for perioperative cardiovascular evaluation for noncardiac surgery. *J Am Coll Cardiol*, in press.

35 Coronary Interventional Procedures

Percutaneous Transluminal Coronary Angioplasty as a First Revascularization Procedure in Single-, Double- and Triple-Vessel Coronary Artery Disease

Weintraub WS, King SB III, Douglas JS Jr, Kosinski AS (Emory Univ, Atlanta, Ga)

J Am Coll Cardiol 26:142–151, 1995 119-96-35–1

Background.—Coronary angioplasty has become the most common form of myocardial revascularization. However, its usefulness in patients with multivessel disease has not been well studied. The long-term outcome of coronary angioplasty was evaluated in patients with single- or multiple-vessel disease.

Subjects.—From June 1980 through December 1991, 10,783 patients without previous angioplasty or coronary surgery, whose diseased vessels could be completely identified, underwent angioplasty at Emory University Hospitals. Patients with acute myocardial infarction were excluded.

Findings.—Of the 10,783 patients, 71% had 1-vessel, 24% had 2-vessel, and 5% had 3-vessel disease. Age, male sex, diabetes, hypertension, history of previous infarction, and angina and congestive failure all increased with disease severity. Complete revascularization was achieved in most patients with 1-vessel disease and rarely in those with 3-vessel disease. The pecentage of those requiring emergency coronary bypass surgery increased from 1.7% of those with 1-vessel disease to 3.2% of those with 3-vessel disease. The mortality rate increased from 0.2% with 1-vessel disease to 1.2% with 3-vessel disease. Multivariate analysis indicated that the number of diseased vessels was correlated with length of hospital stay and long-term mortality. The 1-, 5- and 10-year survival rates were 0.99, 0.93, and 0.86, respectively, for 1-vessel disease; 0.97, 0.89, and 0.76 for 2-vessel disease; and 0.95, 0.85, and 0.70 for 3-vessel disease (Fig 1). There was an increased risk of myocardial infarction, coronary bypass surgery, and repeat angioplasty with an increased number of diseased vessels.

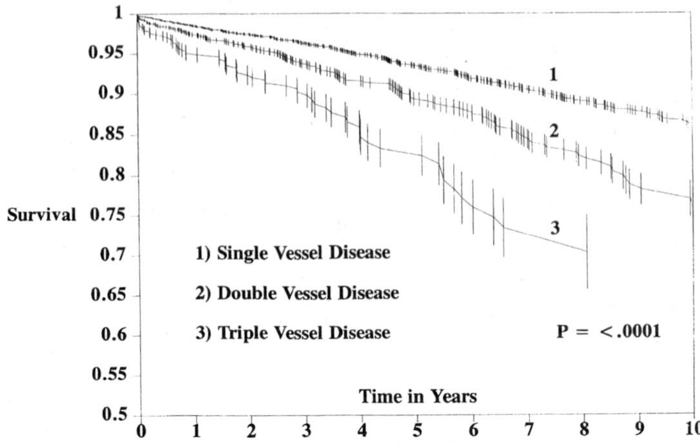

FIGURE 1.—Survival after angioplasty for single-, double-, and triple-vessel disease. (Reprinted with permission from the American College of Cardiology [*Journal of the American College of Cardiology*, 1995, 26:142–151.])

Conclusions.—Increased diseased vessel numbers are correlated with increased hospital stay, long-term mortality, myocardial infarction, and subsequent revascularization. Although angioplasty is a common treatment for patients with 1-vessel disease, it is not a common method of treatment of 3-vessel disease.

► This study would support the concept that symptomatic 3-vessel coronary artery disease remains primarily a surgical disease, although improved medical therapy with careful control of serum levels of lipids as well as improved interventional techniques may further limit coronary bypass surgery. In choosing a form of revascularization, the ability to achieve complete revascularization may be the decisive element in decision-making. In several randomized studies comparing multivessel angioplasty and coronary bypass surgery, there was more complete revascularization in those undergoing surgery initially and at 1- to 5-year follow-up. Complete revascularization has been shown to be important in a surgical series. In deciding whether to perform revascularization, multiple factors must be considered. Clearly, each patient must be considered individually, with clinical features and arteriographic findings taken into account. For example, a recent report from the Bypass Angioplasty Revascularization Investigation (BARI) study indicates that the patients with three-vessel coronary disease who have diabetes have a better prognosis with coronary artery bypass graft surgery than with multivessel coronary angioplasty.

In an important study assessing the immediate and long-term clinical outcome of coronary angioplasty in patients aged 35 years or younger, Kofflard and associates[1] followed 57 patients in this young age group for a median of 4.7 years. During follow-up, 12% of the patients died, 18% sustained a myocardial infarction, and 49% underwent repeat revascularization (coronary artery bypass surgery in 12% and repeat angioplasty in 37%).

The estimated 5-year survival was 87%, and the event-free survival was 50%. Thus, in young patients, coronary angioplasty has a high immediate success rate, but many had repeat revascularization procedures during the follow-up, and long-term survival was not markedly improved. Coronary angioplasty in young patients should be regarded as a palliative procedure.

Concerning the use of coronary angioplasty after myocardial infarction, Miketić and colleagues[2] prospectively evaluated patients with a first myocardial infarction, postinfarction ischemia, and residual high-grade stenosis with reduced flow in the infarct-related artery who underwent successful coronary angioplasty. Global ejection fraction and infarct region function were angiographically measured before coronary angioplasty and on routine follow-up study 6 ±1 months after angioplasty. The global ejection fraction in patients with complete flow at follow-up increased significantly, as did regional wall motion of the infarct area in both patients with anterior and inferior wall infarctions. However, in patients with restenosis at 6 months there was no difference at follow-up in either global ejection fraction or regional wall motion of the infarct area. Therefore, global and regional myocardial dysfunction resulting from postinfarction ischemia decreases significantly after successful coronary angioplasty of the infarct-related coronary artery with long-term sustained normal, complete flow. In contrast, restenosis and reduced flow prevent long-term improvement of left ventricular function.

R.A. O'Rourke, M.D.

References

1. Kofflard MJ, de Jaegere PP, van Domburg R, et al: Immediate and long-term clinical outcome of coronary angioplasty in patients aged 35 years or less. *Br Heart J* 73:82–86, 1995.
2. Miketić S, Carlsson J, Tebbe U: Improvement of global and regional left ventricular function by percutaneous transluminal coronary angioplasty after myocardial infarction. *J Am Coll Cardiol* 25:843–847, 1995.

Directional Atherectomy Versus Balloon Angioplasty for Coronary Ostial and Nonostial Left Anterior Descending Coronary Artery Lesions: Results From a Randomized Multicenter Trial

Topol EJ, for the CAVEAT-I Investigators (Cleveland Clinic Found, Ohio)
J Am Coll Cardiol 25:1380–1386, 1995 119-96-35-2

Background.—Proximal left anterior descending coronary artery stenoses are an important and challenging group of lesions associated with a worse outcome than stenoses at other locations. A subset of these proximal lesions, ostial left anterior descending coronary artery stenoses, are thought to have unique characteristics and lower rates of success after balloon angioplasty. Data from a large multicenter trial were used to test the hypothesis that atherectomy would be superior to balloon angioplasty in the treatment of both ostial and nonostial left anterior descending coronary artery lesions.

Methods.—Thirty-five sites enrolled 1,012 patients in the Coronary Angioplasty Versus Excisional Atherectomy Trial. The stipulated objective of coronary intervention was a value of 20% diameter stenosis; technical success was defined as a residual stenosis less than 50%. Proximal left anterior descending coronary artery lesions were seen in 563 patients, 74 of whom had ostial lesions. Early and 6-month results were compared for ostial and nonostial lesions.

Results.—Among the 489 patients with nonostial lesions, 250 had been randomized to directional atherectomy and 239 were randomized to undergo balloon angioplasty; 41 patients with ostial lesions were randomized to have directional atherectomy and 33 were randomized to receive conventional angioplasty. The 2 treatment groups had similar initial procedural success rates, but atherectomy produced a larger early gain in minimal lumen diameter compared with balloon angioplasty (1.13 vs. .56 mm) and a smaller degree of residual stenosis (26% vs. 39%). Other results were nearly identical for the 2 procedures: rate of restenosis by the binary dichotomous definition, 6-month minimal lumen diameter, 6-month percent stenosis, and rates of most major acute complications. There was a higher rate of adjudicated non–Q-wave myocardial infarction events, however, in the directional atherectomy group (24%) compared with the balloon angioplasty group (13%). Atherectomy did not lower the rate of subsequent coronary artery bypass surgery or of repeat percutaneous coronary intervention.

Conclusion.—Rates of initial success and restenosis were similar for ostial left anterior descending coronary artery lesions treated by atherectomy or balloon angioplasty. Although gains were greater in proximal nonostial lesions treated by atherectomy, the rate of clinical restenosis was not lowered and the incidence of in-hospital myocardial infarction was increased.

▶ These results yield some new therapeutic information concerning patients with proximal left anterior descending coronary artery disease who are candidates for nonsurgical revascularization. An analysis of patients with ostial and proximal left anterior descending coronary lesions who were randomized to undergo treatment with either directional coronary atherectomy or balloon angioplasty indicates no significant advantage for directional atherectomy.

Harrington and the CAVEAT Investigators[1] recently reported on the characteristics and consequences of myocardial infarction after the coronary angioplasty vs. excisional atherectomy trial. Postintervention enzyme levels and ECG findings were obtained from 500 patients receiving balloon angioplasty and 512 patients receiving directional atherectomy. Myocardial infarction was defined as new pathologic Q waves on postintervention ECGs or a threefold increase in creatine kinase–MB values above normal levels. During 6 months of follow-up, the atherectomy group had 78 myocardial infarctions, which is significantly more than the balloon angioplasty group, which had 34. In the atherectomy group, 48 patients had new Q waves or threefold greater than normal increase creatine kinase–MB levels as compared with the balloon angioplasty group of 21 such patients. Patients with myocardial infarction had significantly longer hospital stays and incurred significantly higher costs than did those without myocardial infarction. Myocardial infarction was predictive of death, bypass surgery, or repeat intervention within 30 days and of death within 1 year. This study indicates that the incidence of myocardial infarction is higher after atherectomy than after angioplasty, although short-term outcomes are similar. Patients with postintervention myocardial infarction have a poorer clinical outcome.

Recently, Umans and colleagues[2] examined whether restenosis was related to the extent or mechanism of lumen improvement in patients undergoing atherectomy or balloon angioplasty. They compared 2 similar groups with equal baseline and clinical stenosis characteristics. Although atherectomy and angioplasty resulted in similar immediate mean lumen gain by design, lumen loss was more pronounced after atherectomy; thus, the minimal lumen diameter at follow-up differed significantly between the 2 groups. Therefore, restenosis is a consequence not only of the extent of lumen improvement but also of the mechanism of vessel wall injury (dilating vs. debulking). When atherectomy is performed, the operator should try for an optimal procedural result to accommodate the increased intimal hyperplastic response.

R.A. O'Rourke, M.D.

References

1. Harrington RA, for the CAVEAT Investigators: Characteristics and consequences of myocardial infarction after percutaneous coronary intervention: Insights from the Coronary Angioplasty Versus Excisional Atherectomy Trial (CAVEAT). *J Am Coll Cardiol* 25:1693–1699, 1995.
2. Umans VAWM, Keane D, Foley D, et al: Optimal use of directional coronary atherectomy is required to ensure long-term angiographic benefit: A study with matched procedural outcome after atherectomy and angioplasty. *J Am Coll Cardiol* 24:1652–1659, 1994.

A Multicenter, Randomized Trial of Coronary Angioplasty Versus Directional Atherectomy for Patients With Saphenous Vein Bypass Graft Lesions

Holmes DR Jr, Topol EJ, Califf RM, Berdan LG, Leya F, Berger PB, Whitlow PL, Safian RD, Adelman AG, Kellett MA Jr, Talley JD III, Shani J, Gottlieb RS, Pinkerton CA, Lee KL, Keeler GP, Ellis SG, the CAVEAT-II Investigators (Mayo Clinic and Found, Rochester, Minn; Cleveland Clinic Found, Ohio; Duke Univ, Durham, NC; et al)
Circulation 91:1966–1974, 1995 119-96-35–3

Introduction.—Percutaneous transluminal coronary angioplasty (PTCA) has been used in the treatment of restenosis of grafted vessels, with varying outcomes. Directional coronary atherectomy (DCA) has also been used in the treatment of graft restenosis. It has been suggested that restenosis rates could be decreased with excision and removal of the plaque as compared to balloon dilation. The efficacy of DCA vs. PTCA in reducing the rates of restenosis in de novo bypass grafts was assessed in a multicenter trial.

Methods.—A total of 305 patients with previous coronary artery bypass graft surgery who required revascularization were randomly assigned to undergo either DCA or PTCA. Coronary angiography was obtained before and after the procedure and at a 6-month follow-up. Angiograms taken before the procedure were evaluated in a blinded fashion for degree of coronary artery disease and number, complexity, and morphologic features of the lesions. Vessel caliber, minimum diameter, percent diameter stenosis, and percent stenosis of lesions were measured on all films. Patients were also assessed for procedural success (defined as less than 50% stenosis), development of complications (death, myocardial infarction, abrupt closure), quality of life, and length of hospital stay. At follow-up, rates of restenosis, development of late complications (myocardial infarction, death, need for bypass surgery), and functional and exercise capacity were evaluated.

Results.—One hundred forty-nine patients underwent DCA, and 156 underwent PTCA. Unstable angina and comorbid conditions were common in both groups. Graft age was 9.5 years in patients undergoing DCA and 9.9 years in patients undergoing PTCA. Location of vein grafts and of stenoses within the graft were similar for both groups. Lesion length and morphologic features were also similar. On the basis of site assessment, no significant differences in initial success rates were found between the 2 groups (98.0% for DCA vs. 97.4% for PTCA). However, based on core laboratory assessment, DCA resulted in a significantly higher success rate as compared to PTCA (89.2% vs. 79.0%). Directional coronary atherectomy also achieved a significantly greater increase in diameter than PTCA (1.45 vs. 1.12 mm) and had a significantly smaller percent diameter stenosis (31.5% vs. 37.6%). The incidence of complications was similar between the 2 groups; however, there was a trend for increased incidence of non–Q-wave myocardial infarction and a significantly higher incidence of distal embolization with DCA. At the 6-month follow-up, percent diameter stenosis was 30% to 40% in patients who underwent DCA as compared to 40% to 50% with PTCA, a nonsignificant difference (Fig 2). Although the differences were not significant, rates of restenosis (greater than 50% stenosis) were lower and minimal luminal diameter greater with DCA. There was no significant difference in 6-month survival. Significantly fewer patients who underwent DCA required repeat target vessel intervention for survival as compared to those who underwent PTCA (13.2% vs. 22.4%).

Discussion.—Directional coronary atherectomy resulted in greater success rates and larger initial improvements in graft diameters as compared with PTCA in patients with de novo graft lesions. However, patients who underwent DCA also had a greater incidence of distal embolization and a trend toward more non–Q-wave myocardial infarction after the proce-

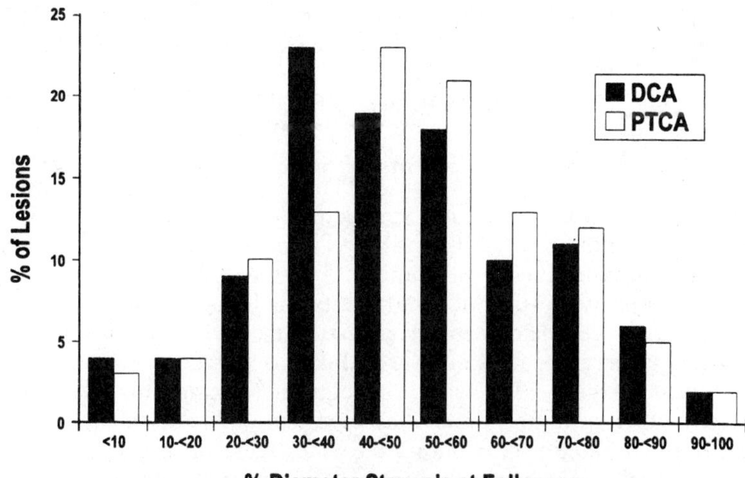

FIGURE 2.—Bar graph showing distribution of follow-up stenoses by treatment group. *Abbreviations: DCA,* directional coronary atherectomy; *PTCA,* percutaneous transluminal coronary angioplasty. (Reproduced with permission [*Circulation*]. Copyright [1995] American Heart Association.)

dure. Six-month restenosis rates were similar for the 2 procedures, but fewer patients who underwent DCA required repeat vessel intervention for survival as compared with PTCA.

▶ Although both forms of coronary revascularization are viable options for patients with saphenous vein bypass graft lesions, each has positive and negative features. Direct coronary atherectomy resulted in a higher initial angiographic success rate and a larger initial increase in graft dimensions than conventional coronary angioplasty. The improved success rate was, in part, offset by the moderate initial increase in distal embolization and non–Q-wave myocardial infarction, which was likely attributable to passage of the large atherectomy device and active debulking and manipulation of the lesion. Importantly, there was no difference in angiographic restenosis rate.

R.A. O'Rourke, M.D.

Stent Implantation of Saphenous Vein Graft Aorto-Ostial Lesions in Patients With Unstable Ischemic Syndromes: Immediate Angiographic Results and Long-Term Clinical Outcome

Rechavia E, Litvack F, Macko G, Eigler NL (Cedars-Sinai Med Ctr, Los Angeles; Univ of California, Los Angeles)

J Am Coll Cardiol 25:866–870, 1995 119-96-35–4

Background.—Few studies have investigated the usefulness, safety, and short- and long-term clinical results of stent implantation in patients with aorto-ostial lesions and unstable angina. The immediate angiographic and long-term clinical findings in patients undergoing such procedures were, therefore, investigated.

Patients and Findings.—Twenty-nine patients (mean age, 70 years) with complex vein graft aorto-ostial lesions and unstable angina were included. Twenty-three of the 29 patients had a previous myocardial infarction, and 13 had undergone bypass operations. The mean graft age in these latter patients was 9 years. A mean left ventricular ejection fraction of 42% was noted. All patients received Palmaz or Palmaz-Schatz stents. Thirty-two stents were implanted in 25 new and in 4 restenotic aorto-ostial lesions; 5 patients also received 10 additional stents for 8 lesions not at ostial sites. The procedures were successful in all patients, and no mortality, Q-wave myocardial infarction, or stent thrombosis occurred within the first 30 days. Bypass surgery also was not required during this period. Mean improvements in minimal lumen diameter, from 0.7 mm to 3.3 mm, and in percent diameter stenosis, from 80% to 1%, were observed after stenting. A mean immediate loss from recoil of 0.2 mm was observed, coinciding with a mean percent recoil of 7%. Patients were followed for a mean period of 11 months. Twenty-seven patients survived, with no evidence of myocardial infarction noted. One patient required bypass surgery and 2 underwent balloon angioplasty. Of the remaining 24 patients, symptoms were reduced by 2 or more symptom classes in 21 (Fig 2).

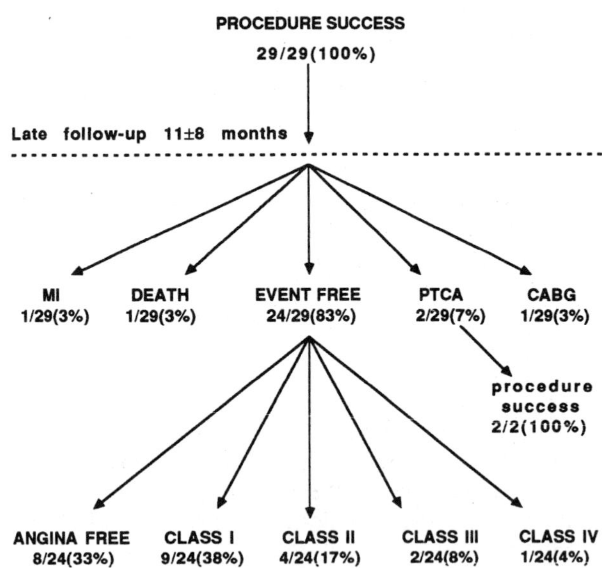

FIGURE 2.—Long-term follow-up and Canadian Cardiovascular Society angina class after stent deployment in 29 patients with unstable angina (angina class IV) with saphenous vein graft aorto-ostial lesions. *Abbreviations: CABG,* coronary artery bypass grafting; *MI,* myocardial infarction; *PTCA,* percutaneous transluminal coronary angioplasty. (Reprinted with permission from the American College of Cardiology [*Journal of the American College of Cardiology,* 1995, 25:866–870].)

Conclusions.—The probability of immediate success and a large immediate gain in lumen diameter is high in patients undergoing Palmaz or Palmaz-Schatz stenting procedures for saphenous vein graft aorto-ostial stenosis. Immediate and long-term complication rates also are low. Thus, stenting of saphenous vein graft aorto-ostial lesions in elderly patients with unstable angina and large-diameter vessels appears to be a feasible therapeutic alternative.

► This study shows that stent implantation in aorto-ostial saphenous vein graft lesions has a high probability of procedural success, a relatively low morbidity, and uncommon adverse clinical events. In view of their current data, the authors recommend that primary stenting be considered for aorto-ostial lesions in vein grafts with a diameter of 3 mm or larger. In vein grafts or native arteries of 3 mm or smaller, they consider treatment with a debulking device (atherectomy) and adjunctive balloon angioplasty.

In a relevant report concerning stent implantation in saphenous vein graft lesions, Leon, Wong, and associates[1] report the multicenter registry experience evaluating the safety and efficacy of the Palmaz-Schatz stent in the treatment of saphenous vein graft disease. The group comprised a total of 589 symptomatic patients (624 lesions) evaluated for treatment of focal vein graft stenosis between January 1990 and April 1992. Follow-up angiography was performed at 6 months, and clinical course data of all study patients were prospectively collected at regular intervals for up to 12 months. Stent delivery was successful in 98.8% of cases, and the procedural success rate was 97.1%. Major in-hospital complications occurred in 2.9% of the patients, with stent thrombosis found in 1.4% and major vascular or bleeding complications in 14.3%. Six-month angiographic follow-up revealed an overall rate of restenosis of 29.7%. Stent implantation in patients with focal saphenous vein graft lesions was achieved with a high rate of procedural success, acceptable major complications, reduced angiographic restenosis, and favorable late clinical outcome as compared with historical balloon angioplasty control series. As expected, the strict anticoagulation regimen required after stent placement resulted in more frequent vascular and other bleeding complications.

Another important study analyzed the outcomes of revascularization procedures in cardiac transplant recipients.[2] Thirteen medical centers retrospectively analyzed their complete experience with coronary angioplasty, direct coronary atherectomy, and coronary bypass graft surgery in allograft coronary heart disease. Sixty-six patients underwent coronary angioplasty with an angiographic success rate of 94%. Forty patients were alive without retransplantation 19 ± 14 months after angioplasty. The consequences of failure in revascularization were severe. Angiographic restenosis occurred in 55% of 76 lesions at 8 ± 5 months after angioplasty. These data suggest that coronary revascularization may be an effective palliative therapy in suitable cardiac transplant recipients. Angioplasty results in acceptable survival in patients with no angiographic evidence of distal arteriopathy, which was defined as the presence of discrete or multiple stenoses, diffuse concentric narrowing, or diseased, diffusely irregular lesions of tertiary vessels.

R.A. O'Rourke, M.D.

References

1. Leon MB, Wong SC, Baim DS, for the Palmaz-Schatz Stent Study Group: Immediate results and late outcomes after stent implantation in saphenous vein graft lesions: The multicenter U.S. Palmaz-Schatz stent experience. *J Am Coll Cardiol* 26:704–712, 1995.
2. Halle AA III, DiSciascio G, Massin EK, et al: Coronary angioplasty, atherectomy and bypass surgery in cardiac transplant recipients. *J Am Coll Cardiol* 26:120–128, 1995.

In-Hospital Cost of Percutaneous Coronary Revascularization: Critical Determinants and Implications

Ellis SG, Miller DP, Brown KJ, Omoigui N, Howell GL, Kutner M, Topol EJ
(Cleveland Clinic Found, Ohio)
Circulation 92:741–747, 1995 119-96-35-5

Background.—Since being introduced nearly 20 years ago, percutaneous balloon angioplasty has become an increasingly popular approach to relieving angina pectoris. Approximately 430,000 procedures were scheduled in 1994. At a hospital charge of $15,000, the overall cost exceeded $6 billion. Not enough information is available on the major components of these costs.

Objective and Methods.—Records were reviewed for 1,258 consecutive patients at a tertiary referral center in whom percutaneous transluminal coronary revascularization was attempted. In general, the patients were typical of those referred for coronary intervention, but 71% had unstable angina. Direct and indirect hospital and physician charges were estimated on the basis of resource utilization using the "top-down" approach. Data were available for 1,086 patients undergoing 1,237 procedures.

Results.—Procedural success was achieved in 89% of cases. The rate of major complications (death, Q-wave infarction, bypass surgery) was 3.8%. Total hospital and physician costs averaged $13,071 but ranged widely, from $3,422 to $193,474. The preoperative variables that most strongly influenced cost included acute myocardial infarction, decisional delay, use of the intra-aortic balloon, an intention to place a stent, a complex lesion, and an increased serum level of creatinine. The time in hospital, urgent bypass surgery, and noncardiac death also were close correlates of cost, as were the use of blood products, the occurrence of Q-wave infarction, and use of the Rotablator. The median unadjusted hospital costs of various techniques are contrasted in the figure from p. 742.

Conclusions.—Hospital costs for percutaneous coronary revascularization are extremely variable. Roughly half the variance comes from patient characteristics, but procedural complications and system delay make im-

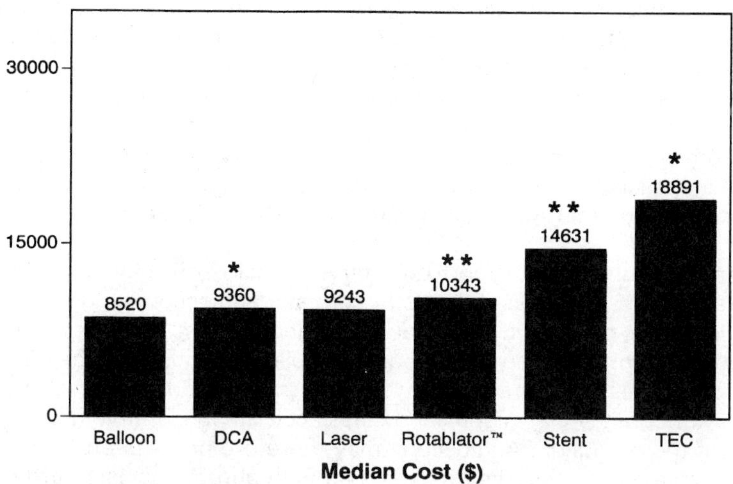

FIGURE p 742.—Bar graph showing median unadjusted in-hospital costs for patients treated with the devices noted. $^{*}P \leq 0.05$, $^{**}P \leq 0.01$ compared with balloon angioplasty in multivariate modeling. *Abbreviations: DCA,* directional coronary atherectomy: *TEC,* transluminal extraction coronary atherectomy. (Reproduced with permission [*Circulation*]. Copyright [1995] American Heart Association.)

portant contributions. Further cost analyses may help develop strategies for limiting resource utilization and promoting economically efficient care.

▶ The data reported extend prior observations by noting the predictive information contained in the variables available before the procedure, which explain nearly one third of the variation in costs; the importance of system-related problems such as delays in treatment because of the unavailability of some hospital services on weekends or protracted decision-making; and the high cost of noncardiac complications such as renal dysfunction, blood transfusion, and peripheral vascular complications. Variables such as baseline creatinine and the need for balloon counterpulsation or heparin therapy appear to be better markers for resource consumption. A reduction in the in-hospital complications should lead to a corresponding reduction in hospitalization costs. The complications of balloon angioplasty are well described, as are those for newer techniques. However, it is not clear whether the use of new nonballoon technologies will decrease or increase complications overall.

Other important considerations relative to the cost of myocardial revascularization are contained in the report by Weintraub and associates,[1] using data from the Emory Angioplasty Versus Surgery Trial (EAST). In this randomized trial, the clinical outcome and costs of percutaneous transluminal coronary angioplasty (PTCA) and coronary surgery for multivessel coronary artery disease from a randomized trial are reported. Costs were assessed for the initial hospitalization and the accumulative costs of the initial hospitalization and additional revascularization procedures for up to 3 years. There was no difference in mortality and the primary end point (death, Q-wave myocardial infarction, and a large reversible thallium defect at 3 years).

Three-year total charges were $25,458 for PTCA and $31,033 for surgery ($P < 0.0001$). Three-year costs were $23,734 for PTCA and $25,310 for coronary surgery ($P < 0.0001$). There were more hospitalizations for angina and more antianginal medication used in the PTCA group, which would further narrow the differences in cost. Although the primary procedural costs for coronary surgery are more than those for coronary angioplasty, the cost advantage is largely lost by 3 years because of the more frequent additional procedures and other resource consumption after a first revascularization by PTCA.

In another interesting report on interventional cardiology, White and associates[2] assessed the usefulness of coronary angioscopy to determine the specific cause of abrupt occlusion after angioplasty. Angioscopy demonstrated the primary cause of the postangioplasty occlusion to be dissection in 82% of cases and intracoronary thrombi in 18%. Compared with angioscopy, arteriography was significantly less accurate in identifying the specific cause of the occlusion. Angioscopy may therefore prove useful in selecting specific treatment strategies for patients with abrupt occlusion after angioplasty such as stent placement, atherectomy, repeat dilation, or thrombolysis.

In another intriguing report, Mehta and associates[3] studied the possibility that spontaneous regression in stenosis severity occurs over time in patients with restenosis after coronary angioplasty. Fifteen asymptomatic patients with coronary artery restenosis after initially successful angioplasty consented to undergo repeat angiography, which was performed 6–25 months later, to assess the possibility of regression. There was a significant mean decrease in lesion severity from 66.9% to 47.5% and a significant mean increase in minimal lumen diameter from 0.91 mm to 1.44 mm. No patients showed progression of stenosis, but regression of restenosis defined as a decrease in minimal lumen diameter of greater than 0.2 mm was noted in 12 of the patients. Although all 15 study patients were asymptomatic, similar changes may occur in symptomatic patients. Therefore, a trial of medical therapy may be appropriate in asymptomatic or mildly symptomatic patients before further interventions. This strategy might avoid unnecessary invasive procedures, preventing a "restenosis cycle" and resulting in significant cost savings.

It had been hypothesized that high-dose angiotensin-converting enzyme (ACE) inhibition might result in a decreased rate of restenosis in patients undergoing coronary angioplasty. Faxon and associates[4] report the results of a multicenter study assessing the incidence of coronary artery restenosis in 1,436 patients randomly assigned to be treated with the ACE inhibitor cilazapril or placebo for 6 months in addition to aspirin daily. Unfortunately, like so many other attempts to prevent coronary artery restenosis after angioplasty, cilazapril in low or high doses was not found to reduce restenosis in patients after coronary angioplasty. Additionally, overall cardiac events were not affected by treatment with the ACE inhibitor.

R.A. O'Rourke, M.D.

References

1. Weintraub WS, Mauldin PD, Becker E, et al: A comparison of the costs of and quality of life after coronary angioplasty or coronary surgery for multivessel coronary artery disease: Results from the Emory Angioplasty Versus Surgery Trial (EAST). *Circulation* 92:2831–2840, 1995.
2. White CJ, Ramee SR, Collins TJ, et al: Coronary angioscopy of abrupt occlusion after angioplasty. *J Am Coll Cardiol* 25:1681–1684, 1995.
3. Mehta VY, Jorgensen MB, Raizner AE: Spontaneous regression of restenosis: An angiographic study. *J Am Coll Cardiol* 26:696–702, 1995.
4. Faxon DP: Effect of high dose angiotensin-converting enzyme inhibition on restenosis: Final results of the MARCATOR study, a multicenter, double-blind, placebo-controlled study of cilazapril. *J Am Coll Cardiol* 2:362–369, 1995.

36 Cardiomyopathy/ Heart Failure

A Clinical Trial of Immunosuppressive Therapy for Myocarditis

Mason JW, O'Connell JB, Herskowitz A, Rose NR, McManus BM, Billingham ME, Moon TE, and the Myocarditis Treatment Trial Investigators (Univ of Utah, Salt Lake City; Univ of Mississippi, Jackson; Johns Hopkins Univ, Baltimore, Md; et al)

N Engl J Med 333:269–275, 1995 119-96-36–1

Introduction.—Immunosuppressive agents appear to be of benefit in myocarditis, but the efficacy of this therapy has not been established. The Myocarditis Treatment Trial was conducted to determine whether immunosuppressive therapy improves left ventricular function and to identify immunologic markers of the severity of the disease.

Methods.—Patients were enrolled at 31 centers in the United States, Canada, and Japan. All had heart failure without coronary artery disease or another specific cause diagnosed during the 2 years preceding enrollment. A total of 111 patients with histologic evidence of myocarditis and left ventricular fractions under 0.45 were randomly assigned to receive azathioprine and prednisone, cyclosporine and prednisone, or no immunosuppressive therapy. All 3 groups received conventional drugs for heart failure. Patients were followed for 1 year with radionuclide ventriculography, echocardiography, exercise testing, endomyocardial biopsies, and blood studies. The primary outcome measure was a change in left ventricular ejection fraction at 28 weeks.

Results.—The 3 treatment groups were similar in clinical characteristics; most were in New York Heart Association class I or II. For the patients as a whole, the mean left ventricular ejection fraction was 0.24 at baseline and improved to 0.34 at 28 weeks. Those receiving immunosuppressive therapy had a mean gain of 0.10 and those given conventional therapy a mean gain of only 0.07, a difference that was not significant. There was continued improvement in left ventricular ejection fraction at 52 weeks, again with no significant difference between groups (Fig 1). Increased left ventricular ejection fraction at 28 weeks was related to a higher left ventricular ejection fraction and less intensive conventional therapy at baseline and to a shorter duration of disease. Immunosuppression and

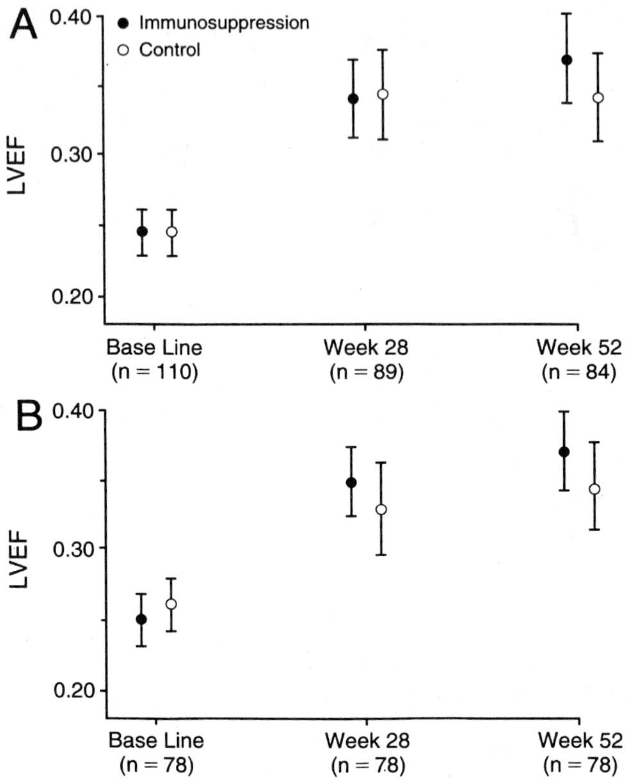

FIGURE 1.—Mean (± standard error) left ventricular ejection fraction (*LVEF*) in the immunosuppression and control groups at baseline, week 28, and week 52. **A,** the mean values for all available studies at each time, with the numbers of patients indicated at the bottom of the panel. There was no difference between the 2 groups in the mean LVEF at baseline, week 28, or week 52 (P = 0.97, P = 0.95, and P = 0.45, respectively). **B,** the mean values for the 78 patients for whom data were available at all 3 times. There was no significant difference between the groups (P = 0.51, P = 0.60, and P = 0.50, respectively). (Reprinted by permission of *The New England Journal of Medicine.* Mason JW, O'Connell JB, Herskowitz A, et al: A clinical trial of immunosuppressive therapy for myocarditis. *N Engl J Med* 333:269–275, Copyright 1995, Massachusetts Medical Society.)

control groups did not differ significantly in survival at 1 year or throughout follow-up. Immunologic variables showed no systematic change during the study period.

Conclusion.—Immunosuppressive therapy, compared with conventional therapy alone, did not significantly increase left ventricular ejection fraction or improve survival in patients with histologically confirmed myocarditis. There remains a possibility that other immunosuppressive regimens may benefit specific subgroups of patients with myocarditis.

► The results of this important clinical study do not support the routine treatment of myocarditis with immunosuppressive drugs. Ventricular function improved regardless of whether patients received immunosuppressive therapy, but long-term mortality was high. In this study, multivariate analysis not surprisingly identified a higher baseline left ventricular ejection fraction, less intense conventional drug therapy at baseline, and a shorter duration of disease as independent predictors of improvement in left ventricular ejection fraction. Left ventricular ejection fraction is a well-known predictor of survival, and more intensive therapy for heart failure would be expected for patients with more severe disease and a poorer prognosis.

In another important study on this topic, Grogan et al.[1] compared the long-term outcome of patients with biopsy-proven myocarditis and those with idiopathic dilated cardiomyopathy who were biopsy negative for myocarditis. Ejection fraction was lower in the 58 patients with idiopathic dilated cardiomyopathy (25 ± 11%) than in the 27 patients with biopsy-proven myocarditis (38 ± 19%; $P = 0.001$). Even though a higher proportion of patients in the myocarditis group were New York Heart Association functional class III or IV compared with patients in the dilated cardiomyopathy group, there was no difference in the 5-year survival between the myocarditis and idiopathic dilated cardiomyopathy groups (56% vs. 54%, respectively). With the current lack of proven effective treatment for lymphocytic myocarditis and no demonstration of survival benefit for patients with myocarditis, endomyocardial biopsy performed to exclude myocarditis may be of limited prognostic value in the routine evaluation of patients with dilated cardiomyopathy. However, it should be noted that this study was limited to idiopathic lymphocytic myocarditis; in patients with some other forms of myocarditis, who are treatable or have a different prognosis, endomyocardial biopsy remains of clinical usefulness.

R.A. O'Rourke, M.D.

Reference

1. Grogan M, Redfield MM, Bailey KR, et al: Long-term outcome of patients with biopsy-proved myocarditis: Comparison with idiopathic dilated cardiomyopathy. *J Am Coll Cardiol* 26:80–84, 1995.

Sudden Cardiac Death in Hypertrophic Cardiomyopathy: Variability in Phenotypic Expression of β-Myosin Heavy Chain Mutations

Marian AJ, Mares A Jr, Kelly DP, Yu Q-T, Abchee AB, Hill R, Roberts R (Baylor College of Medicine, Houston; Washington Univ, St Louis, Mo)

Eur Heart J 16:368–376, 1995 119-96-36–2

Background.—Analysis of the genotype-phenotype correlation in families with hypertrophic cardiomyopathy (HCM) has been made possible by the recent discovery of mutations in the β-myosin heavy chain gene (MYH7). The phenotypic expression of 2 β-myosin heavy chain (βMHC) mutations was investigated in 3 unrelated families with HCM.

Participants and Methods.—History was obtained, and physical examinations, ECG, and two-dimensional echocardiography were performed in living individuals from unrelated HCM families 1, 2, and 3. After blood samples were obtained from all participants, DNA was extracted and polymerase chain reaction, restriction endonuclease digestion, and chemical cleavage were performed. All detected mutations were verified using sequence analysis.

Results.—Seven members of family 1 had HCM, 1 of whom died of sudden cardiac death (SCD) and another of recurrent cerebral emboli. Fifteen individuals in family 2 had HCM. Of these, 9 have died, 7 of SCD. The mean age at SCD was 33 years. In family 3, there were 11 affected individuals and 1 obligate carrier. One patient in this group died of progressive heart failure at age 17 years, and 2 others died of SCD at age 60 years. Various clinical and echocardiographic indications of HCM were observed in each family. The patients with HCM from families 1 and 2 had a missense mutation in exon 13 of the βMHC gene ($Arg^{403}Gln$). Two fragments of 84 and 70 bp were found in normal individuals after polymerase chain reaction amplification of the exon 13 DNA, followed by Ddel digestion of the polymerase chain reaction product and gel electrophoresis. In the patients with HCM, 4 fragments of 84, 70, 52, and 32 bp were detected. The replacement of an adenine for guanine was observed at coding position 1208 on sequence analysis. Among the patients with HMC in family 3, a missense mutation in exon 16 of the βMHC gene was observed ($Val^{606}Met$). An uncleaved product of 337 bp was found on chemical cleavage of the polymerase chain reaction products in normal individuals. In the affected patients, a 90 bp cleaved product was detected in addition to the uncleaved product. This suggested a mismatch in 1 allele. Replacement of an adenine for guanine in coding position 1,817 was noted on sequence analysis. The $Arg^{403}Gln$ mutation was found to be associated with a more unfavorable prognosis in HCM families, compared with $Val^{606}Met$ (Fig 4).

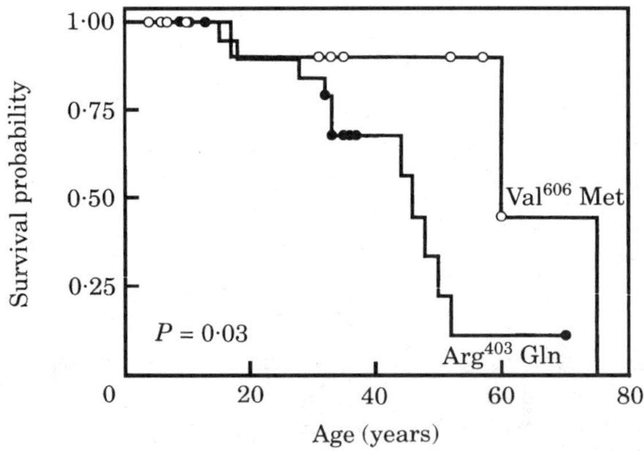

FIGURE 4.—Kaplan-Meier survival curves for members of families 1 and 2 with $Arg^{403}Gln$ mutation and members of family 3 with $Val^{606}Met$ mutation. (Courtesy of Marian AJ, Mares A Jr, Kelly DP, et al: Sudden cardiac death in hypertrophic cardiomyopathy: Variability in phenotypic expression of β-myosin heavy chain mutations. *Eur Heart J* 16:368–376, 1995.)

Conclusions.—β-myosin heavy chain mutations are potent predictors of survival in families with HMC. The Arg^{403}Gln mutation is associated with a worse prognosis and a higher incidence of SCD in comparison with Val^{606}Met.

► A characteristic feature of HCM is the variability of the clinical manifestations, such as the incidence of sudden cardiac death, among families with HCM. The recent identification of several mutations in the β-MHC gene, a major responsible gene for HCM, permits a correlation of the genotypes with the clinical manifestation (phenotypes) of hypertrophic cardiomyopathy. Using molecular biology techniques, the authors were able to identify certain patients who were at high risk for sudden cardiac death. The identification of high-risk individuals in families with HCM by genetic analysis, independent of the development of symptoms and before the occurrence of sudden cardiac death, provides the opportunity to use therapeutic modalities such as the implantation of cardioverter defibrillators to prevent sudden cardiac death. Recent preliminary data support such a role for defibrillators in high-risk patients with HCM.

R.A. O'Rourke, M.D.

Dissociation Between Exertional Symptoms and Circulatory Function in Patients With Heart Failure

Wilson JR, Rayos G, Yeoh TK, Gothard P, Bak K (Vanderbilt Univ, Nashville, Tenn)

Circulation 92:47–53, 1995 119-96-36–3

Objective.—Although exercise intolerance in patients with heart failure is usually attributed to circulatory dysfunction, there is evidence that exercise training can improve exertional symptoms in these patients without compromising hemodynamic function. The relation between exertional symptoms and circulatory function and between hemodynamic function and perceived functional intolerance in ambulatory patients with heart failure was investigated.

Methods.—A total of 52 patients with heart failure (14 women), aged 26–67 years, underwent hemodynamic monitoring during treadmill exercise testing. Severity of dyspnea and fatigue was determined. Perceived functional limitations were assessed using the Minnesota Living With Heart Failure Questionnaire and the Yale Dyspnea-Fatigue Index.

Results.—Average pulmonary wedge pressure increased to 28 mm Hg, lactate concentration to 34.5 mg/dL, and oxygen consumption ($\dot{V}O_2$) increased to 13.4 mL/min^{-1}/kg^{-1} during peak exercise. Mild hemodynamic dysfunction was observed in 11 patients, moderate in 22, and severe in 19. The mean dyspnea and fatigue scores increased to 15.7 and 14.8. Pulmonary artery hemoglobin oxygen saturation decreased to a mean of 30%. There was a small but significant correlation between peak exercise $\dot{V}O_2$

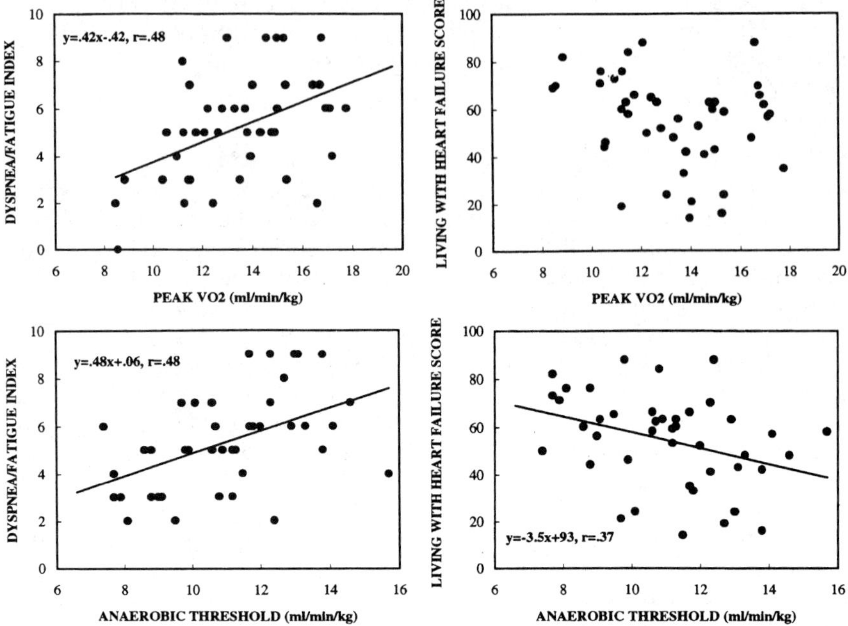

FIGURE 5.—Plots showing relation between questionnaire results and peak exercise oxygen consumption ($\dot{V}O_2$) and the anaerobic threshold during maximal treadmill exercise testing. (Reproduced with permission [*Circulation*]. Copyright [1995] American Heart Association.)

and the Dyspnea-Fatigue exercise (Fig 5). Both the Living With Heart Failure Questionnaire and the Dyspnea-Fatigue Index were weakly correlated with the anaerobic threshold.

Conclusion.—Exercise intolerance is not correlated with circulatory, ventilatory, or metabolic dysfunction. Patients' reports of exercise intolerance should be compared with objective measures of hemodynamic parameters to determine possible circulatory dysfunction.

▶ These findings suggest that physicians should no longer assume that exertional symptoms in patients with heart failure indicate left ventricular dysfunction and, therefore, should no longer depend only on pharmaceutical interventions to treat these symptoms. The possibility that exertional symptoms are related to muscle deconditioning, obesity, and other noncardiac factors should be considered. If necessary, direct hemodynamic monitoring during exercise should be used to interpret exertional symptoms. Conversely, the absence of exertional symptoms should not be considered definite evidence that cardiac pump function is preserved. In this study, several patients with severe hemodynamic dysfunction during exercise and severe exercise impairment denied significant exertional symptoms. Such patients probably might be considered for heart transplantation on the basis of a poor long-term prognosis and probably are best identified by maximal exercise testing.

Because patients with advanced heart failure often undergo cardiopulmonary exercise testing to predict prognosis, DiSalvo and associates[1] assessed exercise and radionuclide ventriculographic variables as prognostic indicators in patients with advanced heart failure. They studied 67 patients with advanced heart failure with 58% in New York Heart Association functional class III and 18% in functional class IV. The mean left ventricular ejection fraction was 22%. Simultaneous upright bicycle ergometric cardiopulmonary exercise testing and first-pass rest/exercise radionuclide ventriculography were performed by all patients. The mean peak oxygen consumption was 11.8 mL/kg per minute. Predictors of overall survival identified by a multivariate analysis were a right ventricular ejection fraction of ≥ 0.35 and a percent predicted oxygen consumption of 45% or higher. The right ventricular ejection fraction of ≥ 0.35 at rest and exercise was a more potent predictor of survival in advanced heart failure than was mean peak oxygen consumption or percent of mean peak oxygen consumption during exercise. Also, percent predicted mean oxygen consumption, rather than peak oxygen consumption, better predicted survival in advanced heart failure.

R.A. O'Rourke, M.D.

Reference

1. DiSalvo TG, Mathier M, Semigran MJ, et al: Preserved right ventricular ejection fraction predicts exercise capacity and survival in advanced heart failure. *J Am Coll Cardiol* 25:1143–1153, 1995.

Mechanism of Hemodynamic Improvement by Dual-Chamber Pacing for Severe Left Ventricular Dysfunction: An Acute Doppler and Catheterization Hemodynamic Study

Nishimura RA, Hayes DL, Holmes DR Jr, Tajik AJ (Mayo Clinic and Found, Rochester, Minn)

J Am Coll Cardiol 25:281–288, 1995 119-96-36–4

Objectives.—For patients with dilated cardiomyopathy and severe heart failure, dual-chamber pacing is proposed as a new therapeutic modality for relief of symptoms. The mechanisms by which this treatment improves hemodynamic variables in patients with left ventricular systolic dysfunction and the selection of patients who could potentially receive the greatest benefit were studied.

Patients.—Fifteen patients with dilated cardiomyopathy were studied. All had symptoms of heart failure, with 11 in New York Heart Association functional classes III and IV and 4 in class II. The mean ejection fraction was 19%. Six patients had grade 3 or 4 mitral regurgitation on Doppler echocardiography or left ventriculography, or both.

Methods.—The patients were studied acutely during atrioventricular (AV) sequential pacing at AV intervals of 60, 100, 120, 140, 180, and 240 ms with use of combined Doppler velocity curves and pressures obtained by high-fidelity manometer-tipped catheters and thermodilution cardiac output.

Results.—No significant changes were found in mean left atrial pressure or cardiac output between the baseline state and the various dual-chamber pacing modes. According to baseline PR interval on the 12-lead ECG, the patients were classified into 2 groups. Group 1 included 8 patients with PR intervals > 200 ms. In these patients, an optimal AV interval was selected as the interval when the increase in left ventricular pressure from left ventricular contraction would begin after the peak of the increase in left ventricular pressure from atrial contraction but before atrial relaxation was complete. When AV sequential pacing was performed at the optimal AV interval, cardiac output increased significantly by 38% when compared with baseline values (Fig 5). The optimal AV interval varied between patients, and pacing at too short AV intervals decreased cardiac output in 5 patients. Furthermore, pacing at the optimal AV interval significantly increased left ventricular end-diastolic pressure and duration of diastolic filling and abolished diastolic mitral regurgitation in 5 patients. Cardiac output did not change in a patient without mechanical atrial contraction. The percent change in cardiac output with AV sequential pacing was directly correlated with the increase in left ventricular pressure at the time of ventricular contraction and percent change in diastolic filling period. In the second group of patients (7 patients with normal AV conduction at rest), cardiac output during AV pacing decreased 23% from baseline value without change in the diastolic filling period.

Conclusion.—Dual-chamber pacing may improve acute hemodynamic variables in selected patients with dilated cardiomyopathy who have a prolonged PR interval, mainly by optimizing the timing of mechanical atrial and ventricular synchrony. Patients with a relatively large increase in left ventricular pressure during atrial contraction obtain the greatest ben-

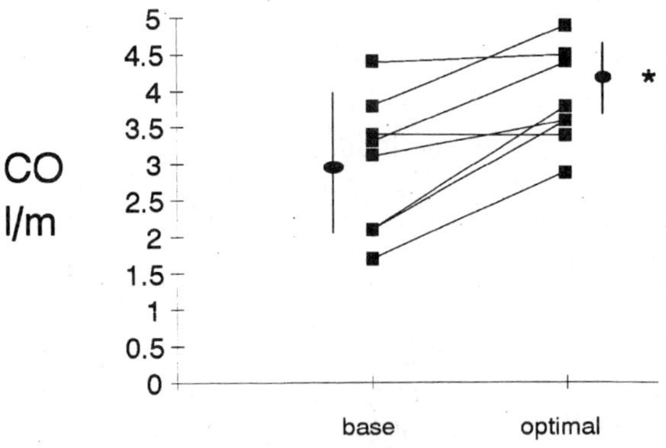

FIGURE 5.—Changes in cardiac output (*CO*) in the 8 group 1 patients when the baseline state (*base*) is compared with the optimal atrioventricular (*AV*) interval. A significant increase in cardiac output ($P < 0.0007$) occurred. *Circle* and vertical *lines* indicate mean values ± standard deviation. *$P < 0.05$ compared with baseline. (Reprinted with permission from the American College of Cardiology (*Journal of the American College of Cardiology,* 1995, 25:281–288.)

efit from dual-chamber pacing. Patients in whom there is already optimally timed mechanical atrial and ventricular synchrony may not benefit from dual-chamber pacing or may even deteriorate with improper timing of atrial synchrony with dual-chamber pacing.

► Dual-chamber cardiac pacing, which has previously been reported to improve hemodynamics in certain patients who have hypertrophic cardiomyopathy, is now being used in several medical centers to improve acute hemodynamic variables in selected patients with dilated cardiomyopathies. Optimizing the timing of mechanical atrial and ventricular systole, reestablishing the optimal diastolic period, and abolishing diastolic mitral regurgitation probably all contribute to the hemodynamic improvement observed in certain patients, particularly those with a prolonged PR interval. In this study, the greatest benefit from dual-chamber pacing was observed in patients who had a relatively large increase in left ventricular pressure during atrial contraction, suggesting that the left ventricle was on the steep portion of the diastolic pressure volume curve with a low effective compliance. The AV interval required to achieve the optimal AV synchrony varies from patient to patient, as demonstrated in this study.

In a less optimistic study concerning the long-term clinical effects of dual-chamber pacing in patients with chronic heart failure, Gold and associates[1] performed a double-blind, randomized, crossover trial in 12 patients with chronic congestive heart failure despite optimal medical therapy. The day after implantation of a dual-chamber pacemaker, invasive hemodynamic measurements were made at AV delays varying between 100 and 200 ms. Patients were then randomized to either dual-chamber pacing with a 100-ms AV delay or backup mode; after 4–6 weeks, crossover to the other pacing mode was programmed. Hemodynamic measurements done on the day after pacemaker implantation demonstrated no benefit of pacing with any AV delay compared with intrinsic conduction. At the optimal AV interval for each patient, neither cardiac output nor wedge pressure improved significantly from baseline measurements during intrinsic conduction. The long-term pacing protocol was completed in 9 patients, and no patient had an increase in ejection fraction greater than 5% with dual-chamber pacing, nor did any patient improve in functional class with short AV delayed dual-chamber pacing. Final conclusions on which patients with heart failure improve hemodynamically or survive longer with dual-chamber pacing are still forthcoming.

In another important study, Krum and associates[2] studied the effects of long-term digoxin therapy on autonomic function in patients with chronic heart failure. They determined sympathetic activity in 26 patients with heart failure by measuring plasma norepinephrine levels and parasympathetic activity from measures of heart rate variability derived from 24-hour ambulatory ECG recordings obtained before and after 4–8 weeks of digoxin therapy. After digoxin therapy, plasma levels of norepinephrine decreased significantly and ECG indicators showed a substantial increase in parasympathetic activity as a result of digitalis treatment. The results indicate that long-term therapy with digitalis acts to ameliorate the autonomic dysfunction of patients with heart failure and that the short-term neurohumoral effects of digoxin are sustained during prolonged treatment with the drug.

R.A. O'Rourke, M.D.

References

1. Gold MR, Feliciano Z, Gottlieb SS, et al: Dual-chamber pacing with a short atrioventricular delay in congestive heart failure: A randomized study. *J Am Coll Cardiol* 26:967–973, 1995.
2. Krum H, Bigger JT Jr, Goldsmith RL, et al: Effect of long-term digoxin therapy on autonomic function in patients with chronic heart failure. *J Am Coll Cardiol* 25:289–294, 1995.

Predictors of Systolic and Diastolic Improvement in Patients With Dilated Cardiomyopathy Treated With Metoprolol

Eichhorn EJ, Heesch CM, Risser RC, Marcoux L, Hatfield B (Dallas VA Hosp; Univ of Texas, Dallas)

J Am Coll Cardiol 25:154–162, 1995 119-96-36–5

Introduction.—Systolic and diastolic function of patients with cardiomyopathy can be significantly improved with β-adrenergic blockade. Selected patients, such as those with dilated cardiomyopathy, high baseline heart rate, and the least fibrosis, respond well to β-blockade, whereas patients with coronary heart disease do not respond as well. Such findings imply that there should be some predictors of successful treatment with β-blockade. To test the hypothesis that those patients with the greatest contractile reserve would achieve the greatest improvement, a retrospective study with metoprolol was done.

Methods.—Data on 24 patients who underwent a double-blind then open-label treatment with metoprolol were reviewed. Cardiac catheterization was performed at baseline, after 3 months of either metoprolol or placebo, and after 3 months of metoprolol treatment. Ventricular volumes, ejection fraction, left ventricular stroke work, end-systolic and arterial elastance, end-diastolic pressure, isovolumetric relaxation, and myocardial respiratory quotient, among others, were all determined on the patients at each catheterization.

Findings.—The best correlations with improvement in ejection fraction were baseline systolic pressure and the first derivative of the peak +dP/dt. Variables that did not predict response included baseline heart rate, ventricular volumes, ejection fraction, and adrenergic activation. The greatest improvement in diastolic pressure occurred in patients with the greatest diastolic impairment. The most marked reduction in left ventricular end-diastolic pressure exhibited the greatest utilization of fatty acids at baseline.

Conclusion.—Patients with the highest peak systolic pressure, left ventricular end-diastolic pressure, and the most prolonged isovolumetric relaxation have the best response to metoprolol. Other patients without these features will also respond to β-blockade.

▶ That certain patients with dilated cardiomyopathy respond favorably hemodynamically and clinically to β-adrenergic blocking agents is an irrefutable fact. However, it is still unclear which patients have the best response to this type of therapy. In this retrospective analysis, improvement in left ventricular ejection fraction in patients with nonischemic dilated cardiomyopathy who were receiving metoprolol was best predicted by baseline peak systolic pressure. Left ventricular volume, ejection fraction, or neurohormonal status did not predict who would best respond to this therapy. Also, patients with the highest left ventricular end-diastolic pressure and the most prolonged isovolumetric relaxation had the most improvement in diastolic function. It is still unclear whether β-blockers prolong survival in patients with heart failure. The Beta Blocker Evaluation of Survival Trial (BEST) and other clinical trials in progress using beta-blockers with and without additional vasodilator properties will evaluate survival and determine whether survival is improved in patients with little hemodynamic improvement.

In a study examining the time course of improved ventricular function in patients with dilated cardiomyopathy who received β-blockers, Hall and associates[1] found that patients with heart failure treated with metoprolol do not demonstrate improvement in systolic performance until after 1 month of therapy and may have a mild reduction in function initially. Long-term therapy with metoprolol apparently resulted (serial echocardiograms) in a reduction in left ventricular volumes, regression of left ventricular mass, and improved ventricular geometry by 18 months.

In a recent double-blind, placebo-controlled study of the vasodilating β-blocker carvedilol, Krum and colleagues[2] followed 33 patients receiving carvedilol and 16 receiving placebo for 14 weeks while background therapy remained constant; hemodynamic and functional variables were measured at the start and end of this study. Compared with the placebo group, patients in the carvedilol group showed improved cardiac performance, as reflected by an increase in left ventricular ejection fraction and stroke volume index and a decrease in pulmonary wedge pressure, mean right atrial pressure, and systemic vascular resistance. In addition, patients treated with carvedilol benefited clinically, as shown by improvements in symptom scores, functional class, and maximal exercise tolerance, all of which were statistically significant. The combined risk of death, worsening heart failure, and life-threatening ventricular tachyarrhythmias was lower in the carvedilol group than in the placebo group ($P = 0.028$). However, carvedilol-treated patients had more dizziness and advanced heart blocks. These data indicate that carvedilol produces clinical and hemodynamic improvement in patients with severe heart failure when it is added to treatment with angiotensin-converting enzyme inhibitors, and a multicenter report at the 1995 American Heart Association Scientific Sessions indicated that it likely decreases the mortality rate as well.

In a less favorable report, the Australia-New Zealand Heart Failure Research Collaborative Group[3] studied the effects of carvedilol in patients with congestive heart failure resulting from ischemic heart disease. Two hundred seven patients were randomized to receive carvedilol treatment and 208 to placebo therapy, all of whom had stable heart failure of ischemic etiology with an ejection fraction less than 45%. After 6 months of therapy, left ventricular ejection fraction had increased by 5.2% in the carvedilol group compared with the placebo group, and left ventricular end-systolic and end-diastolic dimensions had decreased by 2.6 mm and 1.3 mm, respectively (all significant). However, no significant changes in either duration of treadmill exercise or 6-minute walk distance between carvedilol and placebo groups occurred, and symptoms assessed by the New York Heart Association scale and the Specific Activity Scale (SAS) were unchanged in two thirds of the patients in both groups. Therefore, in patients who have cardiac heart failure of ischemic etiology, 6 months of treatment with carvediolol improved left ventricular function and maintained exercise performance at a lower rate-pressure product, but symptoms assessed by functional class were slightly worsened.

R.A. O'Rourke, M.D.

References

1. Hall SA, Cigarroa CG, Marcoux L, et al: Time course of improvement in left ventricular function, mass and geometry in patients with congestive heart failure treated with beta-adrenergic blockade. *J Am Coll Cardiol*, 25:1154–1161, 1995.
2. Krum H, Sackner-Bernstein JD, Goldsmith RL, et al: Double-blind, placebo-controlled study of the long-term efficacy of carvedilol in patients with severe chronic heart failure. *Circulation* 92:1499–1506, 1995.
3. Australia-New Zealand Heart Failure Research Collaborative Group: Effects of carvedilol, a vasodilator–β-blocker, in patients with congestive heart failure due to ischemic heart disease. *Circulation* 92:212–218, 1995.

Characteristics of Patients Surviving More Than Ten Years After Cardiac Transplantation

DeCampli WM, Luikart H, Hunt S, Stinson EB (Stanford Univ, Calif)
J Thorac Cardiovasc Surg 109:1103–1115, 1995 119-96-36–6

Background.—Most studies support the benefits of cardiac transplantation for selected patients with end-stage heart failure. With relatively limited periods of follow-up, many patients have achieved a good postoperative quality of life and a favorable survival rate. To assess the long-term impact of cardiac transplantation, 40 patients from a single institution who are alive or who lived longer than 10 years were reviewed.

Patients and Methods.—Of 661 patients undergoing a first heart transplantation at Stanford University Medical Center since 1970, 40 had survived more than 10 years. Seven underwent cardiac retransplantation, all but 2 more than 10 years after the original operation. Twenty-six patients were alive at the time of review and 14 had died. Clinical status and quality of life of these transplant patients were assessed by means of the transplant database, prospective examinations, cardiac catheterization, exercise testing, and standardized health surveys. A Cox proportional hazards model was used to determine factors associated with longevity.

Results.—The mean age of the patients at transplant was 32.4 years, and the current age or age at death was 46.1 years. All but 8 of the 40 patients had undergone transplantation before cyclosporine was introduced into the program. Compared with those who survived less than 5 years or from 5 to 10 years, long-term survivors had significantly greater freedom from infection, particularly pneumonia. Actuarial freedom from rejection was similar for those surviving less than or more than 10 years. At a mean follow-up of 11.7 years, graft function was well preserved as evidenced by catheterization hemodynamic data. All patients were taking prednisone (mean dose, 12.7 mg/day), and nearly all were treated with azathioprine. Chronic medical problems in the group included hypertension (55%), graft coronary artery disease (CAD) (51%), and osteoporosis (35%). Fourteen of the 26 living patients who underwent maximal exercise testing had a mean exercise duration of 8.7 minutes, a maximum heart rate/expected heart rate value of 77.3%, and maximum systolic blood pressure of 171 mm Hg. Scores on well-being/health surveys were generally in the normal range. Some older (50–64 years) patients, however, reported impairment in mobility, energy level, and sleep quality. Causes of death were CAD in 7 patients, infection in 4, lymphoma in 1, and nonlymphoid cancer in 2 (Fig 5). Variables associated with long-term survival were younger age at transplantation, shorter preoperative duration of illness, absence of postoperative cytomegalovirus infection, and a larger ejection fraction 12 months after operation.

Conclusion.—Long-term survivors of heart transplantation had well-preserved graft function, exercise capacity 80% to 90% of that of age-matched general populations, and perceived health and well-being close to normal values. As in the cardiac transplant population as a whole, CAD continued to develop and was a major cause of death.

▶ This study of long-term survivors of heart transplantation indicates that graft function is well preserved in the second decade after transplantation, as is exercise capacity and patients' perception of well-being. However, the

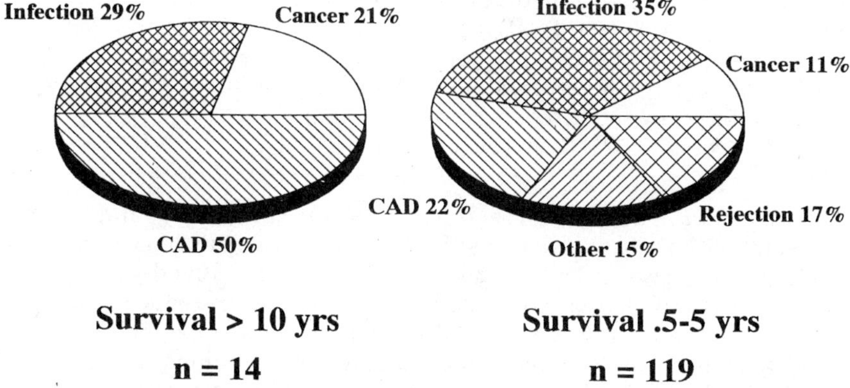

FIGURE 5.—Distribution of causes of death for long-term survivors compared with those of transplant patients surviving only up to 5 years after transplantation. (Courtesy of DeCampli WM, Luikart H, Hunt S, et al: Characteristics of patients surviving more than ten years after cardiac transplantation. *J Thorac Cardiovasc Surg* 109:1103–1115, 1995.)

cumulative incidence of graft CAD is similar to that in the cardiac transplant population as a whole, and CAD continues to develop after 10 years; it is a significant source of mortality. Long-term survival was correlated with younger age at transplantation, shorter preoperative duration of illness, absence of postoperative cytomegalovirus infection, and a larger ejection fraction 12 months after operation. Cardiac transplantation can provide patients with end-stage cardiac failure with an acceptable general medical condition, functional status, and perceived quality of life well into the second decade after operation.

In another important report from the same institution, Rickenbacher and associates[1] describe the incidence and severity of transplant coronary artery disease early and up to 15 years after transplantation, as detected by intravascular ultrasound. A total of 304 intracoronary ultrasound studies were performed in 174 heart transplant recipients at baseline and up to 15 years after transplantation. Compared with findings in patients studied at baseline, the coronary artery mean intimal thickness and intimal index and the mean severity class were significantly higher at year 1 after transplantation. Thereafter, all 3 variables further increased over time and reached highest values between years 5 and 15. Calcification of lesions was detected in 2% to 12% of studies up to 5 years after transplantation with a significant increase to 24% at years 6–10. Thus, the severity of transplant coronary artery disease appears to progress with time after transplantation and is a continuing problem for transplant patients.

R.A. O'Rourke, M.D.

Reference

1. Rickenbacher PR, Pinto FJ, Chenzbraun A, et al. Incidence and severity of transplant coronary artery disease early and up to 15 years after transplantation as detected by intravascular ultrasound. *J Am Coll Cardiol* 25:171–177, 1995.

Effect of Pravastatin on Outcomes After Cardiac Transplantation

Kobashigawa JA, Katznelson S, Laks H, Johnson JA, Yeatman L, Wang XM, Chia D, Terasaki PI, Sabad A, Cogert GA, Trosian K, Hamilton MA, Moriguchi JD, Kawata N, Hage A, Drinkwater DC, Stevenson LW (Univ of California, Los Angeles; Brigham and Women's Hosp, Boston)

N Engl J Med 333:621–627, 1995 119-96-36–7

Background.—Hypercholesterolemia occurs frequently after cardiac transplantation and is associated with the development of coronary vasculopathy in these patients. Inhibitors of 3-hydroxy-3-methylglutaryl coenzyme A (HMG-CoA) reductase have been found to reduce blood cholesterol levels and suppress natural killer cells, which may be involved in the development of acute rejection and coronary vasculopathy. The effects of pravastatin, an HMG-CoA reductase inhibitor, on serum cholesterol, rejection, survival, and the development of coronary vasculopathy were evaluated in a prospective, randomized, open-label trial in patients with cardiac transplants.

Methods.—A total of 97 cardiac transplant recipients were randomly assigned to receive pravastatin or no pravastatin in addition to their immunosuppressive regimen. The patients were regularly monitored for serum levels of cholesterol and for signs of acute rejection. The presence of coronary vasculopathy was determined with coronary angiography and intracoronary ultrasonography performed at baseline and 1 year after transplantation. Peripheral blood natural killer cells were assayed in the last 20 randomized patients to assess immunosuppression in the 2 groups.

Results.—At 1 year after transplantation, the pravastatin group had a significantly lower mean level of cholesterol than did the control group. Although the 2 groups had a comparable average number of episodes of mild or moderate cardiac rejection, the pravastatin group had significantly fewer episodes of cardiac rejection accompanied by hemodynamic compromise. At 1 year, 94% of the pravastatin group and 78% of the control group survived (Fig 2). Three patients in the pravastatin group and 7 patients in the control group had angiographic evidence of coronary vasculopathy 1 year after transplantation. An additional 3 patients from the control group were discovered to have coronary vasculopathy at autopsy. Intracoronary ultrasonography demonstrated less progression in maximal intimal thickness and the intimal index in the pravastatin group, compared with the control group. The pravastatin group had significantly lower natural killer cell cytotoxicity than the control group.

Conclusions.—Inclusion of pravastatin in the immunosuppression regimen after cardiac transplantation reduces cholesterol levels and the incidence of major rejection, improves 1-year survival, and limits the development of coronary vasculopathy. The reduction of natural killer cells also

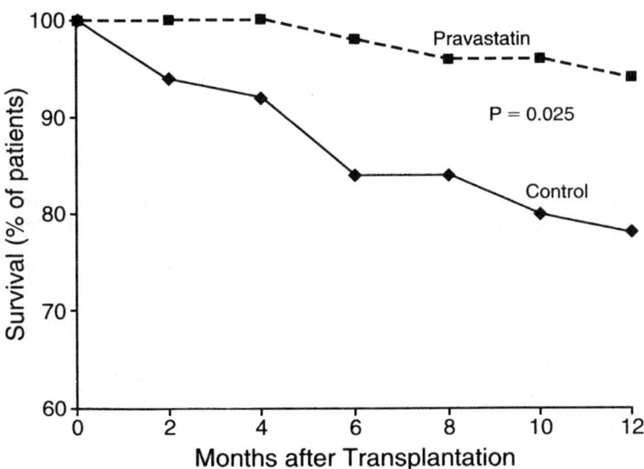

FIGURE 2.—Survival during the first year after cardiac transplantation in the study patients. (Reprinted by permission of The New England Journal of Medicine. Courtesy of Kobashigawa JA, Katznelson S, Laks H, et al: Effect of pravastatin on outcomes after cardiac transplantation. *N Engl J Med* 333:621–627, Copyright 1995, Massachusetts Medical Society.)

suggests that pravastatin increases the immunosuppressive effect of cyclosporine in patients with cardiac transplants.

► Considering the frequency of allograft coronary arteriopathy in patients after transplant, this study assumes significant importance. It suggests that the HMG-CoA reductase inhibitors slow the progression of coronary arteriopathy by more than just the effect of cholesterol reduction. The decrease in natural killer cell cytotoxicity in the pravastatin-treated group suggests that pravastatin may cause an increased state of immunosuppression in addition to its cholesterol-lowering effects. Long-term follow-up studies will be needed to determine whether pravastatin continues to have beneficial effects after 1 year.

In another study concerning cardiac transplantation, Keogh et al.,[1] at the time of cardiac transplantation, randomly assigned 43 patients to receive ketoconazole or no ketoconazole, with the main end points being the dose of cyclosporine required and the incidence of cardiac rejection and infection. The interaction of ketoconazole with cyclosporine results in a delayed metabolism of cyclosporine. Ketoconazole reduced the dose of cyclosporine needed to maintain target levels by 62% in 1 week and by 80% in 1 year with significant cost savings. The mean rate of rejection in the first month was significantly lower in the ketoconazole group than in the control group, and the average number of days to the first rejection was higher. The incidence of infection was lower in ketoconazole-treated patients than in controls during the second and third month of therapy. Transient asymptomatic cholestasis was observed in the ketoconazole group. Therefore, after cardiac transplantation, ketoconazole greatly reduced the need for cyclosporine, resulting in substantial cost savings. It also decreased the rates of rejection and infection without persistent toxic effects. Diltiazem has previously been shown to lessen or prevent cardiac transplant-accelerated coronary vascular disease.[2]

R.A. O'Rourke, M.D.

References

1. Keogh A, Spratt P, McCosker C, et al: Ketoconazole to reduce the need for cyclosporine after cardiac transplantation. *N Engl J Med* 333:628–633, 1995.
2. 1994 Year Book of Medicine, pp 413–415.

37 Valvular Heart Disease

Clinical Outcome of Severe Asymptomatic Chronic Aortic Regurgitation: A Long-Term Prospective Follow-Up Study

Tornos MP, Olona M, Permanyer-Miralda G, Herrejon MP, Camprecios M, Evangelista A, del Castillo HG, Candell J, Soler-Soler J (Hosp Gen Universitari Vall d'Hebron, Barcelona)

Am Heart J 130:333–339, 1995 119-96-37–1

Objective.—The prognosis of severe asymptomatic chronic aortic regurgitation is poor, and delayed surgical replacement of the valve until symptoms or dysfunction appear leads to unsatisfactory results. Predictors of development of left ventricular failure and symptoms that indicate the need for surgery include age, end-systolic dimension and rate of change in end-systolic dimension, and rest ejection fraction. One hundred one patients with asymptomatic severe aortic regurgitation who were free from significant left ventricular dysfunction at the beginning of follow-up were studied prospectively.

Methods.—Echocardiography and radionuclide angiography were performed on 168 patients with severe aortic regurgitation. Left and right catheterization were performed if cardiac symptoms developed or if rest ejection fraction fell below 50%.

Results.—Surgery was performed in 58 patients with cardiac symptoms and in 9 asymptomatic patients with a baseline ejection fraction less than 50%. The remaining 101 patients (20 women, average age 41 years) were monitored for 6–126 months. Eight patients had surgery because cardiac symptoms developed, and 6 had surgery because their ejection fraction fell below 50%. The risk of surgery at 5 years was 12% and at 10 years was 24% (Fig 1). Multivariate analysis showed that end-systolic diameter and radionuclide ejection fraction were significant predictors of the need for surgery. An increase in left ventricular end-diastolic diameter over time was found in patients who needed surgery. There were no perioperative deaths, and left ventricular function and ejection fraction normalized within a year.

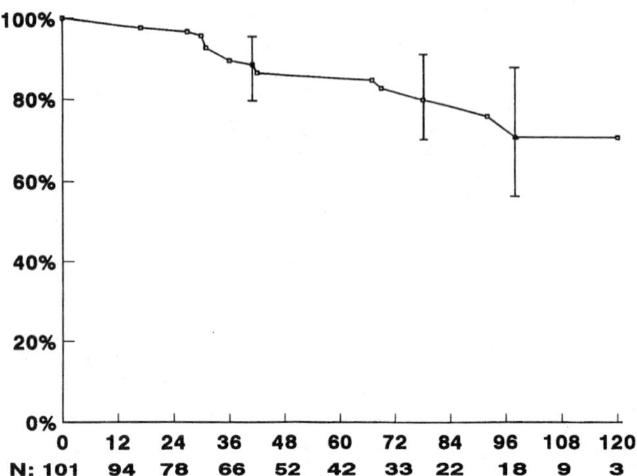

FIGURE 1.—Kaplan-Meier survival curves for the need for surgery during follow-up. (Courtesy of Tornos MP, Olona M, Permanyer-Miralda G, et al: Clinical outcome of severe asymptomatic chronic aortic regurgitation: A long-term prospective follow-up study. *Am Heart J* 130:333–339, 1995.)

Conclusion.—The prognosis of patients with severe asymptomatic aortic regurgitation is good. Surgery can be postponed until the appearance of left ventricular dysfunction or cardiac symptoms at rest.

► The data from this long-term prospective follow-up study of patients with severe asymptomatic chronic aortic regurgitation confirm the important studies by Bonow.[1] The prognosis of aortic regurgitation in patients with no symptoms is good, and the occurrence of asymptomatic left ventricular dysfunction is not a common event. Surgery can be safely postponed until the appearance of cardiac symptoms or the documentation of left ventricular systolic dysfunction at rest. There were no deaths during surgery, and echocardiographic and radionuclide parameters of left ventricular function improved during the first year of follow-up.

Concerning the progression of aortic stenosis, Brener et al.[2] performed serial Doppler echocardiography on 394 consecutive patients with valvular aortic stenosis at baseline and after mean follow-up of 37 ± 16 months. Peak gradients increased by an average of 8.3 mm Hg/yr and mean gradient by 6.3 mm Hg/yr. End-systolic diameter increased by 1.9 mm/yr, end-diastolic diameter increased by 1.6 mm/yr, and the aortic valve area decreased by 0.14 cm^2/yr during the follow-up interval (all $P < 0.001$) indicating progression of aortic stenosis and ventricular dilatation. Patients with more mitral regurgitation at follow-up than at baseline had higher percent increases in mean and peak gradients as well as more progression of ventricular dilatation and worsening of systolic function compared with those with stable or improved mitral regurgitation. Patients with worsening left ventricular hypertrophy had larger percent increases in mean and peak gradients than did those with stable left ventricular hypertrophy, but they maintained stable ventricular volumes and function. Although stenosis progresses over time, systolic dysfunction is an inconsistent marker of the hemodynamic sequelae. Progression of pressure overload hypertrophy appears to prevent ventricular dilatation and development or worsening of mitral regurgitation.

R.A. O'Rourke, M.D.

References

1. Bonow RO, Lakatos E, Maron BJ, et al: Serial long-term assessment of the natural history of asymptomatic patients with chronic aortic regurgitation and normal left ventricular systolic function. *Circulation* 84:1625–1635, 1991.
2. Brener SJ, Duffy CI, Thomas JD, et al: Progression of aortic stenosis in 394 patients: Relation to changes in myocardial and mitral valve dysfunction. *J Am Coll Cardiol* 25:305–310, 1995.

Effects of Valve Surgery on Left Ventricular Contractile Function in Patients With Long-Term Mitral Regurgitation

Starling MR (Univ of Michigan, Ann Arbor; VA Med Ctrs, Ann Arbor, Mich)

Circulation 92:811–818, 1995 119-96-37–2

Introduction.—Both clinical studies and animal models indicate that left ventricular contractile function may be impaired in long-term mitral regurgitation, despite preservation of left ventricular ejection fraction. To determine whether surgery for long-term mitral regurgitation improves left ventricular contractile function, patients were studied both before and 1 year after successful surgery.

Methods.—The patient group included 14 men and 1 woman with a mean age of 57 years. All had received a diagnosis of severe, long-term mitral regurgitation. Micromanometer left ventricular pressures and radionuclide angiograms for left ventricular volumes were acquired before and 1 year after valve surgery, confirmed successful by physical examination and 2-dimensional Doppler echocardiography.

Results.—A year after surgery, significant decreases were observed in average right atrial and pulmonary capillary wedge pressures and left ventricular end-diastolic pressure. Changes in left ventricular peak systolic pressure, mean aortic pressure, and average cardiac index were not significant. The average radionuclide regurgitant index decreased significantly, from 2.70 to 1.28. The average fall in left ventricular ejection fraction, from 0.58 to 0.53, was not significant. Left ventricular contractility was assessed by calculating left ventricular chamber elastance (E_{es}), correcting this value for corresponding changes in heart size. Both the average E_{es} values and the corrected E_{es} values were increased significantly 1 year after successful valve surgery (Fig 2). These increases were in excess of those that might be expected solely as a result of interval changes in left ventricular end-diastolic volume. Left ventricular pump efficiency was improved significantly by surgery, from a mean preoperative value of 0.23 to 0.55.

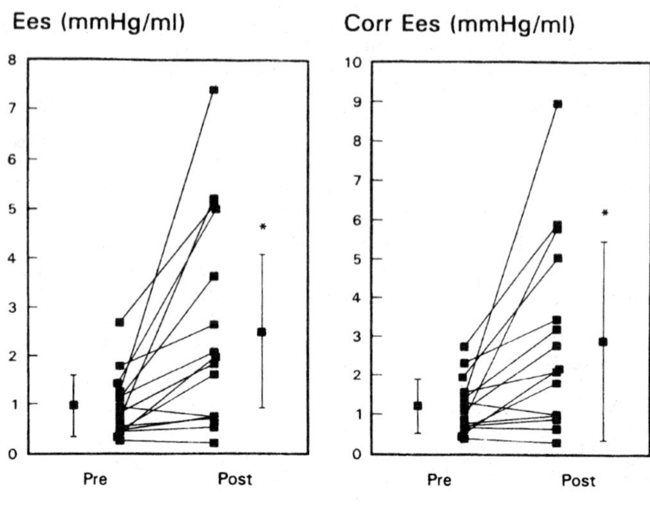

FIGURE 2.—**Left,** plot of individual and mean left ventricular chamber elastance (*Ees*) values. **Right,** plot of individual and mean heart size–corrected E_{es} values. Significant differences are noted. (Reproduced with permission [*Circulation*]. Copyright [1995] American Heart Association.)

Conclusion.—Left ventricular contractile impairment is obscured by favorable left ventricular loading conditions in patients with long-term mitral regurgitation. Successful valve surgery improves this impairment in many patients. To reverse left ventricular contractile impairment, mitral valve surgery should be undertaken before the development of left ventricular dilatation and pump dysfunction.

► This study shows that left ventricular contractile impairment is not irreversible in all patients with long-term severe mitral regurgitation. In fact, left ventricular contractility improves in many patients who are undergoing successful valve surgery for mitral regurgitation; both left ventriculo-arterial coupling and pump efficiency often improve. Depressed left ventricular contractility and pump efficiency can improve, however, only if mitral valve surgery is undertaken before the onset of left ventricular dilatation and pump dysfunction. Many patients with long-term mitral regurgitation are undergoing left ventricular contractile impairment and a reduction in forward pump efficiency despite the measurement of a normal left ventricular ejection fraction resulting from the favorable alterations in loading conditions and uncoupling of end systole from end ejection. Mitral valve surgery and particularly mitral valve repair should be considered earlier in patients with less severe left ventricular dilatation and normal pump performance to preserve left ventricular contractility and improve pump efficiency.

Enriquez-Sarano and associates[1] performed a long-term evaluation of congestive heart failure after surgical correction of mitral regurgitation. They analyzed the long-term outcome of 576 survivors of surgical correction of mitral regurgitation performed between 1980 and 1989. The cumulative incidence of postoperative congestive heart failure was 23 ± 2% at 5 years, 33 ± 3% at 10 years, and 37 ± 3% at 14 years. Survival after the first episode of congestive heart failure was poor (44 ± 4% at 5 years). Independent predictors of postoperative heart failure were preoperative ejection fraction, coronary artery disease, and New York Heart Association functional class. The performance of valve repair was independently predictive of a lower incidence of the combined end point of death and heart failure, compared with valve replacement. Therefore, congestive heart failure frequently occurs late after surgical correction of mitral regurgitation and has a poor prognosis.

Recently, Bach and Bolling[2] assessed the effects of mitral valve reconstruction in 9 consecutive patients with severe mitral regurgitation resulting from end-stage dilated cardiomyopathy. Clinical and echocardiographic follow-up studies were obtained at 17 ± 5 and 16 ± 6 weeks, respectively, after surgery. There were no operative or early deaths. All patients noted symptomatic improvement postoperatively and there was an improvement by at least 1 New York Heart Association functional class. Quantitative echocardiography demonstrated a small, but significant decrease in left ventricular end-diastolic volume and increases in ejection fraction and forward cardiac output during follow-up. Therefore, mitral valve reconstruction for severe mitral regurgitation in certain patients with dilated cardiomyopathy may improve symptomatic status and left ventricular function on early follow-up. However, the long-term prognosis is still dismal, and long-term follow-up of larger numbers of patients will be required to confirm a sustained improvement in symptomatic status with an acceptable 5-year mortality rate.

R.A. O'Rourke, M.D.

References

1. Enriquez-Sarano M, Schaff HV, Orszulak TA, et al: Congestive heart failure after surgical correction of mitral regurgitation: A long-term study. *Circulation* 92:2496–2503, 1995.
2. Bach DS, Bolling SF: Early improvement in congestive heart failure after correction of secondary mitral regurgitation in end-stage cardiomyopathy. *Am Heart J* 129:1165–1170, 1995.

Influence of Mitral Regurgitation on Left Atrial Thrombus and Spontaneous Echocardiographic Contrast in Patients With Rheumatic Mitral Valve Disease

Karatasakis GT, Gotsis AC, Cokkinos DV (Onassis Cardiac Surgery Ctr, Athens, Greece; Tzanio Gen Hosp, Piraeus, Greece)

Am J Cardiol 76:279–281, 1995 119-96-37–3

Objective.—Although patients with rheumatic mitral valve disease are at increased risk of left atrial thrombi and spontaneous echocardiographic contrast, some studies indicate that coexisting mitral regurgitation (MR) lowers the risk of thrombus or spontaneous contrast. Because MR studies

TABLE 1.—Characteristics of Patients With and Without Thrombus

	Thrombus Present (n = 13)	Thrombus Absent (n = 42)	P Value
Age (yr)	58 ± 11	54 ± 13	NS
INR	2.5 ± 0.4	2.6 ± 0.3	NS
Mitral valve area (cm^2)	1.07 ± 0.42	1.36 ± 0.6	NS
Fractional shortening (%)	32.4 ± 8.8	33.5 ± 7.0	NS
Left atrial diameter (cm)	58.2 ± 8.4	55.3 ± 10.7	NS
Atrial fibrillation (%)	12/13 (92)	25/42 (60)	< 0.05
Spontaneous contrast (%)	13/13 (100)	21/42 (50)	< 0.0002
Embolic events (%)	6/13 (46)	4/42 (9.5)	< 0.003
Significant mitral regurgitation (%)	1/13 (8)	18/42 (43)	< 0.03
Regurgitant jet area (cm^2)	1.6 ± 2.1	4 ± 4	< 0.02

Note: Values are expressed as mean ± 1 SD or number (%).
Abbreviations: INR, international normalized ratio; *NS*, not significant.
(Courtesy of Karatasakis GT, Gotsis AC, Cokkinos DV: Influence of mitral regurgitation on left atrial thrombus and spontaneous echocardiographic contrast in patients with rheumatic mitral valve disease. *Am J Cardiol* 76:279–281, 1995. Reprinted with permission from American Journal of Cardiology.)

are controversial, a prospective investigation was conducted to examine the relationship between the incidence of embolism, atrial thrombi, and spontaneous contrast and the degree of MR in patients with rheumatic valve disease.

Methods.—Echocardiography and cardiac catheterization were performed in 55 patients (12 men) aged 27–74 years, 22 with mitral valve stenosis and 33 with combined mitral stenosis. All were receiving warfarin therapy, and 37 had atrial fibrillation.

Results.—Transesophageal echocardiography detected left atrial thrombi in 13 patients, 6 of whom had a history of embolization (Table 1). Significant MR was detected in 1 of these patients and in 18 patients without thrombi. No patients with significant MR had a history of embolization. Absence of significant MR, presence of atrial fibrillation, and smaller regurgitant jet were significant predictors of thrombi. Transesophageal echocardiography detected spontaneous contrast in 34 patients, 9 of whom had a history of embolization. Only 1 patient without spontaneous contrast had such a history. Atrial fibrillation, significant MR, smaller mitral valve area, and smaller regurgitant jet were significantly associated with spontaneous contrast.

Conclusion.—In this study, all patients received anticoagulation therapy. Those with significant MR have a lower risk for left atrial thrombus formation and embolization events. Patients without significant MR, who have spontaneous contrast and atrial fibrillation, are at high risk of thrombus formation and should receive anticoagulant therapy.

► The authors showed that significant mitral regurgitation in patients with rheumatic mitral disease who were receiving anticoagulation therapy was associated with an almost tenfold decrease in the relative risk of thrombus formation and a 20-fold decrease in spontaneous contrast by echocardiography (TEE). Left atrial thrombus, when present, was frequently associated with embolization, and patients with spontaneous contrast on echocardiography also had a higher incidence of thrombotic events than did those without. The possibility that patients with significant mitral regurgitation as a result of rheumatic heart disease may have fewer left atrial thrombi and embolic events, even with low-intensity anticoagulation, remains to be proved. Moreover, patients without mitral regurgitation seen with spontaneous contrast on TEE or with left atrial fibrillation must be considered at high risk for left atrial thrombus formation and should undergo anticoagulation therapy.

R.A. O'Rourke, M.D.

Carcinoid Heart Disease: Correlation of High Serotonin Levels With Valvular Abnormalities Detected by Cardiac Catheterization and Echocardiography

Robiolio PA, Rigolin VH, Wilson JS, Harrison JK, Sanders LL, Bashore TM, Feldman JM (Duke Univ Med Ctr, Durham, NC; Durham VA Med Ctr, NC)

Circulation 92:790–795, 1995 119-96-37–4

Objective.—Although carcinoid tumors are rare, the prevalence of carcinoid heart disease in patients with these tumors is 57% to 77%. Methods have been sought to measure ambient serotonin levels directly, because serotonin has been implicated as an etiologic agent in the development of carcinoid heart disease. The results of measurement of urinary 5-hydroxyindole acetic acid (5-HIAA) and circulating levels of serotonin in patients with carcinoid heart disease were assessed.

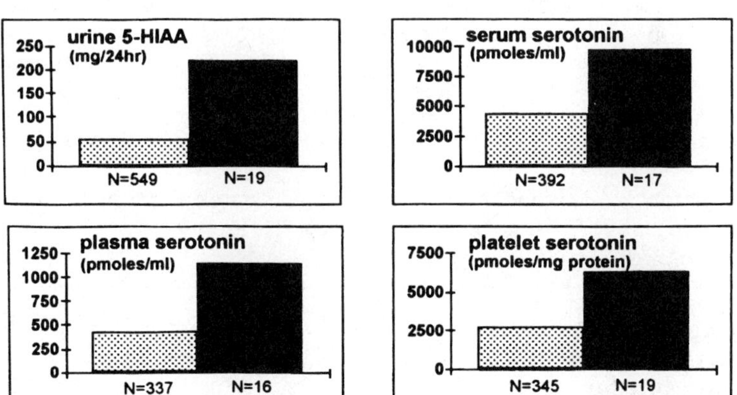

FIGURE 2.—Bar graphs comparing cardiac and noncardiac patients. Cardiac patients demonstrated higher ($P < 0.0001$) mean levels of urine 5-hydroxyindole acetic acid (*5-HIAA;* 219 ± 124 vs. 55.3 ± 141 mg/24 hr), serum serotonin (9,750 ± 4,130 vs. 4,350 ± 6,460 pmol/mL), plasma serotonin (1,130 ± 1,210 vs. 426 ± 1,130 pmol/mL), and platelet serotonin (6,240 ± 4,030 vs. 2,700 ± 2,880 pmol/mg protein). *Stippled box* indicates no heart disease; *solid box,* heart disease. (Reproduced with permission [*Circulation*]. Copyright [1995] American Heart Association.)

Methods.—Tumor secretory products were prospectively measured in 604 patients with carcinoid tumor; 19 of them had carcinoid heart disease.

Results.—Flushing and diarrhea were 3 times more common in patients with carcinoid heart disease than in other patients with carcinoid tumors. Patients with carcinoid heart disease had significantly higher serum, plasma, and platelet levels of serotonin and fourfold higher levels of 5-HIAA (Fig 2). Of the 16 patients with carcinoid heart disease who underwent echocardiography, 13 had enlarged right atria and ventricles and 9 had thickened or immobile tricuspid valves. There was 91% agreement between echocardiography and cardiac catheterization on valvular lesions.

Conclusion.—Patients with carcinoid heart disease exhibit higher circulating levels of serotonin than do patients with carcinoid tumor without heart disease, suggesting a pathogenic role for serotonin.

▶ Although the ultrastructure of the carcinoid plaque has been well delineated for many years, the biochemical basis of carcinoid heart disease has been poorly defined. This study is the first to directly demonstrate increases of circulating serotonin in cardiac patients compared with patients without heart disease. Thirteen of the 16 cardiac patients who had echocardiograms performed had evidence of right atrial and right ventricular enlargement and 9 had evidence of a thickened or immobile tricuspid valve. Tricuspid valve disease, as in previous studies, was most prevalent. Left-sided lesions tend to be less common and of milder severity. Therefore, the carcinoid syndrome continues to be a differential diagnostic consideration in patients who are seen with moderate-to-severe tricuspid or pulmonic valvular heart disease. In this study of a relatively small number of patients, there was no survival difference between the cardiac and noncardiac patients, regardless of whether survival was measured from the time of onset of the first carcinoid symptoms or from the time of diagnosis of carcinoid tumors.

R.A. O'Rourke, M.D.

Optimal Oral Anticoagulant Therapy in Patients With Mechanical Heart Valves

Cannegieter SC, Rosendaal FR, Wintzen AR, van der Meer FJM, Vandenbroucke JP, Briët E (Univ Hosp Leiden, The Netherlands)

N Engl J Med 333:11–17, 1995 119-96-37–5

Background.—In patients with mechanical heart valves, the level at which thromboembolic complications are effectively prevented without excessive bleeding has not been established. A method to determine the optimal intensity of anticoagulation was developed and applied in a study of the dose-effect relation between anticoagulation intensity and the benefits and risks of treatment.

Methods.—All patients with mechanical heart valves treated at 4 regional Dutch anticoagulation clinics since 1985 were included in the data analysis. The intensity-specific incidence of each type of event was defined

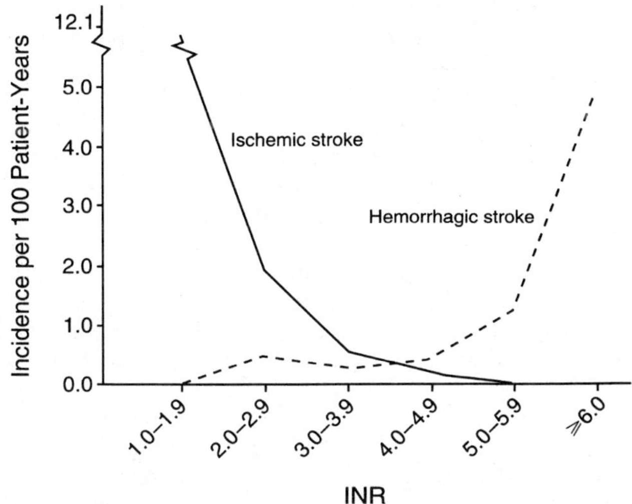

FIGURE 2.—Incidence of ischemic and hemorrhagic stroke according to international normalized ratio category. *Abbreviation: INR,* international normalized ratio. (Reprinted by permission of *The New England Journal of Medicine.* Courtesy of Cannegieter SC, Rosendaal FR, Wintzen AR, et al: Optimal oral anticoagulant therapy in patients with mechanical heart valves. *N Engl J Med* 333:11–17, Copyright 1995, Massachusetts Medical Society.)

as the number of events occurring at a certain anticoagulation intensity divided by the number of patient-years during which the international normalized ratio (INR) was at this level in all patients.

Findings.—A total of 1,608 patients were followed for 6,475 patient-years. Forty-three patients had cerebral embolism, yielding an incidence of 0.68 per 100 patient-years, and 2 had peripheral embolism, for an incidence of 0.03 per 100 patient-years. Thirty-six patients had intracranial and spinal bleeding, and 128 had major extracranial bleeding, yielding incidences of 0.57 and 2.1 per 100 patient-years, respectively. The optimal anticoagulation intensity occurred when the INR decreased to between 2.5 and 4.9. In this range, the incidence of both complications was at its lowest (Fig 2).

Conclusions.—The optimal intensity of anticoagulation can be achieved with a recommended target INR of 3 to 4. An INR between 2.5 and 4.9 is optimal for patients with prosthetic heart valves.

► Although there is no debate as to whether oral anticoagulant therapy is necessary for patients with mechanical heart valve prostheses, the optimal intensity of anticoagulation has been a matter of considerable disagreement. The optimal intensity of anticoagulation for preventing thromboembolic complications without excessive bleeding is not known, even though anticoagulant therapy has been given as a lifetime therapy to a very large number of patients. It was not feasible to present the intensity of anticoagulation in a standardized manner until 1985, when the INR was introduced.

In this study of more than 1,600 patients, the optimal intensity of anticoagulation in patients with mechanical heart valves that produced the fewest thromboembolism and bleeding events occurred between measured INR values of 2.5 and 4.9. As a result, a target range in INR of 3.0–4.0 was recommended. The risk of embolism sharply increased with an INR below 2.5, and the actual INR achieved usually was somewhat lower than the target level. As in prior studies, a lower risk of thromboembolism occurred in those younger than age 50 years who had prostheses in the aortic position and with a bileaflet prosthetic valve.

Since the first report of pregnancy in a woman with a prosthetic valve, many studies have analyzed the maternal and fetal risk associated with the type of prostheses implanted, the anticoagulation prescribed, and its mode of administration. In a French cooperative, retrospective study of pregnant patients with prosthetic heart valves, Hanania and associates[1] reported on 155 pregnancies and 103 patients with prosthetic heart valves, 35 having mechanical prostheses and 60 bioprostheses. Among the 108 mechanical prostheses–bearing patients, 16 thromboembolic events were recorded. They were 4 times more frequent with *oral* anticoagulant therapy. Among the 74 patients with bioprostheses, 7 had premature valve failure and 20 had miscarriages; the miscarriages occurred significantly more often with anticoagulation treatment (17%) than without it (4%). Warfarin-induced embryopathies were rare.

Therefore, pregnancy in a mechanical prostheses–bearing patient is often associated with maternal and fetal complications that lead to a low success rate (53%). In contrast, pregnancy with a bioprostheses without anticoagulants had an 84% rate of normal births; however, this better result is obtained with the likely need of surgical reintervention in the subsequent 5–15 years.

One approach when valve replacement surgery is indicated in young women is as follows: For aortic valve disease, replacement with a mechanical valve for which the thromboembolic risk does not seem to be excessive, but the risks associated with anticoagulation therapy remain. For mitral valve disease, conservative procedures, such as percutaneous mitral commissurotomy for stenosis and reconstructive valvuloplasty for regurgitation or for slightly altered valvular or subvalvular apparatus disease, should be recommended when possible. If these conservative techniques are not applicable, a mechanical prostheses should be implanted in women who already have had children and for whom a new pregnancy should be strongly discouraged, and oral contraception should be prescribed.

There have been few reports concerning the natural history of vegetations during and after successful medical treatment of endocarditis. Vuille and associates[2] followed the evolution of vegetation size, mobility, consistency, the extent of the disease, and the severity of valvular regurgitation as related to late complications such as embolism, valve replacement, or death occurring after the end of therapy in 32 patients with 41 vegetations on initial echocardiograms. At the end of treatment, 29 vegetations were still present, 59% had no significant change in size, and 52% appeared to be more dense in consistency. Morphologic changes did not correlate with late complications, but the presence of severe valvular regurgitation often resulted in subsequent late valve replacement. Without severe valvular dysfunction, persistent vegetations by echocardiography were not independently associated with late complications. These data are consistent with postmortem studies performed in many patients years after the successful treatment of an episode of infective endocarditis where pathologic evidence of "healed" valvular vegetations remains unrelated to the cause of the patient's death.

R.A. O'Rourke, M.D.

References

1. Hanania G, Thomas D, Michel PL, et al: Pregnancy and prosthetic heart valves: A French cooperative retrospective study of 155 cases. *Eur Heart J* 15:1651–1658, 1994.
2. Vuille C, Nidorf M, Weyman AE, et al: Natural history of vegetations during successful medical treatment of endocarditis. *Am Heart J* 128:1200–1209, 1994.

38 Noninvasive Testing

Significance of Silent Myocardial Ischemia During Exercise Testing in Women: Report From the Coronary Artery Surgery Study
Weiner DA, Ryan TJ, Parsons L, Fisher LD, Chaitman BR, Sheffield LT, Tristani FE (Boston Univ; Univ of Washington, Seattle; St Louis Univ, Mo; et al)
Am Heart J 129:465–470, 1995 119-96-38–1

Background.—Both men and women frequently experience transient myocardial ischemia without having symptoms. Silent ischemia is known to compromise survival in men with coronary artery disease (CAD), but prognostic data are not available for women.

Study Population.—The prognostic importance of silent ischemia was examined in 1,087 women and 3,834 men participating in the Coronary Artery Surgery Study who underwent both exercise testing and coronary angiography. Exercise testing distinguished 3 groups of individuals: those with silent ischemia (group 1), defined as 1 mm or more of ST-segment depression as measured 0.08 second after the J-point; symptomatic patients with ischemia (group 2); and those lacking evidence of ischemia (group 3). Men were more likely than women to not have congestive failure, but they also were more likely to have had myocardial infarction and more marked CAD. Women were more likely than men to be free of anginal symptoms.

Findings.—In both women and men, silent and symptomatic ischemia adversely affected survival when 12-year rates were analyzed. This remained the case after multivariate analysis. The extent of CAD was a significant factor in both men and women with silent ischemia. Bypass surgery was demonstrably beneficial to men with silent ischemia who had triple-vessel CAD. In contrast, women with silent ischemia did not benefit significantly from bypass surgery regardless of the extent of disease.

Implications.—Although silent myocardial ischemia lessens the chance of both men and women with CAD surviving over the long term, men with triple-vessel disease may benefit more than women from coronary bypass surgery.

▶ This study indicates that both silent and symptomatic ischemia during exercise ECG testing have an adverse effect on the 12-year survival rate in women and in men. The survival of both men and women with silent ischemia during ECG exercise testing was influenced by the severity of CAD. Silent ischemia occurs less frequently when patients are evaluated by exercise testing than by ambulatory ECG monitoring, and asymptomatic ischemia during exercise testing occurs more frequently with increasing age. In the Coronary Artery Surgical Study (CASS) registry study, the decision to perform coronary bypass graft surgery among men and women with silent ischemia was not randomized, and the number of patients undergoing surgery was small, especially in the female group. However, the data suggest a benefit of coronary artery bypass graft surgery overall and that men may benefit more than women when 3-vessel CAD is present.

Launbjerg et al.[1] studied 257 consecutive noninfarction patients without other severe disease and younger than 76 years of age to identify the long-term risk factors for cardiac events (cardiac death and nonfatal acute myocardial infarction) and for the development of angina pectoris among patients admitted with acute chest pain but no acute myocardial infarction. The patients were followed for 7 years.

The results indicate that patients with nonacute myocardial infarction hospitalized in a critical care unit with chest pain are at an increased risk for later cardiac events. When data from noninvasive testing are included in a multivariate analysis, the strongest prognostic markers are a small increase in the heart rate blood pressure product during exercise and ST abnormalities on the ECG at rest. Thallium scintigrams and, less often, Holter monitoring, may provide further information. Even in patients without prior CAD, exercise testing and the ECG at rest provide significant prognostic information. An exercise test should be considered for all patients with nonacute myocardial infarction who are hospitalized with chest pain to: (1) identify low-risk patients who can be reassured of their excellent long-term prognosis and (2) identify high-risk patients in whom further evaluation, treatment, and follow-up are deemed justified.

Taylor and associates[2] prospectively studied 144 consecutive patients who were referred to an exercise laboratory for combined symptom-limited ECG exercise testing and quantitative thallium-201 scintigraphy. Fifty-four patients with exercise-induced ST-segment depression were identified, and in this group, the magnitude of ST-segment depression on symptom-limited exercise testing did not correlate with the extent of ischemia as assessed by quantitative thallium-201 scintigraphy. However, those with more than 2.0 mm of ST-segment depression had comparable exercise capacity and comparable ischemic burden by thallium-201 scintigraphic assessment. Nevertheless, the presence of 2 mm or less of ST-segment depression did not reliably indicate an increased ischemic burden by thallium-201 scintigraphic assessment over patients with lesser degrees of ST-segment depression. Therefore, in patients with known or suspected CAD combined exercise testing and perfusion imaging should be considered for assessing the ischemic burden.

In another study of 321 patients with an intermediate-to-high pretest likelihood of CAD who underwent exercise testing and coronary arteriography,[3] the diagnostic accuracy of exercise thallium-201 single-photon emission computed tomography (SPECT) was superior to the ECG response in detecting coronary artery disease. In addition, SPECT imaging provided incremental power to ECG exercise testing in identifying patients with left main or 3-vessel CAD.

R.A. O'Rourke, M.D.

References

1. Launbjerg J, Fruergaard P, Jacobsen HL, et al: Long-term risk factors from noninvasive evaluation of patients with acute chest pain, but without myocardial infarction. *Eur Heart J* 16:30–37, 1995.
2. Taylor AJ, Sackett MC, Beller GA: The degree of ST-segment depression of symptom-limited exercise testing: Relation to the myocardial ischemic burden as determined by thallium-201 scintigraphy. *Am J Cardiol* 75:228–231, 1995.
3. Nallamothu N, Ghods M, Heo J, et al: Comparison of thallium-201 single-photon emission computed tomography and electrocardiographic response during exercise in patients with normal rest electrocardiographic results. *J Am Coll Cardiol* 25:830–836, 1995.

Role of Adenosine Thallium-201 Tomography for Defining Long-Term Risk in Patients After Acute Myocardial Infarction

Mahmarian JJ, Mahmarian AC, Marks GF, Pratt CM, Verani MS (Baylor College of Medicine, Houston; Methodist Hosp, Houston)

J Am Coll Cardiol 25:1333–1340, 1995 119-96-38–2

Background.—A significant subset of patients is at increased risk for subsequent cardiac events after myocardial infarction. Cardiac risk is related to the infarct size and the extent of residual ischemia, and these parameters can be accurately quantified with tomographic imaging. The potential of combining the absolute extent of myocardial ischemia, as assessed by quantitative adenosine tomography, with the left ventricular ejection fraction for defining long-term cardiac risk was examined in postinfarction patients for the first time.

Methods.—One hundred forty-six patients underwent thallium-201 adenosine tomography within a mean of 5 days after acute myocardial infarction. The left ventricular function was assessed by gated radionuclide angiography, echocardiography, or contrast cineangiography. Statistical risk models were generated for 92 patients, after excluding 51 who underwent revascularization after scintigraphy and 3 lost to follow-up.

Results.—During a mean follow-up of 15.7 months, 33% of patients had a nonfatal reinfarction, unstable angina, congestive heart failure, or they died. The mean time from hospital discharge to all events was 7.9 months, and 53% occurred within the first 6 months. Univariate predictors of all events included the quantified perfusion defect size, the absolute extent of left ventricular ischemia, and the ejection fraction. The absolute extent of scintigraphic ischemia was the best defined risk. More than 50% of patients with a greater than 10% ischemic defect had an event by 1 year vs. 10% of patients with a defect of 10% or less. Similar results were observed for infarct-free survival (Fig 1C). In patients with a low predicted risk with an ejection fraction more than 40% and scintigraphic ischemia of

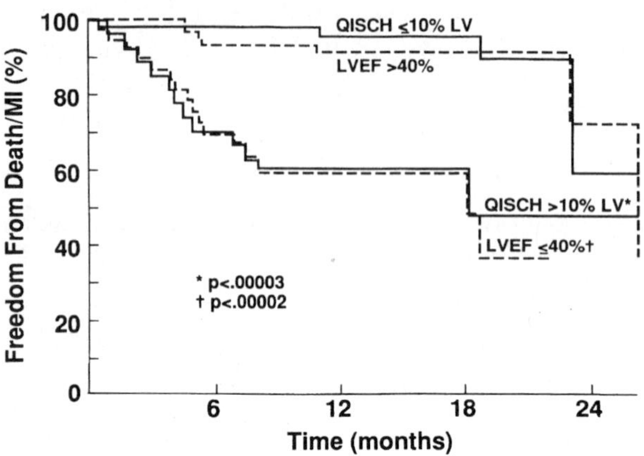

FIGURE 1C.—The quantified extent of ischemia predicted risk, irrespective of the initial therapy during acute infarction. *Solid lines* represent early reperfusion therapy; *dashed lines,* no early reperfusion therapy. *Abbreviations: MI,* myocardial infarction; *QISCH,* quantified extent of left ventricular ischemia; *LVEF,* left ventricular ejection fraction. (Reprinted with permission from the American College of Cardiology [*Journal of the American College of Cardiology,* 1995, 25:1333–1340.])

10% or less, the 1-year infarct-free survival rate was 94% and that for any cardiac event was 88%. Stepwise Cox regression analysis showed 3 models that best predicted individual patient risk. The most powerful model was based on the absolute extent of scintigraphic ischemia and the ejection fraction. For every 10% increment in these variables, the risk increased by 82% or decreased by 32%, respectively. Model 2 was based on the percent of infarct zone ischemia and the ejection fraction, and model 3 was based on the total perfusion defect size and the percent of infarct zone ischemia. The absolute extent of scintigraphic ischemia, the ejection fraction, and the percent of infarct zone ischemia were equally powerful in predicting infarct-free survival and nonfatal reinfarction, whereas death was best predicted by the total perfusion defect size.

Summary.—Adenosine tomography can effectively evaluate cardiac risk in patients in stable condition early after infarction. The absolute extent of scintigraphic ischemia is a strong predictor of overall cardiac risk, particularly when combined with the ejection fraction. Further studies are needed to prospectively validate the risk models in postinfarction patients and to determine whether reducing the extent of scintigraphic ischemia in high risk patients can be beneficial.

▶ This study indicates that the quantitative extent of myocardial ischemia induced by pharmacologic stress with adenosine combined with the left ventricular ejection fraction defines the long-term risk in patients after acute myocardial infarction. The absolute extent of scintigraphic myocardial ischemia, as determined by ^{201}Tl-SPECT, is a strong predictor of overall cardiac risk, particularly when combined with a low ejection fraction.

Importantly, this study indicated that the statistical models generated for predicting risk appeared equally valid for patients who did or did not receive reperfusion therapy. This is particularly important considering the controversy regarding the ability to risk-stratify post–myocardial infarction patients who have been treated with thrombolytic drugs. Many of the previous myocardial perfusion imaging studies assessed only the presence or absence of reversible defects in evaluating postthrombolytic patients for high risk; the subgroup of postthrombolytic patients in this study had a *quantitative* analysis of the extent of adenosine-induced myocardial ischemia.

In a study from the Multicenter Myocardial Ischemia Research Group, Bodenheimer and associates[1] reported the prognostic significance of a fixed thallium defect at 1–6 months after the onset of acute myocardial infarction or unstable angina. They studied 896 patients, 70% of whom had a previous acute myocardial infarction and 30% of whom had previous unstable angina. With follow-up averaging 23 months, the likelihood of cardiac death, nonfatal infarction, and unstable angina was similar in patients who had a normal exercise thallium test result or showed only a fixed defect. Moreover, cardiac events were not related to the size of a fixed defect. In contrast, both cardiac death and nonfatal infarction were increased in patients with the largest areas of reversible defects, although the sensitivity for nonfatal infarction was suboptimal. The results of this study are not surprising, because many patients with a fixed thallium defect and no reversible ischemia do well long term; in some of these, a fixed thallium defect represents a photon attenuation artifact rather than an old scar.

R.A. O'Rourke, M.D.

Reference

1. Bodenheimer MM, and the Multicenter Myocardial Ischemia Research Group: Prognostic significance of a fixed thallium defect one to six months after onset of acute myocardial infarction or unstable angina. *Am J Cardiol* 74:1196–1200, 1994.

Prediction of Improvement of Regional Left Ventricular Function After Surgical Revascularization: A Comparison of Low-Dose Dobutamine Echocardiography With ^{201}Tl Single-Photon Emission Computed Tomography

Arnese M, Cornel JH, Salustri A, Maat APWM, Elhendy A, Reijs AEM, Cate FJT, Keane D, Balk AHMM, Roelandt JRTC, Fioretti PM (Univ Hosp Rotterdam-Dijkzigt, The Netherlands; Erasmus Univ, Rotterdam, The Netherlands)
Circulation 91:2748–2752, 1995 119-96-38–3

Objective.—Coronary artery bypass graft surgery improves left ventricular function possibly by restoring myocardial viability. Although both thallium-201 single-photon emission computed tomography (SPECT) and low-dose dobutamine echocardiography (LDDE) have been used to evaluate myocardial viability, comparative reliability and efficacy studies have not been conducted. The 2 imaging techniques were compared in 38 patients with left ventricular dysfunction undergoing coronary artery by-

TABLE 2.—Diagnostic Accuracy With 95% Confidence Intervals of Low-Dose Dobutamine Echocardiography and High-Dose Dobutamine-Reinjection Thallium-201 SPECT for Prediction of Postoperative Improvement of Wall Motion in Severely Dyssynergic Segments

Method	Sensitivity	Specificity	PPV	NPV
LDDE, %	74	95	85	93
95% CI	67 to 81	92 to 98	80 to 90	89 to 97
TL SPECT, %	89	48	33	94
95% CI	84 to 94	40 to 56	26 to 40	90 to 98

Abbreviations: PPV, positive predictive value; *NPV*, negative predictive value; *LDDE*, low-dose dobutamine echocardiography; *SPECT*, single-photon emission computed tomography; *CI*, confidence interval.

pass graft surgery, and their recovery prediction value was assessed using 3-month postoperative echocardiographic analyses of ventricular improvement.

Methods.—Simultaneous dobutamine stress echocardiography and poststress reinjection ^{201}Tl SPECT were performed on 38 symptomatic patients (12 women) aged 36–73 years before surgery. Echocardiographic left ventricular (LV) segments were classified as akinetic (Ak) or severely hypokinetic (SH). Postoperative improvement of dyssynergic segments was determined with rest echocardiography 3 months after surgery.

Results.—Preoperatively 169 of 608 LV segments were classified as Ak and 51 as SH. During low-dose dobutamine infusion (5 μ/kg/min), 14 of 126 Ak segments and 19 of 44 SH segments showed wall thickening. At high dobutamine doses (10 μ/kg/min), 32 of 36 patients showed wall motion abnormalities, 28 of whom had episodes of angina. Thallium-201 SPECT detected viable myocardium in 14 of 14 Ak regions and 18 of 19 SH regions responding to dobutamine and 49 of 112 Ak and 22 of 25 SH regions not responding to dobutamine. Low-dose dobutamine echocardiography had a higher positive predictive value than did SPECT (Table 2). Although 36 patients had angina before surgery, only 1 complained of angina 3 months after surgery; 10 patients still had dyspnea. After surgical revascularization, stress-induced ischemia was significantly reduced as demonstrated by high-dose dobutamine echocardiography.

Conclusion.—Low-dose dobutamine echocardiography is a good predictor of improvement of regional left ventricular function after surgical revascularization, and it is preferred over SPECT as a preoperative imaging technique.

▶ Reliable preoperative prediction of patients with regional and/or global LV dysfunction that will improve after revascularization would present several clinical advantages, including the appropriate referral for cardiac surgery of patients who would otherwise be considered unsuitable for revascularization on the basis of a very low LV ejection fraction. In this study of a group of patients with severe chronic LV dysfunction who were candidates for surgical revascularization, LDDE and ^{201}Tl SPECT imaging were compared for predicting improvement. This study indicates that improvement of akinetic and hypokinetic myocardial segments with low-dose dobutamine is both a specific and a sensitive predictor of postrevascularization improvement in LV function. Compared with LDDE, ^{201}Tl SPECT imaging has an equivalent sensitivity for the prediction of postoperative myocardial function but a lower specificity. It must be emphasized that, in this study, simultaneous dobutamine stress echocardiography and post–stress reinjection ^{201}Tl SPECT were compared before surgery. The results might be different if dobutamine stress echocardiography and exercise stress ^{201}Tl SPECT and postexercise reinjection with ^{201}Tl SPECT were compared as indicators of viable myocardial segments.

In another recent study, Ho and associates[1] compared dobutamine stress echocardiography with dipyridamole ^{201}Tl SPECT for detecting coronary artery disease. Both tests were performed on 54 patients who also underwent coronary arteriography. Dobutamine stress echocardiography detected 93% of the 43 patients with significant coronary artery disease, and dipyridamole ^{201}Tl SPECT detected 98% of the patients with significant stenosis. The specificity was 73% for both tests. For detecting individual coronary artery stenosis, the sensitivity of the 2 tests varied between 61% and 97% for individual coronary artery stenosis. Therefore, both dobutamine tests appear highly sensitive for detection and localization of coronary artery disease. In this study, the sensitivity of dobutamine stress was affected by the level of stenosis severity.

Dagianti and colleagues[2] compared the specific effects of exercise, dipyridamole, and dobutamine as 3 types of stress echocardiography. In 60 patients who had suspected coronary artery disease, the sensitivity of exercise echocardiography averaged 76%; that of dobutamine echocardiography, 72%; and that of dipyridamole echocardiography, only 52%. Specificity did not differ significantly among the tests (94% for exercise, 97% for dipyridamole, and 95% for dobutamine). In 40 patients with known coronary artery disease, the accuracy of predicting the extent of disease was 71% for exercise, 33% for dipyridamole, and 75% for dobutamine. Therefore, dobutamine and exercise echocardiography are superior to dipyridamole echocardiography for the diagnosis of coronary artery disease and the estimation of its extent. Exercise echocardiography could be the first diagnostic approach in many patients because it has high diagnostic efficacy and provides additional information on exercise capacity. Pharmacologic stress, particularly dobutamine, is a useful diagnostic test when adequate exercise is not feasible or its results are nondiagnostic.

In certain patients, the transthoracic echocardiographic images are suboptimal for a comprehensive assessment of the effect of dobutamine stress on wall motion and thickening. In a recent study, Frohwein and associates[3] studied 51 patients using dobutamine stress transesophageal echocardiography to assess the presence or absence of coronary artery disease. They demonstrated this to be a feasible, safe, and accurate technique for the detection of myocardial ischemia in patients with inadequate transthoracic echocardiographic imaging.

Left ventricular dilatation and multivessel coronary artery disease on ^{201}Tl SPECT imaging are important prognostic indicators in patients who have large defects in the left anterior descending coronary artery (LAD) distribution. Krawczynska et al.[4] identified a large perfusion defect in 291 patients examined with ^{201}Tl SPECT initial and 3-hour redistribution studies. Three-year survival for patients with left ventricular dilatation was 73% vs. 89% without LV dilatation; in patients with 1-vessel disease ("LAD only"), 3-year survival was 94% vs. 78% for multivessel disease. Not surprisingly, ^{201}Tl SPECT findings of a large perfusion defect in the LAD coronary artery distribution accompanied by LV dilatation and/or a thallium-derived diagnosis of multivessel coronary artery disease are strong prognostic indicators of a diminished survival at 3 years.

To evaluate the prognostic role of exercise ^{201}Tl SPECT imaging in patients with known or suspected coronary artery disease, Marie et al.[5] studied 217 such patients who underwent ^{201}Tl SPECT, coronary angiography, and rest radionuclide angiography, and who initially received medical therapy. During a mean follow-up of 70 months, 29 patients had a major ischemic event (cardiac death or myocardial infarction). Total extent of exercise defects was the best predictor, by ^{201}Tl SPECT, of major events, and it provided additional prognostic information compared with clinical exercise testing and catheterization variables. The extent of reversible ^{201}Tl SPECT perfusion defects was the only ^{201}Tl SPECT variable providing additional prognostic information.

R.A. O'Rourke, M.D.

References

1. Ho F-M, Huang P-J, Liau C-S, et al: Dobutamine stress echocardiography compared with dipyridamole thallium-201 single-photon emission computed tomography in detecting coronary artery disease. *Eur Heart J* 16:570–575, 1995.
2. Dagianti A, Penco M, Agati L, et al: Stress echocardiography: Comparison of exercise, dipyridamole and dobutamine in detecting and predicting the extent of coronary artery disease. *J Am Coll Cardiol* 26:18–25, 1995.
3. Frohwein S, Klein JL, Lane A, et al: Transesophageal dobutamine stress echocardiography in the evaluation of coronary artery disease. *J Am Coll Cardiol* 25:823–829, 1995.
4. Krawczynska EG, Weintraub WS, Garcia EV, et al: Left ventricular dilatation and multivessel coronary artery disease on thallium-201 SPECT are important prognostic indicators in patients with large defects in the left anterior descending distribution. *Am J Cardiol* 74:1233–1239, 1994.
5. Marie P-Y, Danchin N, Durand JF, et al: Long-term prediction of major ischemic events by exercise thallium-201 single-photon emission computed tomography: Incremental prognostic value compared with clinical, exercise testing, catheterization and radionuclide angiographic data. *J Am Coll Cardiol* 26:879–886, 1995.

Enhanced Detection of Myocardial Ischemia by Stress Dobutamine Echocardiography Utilizing the "Biphasic" Response of Wall Thickening During Low and High Dose Dobutamine Infusion

Senior R, Lahiri A (Northwick Park Hosp and Inst of Med Research, Harrow, England)

J Am Coll Cardiol 26:26–32, 1995 119-96-38–4

Introduction.—If there is a wall motion abnormality present at rest, exercise echocardiography cannot identify areas of reversible myocardial ischemia. In these cases, radionuclide perfusing imaging is the method of choice. Regional myocardial viability can be detected using dobutamine echocardiography because the medication improves wall thickening. This response decreases with a higher dose of dobutamine. Because of this biphasic response, dobutamine may be used on a wide range of patients with stable coronary disease and abnormal wall motion.

Methods.—A total of 54 patients who had contrast angiography for determination of coronary disease had wall motion abnormalities and were evaluated by echocardiography. Baseline echocardiograms were performed and then followed by infusion of increasing doses of dobutamine (5 µg/kg/min + 5 µg/kg/min every 3 minutes). At the peak dose (40 µg/kg/min) technetium-99 sestamibi or ^{99m}Tc tetrofosmin was injected and scintigraphic images were obtained. Resting scintigraphy was performed on a separate day. Other infusion end points included increasing ischemia or intolerable side effects. Parasternal long and short axis and apical 2- and 4-chamber views were obtained via echocardiography. Wall motion of the left ventricle was determined on 11 segments. Each segment was graded as 1 (normal) to 5 (dyskinetic). Collateral circulation was graded using coronary arteriography. Vessels with a score of 1 had a well-developed collateral circulation. Significant ischemia was defined as a narrowing of a coronary artery by greater than 50%.

Results.—At the peak dose of dobutamine, the mean heart rate was 134 bpm and the systolic blood pressure was 165 mm Hg. Maximal ST-segment depression was 0.9 mm. The maximal dose of dobutamine was achieved in 18 patients. Of the 162 myocardial regions examined, 48 regions were akinetic, 13 were severely hypokinetic, and 7 were mildly hypokinetic. Forty patients had 1 region with a wall motion abnormality. Nine patients showed fixed defects and the remaining had fully or partially reversible defects. A biphasic response was evident in 98% of the patients. Ischemia by radionuclide imaging and findings by biphasic dobutamine echocardiography were in agreement 89% of the time, but only 56% of the time when only the data from the peak dobutamine dose were used. The sensitivity for detecting reversible ischemia using perfusion imaging was 67% for 1-vessel disease, 55% for 2-vessel disease and 29% for 3-vessel disease. For dobutamine echocardiography, the sensitivities were 71% for 1-vessel disease, 52% for 2-vessel disease and 26% for 3-vessel disease.

Conclusion.—Echocardiographic stress testing with dobutamine has value in detecting myocardial ischemia. Knowledge of the biphasic response can enhance the detection of ischemia and the agreement with the findings of radionuclide perfusion imaging.

► The frequent biphasic response to low- and high-dose IV dobutamine infusion using echocardiographic assessment of wall motion and thickening has been well documented. At low doses (2.5–20 mg/kg), areas of abnormal wall motion frequently improve, as does wall thickening in areas of ischemic but viable myocardium. At high doses (30–40 mg/kg/min), the ventricular function deteriorates, as does segmental wall thickening in areas that originally were dyskinetic. Because wall motion and thickening in multisegments can be better evaluated during dobutamine echocardiography than during exercise echocardiography, it would appear to be a better method of stress echocardiography for assessing areas with initial regional wall motion abnormalities. In this study, the biphasic response to dobutamine, using echocardiography for wall motion assessment, was equivalent to positive results with SPECT imaging using either ^{99m}Tc sestamibi or ^{99m}Tc tetrofosmin. The 89% agreement in the detection of ischemia between the 2 techniques when the biphasic response was observed during stress dobutamine echocardiography is encouraging.

The absence of clinical risk factors such as angina, diabetes, Q waves on ECG, symptomatic ventricular tachyarrhythmias, and age older than 70 years identifies a low-risk group of patients being evaluated for major vascular surgery. In a study by Poldermans and associates,[1] the positive predictive value for a cardiac event in the perioperative period with dobutamine-atropine stress echocardiography was 38%, and the negative predictive value was 100%. Those individuals having ischemia at a relatively low heart rate during infusion of dobutamine represented a very small high-risk group with a low ischemic threshold. In the assessment of perioperative cardiac risk using noninvasive testing, imaging techniques should be preserved for patients who, on the basis of their clinical characteristics, a low functional capacity, or a high-risk noncardiac surgical procedure, would benefit from further risk stratification. Patients at low risk benefit little from noninvasive testing for inducible myocardial ischemia; however, dobutamine echocardiography is a useful test for patients at intermediate risk and for patients with a low functional capacity in whom high-risk noncardiac surgery is necessary.

R.A. O'Rourke, M.D.

Reference

1. Poldermans D, Arnese M, Fioretti PM, et al: Improved cardiac risk stratification in major vascular surgery with dobutamine-atropine stress echocardiography. *J Am Coll Cardiol* 26:648–653, 1995.

Magnetic Resonance Imaging Assessment of the Severity of Mitral Regurgitation: Comparison With Invasive Techniques

Hundley WG, Li HF, Willard JE, Landau C, Lange RA, Meshack BM, Hillis LD, Peshock RM (Univ of Texas Southwestern Med Ctr, Dallas)
Circulation 92:1151–1158, 1995 119-96-38–5

Background.—Cardiac catheterization is usually done in candidates for valvular surgery to determine the severity of mitral regurgitation and its effect on left ventricular volumes and systolic function. There have been no rigorous examinations of the accuracy and cost-effectiveness of MRI assessment of mitral valvular regurgitation.

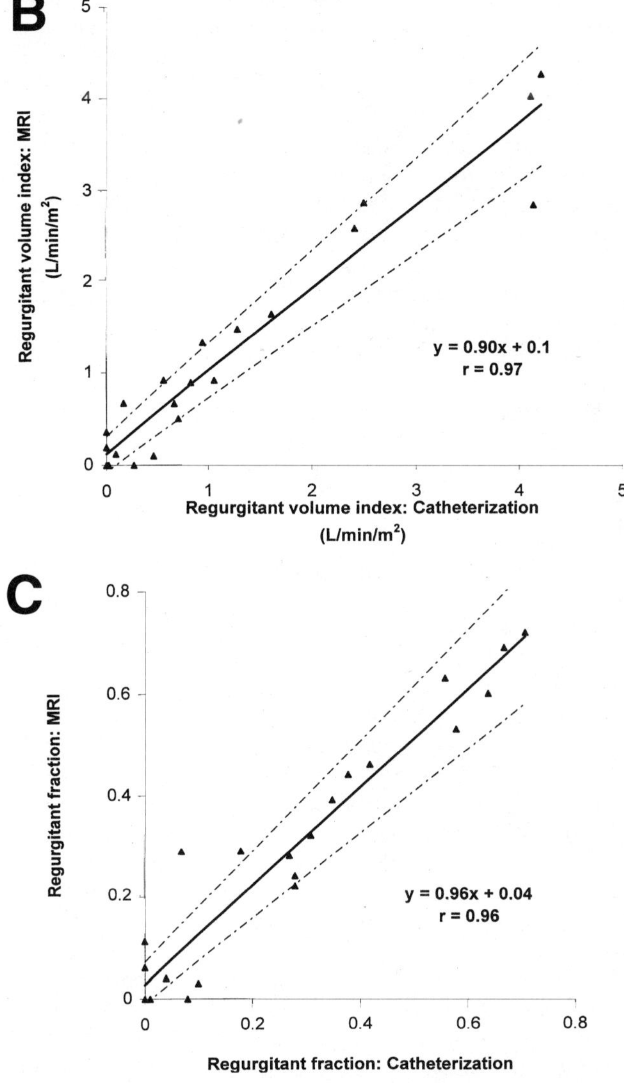

FIGURE 3B and 3C.—Scatterplots showing catheterization (*horizontal axes*) and MRI (*vertical axes*) measurements of (**B**) regurgitant volume index and (**C**) regurgitant fraction for 23 patients. Shown are the regression lines (*solid lines*) and equations; *dashed lines* represent ± 95% confidence intervals for the regression equations. (Reproduced with permission [*Circulation*]. Copyright [1995] American Heart Association.)

Methods.—Fourteen females and 9 males, aged 15–72 years, were enrolled in a study. Seventeen had mitral regurgitation, and 6 did not. Immediately after MRI was performed in each patient, cardiac catheterization was done. Left ventricular volumes and regurgitant fractions were quantified.

Findings.—Regurgitant jets were visible on the MRI long-axis view of the left ventricle in all 17 patients with angiographic evidence of mitral regurgitation. The correlation between invasive and MRI evaluations of left ventricular end-diastolic and end-systolic volumes was excellent, the coefficient being 0.95 for each. The correlation coefficient between these 2 modalities for regurgitant fraction was 0.96 (Fig 3B and C). In each patient, MRI examination was completed in less than 28 minutes. Magnetic resonance imaging was also found to be cost-effective.

Conclusions.—Cine gradient-echo and velocity-encoded phase-difference MRI accurately determines the magnitude of regurgitation in surgical candidates with mitral regurgitation. This modality can help physicians determine suitability for surgical correction and estimate perioperative mortality by quantifying left ventricular systolic function. Magnetic resonance imaging is a safe, efficient, widely available, and cost-effective technique well suited for repetitive assessments to determine the correct timing for surgery.

▶ In this study, MRI compared favorably with cardiac catheterization and left ventricular (LV) cineangiography for assessing the severity of mitral regurgitation and its influence on LV volumes and systolic function. It is an alternate technique to transthoracic and transesophageal echocardiography for assessing the severity of mitral regurgitation and its effect on LV function. When performed in properly skilled laboratories, it is probably more accurate than echocardiographic techniques for assessing the extent of mitral regurgitation. Magnetic resonance imaging will be used more frequently in the future for the initial determination of the severity of mitral regurgitation and for follow-up studies before surgical intervention. Confirmatory studies in a larger number of patients are required before this technique is routinely utilized in clinical laboratories across the country. Also, this technique does not include the ability to estimate pulmonary artery pressure, such as by transthoracic echo continuous waveform assessment of the tricuspid regurgitation jet or by cardiac catheterization. This is important, because the pulmonary artery pressure at rest or during exercise is frequently considered when making decisions concerning surgery in patients who are relatively asymptomatic but have severe mitral regurgitation.

In another report concerning gradient echo MRI of the heart, Dendale and his collaborators[1] studied 37 patients with recent myocardial infarction, assessing images of wall motion and the reaction to low-dose dobutamine stimulation and comparing the results with those of 2-dimensional echocardiography. A concordant diagnosis of viability between the 2-dimensional echocardiography and MRI techniques was obtained in 30 of 37 patients. The MRI correctly predicted evolution of wall motion after myocardial infarction in 19 of 24 patients. Thus, low-dosage dobutamine MRI is a safe alternative to dobutamine echocardiography for predicting recovery of wall motion abnormalities after myocardial infarction.

The diagnostic role of echocardiography in the assessment of patients with known or suspected infective endocarditis has been firmly established during the past 20 years. Although the detection of valvular vegetations by transthoracic echocardiography has improved significantly, and transesophageal echocardiography provides additional information in selected cases, the prognostic significance of these lesions remains unclear. Recently, Heinle and associates[2] reported on the value of transthoracic echocardiography in predicting embolic events in active infective endocarditis in 41 patients whose echocardiograms were reviewed by 4 echocardiographers blinded to the clinical data. Interobserver agreement was 98% with regard to echocardiographic vegetation presence and 97% with regard to the involved site. However, interobserver variability was great, with respect to vegetation shape, mobility, and attachment characteristics.

Echocardiographic vegetation characteristics were not useful in defining the risk of embolic complications in patients with endocarditis. Systolic embolic events occurred in 20 of the 41 patients with infected endocarditis and did not correlate with a vegetation size greater or less than 10 mm.

R.A. O'Rourke, M.D.

References

1. Dendale PAC, Franken PR, Waldman G-J, et al: Low-dosage dobutamine magnetic resonance imaging as an alternative to echocardiography in the detection of viable myocardium after acute infarction. *Am Heart J* 130:134–140, 1995.
2. Heinle S, Wilderman N, Harrison JK, et al: Value of transthoracic echocardiography in predicting embolic events in active infective endocarditis. *Am J Cardiol* 74:799–801, 1994.

39 Arrhythmias

The Natural History of Atrial Fibrillation: Incidence, Risk Factors, and Prognosis in the Manitoba Follow-Up Study

Krahn AD, Manfreda J, Tate RB, Mathewson FAL, Cuddy TE (Univ of Manitoba, Winnipeg, Canada)

Am J Med 98:476–484, 1995 119-96-39–1

Introduction.—Atrial fibrillation has been associated with increased morbidity and mortality, especially when other cardiovascular diseases are present. Most studies demonstrating an increased risk of stroke and cardiovascular mortality in patients with atrial fibrillation have used a case-control design. The incidence, risk factors, and prognosis of atrial fibrillation were determined from cohort data in a prospective study.

Methods.—The Manitoba Follow-Up Study involved 3,983 male air crew recruits who were observed for 44 years. Physical examination (including a resting ECG) was performed at baseline and at regular intervals during the study. Atrial fibrillation was diagnosed by the interpretation of ECGs or by a physician's report. The risk factors for atrial fibrillation (cardiac, noncardiac, lifestyle-related, and ECG abnormalities) were evaluated, and their association with the development of atrial fibrillation was determined. Total, cardiovascular, and noncardiovascular mortality was assessed and related to the prognosis for atrial fibrillation. The Cox proportional hazard model with time-dependent covariates was used for the analyses of risk factors and outcome.

Results.—Three hundred study participants (7.5%) had atrial fibrillation, documented by an ECG in 85% and by a physician's report in 15%. The incidence of atrial fibrillation increased with age (Fig 1). At age 50 years or younger, the age-specific incidence was 0.5 per 1,000 person-years; by age 60 years the incidence increased to 2.3 per 1,000 person-years, and by age 85 years it increased to 16.9 per 1,000 person-years. The age-adjusted relative risk for atrial fibrillation was significantly increased with all cardiac conditions (ischemic heart disease, valvular disease, congestive heart failure, cardiomyopathy, hypertension, murmur, or palpitations). Most noncardiac conditions, with the exception of smoking and obesity, were uncommon in subjects with atrial fibrillation. Pulmonary embolism had the greatest relative risk (RR, 3.67) for the development of atrial fibrillation, compared to other noncardiac risk factors. The ST- or T-wave abnormalities carried a relative risk of 3.11. Based on multivariate

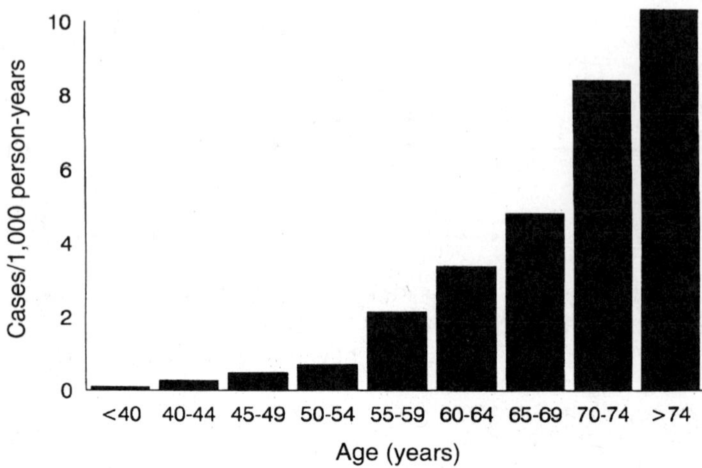

FIGURE 1.—Incidence of atrial fibrillation by age in the Manitoba Follow-Up Study, 1948–1982. (Courtesy of Krahn AD, Manfreda J, Tate RB, et al: *Am J Med* 98:476–484, 1995. Adapted with permission from *American Journal of Medicine.*)

analysis, all cardiac risk factors (except murmur and miscellaneous factors), obesity, ST- or T-wave changes, and supraventricular and ventricular arrhythmias, were significant risks for atrial fibrillation. Total mortality was increased by 1.31 in the presence of atrial fibrillation. The risk of death for study members with both myocardial infarction, and atrial fibrillation was 4.28 times greater than for study members free of both conditions. The risk of fatal stroke was increased by 2.48.

Conclusions.—Cardiac risk factors had the greatest effect on the risk of atrial fibrillation, with ischemic heart disease and hypertension commonly preceding atrial fibrillation. The ST- or T-wave changes in ECG also increased the risk for atrial fibrillation, but to a lesser degree. Age was a risk factor for atrial fibrillation, with increases in age associated with an increased risk. An increase in mortality was observed in association with atrial fibrillation and was increased in the presence of underlying cardiac diseases.

▶ The data from the present cohort reflect the incidence of atrial fibrillation in a selected healthy male population and are consistent with published series reporting a low prevalence of atrial fibrillation before age 65 in both sexes. This report, like others, draws attention to the importance of the higher frequency of this arrhythmia with advancing age. All cardiac conditions examined had a significantly increased relative risk for atrial fibrillation. Except for smoking and obesity, noncardiac conditions examined were uncommon among patients with atrial fibrillation. Of interest, unlike the Framingham Study, diabetes was not significant in the multivariate model for relative risk and its association with atrial fibrillation may not be independent of the effect of ischemic heart disease, hypertension, or congestive heart failure on the development of atrial fibrillation. This report is one of the first to document the association of atrial fibrillation with subsequent congestive heart failure, independent of the effect of ischemic heart disease or hypertension. Although ischemic heart disease often preceded atrial fibrillation and was an independent risk factor, myocardial infarction was not increased following atrial fibrillation after adjusting for preexisting risk factors for ischemic heart disease.

R.A. O'Rourke, M.D.

Cardioversion of Nonrheumatic Atrial Fibrillation: Reduced Thromboembolic Complications With 4 Weeks of Precardioversion Anticoagulation Are Related to Atrial Thrombus Resolution

Collins LJ, Silverman DI, Douglas PS, Manning WJ (Harvard Med School, Boston; Beth Israel Hosp, Boston; Univ of Connecticut, Farmington)

Circulation 92:160–163, 1995 119-96-39–2

Introduction.—Several weeks of anticoagulation with warfarin is recommended for patients with atrial fibrillation scheduled for cardioversion to sinus rhythm, for this treatment is reported to reduce the incidence of clinical thromboembolism from 5% to 7% to 0% to 1.6%. Although the mechanism by which warfarin accomplishes its effect is unknown, the effect is often attributed to enhanced thrombus organization. Serial transesophageal echocardiography was performed in 14 patients with nonrheumatic atrial fibrillation to better describe the mechanism by which warfarin acts.

Patients and Methods.—All patients underwent transesophageal echocardiography before and after warfarin therapy (Fig p 162). Warfarin anticoagulation was administered to maintain a prothrombin time of 1.5 –1.8 times control. The patients, 7 men and 7 women, had a mean age of 69 years. Duration of atrial fibrillation before transesophageal echocardiography was estimated at a mean of 6.1 weeks; the median interval between the echocardiographic studies was 4 weeks. Patients were followed clinically for signs of thromboembolism.

Results.—The initial transesophageal echocardiographic study identified 18 atrial thrombi, including 14 confined to the left atrial appendage. Thrombi ranged in size from 5 to 20 mm in longest dimension; one third were considered mobile. After a median of 4 weeks of warfarin therapy, all but 2 of the 18 atrial thrombi had completely resolved and no new thrombi were identified on repeat transesophageal echocardiography. No patient had clinical evidence of a thromboembolic event during this period.

Conclusion.—Warfarin anticoagulation was found to resolve atrial thrombi in patients awaiting cardioversion from nonrheumatic atrial fibrillation to sinus rhythm. The primary mechanisms by which warfarin achieves its benefits are thrombus resolution and prevention of new thrombus formation rather than thrombus organization. Cardioversion for patients with thrombi should be undertaken only after follow-up transesophageal echocardiography is performed.

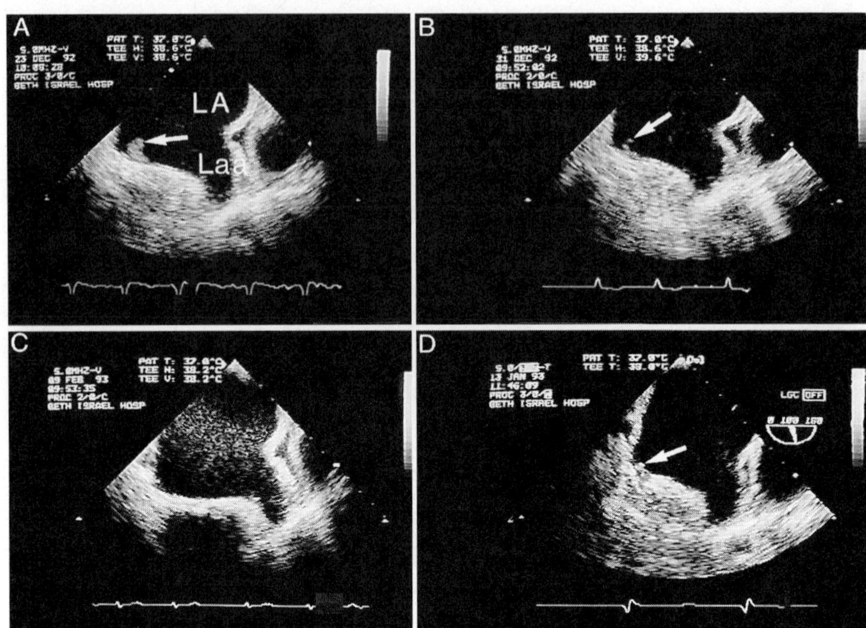

FIGURE p 162.—Serial transesophageal echocardiograms showing the left atrium (*LA*) and left atrial appendage (*Laa*) viewed in the vertical plane with a 5-MHz biplane transesophageal probe. The thrombus (*arrow*) is in the body of the atrium, closely associated with the mitral annulus in the posterior portion of the left atrium. **A,** initial study showing a mobile 12-mm thrombus; **B,** thrombus persists (*arrow*) but is smaller after 1 week of warfarin therapy; **C,** after 3 weeks of warfarin, the thrombus continues to be seen (*arrow*); **D,** complete thrombus resolution after 5.5 weeks of warfarin. (Reproduced with permission [*Circulation*]. Copyright [1995] American Heart Association.)

► Transesophageal echocardiography is both sensitive and specific for the noninvasive identification of left atrial thrombi. However, transesophageal echocardiography is not a necessary requirement for the precardioversion evaluation of all patients with chronic atrial fibrillation being selected for cardioversion. Many will receive anticoagulants routinely for 4 weeks, as has been done in the past, with a very low risk of thromboembolic events at the time of cardioversion. The authors of this study used serial transesophageal echocardiography to assess the course of left atrial thrombi in patients with positive transesophageal echocardiography results at the initial study. Their data demonstrate that in the majority of patients with nonrheumatic atrial fibrillation, left atrial thrombi are resolved after 4 weeks of warfarin therapy without clinical evidence of thromboembolism. Therefore, thrombus resolution rather than thrombus organization, and prevention of new thrombus formation during the period of anticoagulation appear to be the primary benefits of this approach.

Stoddard and colleagues[1] performed 2-dimensional transesophageal echocardiography in 143 patients with acute atrial fibrillation (i.e., less than 3 days) and 147 patients with chronic atrial fibrillation. They found a left atrial thrombus in 14% of patients with acute and 27% of patients with chronic atrial fibrillation. In patients with a recent embolic event, the frequency of left atrial appendage thrombus did not differ between those with acute and those with chronic atrial fibrillation. Thus, patients with acute atrial fibrillation for less than 3 days require anticoagulation prophylaxis or evaluation by transesophageal echocardiography before cardioversion and should not be assumed to be free of left atrial thrombus.

Recently, Manning et al.[2] reported on 233 patients with atrial fibrillation for 2 days or more or of unknown duration. Patients received anticoagulation with heparin or warfarin and underwent conventional transthoracic echocardiography followed by a transesophageal study. Patients in whom transesophageal echocardiography revealed no atrial thrombus underwent pharmacologic or electric cardioversion followed by warfarin therapy for 1 month. Cardioversion was deferred for patients with evidence of atrial thrombi and they received prolonged warfarin treatment. Importantly, 186 (95%) of 196 patients without thrombi had successful cardioversion to sinus rhythm, all without prolonged anticoagulation, and none experienced a clinical thrombi or embolic event. Eighteen patients with atrial thrombi underwent uneventful cardioversion after prolonged anticoagulation. Thus, one strategy for the electric reversion from atrial fibrillation to sinus rhythm consists of transesophageal echocardiography followed by earlier cardioversion in conjunction with short-term anticoagulation for those with no evidence of thrombi on transesophageal echocardiography evaluation.

Several additional reports[3–6] concern the efficacy of various drug therapies in patients with supraventricular tachyarrhythmias. Ellenbogen and associates[3] studied the efficacy of various doses of IV diltiazem to control the ventricular response during atrial fibrillation or atrial flutter. Eighty-four patients with atrial fibrillation or flutter or both received an IV bolus of diltiazem followed by a continuous infusion of diltiazem at 5, 10, and 15 mg/hr. A bolus dose of 20–25 mg, followed by titration of continuous infusion, was a safe and effective regimen to rapidly lower the heart rate in patients with atrial fibrillation and atrial flutter. By the end of the infusion, 18% of patients had reverted to sinus rhythm; symptomatic hypotension occurred in 3.9% of cases but responded to normal saline solution in all cases.

In a randomized, double-blind control study of 98 patients with atrial fibrillation present for more than 30 minutes but less than 72 hours and a ventricular response greater than 100 beats/min, Donovan compared the results of IV flecainide with IV amiodarone and placebo. Twenty of 34 patients who were (59%) given flecainide, 11 of 32 (34%) given amiodarone, and 7 of 32 (22%) given placebo reverted to a stable sinus rhythm in less than 2 hours after starting medication. After 8 hours, there were no significant differences in reversion between the treatment groups: flecainide, 68%; amiodarone, 59%; and placebo, 56%. Amiodarone promptly reduced the ventricular rate, and this effect was maintained for 8 hours in those in whom reversion to stable sinus rhythm was unsuccessful. Flecainide was no more effective than placebo in controlling the ventricular rate. Nearly 60% of patients with atrial fibrillation of *recent* onset reverted to sinus rhythm within a few hours without any treatment whatsoever.

Recently, a double-blind, placebo-controlled trial of the efficacy and tolerability of propafenone[5] was undertaken in 100 patients with paroxysmal supraventricular tachycardia or atrial fibrillation/flutter who had recorded 2 or more symptomatic arrhythmia recurrences by transtelephonic ECG monitoring during a 3-month drug-free observation. Recurrent paroxysmal tachycardia was documented by ECG and symptom diary. Data from this study indicate that propafenone is of value in the prophylaxis of both paroxysmal supraventricular tachycardia and paroxysmal atrial fibrillation. A dose of 300 mg twice daily was effective and well tolerated. A larger dose of 300 mg given 3 times daily caused more adverse effects but may be more effective in those who can tolerate it.

Recently, a retrospective survey was conducted to determine the safety and efficacy of IV adenosine when used for the treatment of supraventricular arrhythmias during pregnancy.[6] The results of the study suggest that the use of IV adenosine for determination of maternal supraventricular tachycardia during the second and third trimester of pregnancy is safe and effective. However, the development of fetal bradycardia after administration of multiple antiarrhythmic drugs emphasizes the importance of fetal heart rate monitoring during acute antiarrhythmic therapy.

R.A. O'Rourke, M.D.

References

1. Stoddard MF, Dawkins PR, Prince CR, et al: Left atrial appendage thrombus is not uncommon in patients with acute atrial fibrillation and a recent embolic event: A transesophageal echocardiographic study. *J Am Coll Cardiol* 25:452–459, 1995.
2. Manning WJ, Silverman DI, Keighley CS, et al: Transesophageal echocardiographically facilitated early cardioversion from atrial fibrillation using short-term anticoagulation: Final results of a prospective 4.5-year study. *J Am Coll Cardiol* 25:1354–1361, 1995.
3. Ellenbogen KA, Dias VC, Cardello FP, et al: Safety and efficacy of intravenous diltiazem in atrial fibrillation or atrial flutter. *Am J Cardiol* 75:45–49, 1995.
4. Donovan KD, Power BM, Hockings BEF, et al: Intravenous flecainide versus amiodarone for recent-onset atrial fibrillation. *Am J Cardiol* 75:693–697, 1995.
5. UK Propafenone PSVT Study Group: A randomized, placebo-controlled trial of propafenone in the prophylaxis of paroxysmal supraventricular tachycardia and paroxysmal atrial fibrillation. *Circulation* 92:2550–2557, 1995.
6. Elkayam U, Goodwin TM. Adenosine therapy for supraventricular tachycardia during pregnancy. *Am J Cardiol* 75:521–523, 1995.

Spontaneous Sustained Ventricular Tachycardia in the Electrophysiologic Study Versus Electrocardiographic Monitoring (ESVEM) Trial

Anderson KP, for the ESVEM Investigators (Presbyterian Univ Hosp, Pittsburgh, Pa)

J Am Coll Cardiol 26:489–496, 1995 119-96-39–3

Background.—An appropriately timed premature ventricular complex may lead to ventricular tachyarrhythmias and sudden death in patients with myocardial damage. The "premature ventricular complex-trigger" theory also posits the idea that pathologic changes in the myocardium produce a stable substrate. Drugs that eliminate premature ventricular complex triggers or disable the substrate might therefore prevent arrhythmias and sudden death, yet recent clinical trials have not confirmed this paradigm. A review of 1,102 episodes of spontaneous, sustained monomorphic ventricular tachycardia sought to determine whether premature ventricular complexes were required for their initiation and whether tachycardia induced at electrophysiologic study reproduced the spontaneous arrhythmia.

Methods.—Holter monitor tapes were obtained in the course of the Electrophysiologic Study Versus Electrocardiographic Monitoring trial. Enrolled patients had at least 10 premature ventricular complexes per hour and inducible, sustained ventricular tachyarrhythmias. Tapes with episodes of ventricular tachycardia of 30 seconds or longer were examined further. Digital waveform analysis distinguished episodes initiated by configurationally distinct, possibly triggering, complexes (type 1) from those in which the initial QRS waveforms were identical to subsequent complexes, suggesting no requirement for premature ventricular beats (type 2).

Results.—Of the 1,102 episodes of ventricular tachycardia analyzed, only 73 (7%) were of type 1 onset. Thirty-seven of these were preceded by a single premature ventricular complex of differing configuration, and 22 were preceded by 2 or more ventricular complexes with configurations different from ventricular tachycardia. Type 1 and 2 events did not differ significantly in mean duration (17 and 14 minutes, respectively), but mean cycle length was significantly shorter in type 1 (367 ms) than in type 2 events (407 ms). Of 59 patients represented by the episodes analyzed, 24% had only type 1 episodes and 63% had predominantly type 2 episodes. Sustained ventricular tachycardia could be induced in all group 1 patients, and in 57% the induced rhythm was similar to the spontaneous rhythm. Induced and spontaneous rhythms differed in half of the patients in group 2. Group 2 patients who received therapy guided by Holter monitoring

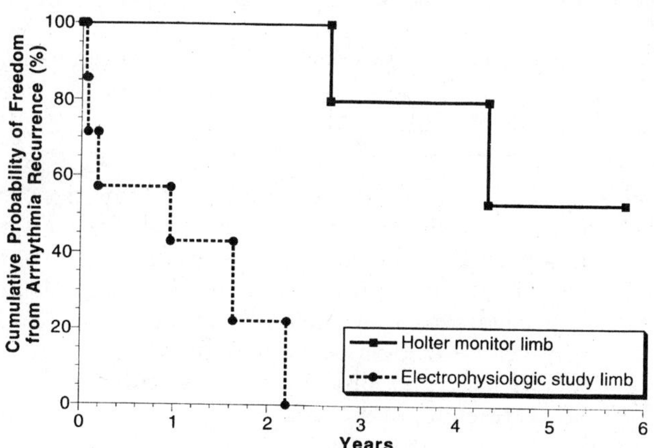

FIGURE 2.—Kaplan-Meier plot indicating cumulative probability of remaining free of arrhythmia recurrence in group 2 patients discharged with medical therapy predicted to be effective by Holter monitoring (n = 10) or by electrophysiologic testing (n = 7). The difference in arrhythmic event-free survival was significant (P = 0.001) by the log-rank test. (Reprinted with permission from the American College of Cardiology [*Journal of the American College of Cardiology*, 1995, 26:489–496.])

were significantly more likely to be free of arrhythmia recurrences during follow-up than were those assigned to electrophysiologic study (Fig 2).

Conclusion.—Mechanisms other than classically conceived reentry could be responsible for the majority of spontaneous ventricular tachyarrhythmias analyzed in this study. The properties of spontaneous arrhythmias observed in this patient group were not readily accounted for by the paradigm of a premature ventricular complex activating a stable substrate for reentry.

▶ Although premature beats were not required for the initiation of ventricular tachycardia in this study, this finding does not prove or exclude the presence of a particular arrhythmia mechanism. Therefore, any of the 3 major categories of arrhythmia mechanisms—reentry, triggered activity, or automaticity—could be responsible for the observed rhythms. These findings could have clinical importance if many of the patient population behave as group 2 patients and have a significantly better outcome with treatment selected by continuous ambulatory ECG recordings and a worse outcome with therapy identified by electrophysiologic study. Importantly, the pattern of initiation of spontaneous ventricular tachycardia may separate patients with different responses to programmed stimulation and treatment. These findings plus the high rate of sudden death and arrhythmia recurrences observed in recent clinical trials, despite accepted therapy and the inability to predict and prevent proarrhythmic effects, indicate that current models of arrhythmogenesis are inadequate.

R.A. O'Rourke, M.D.

Relations Between Heart Failure, Ejection Fraction, Arrhythmia Suppression and Mortality: Analysis of the Cardiac Arrhythmia Suppression Trial

Hallstrom A, for the Cardiac Arrhythmia Suppression Trial Investigators (Univ of Washington, Seattle)

J Am Coll Cardiol 25:1250–1257, 1995 119-96-39-4

Introduction.—The degree of left ventricular dysfunction has been associated with post–myocardial infarction mortality. The presence of ventricular arrhythmia has also been shown to be prognostic of sudden death and cardiovascular mortality in these patients. Death resulting from arrhythmia and other cardiovascular causes was found to be less frequent in patients with preserved ventricular function during the Cardiac Arrhythmia Suppression Trial (CAST). Clinical outcomes and mortality in patients in the CAST trial were evaluated for associations between ejection fraction, heart failure, and arrhythmia suppression.

Methods.—Data from 3,549 patients in CAST were evaluated, including ejection fraction measurements and congestion heart failure syndromes. Three definitions of heart failure syndrome were used: history of symptomatic heart failure; history of or evidence of congestive heart failure by physical examination; or any congestive heart failure. Study end points were defined as death or cardiac arrest, arrhythmic death or cardiac arrest, definite congestive heart failure, or evidence (worsening or new) of congestive heart failure. Arrhythmia suppression required a greater than 80% reduction, with partial suppression considered a 1% to 79% reduction.

Results.—Suppression of arrhythmia was significantly less likely in patients who had congestive heart failure as compared with those patients who did not have congestive heart failure. Similarly, for an ejection fraction less than 30%, the likelihood of suppression of arrhythmia was significantly less as compared with patients with ejection fraction greater than 30%. Stepwise logistic regression determined a significant association with failure of suppression of arrhythmia and the presence of both congestive heart failure and a low ejection fraction. Both ejection fraction and history of heart failure were predictive of failure of arrhythmia suppression, with a stronger association for heart failure. A strong association between ejection fraction and mortality outcome was also found, with an ejection fraction of less than 20% associated with a significantly greater mortality as compared to an ejection fraction greater than 50%. Congestive heart failure was also associated with mortality, with a twofold higher mortality observed in patients with congestive heart failure as compared to those without heart failure.

Conclusion.—Congestive heart failure has a significant effect on arrhythmia suppression, with only 58% of patients with congestive heart failure in this study achieving suppression as compared to 75% of patients without heart failure. Ejection fraction was also found to be a significant predictor of arrhythmia suppression. These data indicate that patients at higher risk for mortality from arrhythmias have a significant loss of antiarrhythmic drug effect.

► The information from this report on the relation between heart failure status and suppression of arrhythmia in a population with mild-to-moderate left ventricular dysfunction complements prior published observations on the relation of ejection fraction to arrhythmia suppression. In the CAST population at highest risk (those with both congestive heart failure syndrome and an ejection fraction less than 30%), almost 50% of the patients did not achieve arrhythmia suppression. Therefore, a significant loss of drug efficacy occurs in the subset of CAST patients known to be at high risk for death from arrhythmia. The data from CAST suggest that baseline heart failure status is a more significant predictor of the failure to suppress ventricular arrhythmias than election fraction.

R.A. O'Rourke, M.D.

Dispersion of QT Interval in Patients With and Without Susceptibility to Ventricular Tachyarrhythmias After Previous Myocardial Infarction

Perkiömäki JS, Koistinen MJ, Yli-Mäyry S, Huikuri HV (Univ of Oulu, Finland)

J Am Coll Cardiol 26:174–179, 1995 119-96-39–5

Background.—It has been suggested that the nonhomogeneity of ventricular recovery times can be demonstrated by measuring the variation in duration of the QT interval for different ECG leads. So-called QT dispersion reportedly is increased after acute myocardial infarction, as well as in patients with the long QT syndrome or hypertrophic cardiomyopathy. In the 2 latter groups, prolonged QT dispersion is associated with a greater likelihood of serious ventricular arrhythmia.

Objective.—A study was planned to determine whether QT dispersion measurements are able to identify those patients who are at risk of life-threatening arrhythmia after myocardial infarction.

Patients.—Thirty healthy individuals were compared with 40 patients who had had myocardial infarction but no spontaneous or inducible ventricular tachyarrhythmia, and 30 others who had had sustained either ventricular tachycardia or (in 12 cases) cardiac arrest after infarction.

Methods.—Electrophysiologic testing was performed, including programmed ventricular stimulation with up to 3 extrastimuli at basic drive cycle lengths of 600 and 400 msec. The QT and QT apex (QTa) intervals and the duration of the QRS complex were estimated at each of the 12 surface ECG leads over 2 consecutive cycles.

Results.—The maximum corrected QTc interval (QTc) was longest in patients with tachyarrhythmia. Both patient groups had a significantly longer maximum QTac interval and QRS duration than did control subjects. Interval dispersions were broadest in patients with ventricular

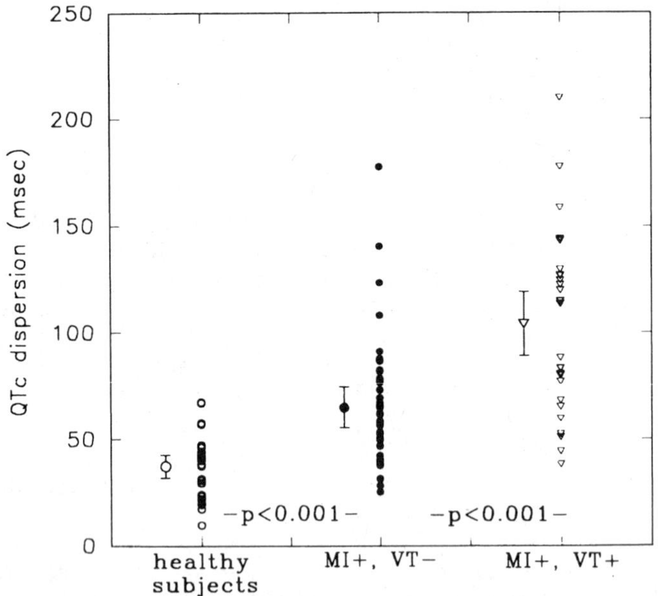

FIGURE 1.—Corrected QT dispersion in the 3 study groups. *Vertical bars* represent 95% confidence intervals of mean values. *Abbreviations: MI,* myocardial infarction; *VT,* ventricular tachyarrhythmia; *plus* (*minus*), presence (absence). (Reprinted with permission from the American College of Cardiology [*Journal of the American College of Cardiology,* 1995, 26:174–179.])

tachyarrhythmia and narrowest in control subjects (Fig 1). On multiple regression analysis, QTc dispersion was the best predictor of vulnerability to ventricular tachyarrhythmia. Taking 80 msec as the upper normal limit for QTc dispersion, this parameter was 70% sensitive and 78% specific in distinguishing between postinfarction patients with and without susceptibility to tachyarrhythmia. Its positive predictive accuracy was 70%.

Conclusion.—Abnormal variability in QT duration among different ECG leads is a marker for an increased risk of reentrant ventricular arrhythmia in patients who have had myocardial infarction.

► Increased QT dispersion appears to be related to the susceptibility to reentrant ventricular tachyarrhythmias independent of the extent of left ventricular dysfunction or patient clinical characteristics; therefore, the simple, noninvasive measurement of this interval from a standard 12-lead ECG may help identify patients at risk for life-threatening arrhythmias after a previous myocardial infarction. However, there is considerable overlap of QT corrected dispersion values between healthy subjects and patients with myocardial infarction but no ventricular tachycardia, and there is even more so between patients with myocardial infarction without ventricular tachycardia and those with ventricular tachycardia. A large prospective study would be necessary to define the true clinical usefulness of what appears to be a simple noninvasive measure of increased risk of ventricular tachyarrhythmias in postinfarction patients.

R.A. O'Rourke, M.D.

Definition of the Best Prediction Criteria of the Time Domain Signal-Averaged Electrocardiogram for Serious Arrhythmic Events in the Postinfarction Period

El-Sherif N, for the Cardiac Arrhythmia Suppression Trial/Signal-Averaged Electrocardiogram (CAST/SAECG) Substudy Investigators (State Univ of New York Health Science Ctr, Brooklyn; et al)

J Am Coll Cardiol 25:908–914, 1995 119-96-39–6

Background.—Former studies investigating the prognostic use of the time domain signal-averaged ECG after myocardial infarction have been limited by small study groups, empiric definitions of an abnormal recording and possible bias of selection of high-risk groups or classification of arrhythmic events, or both. A substudy with correction for these limitations was conducted in association with the Cardiac Arrhythmia Suppression Trial to identify guidelines for the prognostic use of the signal-averaged ECG in postinfarction patients.

Patients and Methods.—Ten participating centers enrolled patients with acute myocardial infarction without applying specific Cardiac Arrhythmia Suppression Trial Holter and ejection fraction study criteria. Analysis of various clinical variables, ventricular arrhythmias on Holter recordings, and 6 signal-averaged ECG variables, including the filtered QRS duration, root-mean-square voltage in the last 40 msec, and duration of late potentials of ≤ 40-μV amplitude recorded at both 25- to 250- and 40-Hz bandpass filter settings, was performed. Of the 1,211 patients initially recruited, 53 with bundle branch block were excluded from the analysis. The remaining 1,158 patients were followed for 12 months after infarction. The Cardiac Arrhythmia Suppression Trial Events Committee independently reviewed the classification of arrhythmic events.

Results.—Forty-five patients had a serious arrhythmic event, including nonfatal ventricular tachycardia or sudden cardiac arrhythmic death, at an average of 10.3 months of follow-up. When Cox regression analysis was applied to the 6 signal-averaged ECG variables, the filtered QRS duration at 40 Hz ≥ 120 msec (QRSD-40 Hz) at a cutpoint of ≥ 120 msec was found to be most predictive of arrhythmic events. When all clinical, Holter, and ejection fraction variables were considered in a regression analysis, the most significant predictor was QRSD-40 Hz ≥ 120 msec. In patients with QRSD-40 Hz < 120 msec, the probability of remaining free of a serious arrhythmic event during the first 12 months postinfarction was significantly higher compared with patients with QRSD-40 Hz ≥ 120 msec (Fig 1). A positive predictive accuracy of 17%, negative predictive accuracy of 98%, total predictive accuracy of 88%, and odds ratio of 8.4 were observed for QRSD-40 Hz ≥ 120 msec. After combining this parameter with an ejection fraction of 40% or less and the presence of complex ventricular arrhythmia on the Holter record, positive predictive accuracy improved to 32% and overall predictive accuracy to 94%. The odds ratio approxi-

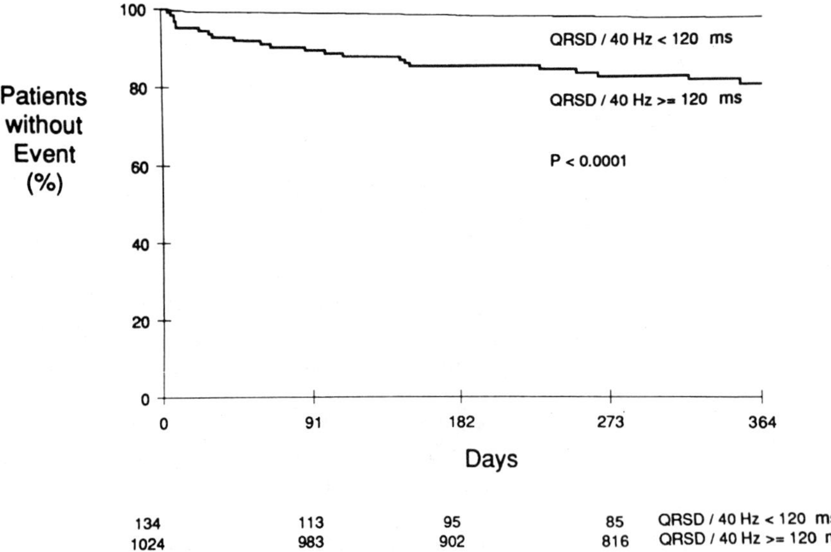

FIGURE 1.—Probability of remaining free of arrhythmic events in patients with filtered QRS duration at 40 Hz (QRSD/40 Hz) < 120 msec (normal signal-averaged ECG results) and ≥ 120 msec (abnormal signal-averaged ECG results). (Reprinted with permission from the American College of Cardiology [*Journal of the American College of Cardiology,* 1995, 25:908–914.])

mately doubled at the same time. Nevertheless, only 4% of patients with acute infarction had all 3 abnormalities.

Conclusions.—During the first 12 months after infarction, signal-averaged ECG is better able to predict serious arrhythmic events than are clinical, ejection fraction, and ventricular arrhythmia variables. The best predictor in this clinical setting is QRSD-40 Hz ≥ 120 msec.

► This large patient study confirms the results of others indicating the high negative predictive value for ventricular tachycardia or sudden death during follow-up in patients with absence of late potentials on a signal-averaged ECG obtained in the first 2 weeks after an acute myocardial infarction. However, a positive signal–averaged ECG has greater significance in identifying patients at risk for these events when it is obtained in patients with a left ventricular ejection fraction less than 40% and in patients with ambulatory ECG evidence of frequent ventricular ectopy or tachyarrhythmias. The negative predictive accuracy in these patients remains at the level of 97%, but the sensitivity for identifying patients likely to have ventricular tachycardia or sudden death during follow-up has a positive predictive accuracy that almost doubled, from 17% to 32%, using a filter-QRS duration of 40 Hz ≥ 120 msec as a cutpoint as the most positive criterion of arrhythmic events from the signal-averaged time domain ECG.

Reduced heart rate variability after acute myocardial infarction is an important risk factor for mortality and life-threatening ventricular arrhythmias after discharge from the hospital. Recently, Dambrink and colleagues[1] investigated the association between heart rate variability assessed before hospital discharge and at 3 months, and left ventricular dilatation at 1 year of follow-up after a first anterior myocardial infarction. They found that a reduced heart rate variability index before discharge was an independent risk factor for left ventricular dilatation during follow-up.

In another report, Kristal-Boneh and associates[2] reviewed the significance of heart rate variability in health and disease. Despite the need for standardization of methodology to facilitate the interpretation and comparison of results, the data presented in this review clearly show that there are individual differences in heart rate variability and that these differences partly reflect differences in the degree of parasympathetic and sympathetic stimulation of the heart. Heart rate variability and its spectral components can be easily and noninvasively assessed and can provide valuable information to the physician as indicated in the study by Dambrink.[1]

R.A. O'Rourke, M.D.

References

1. Dambrink J-HE, Tuininga YS, van Gilst WH, et al: Association between reduced heart rate variability and left ventricular dilatation in patients with a first anterior myocardial infarction. *Br Heart J* 72:514–520, 1994.
2. Kristal-Boneh E, Raifel M, Froom P, et al: Heart rate variability in health and disease. *Scand J Work Environ Health* 21:85–95, 1995.

Amiodarone in Patients With Congestive Heart Failure and Asymptomatic Ventricular Arrhythmia

Singh SN, for the Survival Trial of Antiarrhythmic Therapy in Congestive Heart Failure (Veterans Affairs Med Center, Washington, DC)
N Engl J Med 333:77–82, 1995 119-96-39–7

Background.—The combination of drugs used to treat most patients with heart failure provides symptomatic relief, but it is uncertain whether this regimen improves survival. There is a particularly high risk for fatal cardiovascular events among patients with congestive heart failure and ventricular arrhythmias. In a double-blind, placebo-controlled trial, the effect of amiodarone, a powerful antiarrhythmic agent, on survival of patients with congestive heart failure and asymptomatic ventricular arrhythmias, was investigated.

Methods.—Patients at 24 centers were screened for entry into the trial. The 674 patients who met eligibility criteria had symptoms of congestive heart failure, cardiac enlargement, ≥ 10 premature ventricular contractions per hour, and a left ventricular ejection fraction ≤ 40%. There were 333 patients randomized to receive amiodarone and 338 to receive placebo. All but 7 patients were men. Approximately 70% of patients in each group had an ischemic cause of heart failure. Monitoring included 24-hour continuous ECGs at regular intervals, chest films, blood gas values, and pulmonary function values. The end points of the study were overall mortality and sudden death of cardiac causes.

Results.—The median follow-up was 45 months. Of the 274 deaths during the study, 131 were in the amiodarone group and 143 were in the placebo group. Overall actuarial survival at 2 years was 69.4% in the amiodarone group and 70.8% in the placebo group (Fig 1). Approximately half of the deaths in each group were classified as sudden. Coronary heart disease was diagnosed in 72% of the amiodarone group and 71% of the placebo group. A trend toward reduced mortality was observed in patients with nonischemic heart disease treated with amiodarone. Amiodarone increased the left ventricular fraction by 42% at 2 years and was significantly more effective than placebo in suppressing ventricular arrhythmias. There were more side effects in the amiodarone group, but the difference was not significant.

Conclusion.—Despite its beneficial effects on left ventricular ejection fraction and ventricular arrhythmias, amiodarone was no more effective than placebo in reducing overall mortality or the incidence of sudden death in these patients with congestive heart failure. The drug was well tolerated and may benefit patients with nonischemic cardiomyopathy.

▶ The results of several smaller studies have suggested that amiodarone may be beneficial in the treatment of patients with recent myocardial infarction. Amiodarone markedly suppresses complex premature ventricular contractions and unsustained ventricular tachycardia with little depressant effect on hemodynamic function. The drug does not have important proar-

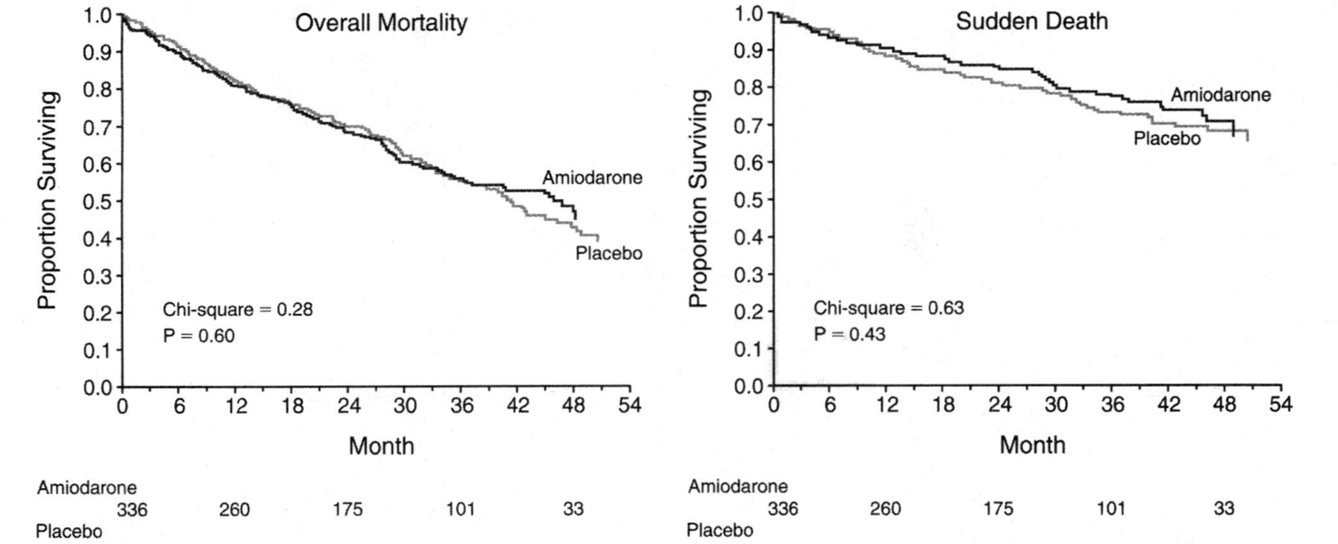

FIGURE 1.—Kaplan-Meier estimates of overall mortality and sudden death resulting from cardiac causes. Amiodarone had no significant effect, as compared with placebo, on either overall mortality or the incidence of sudden death. The numbers below the figures are the numbers of patients at risk. (Reprinted by permission of *The New England Journal of Medicine*. Singh SN, for the Survival Trial of Antiarrhythmic Therapy in Congestive Heart Failure: Amiodarone in patients with congestive heart failure and asymptomatic ventricular arrhythmia. *N Engl J Med* 333:77–82, Copyright 1995, Massachusetts Medical Society.)

rhythmic effects, unlike that which is possibly responsible for the increased mortality rate in the Cardiac Arrhythmia Suppression Trial in patients treated with encainide or flecainide for the suppression of arrhythmias. Amiodarone is known to be effective in controlling life-threatening arrhythmias. These data on amiodarone indicate a disparity between the suppression of arrhythmias and sudden death or overall mortality. No difference in overall mortality was found between the group of patients in whom the ventricular arrhythmias were suppressed (those with 80% or greater suppression of premature ventricular contractions) and the group in whom arrhythmias were not suppressed. Therefore, in this large multicenter trial, amiodarone was well tolerated and effective in suppressing arrhythmias and improving ventricular function, but it did not reduce the frequency of sudden death or prolong survival.

Recently, Ammar and associates[1] studied the effects of chronic administration of amiodarone on systolic and diastolic function in patients with cardiac disease who were undergoing treatment for resistant ventricular arrhythmias. In their study of 12 patients, amiodarone significantly increased left ventricular ejection fraction by 16% at 8 weeks, as well as other ejection phase indices of myocardial contractility. However, amiodarone decreased the mitral valve in-flow peak velocity (Doppler) and increased deceleration and isovolumetric relaxation times incrementally by 12 weeks. The drug is well tolerated even in those with heart failure, but pulmonary congestion may worsen in some patients as a result of negative effects on diastolic function. A more comprehensive study in a larger number of patients assessing the effects of amiodarone on diastolic left ventricular function appears indicated.

The safety aspect of therapy with pure class III antiarrhythmic agents has been emphasized in a large trial of *d*-sotalol in patients post infarction.[2] Preliminary data from this trial are compelling and show an increased mortality in patients receiving *d*-sotalol compared with placebo controls. Accordingly, the use of *d*-sotalol is prohibited in patients post infarction because of the increased mortality demonstrated in this recent report.

In another article, Gonska et al.[3] report the results and long-term follow-up of catheter ablation of ventricular tachycardia in patients with coronary artery disease. One hundred thirty-six patients who had coronary artery disease and monomorphic sustained ventricular tachycardia underwent radiofrequency or direct-current catheter ablation. The procedure to localize an adequate site for ablation included pace mapping during sinus rhythm, endocardial activation mapping, identification of isolated middiastolic potentials, and pacing interventions during ventricular tachycardia. Primary success was achieved in 102 (75%) of the patients. Complications were noted in 12%. During a mean follow-up of 44 months, ventricular tachycardia occurred in 16% of patients. Therefore, catheter ablation of ventricular tachycardia in coronary artery disease is feasible in patients with monomorphic sustained ventricular tachycardia. In a selected group of patients with coronary artery disease, catheter ablation offers an alternative to drug therapy.

R.A. O'Rourke, M.D.

References

1. Ammar A, Wong M, Singh BN: Divergent effects of chronic amiodarone administration on systolic and diastolic function in patients with heart disease. *Am J Cardiol* 75:465–469, 1995.
2. Waldo AL, and the SWORD Investigators: Preliminary mortality results from the survival with oral *d*-sotalol (SWORD) trial. *J Am Coll Cardiol* 25:15A, 1995.
3. Gonska B-D, Cao K, Schaumann A, et al: Catheter ablation of ventricular tachycardia in 136 patients with coronary artery disease: Results and long-term follow-up. *J Am Coll Cardiol* 24:1506–1514, 1994.

Results of the International Study of the Implantable Pacemaker Cardioverter-Defibrillator: A Comparison of Epicardial and Endocardial Lead Systems

Zipes DP, for the Pacemaker-Cardioverter-Defibrillator Investigators
(Krannert Inst of Cardiology, Indianapolis, Ind)
Circulation 92:59–65, 1995 119-96-39–8

Background.—Implantable cardioverter-defibrillators (ICDs) are effective and safe in patients with recurrent ventricular tachycardia and ventricular fibrillation. Third-generation ICDs have been developed to incorporate programmability, multiple detection, and treatment options. A nonthoracotomy lead system that reduces potential perioperative death associated with current epicardial system implantation approaches has been combined with the new ICD technology. The Pacer-Cardioverter-Defibrillator device was studied in an international, multicenter comparison of the epicardial lead and nonthoracotomy systems.

Methods.—Data on 2,834 epicardial and endocardial ICDs implanted in 2,807 patients were analyzed. The patients were followed for nearly 1 year. Patients in the epicardial ICD group and those in the endocardial ICD group had similar clinical characteristics.

Findings.—Nearly 50,000 spontaneous ventricular tachyarrhythmias occurred in more than half of all patients. Epicardial and endocardial ICDs terminated these events with equal success rates of about 98%. Lead dislodgement and pocket infection were more common with the endocardial ICD than with the epicardial device. The perioperative death rate was greater with the epicardial ICD than with the endocardial ICD. Sudden cardiac death occurred in 1.4% of the patients with epicardial ICDs and in 0.6% of those with endocardial ICDs. Overall 1-year mortality was 12.2% in the epicardial ICD group and 6.9% in the endocardial ICD group; this rate reflected the greater surgery-related mortality associated with the epicardial system.

Conclusions.—The endocardial and epicardial ICD systems are equally effective in terminating spontaneous ventricular tachyarrhythmias in patients with ventricular tachycardia and ventricular fibrillation. However, the epicardial ICD is associated with a lower perioperative mortality rate.

► This report confirms that the ICD is an extremely effective device that accurately detects and successfully terminates ventricular tachyarrhythmias. Furthermore, it provides information validating the effectiveness of a nonthoracotomy lead system that is comparable to the thoracotomy implant but is associated with lower perioperative mortality rates. Another important observation is that antitachycardia pacing terminated ventricular tachycardia in more than 90% of episodes. Furthermore, among patients who received an ICD for sudden cardiac death alone, approximately 20% also had ventricular tachycardia. Before implanting a "shock-only" device, one should be certain that the patient has only ventricular fibrillation or ventricular tachycardia that cannot be terminated by pacing. An unanswered question from this study is how the use of the ICD compares with other forms of therapy.

The Antiarrhythmias Versus Implantable Defibrillators (AVID) study[1] is comparing a strategy of initial treatment with an ICD with a strategy of initial treatment with an antiarrhythmic drug for preventing death in patients with a history of ventricular fibrillation, hemodynamically compromising ventricular tachycardia, or both. Antiarrhythmic drug therapy includes empiric amiodarone and guided (electrophysiologic or ambulatory ECG recordings) sotalol. The ICDs are advanced-generation devices, and most are implanted transvenously. The primary end point of the study is total mortality. A secondary end point is cost and quality of life. It is anticipated that 1,200 patients will be followed until September 1998 and will be included in the intention-to-treat analysis.

R.A. O'Rourke, M.D.

Reference

1. The AVID Investigators: Antiarrhythmics Versus Implantable Defibrillators (AVID): Rationale, design, and methods. *Am J Cardiol* 75:470–475, 1995.

40 Other Topics

Effect of Cocaine on Left Ventricular Function: Relation to Increased Wall Stress and Persistence After Treatment

Mehta PM, Grainger TA, Lust RM, Movahed A, Terry J, Gilliland MGF, Jolly SR (East Carolina Univ, Greenville, NC)

Circulation 91:3002–3009, 1995 119-96-40–1

Background.—Although cocaine abuse has been identified as an independent risk factor for heart disease, controlled clinical trials of cocaine cardiotoxicity in humans have been difficult to conduct. The cardiotoxic effects of cocaine may also result from differences in administration route, drug purity, and other factors. To study the relation of left ventricular (LV) function to increased wall stress and persistence after treatment, cocaine in 3 doses or saline was infused into closed-chest, sedated dogs.

Methods.—Thirty dogs were studied. Data on LV fractional shortening and end-systolic wall stress were obtained by 2-dimensional ECG and hemodynamic testing. Radionuclide ventriculography was also done. Cocaine was infused in doses of 10, 30, or 100 µg/kg of body weight^{-1} per min^{-1} for 90 minutes with ECG and arterial pressure monitoring. At the end of infusion, the dogs were monitored for another 2 hours.

Findings.—In all 4 groups, arterial pressure increased during the course of the experiment. However, saline and the lowest dose of cocaine did not significantly alter ejection fraction. The medium and high doses of cocaine acutely raised arterial pressure and heart rate but reduced ejection fraction from a mean of 0.64–0.45 and from a mean of 0.65–0.46, respectively. High-dose cocaine also reduced fractional shortening from 36% to 23%. At medium doses, cocaine also increased wall stress from 42 to 65 g/cm^2 and at high doses, from 37 to 90 g/cm^2. After cocaine infusion, fractional shortening was displaced downward because of increased wall stress, not changes in contractility. Changes in afterload with phenylephrine, 6 µg/kg, and sodium nitroprusside, 10 µg/kg, before and during high-dose cocaine infusion showed similar regression lines for wall stress to fractional shortening (Fig 1).

Conclusions.—In this canine model, ejection-phase indices of LV function were decreased by cocaine. However, the effects were caused by increased wall stress, not decreased myocardial contractility. The effects were evident for at least 2 hours after infusion ended.

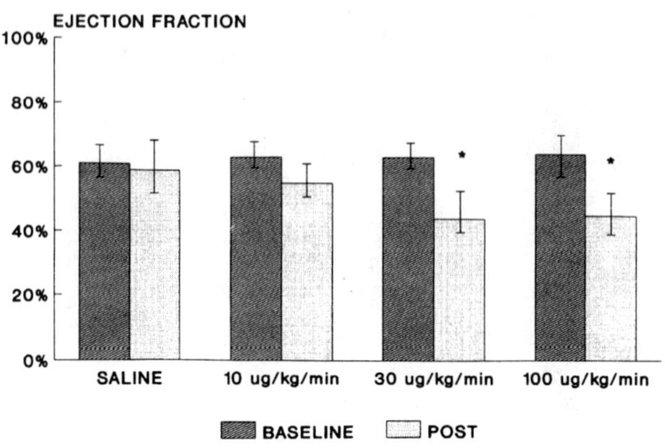

FIGURE 1.—Bar graph showing left ventricular ejection fractions determined from radionuclide angiograms at baseline and 2 hours after infusion of saline or cocaine, 10, 30, or 100 μg • kg^{-1} • min^{-1}. Mean ± SEM of each group is given. *Asterisks* indicate a significant difference between baseline and 2 hours after infusion. $P < 0.05$ compared with baseline. (Reproduced with permission. [*Circulation*] Copyright [1995] American Heart Association.)

► Cocaine abuse may precipitate myocardial infarction, ventricular arrhythmias, and left ventricular (LV) dysfunction; it has been recognized as an independent risk factor for heart disease. However, stringent investigation of cocaine cardiotoxicity in humans, accomplished by controlled clinical trials, has been difficult. Differences in route of administration, drug purity, and other factors may also contribute to the cardiotoxic effects of cocaine. In this study done in closed-chest, sedated dogs, cocaine reduced the ejection phase indices of LV function as a result of increased wall stress without a change in the relation between wall stress and LV fractional shortening. Therefore, the primary effects of cocaine are caused by an increase in afterload and not a persistent reduction in myocardial contractility. Increases in mean arterial pressure and the heart rate–pressure product, and the reduction of fractional shortening and ejection persisted for 2 hours after the cocaine infusion was stopped. Regional myocardial blood flow data obtained in these dogs showed no important myocardial depression as a consequence of local myocardial ischemia.

Recently, Hollander[1] reviewed the management of cocaine-associated myocardial ischemia among patients seen in hospital emergency departments after use of the illicit drug. Chest pain is the most common cocaine-related medical problem. The initial effect of cocaine on the cardiovascular system is vagotonia producing a transient bradycardia. This is rapidly followed by an increased sympathetic simulation that produces tachycardia and hypertension. The ability of cocaine to increase myocardial oxygen demand while decreasing coronary blood flow through vasoconstriction as well as enhancing platelet aggregation, in situ thrombus formation, premature atherosclerosis, left ventricular hypertrophy, hypertension, and tachycardia makes the drug an important cause of clinically important myocardial ischemia.

Cessation of cocaine use prevents recurrent chest pain, which is less common in patients who stop using cocaine and in whom fatal or nonfatal myocardial infarction is rare. Because tobacco smoking enhances cocaine-induced coronary artery vasoconstriction, the combination should be avoided. Aspirin prophylaxis may be useful to prevent platelet aggregation and the formation of thrombi. The value of treatment with oral nitrates or calcium blockers remains unproved. Beta-blocking drugs, although useful in other patient populations with chest pain, should be avoided in patients who continue to use cocaine.

R.A. O'Rourke, M.D.

Reference

1. Hollander JE: The management of cocaine-associated myocardial ischemia. *N Engl J Med* 333:1267–1272, 1995.

Relationship of the Third Heart Sound to Transmitral Flow Velocity Deceleration

Manson AL, Nudelman SP, Hagley MT, Hall AF, Kovács SJ (Washington Univ Med Ctr, St Louis, Mo)

Circulation 92:388–394, 1995 119-96-40–2

Background.—The third heart sound, S_3, is a soft sound with a frequency of 10–50 Hz that accompanies the deceleration of early, rapid ventricular filling and occurs shortly after the E-wave peak of the transmitral diastolic Doppler velocity profile (DVP). Presumably blood flowing through the mitral valve and decelerating in the ventricle produces vibrations of the entire heart and its blood pool. An S_3 reportedly is associated with a steeper rise in early left ventricular filling.

Objective and Methods.—A kinematic study of S_3 was carried out to relate the effects of fluid deceleration in the left ventricle to oscillations of the cardiohemic system. The system was modeled as a forced, damped, nonlinear harmonic oscillator. A closed-form mathematical expression was used to represent the deceleration part of the DVP. Predictions of the amplitude, timing, and frequency of S_3 were compared with transthoracic phonocardiographic findings and with simultaneous recordings of the transmitral Doppler E wave. Records were obtained from patients having a pathologic or physiologic S_3 that was audible and from others lacking an audible sound.

Correlations.—In all subject groups the recorded data correlated very closely with the predictions made by model analysis. The oscillations predicted by the model were very close to what was observed with regard to the timing, duration, frequency, and relative amplitude of S_3. It was not possible to acquire a calibrated or absolute estimate of the recorded S_3 amplitude.

Conclusion.—The cardiohemic system normally oscillates during E-wave deceleration, but the oscillations may not be audible as an S_3 unless deceleration is rapid enough and there is adequate cardiohemic coupling.

► The audible third heart sound is frequently present in young individuals who have no evidence of cardiac disease. Its presence in patients with cardiac disease usually indicates a left ventricular volume load, such as in aortic or mitral regurgitation, or the presence of left ventricular dysfunction. The timing, presence, and clinical correlates of the S_3 have been studied extensively. It has been shown that S_3 is associated with Doppler E-waves that have a more rapid than normal deceleration. It has been suggested that S_3 oscillation is initiated when the rate of ventricular filling exceeds ventricular diastolic distensibility causing a sudden deceleration of the E wave during diastole. The presence of an S_3 in older patients with left ventricular failure can be a poor prognostic sign, whereas in young healthy individuals with S_3, the mechanism of S_3 generation is slightly different. In young subjects the steeper rate of deceleration is caused by a higher maximum E-wave velocity while the duration of deceleration remains the same, whereas in patients with heart disease the steeper rate of deceleration is explained by a normal E-wave amplitude with a shorter deceleration time.

R.A. O'Rourke, M.D.

Efficacy of Different Treatment Strategies for Neurocardiogenic Syncope

Natale A, Sra J, Dhala A, Wase A, Jazayeri M, Deshpande S, Blanck Z, Akhtar M (Univ of Wisconsin, Milwaukee)

PACE 18(Pt I):655–662, 1995 119-96-40–3

Introduction.—Patients with syncope who have positive findings on head-up tilting are considered to have neurally mediated vasodepressor syncope. Most such patients are not in danger of dying, but they nevertheless may have disabling symptoms that limit them physically and psychosocially. A number of treatments have been tried, with uncertain results.

Objective.—The effects of a number of treatments were examined in 303 patients having a history of unexplained syncope who had a positive upright tilt test. Those found to have structural heart disease were excluded. All patients had been followed for 6 months or longer. On average, patients had had 10 episodes of syncope over a mean interval of 7½ years.

Management.—Forty-four of the 303 patients received pharmacotherapy empirically. Another 210 received drugs that proved effective on repeat head-up tilt testing. Forty-nine patients either refused medical treatment or withdrew. All groups were similar with respect to age, gender, and clinical presentation. Follow-up averaged nearly 3 years.

Results.—Nearly all patients given test-guided treatment received metoprolol in a dose of 50 mg given twice daily. A majority of them became test-negative within 7–10 days. Fifty-five unresponsive patients subsequently received theophylline, and 27 of them responded. Six of 15 patients responded to ephedrine. An extended-release preparation of disopyramide, in a dose of 150–200 mg given 2 or 3 times per day, prevented tilt-induced syncope in all but 2 of 35 patients who failed to respond to other medications. Most of the empirically treated patients received metoprolol. Symptoms recurred during follow-up in 6% of the patients given test-guided treatment. More than one third of the empirically treated patients and two thirds of those who were not treated continued to have syncope or presyncopal symptoms.

Conclusion.—It appears worthwhile to use the head-up tilt test to select treatment for patients with neurocardiogenic syncope.

▶ The recurrent rate of symptoms in severely symptomatic head-up tilt test–positive patients treated with head-up tilt-guided pharmacologic therapy is lower than that of those treated with either empiric therapy or no medication. Because negative head-up tilt testing after drug intervention is associated with fewer clinical recurrences during follow-up, this procedure can be useful for guiding long-term management. Also, empiric therapy with β-blockers can be tried in patients with positive head-up tilt testing during isoproterenol infusion. However, all patients in this series who had a prominent bradycardia or asystole were treated with head-up tilt-guided therapy, and only a minority responded to β-blockers. Finally, this study indicates that esmolol, a short-acting β-blocker, can be used to predict the response to oral β-blockers.

Recently, Morillo and associates[1] assessed the incidence of positive results, the specificity, and the same-day reproducibility of a head-up tilt at 60 degrees combined with a low-dose isoproterenol infusion in 120 consecutive patients who had recurrent unexplained syncope, 30 healthy patients in a control group, and 30 patients who had documented syncope not related to a vasodepressor reaction. Head-up tilt testing was positive in 61% of patients with unexplained syncope. The false positive rate in both the control and documented syncope groups was 6.6%. Head-up tilt was positive during the drug-free stage in 25% of 120 patients, and isoproterenol infusion was required in the remaining 36% of patients. Overall sensitivity was 61%, specificity was 93%, and reproducibility was 86%. The clinical variables that increased the probability of a positive outcome were age of 50 years or younger and 2 or more syncopal episodes in the preceding 6 months in the absence of structural heart disease.

Concerning another topic, Pasque[2] reported on a single institution's experience in 34 patients undergoing single lung transplantation for pulmonary hypertension. The limited success and applicability of other treatment options for patients with end-stage pulmonary hypertension led to the use of single lung transplantation in this high-risk patient subset. Operative survival from the entire group of patients was reasonable, with 91% (31 of 34 patients) surviving and being discharged from the hospital after transplantation. The actuarial survival for these 34 patients was 78% at 1 year, 66% at 2 years, and 61% at 3 years. In the subgroup of 24 patients with primary pulmonary hypertension, 96% (23 of 24) were successfully discharged from the hospital after transplantation. The actuarial survival for this isolated primary pulmonary hypertension subgroup was 87% at 1 year, 76% at 2 years, and 68% at 3 years. The early posttransplant normalization of pulmonary vascular resistance and right ventricular ejection fraction appears to persist during follow-up. Although the incidence of bronchiolitis obliterans is high, most of the survivors remain in the New York Heart Association functional class I or II and are employed.

R.A. O'Rourke, M.D.

References

1. Morillo CA, Klein GJ, Zandri S, et al: Diagnostic accuracy of a low-dose isoproterenol head-up tilt protocol. *Am Heart J* 129:901–906, 1995.
2. Pasque MK, Trulock EP, Cooper JD, et al: Single lung transplantation for pulmonary hypertension: Single institution experience in 34 patients. *Circulation* 92:2252–2258, 1995.

PART FIVE

THE DIGESTIVE SYSTEM

NORTON J. GREENBERGER, M.D.

Introduction

The 52 articles selected for the Gastroenterology section of the 1996 YEAR BOOK OF MEDICINE were chosen from more than 3,000 articles reviewed. This year, as in previous years, I have tried to achieve a balance between articles dealing with basic mechanisms of diseases and those providing important useful clinical information. I would like to comment on some of the key articles selected.

The chapter on the esophagus deals primarily with the pathophysiology and treatment of gastroesophageal reflux. Recognition of atypical symptoms and signs of gastroesophageal reflux is very important. Therefore, patients with reflux may experience nocturnal cough and frequent clearing of the throat, and there may also be evidence of dental erosion and loss of enamel. The latter findings should always raise the question of whether either an eating disorder, such as bulimia, or gastroesophageal reflux disease is present. Many patients with gastroesophageal reflux symptoms have a negative workup in that esophagogastroduodenoscopy, gastric emptying studies, and 24-hour pH monitoring studies may all be normal. The vexing problem of endoscopy-negative gastroesophageal reflux disease (GERD) is now better understood in that such patients may well have a decreased esophageal sensory threshold and thus may experience disproportionately severe symptoms with reflux. Virtually all adults have reflux during the day because of inappropriate relaxation of the lower esophageal sphincter, and in many patients, such reflux, albeit less than 4% of the time in a 24-hour period, may nonetheless provoke significant symptoms.

The chapter on the stomach and duodenum provides up-to-date information on the critical role of *Helicobacter pylori* in duodenal ulcer disease. Why *H. pylori* infection results in abnormalities in gastric acid secretion remains incompletely defined. Treatment regimens for *H. pylori*–associated peptic ulceration continue to undergo refinement, and any regimens used should provide an *H. pylori* eradication rate of at least 90%. Quadruple therapy with omeprazole, tetracycline, bismuth, and metronidazole does provide an eradication rate greater than 95%. The search continues for optimal treatment regimens. There is much current interest in a 1-week treatment regimen that includes metronidazole, omeprazole, and clarithromycin.

The section on the small bowel contains a seminal article on symptoms after milk ingestion in patients with self-reported lactose intolerance. The status of home parenteral and enteral nutrition is discussed in detail. Treatment of Crohn's disease continues to evolve, and there are several drugs that are effective in the treatment of this disorder. Effective drugs include sulfasalazine, 5-aminosalicylic analogues, metronidazole, corticosteroids, azathioprine and 6-mercaptopurine, and methotrexate. Treatment with many of these agents is discussed in detail, and there is the provocative report of treatment of Crohn's disease with anti–tumor necrosis factor.

The selections in the chapter on the colon include articles on the incidence and recurrence rates of colorectal adenomas, the emerging chemoprotective role of aspirin in colorectal cancer, and the important new concept of altered rectal perception and enhanced visceral hyperalgesia in patients with irritable bowel syndrome.

Recurrent themes characterize the section on the liver, in which 10 articles are devoted to hepatitis C. It is currently estimated that between 3½ and 4 million Americans have hepatitis C. Furthermore, 60% to 65% of such patients will develop chronic hepatitis, 20% to 25% will develop cirrhosis, and as many as 5% to 10% may develop hepatoma. It is now appreciated that asymptomatic patients who are positive for hepatitis C antibody and have normal aminotransferase levels may have evidence of significant chronic liver disease. This appears to be related to the persistence of hepatitis C virus (HCV) in the blood as evidenced by positive tests for HCV RNA. The persistence of HCV RNA after interferon therapy is also an important predictor of response to various regimens. The titer of HCV RNA, HCV genotypes, and several other factors appear to predict the likelihood of response to interferon. In addition, patients with latent autoimmune hepatitis may have this disorder triggered by interferon therapy. Finally, there are exciting reports of a new hepatitis virus, i.e., hepatitis G. Other topics covered in the Liver section include acetaminophen hepatoxicity, treatment of bleeding esophageal varices, transjugular intrahepatic portal systemic shunt (TIPS) for treatment of refractory ascites, and treatment regimens for spontaneous bacterial peritonitis.

The section on biliary tract disorders includes a provocative article on the use of ursodeoxycholic acid (Ursodiol) in gallstone prevention in patients undergoing weight loss, an important article on the natural history of gallstones, and a discussion of disorders that may mimic primary sclerosing cholangitis.

The section on the pancreas includes an article on early antibiotic treatment in acute necrotizing pancreatitis and an article on the risk of cancer in cystic fibrosis.

Norton J. Greenberger, M.D.

41 Esophagus

Importance of Reflux Symptoms in Functional Dyspepsia

Small PK, Loudon MA, Waldron B, Smith D, Campbell FC (Ninewells Hosp, Dundee, Scotland)

Gut 36:189–192, 1995 119-96-41-1

Background.—An endoscopic diagnosis of gastroesophageal reflux disease (GERD) requires gross damage, which is evident in only 50% to 60% of patients who are symptomatic. Some patients have negative pH monitoring studies as well yet continue to have symptoms.

Objective and Methods.—The sensitivity of the conventional diagnostic threshold of esophageal acid exposure as assessed by ambulatory pH monitoring was prospectively examined in 100 patients with dyspeptic symptoms who did not have peptic ulcer disease or gallstones. Ambulatory pH monitoring was performed for 24 hours, and the profiles were analyzed in connection with symptom scores.

Results.—On the basis of their pH profiles, 20 patients were considered to have GERD. Forty-four others were believed to have reflux-like functional dyspepsia (RFD), whereas 36 had nonreflux dyspepsia (NFD). The groups were similar with respect to age and sex distribution. Symptoms of reflux, including heartburn and regurgitation, were similar in the groups with GERD and RFD, but they were less marked in the NFD group. All parameters of acid reflux were significantly greater in patients with GERD than in those with RFD (Table 2). Acid exposure was more pronounced for patients with RFD, especially for those with a high degree of correlation between pain and reflux compared with those in the NFD group (Fig 1).

TABLE 2.—Comparison of pH Measurements Between Patients With Gastroesophageal Reflux (GORD) Using Current Criteria and Patients With Reflux-Like Dyspepsia

	GORD	*RFD*	P *Value**
Total acid exposure (min)	130·08 (19·5)	16·2 (2·6)	< 0·001
DeMeester score	31·3 (2·9)	12·8 (0·5)	< 0·001
Pain/reflux correlation	52 (9·7)	24 (5·3)	< 0·03
% time pH < 4	10·8 (1·5)	1·4 (0·2)	< 0·001

* Mann-Whitney U test.

Note: Values are mean (SEM).

(Courtesy of Small PK, Loudon MA, Waldron B, et al: Importance of reflux symptoms in functional dyspepsia. *Gut* 36:189–192, 1995.)

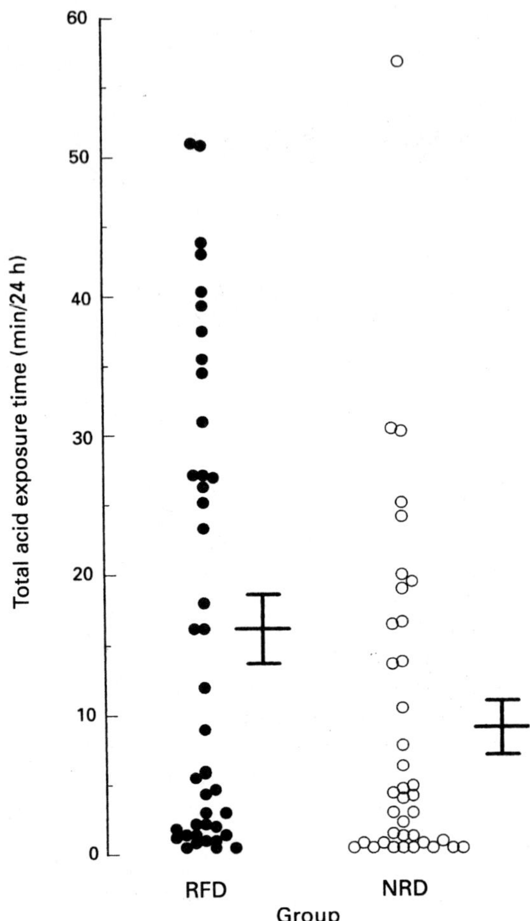

FIGURE 1.—Comparison of total acid exposure (min/24 hr) in reflux-like functional dyspepsia (*RFD*) and nonreflux functional dyspepsia (*NFD*) groups. Mean (SEM) RFD 16.2 (2.6) and NFD 9.05 (2.0). (Courtesy of Small PK, Loudon MA, Waldron B, et al: Importance of reflux symptoms in functional dyspepsia. *Gut* 36:189–192, 1995.)

Conclusion.—Conventional criteria of acid exposure may not be sufficiently sensitive to detect symptomatic esophageal acid reflux. Subthreshold exposure from brief or infrequent episodes of reflux might produce troublesome symptoms of reflux.

► Clinicians are often faced with the difficult problem of patients with persistent reflux symptoms who have negative results from both endoscopy and pH monitoring studies and an incomplete response to antisecretory drugs. Indeed, symptoms may prove recalcitrant to high-dose therapy with proton pump inhibitors such as omeprazole or lansoprazole. The study by Small et al. provides insight into this subset of patients with endoscopy-negative GERD (Americanized terminology for gastroesophageal reflux disease) and a poor response to conventional treatment. Many such patients have subthreshold acid exposure which, although representing infrequent or brief episodes of acid reflux, nonetheless contributes to troublesome symptoms. The following article provides at least a partial explanation of this.

Another treatment option for patients with endoscopy-negative GERD is to use a promotility drug such as cisapride either as monotherapy or in combination with an antisecretory drug. Recent studies[1] have indicated that cisapride is effective in reducing symptoms in GERD patients. Furthermore, cisapride in a dosage of 20 mg qid was superior to 10 mg qid.

Finally, I would like to comment on long-term omeprazole usage. In previous studies,[2] it was noted that 11% of patients on long-term (5 years) omeprazole therapy had serum gastrin levels greater than 500 pg/mL. Wright and Sarich[3] suggest that hypergastrinemia in most, if not all, of such patients could be genetically determined and related to the reduced activity of the major enzyme responsible for metabolizing omeprazole (CXP II C19).

N.J. Greenberger, M.D.

References

1. Richter JE, Long JF: Cisapride for gastroesophageal reflux disease: A placebo-controlled double-blind study. *Am J Gastroenterol* 90:423–429, 1995.
2. Klinkenberg-Knol EC et al: Long term treatment with omeprazole for refractory reflux esophagitis: Efficacy and safety. *Ann Intern Med* 121:161–167, 1994.
3. Wright JM, Sarich TC: Omeprazole therapy in resistent reflux disease. *Ann Intern Med* 122:236, 1995.

Lowered Oesophageal Sensory Thresholds in Patients With Symptomatic But Not Excess Gastro-Oesophageal Reflux: Evidence for a Spectrum of Visceral Sensitivity in GORD

Trimble KC, Pryde A, Heading RC (Royal Infirmary, Edinburgh, Scotland)
Gut 37:7–12, 1995 119-96-41–2

Introduction.—Some patients with suspected gastroesophageal reflux disease (GERD) who undergo ambulatory esophageal pH monitoring show a close correlation between symptoms and reflux episodes but have total acid exposure within the normal range. Whether such patients have enhanced esophageal sensation was tested by measuring sensory thresholds for esophageal balloon distention and discomfort in 20 patients.

Patients and Methods.—The patients, 11 men and 9 women, had a median age of 37.5 years. All had typical symptoms of GERD and a positive symptom index, normal static esophageal manometry, no evidence of esophagitis, and normal total acid exposure time during 23-hour ambulatory pH monitoring. Three groups of controls were also studied: 11 patients with a positive symptom index and excess esophageal acid exposure, 9 patients with histologically confirmed Barrett's esophagus, and 15 healthy volunteers.

Results.—Compared with healthy controls, the study group had lower thresholds for initial perception of esophageal distention and for discomfort. Sensory thresholds were also significantly lower in the study group than in patients with excess reflux and those with Barrett's esophagus (Fig 3). Sensory thresholds for somatic nerve stimulation were similar for the study group and the healthy control group. Study participants described the sensation produced by esophageal distention as tightness or pressure, heartburn, a lump, nausea, and warmth. Patients and controls were similar in their choice of descriptive terms. Eleven of the 20 patients in the study group reported the sensation as being identical to their GERD symptoms.

Conclusion.—Patients with GERD have a wide variety of symptoms, and the severity of symptoms may not correlate well with other measures

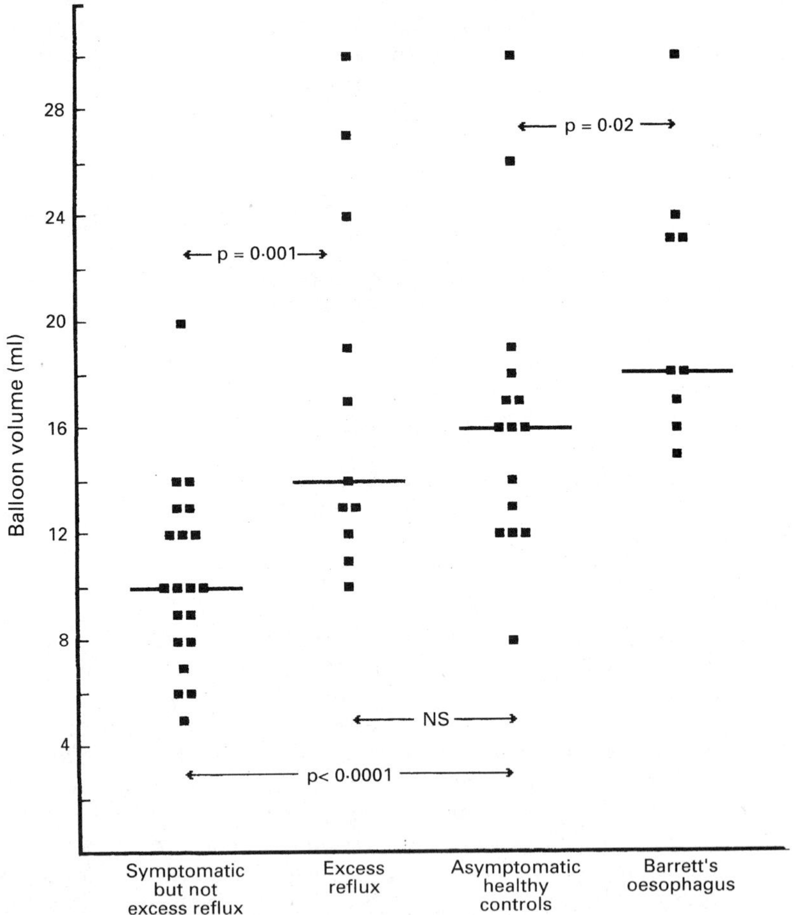

FIGURE 3.—Individual subject data (with medians) for sensory thresholds for discomfort evoked by esophageal balloon distention. (Courtesy of Trimble KC, Pryde A, Heading RC: Lowered oesophageal sensory thresholds in patients with symptomatic but not excess gastro-oesophageal reflux: Evidence for a spectrum of visceral sensitivity in GORD. *Gut* 37:7–12, 1995.)

of esophageal reflux. Those in the study group, with normal acid exposure times, had enhanced esophageal sensation. Thus, their symptoms appear to result from a heightened perception of normal reflux events, similar to the enhanced perception of intestinal physiologic events described in patients with irritable bowel syndrome.

► Mehta and colleagues[1] have also studied the mechanism of abnormal sensory perception in 25 patients with unexplained chest pain. All patients underwent (1) esophageal monitoring; (2) provocation tests with balloon distention of the esophagus, and esophageal perfusion with 0.1 N hydrochloric acid or saline; and (3) 24-hour pH monitoring. Two key observations were made. First, the basal balloon threshold was lower in patients with positive results of esophageal acid perfusion compared with healthy controls and patients with negative results for acid perfusion. Second, after acid perfusion, balloon perception and pain thresholds actually decreased in patients with previous negative results of esophageal tests. The authors conclude that (1) the pain threshold to esophageal balloon distention can be lowered by acid exposure; and (2) positive esophageal provocation tests such as acid perfusion may be markers of abnormal sensory perception.

N.J. Greenberger, M.D.

Reference

1. Mehta AJ, De Caestecker JS, Camm AJ, et al: Sensitization to painful distention and abnormal sensory perception in the esophagus. *Gastroenterology* 108:311–319, 1995.

Dental Erosion and Acid Reflux Disease

Schroeder PL, Filler SJ, Ramirez B, Lazarchik DA, Vaezi MF, Richter JE (Univ of Alabama, Birmingham)

Ann Intern Med 122:809–815, 1995 119-96-41–3

Introduction.—Dental erosion differs from dental caries because the chemical process resulting in loss of tooth substance does not involve bacteria. The factors contributing to dental erosion can be extrinsic, such as acidic beverages and exposure to aerosolized industrial acids in the workplace, or intrinsic, such as exposure to acidic gastric acid contents. Ambulatory 24-hour esophageal pH testing was used to determine the relationship between gastroesophageal reflux and dental erosion.

Patients and Methods.—The study participants were 12 patients with idiopathic dental erosion who were screened for gastroesophageal reflux disease and 30 patients with suspected reflux disease who were referred for dental evaluation. All underwent 24-hour esophageal pH monitoring using a pH probe in the distal and proximal esophagus. Both groups also completed a questionnaire designed to identify the possible causes of erosion. Erosion was graded on every tooth by 2 dental school faculty members. Saliva was analyzed for pH, flow rates, buffering capacity, and levels of calcium and phosphorus.

Results.—Esophageal pH monitoring identified gastroesophageal reflux in 10 of 12 patients in the dental group. Reflux was distal in 9 cases and proximal in 7, and it occurred in the upright position in only 7 patients, in the supine position in only 1, and in both positions in 2. There were no saliva abnormalities in the dental group. Ten patients in the gastroenterology group had distal reflux, 10 had proximal reflux, and 10 did not have reflux. Dental erosion was present in 40% of those with distal reflux, 70% of those with proximal reflux, and 10% of those without reflux. When all 24 patients with dental erosions were analyzed, a correlation was seen between the cumulative dental erosion score and proximal upright reflux. The correlation was even stronger for the 12 patients with abnormal amounts of proximal upright reflux.

Conclusion.—This is the first study to document a relationship between dental erosion and gastroesophageal reflux disease using ambulatory pH monitoring. Dietary factors did not appear to contribute to dental erosion in these individuals, and none appeared to have any relevant occupational exposures. Nearly all had normal salivary flow rates, pH, buffering capacity, and calcium and phosphate levels. Because of the high prevalence of reflux disease in the general population, dental erosion could be a frequently overlooked problem.

▶ This study indicates that dental erosion is a common finding in patients with gastroesophageal reflux disease (GERD) and should be considered an atypical manifestation of this disorder. The high prevalence of GERD in the general population suggests that this could be a frequently overlooked problem.

Dental erosion is also a cardinal finding in patients with an eating disorder such as bulimia. The diagnostic triad for bulimia includes dental erosions with loss of tooth enamel; parotid enlargement; and a rash on the fingers and wrists resulting from frequent induction of emesis.

N.J. Greenberger, M.D.

Esophageal Ulceration in Human Immunodeficiency Virus Infection: Causes, Response to Therapy, and Long-Term Outcome

Wilcox CM, Schwartz DA, Clark WS (Emory Univ, Atlanta, Ga)

Ann Intern Med 123:143–149, 1995 119-96-41–4

Introduction.—Esophageal disease occurs in approximately one third of patients with HIV infection. The causes of esophageal ulceration are varied, response to current therapies is inadequately characterized, and little is known about long-term outcome. Therefore, patients with HIV infection and endoscopically detected esophageal ulceration were prospectively studied.

Patients and Methods.—During a 4-year period, 100 consecutive patients at an urban city-county hospital were identified as having esophageal ulceration and entered into the study. The patient group was primarily male (82%) and black (70%). In 38 cases, esophageal disease was the index diagnosis of HIV infection or the AIDS-defining diagnosis. At least 6 biopsy specimens were obtained from identified ulcers and submitted for pathologic examination. Once causes of the ulcers were determined from clinical, endoscopic, and pathologic findings, standard medical therapies were initiated. The patients were followed for symptomatic and endoscopic response to therapy and long-term outcome.

Results.—Odynophagia was the primary symptom in 89 of the 100 patients; additional symptoms frequently reported were spontaneous substernal chest pain, dysphagia, and heartburn. Fifty-four patients had an empiric trial of oral systemic antifungal therapy that failed to relieve their symptoms. The most common cause of ulceration was cytomegalovirus esophagitis, identified in 51 patients. Ulceration was idiopathic in 41 patients, the result of herpes simplex virus in 5, and of gastroesophageal reflux disease in 4 (Fig 1). Five patients had several potential causes of ulcer, and 10 had more than 1 cause during follow-up. The overall response rate among the 85 patients who had specific medical therapy was 98%. The agents most commonly administered were ganciclovir or foscarnet in patients with cytomegalovirus alone, and prednisone in those with idiopathic esophageal ulcer. The overall median survival from the time esophageal ulceration was diagnosed was 8.9 months. Patients with cytomegalovirus esophagitis had a significantly shorter median survival (7.6 months) than did those with idiopathic esophageal ulcer (13.1 months), a difference that appeared to be related to CD4 lymphocyte count.

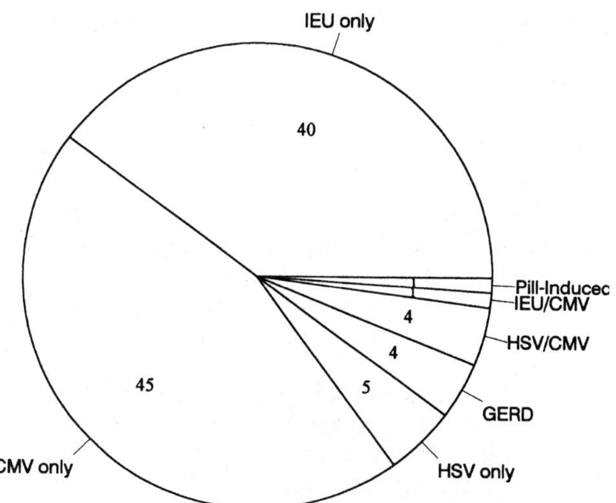

FIGURE 1.—Causes of esophageal ulcer in 100 patients. *Abbreviations: CMV,* cytomegalovirus; *GERD,* gastroesophageal reflux disease; *HSV,* herpes simplex virus; *IEU,* idiopathic esophageal ulcer. (Courtesy of Wilcox CM, Schwartz DA, Clark WS: Esophageal ulceration in human immunodeficiency virus infection: Causes, response to therapy, and long-term outcome. *Ann Intern Med* 122:143–149, 1995.)

Conclusion.—Both opportunistic and nonopportunistic causes of ulcer were identified in patients with HIV infection and esophageal ulceration. Patients responded well to specific therapies once the cause of ulceration was determined; however, long-term survival was poor. Idiopathic esophageal ulcer was common, responded to corticosteroid therapy, and should probably be considered an AIDS-defining illness.

▶ The authors emphasize a key point: all symptomatic HIV-positive patients in whom an esophageal ulceration is identified endoscopically or radiographically should have actual endoscopic biopsies of the lesion so that a firm diagnosis may be established and appropriate therapy initiated. This recommendation is supported by their findings, which can be summarized as follows: 29 of 37 patients (78%) with cytomegalovirus (CMV) esophagitis responded to treatment with ganciclovir or foscarnet; 4 of 4 patients (100%) with herpes simplex (HSV) esophagitis responded to acyclovir; 2 of 4 patients (50%) with both CMV and HSV esophagitis responded to ganciclovir and acyclovir; and 34 of 35 patients (97%) with idiopathic esophageal ulceration responded to prednisone.

Another key finding in this study was that although quality of life can be improved with effective therapy, long-term survival remains poor. Nonetheless, long-term remission and survival may occur in some patients but especially in those with idiopathic esophageal ulceration (IEU). In this regard, 25% of such patients were alive 900 days after the diagnosis of IEU.

N.J. Greenberger, M.D.

The Rumination Syndrome: Clinical Features Rather Than Manometric Diagnosis

O'Brien MD, Bruce BK, Camilleri M (Mayo Clinic and Found, Rochester, Minn)

Gastroenterology 108:1024–1029, 1995 119-96-41–5

Objectives.—The clinical characteristics, diagnosis, treatment, and outcome of rumination are poorly understood. This underdiagnosed condition was evaluated in 38 adults and adolescents to better describe the symptoms of the condition, to determine whether gastroduodenal manometry is useful for diagnosis, and to note whether any particular treatment is successful.

Methods.—The 38 adults and adolescents studied were of normal mental capacity and exhibited symptoms of rumination for a mean of 2.75 years before diagnosis. Thirty-six of the patients underwent upper gastrointestinal manometry, during which pH and times of regurgitation were recorded. Biochemical and hematologic indices and radiographic and endoscopic evaluations from the patients' medical records were analyzed retrospectively. Sixteen patients responded to a follow-up questionnaire to assess improvement.

Results.—The clinical feature most often reported by these patients was daily, effortless regurgitation of food within minutes of meals. The regurgitant was always described as lacking any acidic, bitter, or sour taste. Another prominent feature was weight loss (an average of 29 lb in 42% of the patients). Other symptoms were rare. Analysis of medical records of these patients revealed normal biochemical and hematologic function and no structural abnormality of the upper gastrointestinal tract. The results of gastrointestinal manometry indicated that R waves were present in 17 of 36 patients, but the R waves were associated with regurgitation or changes in pH in only 12 of the 36 patients. Upper gastrointestinal and esophageal manometry results indicated no abnormalities of gastric, proximal small bowel, esophageal sphincter, or esophageal body function. Of the 16 patients who responded to the follow-up questionnaire, only 2 reported cessation of rumination; however, 12 reported subjective improvement in symptoms after diagnosis and explanation of the disorder, and after a variety of treatments, including prokinetics, antacid therapy, behavioral therapy, and psychotherapy.

Conclusions.—Although the clinical symptoms of the rumination syndrome are typically repetitive regurgitation of gastric contents within minutes of a meal, this disorder is underdiagnosed in adolescents and adults of normal mental capacity. The clinical symptoms are sufficient for diagnosis, and the use of gastrointestinal manometry is unfounded.

► This paper calls attention to the rumination syndrome (also termed merycism or merycasm), which is an underdiagnosed condition in adults and adolescents with normal intelligence. Features that suggest rumination include (1) repetitive regurgitation of gastric contents starting within minutes of a meal; (2) a regurgitant that consists of undigested or partially digested food but is not sour or bitter; (3) effortless rumination; (4) rumination that is typically an everyday occurrence; (5) patients making a conscious decision to reswallow the food or spit it out, with the former being more common; and (6) weight loss may be prominent. Rumination appears to be more common in young adults and more frequent in females.

As the authors point out, the diagnoses most often confused with rumination are gastroesophageal reflux, chronic vomiting of undetermined etiology, hiatal hernia, and gastric emptying disorder. Patients were seen by an average of 5 physicians before diagnosis, and they reported having symptoms for an average of 3.5 years.

The authors also emphasize that excessive testing, especially gastrointestinal manometry, is not indicated because the correct diagnosis can be established clinically. Treatment options remain incompletely defined. Patient education and reassurance regarding the benign nature of the condition is important. A wide range of therapies have been used, including behavioral therapy, prokinetic drugs, and antacids, which have resulted in symptomatic improvement but only relatively rare complete symptomatic remissions.

N.J. Greenberger, M.D.

Intrasphincteric Botulinum Toxin for the Treatment of Achalasia

Pasricha PJ, Ravich WJ, Hendrix TR, Sostre S, Jones B, Kalloo AN (Johns Hopkins Med Insts, Baltimore, Md)

N Engl J Med 322:774–778, 1995 119-96-41-6

Introduction.—A local injection of botulinum toxin has been used with good results and few side effects in the treatment of disorders characterized by skeletal muscle spasm. A double-blind trial was undertaken to determine whether intrasphincteric injection of botulinum toxin is effective in the treatment of achalasia, a disorder in which the lower esophageal sphincter fails to relax.

Methods.—Twenty-one patients with achalasia were randomly assigned to receive botulinum toxin (11 patients) or normal saline placebo (10 patients). The patients were evaluated at baseline and 1 week after injection by clinical examination and diagnostic testing and on the basis of changes in symptom scores that ranged from 0 to 9 points. Those receiving

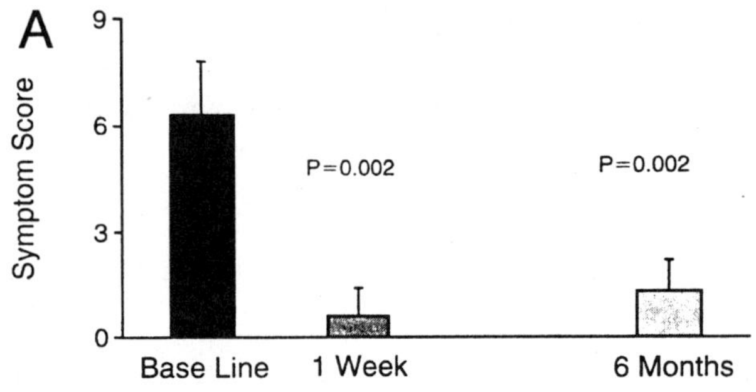

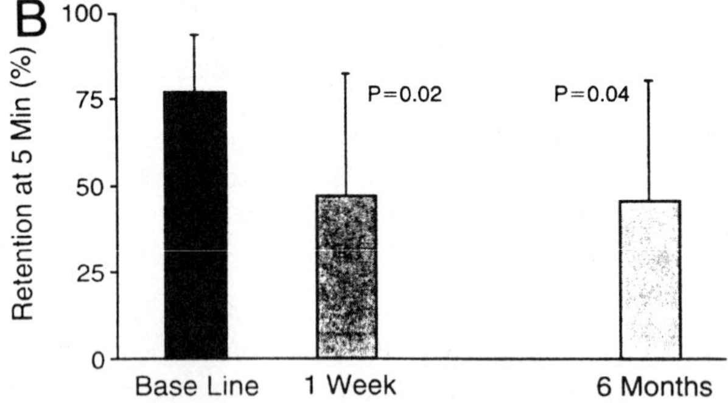

FIGURE 3.—The long-term results in 10 patients treated with botulinum toxin. **A,** the mean (± standard deviation) symptom scores at baseline, 1 week after the injection of botulinum toxin, and 6 months after the injection. A score of 3 or less indicated clinical remission. **B,** the mean values for esophageal retention. The *P* values are for comparisons with baseline values. (Reprinted by permission of *The New England Journal of Medicine.* Pasricha PJ, Ravich WJ, Hendrix TR, et al: Intrasphincteric botulinum toxin for the treatment of achalasia. *N Engl J Med* 322:774–778, Copyright 1995, Massachusetts Medical Society.)

normal saline injection later received an intrasphincteric injection of botulinum toxin. Those patients who did not have a remission after the injection were given a second injection within 6 weeks.

Results.—One week after the initial injection, the mean symptom score decreased in the treatment group from 7.1 to 1.6, and in the placebo group from 5.9 to 5.4. Nine of 11 patients in the treatment group were clinically improved compared with 1 in the placebo group. At 1 week after the injection, the mean decrease in the pressure of the lower esophageal sphincter was 33% in the treatment group compared with a mean increase of 12% in the placebo group. The mean decrease in esophageal retention 5 minutes after ingestion of food was 35% in the treatment group and 3% in the placebo group. The mean increase in the width of the opening of the lower esophageal sphincter was 204% in the treatment group compared with a mean decrease of 14% in the placebo group. Patients in the placebo group who later received botulinum toxin had a significant decrease in symptom scores and improvement in esophageal retention. At 6 months, 14 patients were still in remission. The mean symptom score at 6 months was significantly lower than at baseline (Fig 3).

Conclusions.—Ninety percent of patients treated with botulinum toxin had initial improvement. Two thirds were still in remission at 6-month follow-up. This compares well with a 65% to 90% rate of improvement in patients undergoing pneumatic dilation.

▶ This study indicates that the injection of botulinum toxin into the lower esophageal sphincter is an effective and safe treatment for achalasia, with results that are sustained for several months. However, as the authors and an accompanying editorial[1] emphasize, the role of intrasphincteric botulinum toxin in the treatment of achalasia requires further definition.

Cohen and Parkman[1] suggest that botulinum toxin be considered the initial therapy for symptomatic patients with idiopathic achalasia who are at high risk for the complications of pneumatic dilation or surgical myotomy, including patients who have not had a response to prior myotomy and those who have had a dilation-induced perforation. They also point out that if chemical denervation is to become the first-line therapy in all patients, the technique may need to be improved so that the benefits are longer lasting, if not permanent.

N.J. Greenberger, M.D.

Reference

1. Cohen S, Parkman HP: Treatment of achalasia: From whole bone to botulinum toxin. *N Engl J Med* 322:815–816, 1995.

Long-Term Survival After Photodynamic Therapy for Esophageal Cancer

Sibille A, Lambert R, Souquet J-C, Sabben G, Descos F (Edouard Herriot Hosp, Lyon, France)

Gastroenterology 108:337–344, 1995 119-96-41-7

Background.—Several reports have described the use of photodynamic therapy (PDT) to destroy superficial esophageal and gastric cancers. However, most reported series have been small and had short follow-up, so the efficacy of PDT remains unproven. The long-term results of PDT in the treatment of small esophageal tumors in 123 patients were reviewed.

Methods.—The patients were treated from 1983 to 1991 on a PDT-based nonsurgical therapeutic protocol. The mean age was 66 years. One hundred four had squamous-cell carcinoma and 19 had adenocarcinoma. The tumors ranged in diameter from 0.5 to 4.0 cm and did not extend past the muscular layer or invade adjacent organs. Eighty-eight more recent patients underwent endoscopic ultrasonography; staging was uT1 in 61 patients and uT2 in 27. The patients were injected with a hematoporphyrin derivative 72 hours before laser irradiation, which was delivered with a 630-nm dye laser. Fifty-six patients received PDT alone, including all of those with adenocarcinoma. The remaining 67 patients received other modes of therapy as well, i.e., radiotherapy or chemotherapy. Disease-specific survival was calculated by omitting patients who died of intercurrent disease that was unrelated to the esophageal tumor or its treatment.

Results.—The complete response rate at 6 months was 87%, although 36% of these patients had a local recurrence 12–18 months later. If detected at a superficial stage, the recurrent tumors responded to additional PDT. There was no significant difference in response rates for patients with squamous cell carcinoma vs. adenocarcinoma, and additional modes of treatment had no apparent benefit. The overall actuarial 5-year survival was only 25%, but disease-specific survival was 74%. Relative 5-year survival was 95% for patients with uT1, N0 squamous cell cancers. Complications included nonsevere cutaneous photosensitization in 16 patients and esophageal stenosis requiring dilation in 43.

Conclusions.—Photodynamic therapy achieves effective local destruction of small flat or sessile esophageal tumors. The complete response rate and disease-specific survival are good. For patients with esophageal cancer who are not good candidates for surgery—particularly those with uT1, N0 tumors—PDT may be a reasonable treatment alternative.

▶ For an authoritative yet brief review of photodynamic therapy for early esophageal cancer, see the editorial by Wang and Giller.[1] Sibille et al. provide a rationale for the endoscopic treatment of small superficial esophageal malignancies. Surgical resection is the most accepted form of therapy for esophageal carcinomas and can offer a very good chance for cure. Although the overall survival of patients after esophagectomy for esophageal cancer is only 22%, this rate markedly improves to 90% to 100% at 5 years when only studies of superficial squamous-cell cancers confined to either the mucosa or muscularis mucosa are considered.

Given the slow growth of these early tumors and the high mortality and morbidity rates of esophagectomy, localized treatment using PDT of early carcinomas, as proposed by Sibille et al., seems to be a reasonable option in *selected* patients. It would seem that criteria for selection need to be more clearly defined.

The use of photodynamic therapy for obstructing esophageal cancer has also been reported. Heier et al.[2] have demonstrated that PDT can relieve esophageal obstruction caused by squamous-cell and adenocarcinoma and is an alternative to neodymium: yttrium-aluminum-garnet (Nd:YAG) thermal necrosis with a longer duration of response.

N.J. Greenberger, M.D.

References

1. Wang KK, Giller A: Photodynamic therapy for early esophageal cancers: Light versus surgical might. *Gastroenterology* 108:593–607, 1995.
2. Heier SK, Rothman KA, Heier LM, et al: Photodynamic therapy for obstructing esophageal cancer: Light dosimetry and randomized comparison with Nd:YAG laser therapy. *Gastroenterology* 109:63–72, 1995.

42 Stomach and Duodenum

Accuracy of Invasive and Noninvasive Tests to Diagnose *Helicobacter pylori* Infection

Cutler AF, Havstad S, Ma CK, Blaser MJ, Perez-Perez GI, Schubert TT (Henry Ford Hosp, Detroit; Vanderbilt Univ, Nashville, Tenn)

Gastroenterology 109:136–141, 1995 119-96-42–1

Background.—There are various invasive and noninvasive tests to detect *Helicobacter pylori* infection, none of which is universally accepted. Problems associated with invasive tests include patchy infection, difficult culture, and human errors in interpretation. Global measurement with urea breath tests (UBTs) and serologic studies may be more accurate. The accuracy of the most widely available invasive and noninvasive tests for *H. pylori* was determined.

Methods.—A total of 268 previously untreated patients were studied. *Helicobacter pylori* infection was tested by Warthin-Starry stain, CLO test, and histology of antral biopsy specimens, and by [carbon-13]UBT and evaluation of serum levels of IgG and IgA antibodies to *H. pylori*. Infection was established by concordance of at least 4 of 7 tests.

Results.—Warthin-Starry staining of antral biopsy specimens had the best sensitivity and specificity. There were no significant differences among the CLO test, UBT, and IgG serology. Chronic antral inflammation had the highest sensitivity at 100% and the lowest specificity at 66.3%. Serologic testing for IgA had the lowest combined sensitivity and specificity. The CLO test had a positive predictive value of 100% (Table 2). In patients older than 60 years, the best predictors were UBT and chronic inflammation. In white patients, IgA was a better predictor.

Discussion.—The noninvasive UBT and IgG serology are as accurate as the invasive CLO test and Warthin-Starry stain in determining *H. pylori* infection. In half of these patients, all 7 tests were in agreement. The most valuable information on the accuracy of these tests was furnished by 44% of patients with 1 or 2 tests with false results.

► Many clinicians use serologic testing for *H. pylori* to screen dyspeptic patients for upper gastrointestinal endoscopy. In this regard, Mendall et al.[1]

TABLE 2.—Sensitivity, Specificity, and Negative and Positive Predictive Value of 7 Diagnostic Assays for *Helicobacter pylori* Infection Among 268 Patients Undergoing Esophagogastroduodenoscopy

Parameter	Sensitivity (%)	Specificity (%)	Positive predictive value (%)	Negative predictive value (%)
Invasive				
Chronic inflammation*	100	66.3	84.4	100
Acute inflammation†	86.7	93.7	96.2	79.5
Warthin-Starry stain‡	93.1	99.0	99.4	88.7
CLO test§	89.6	100	100	84.1
Noninvasive				
UBT‖	90.2	95.8	97.5	84.3
Serum IgG¶	91.3	91.6	95.2	85.3
Serum IgA¶	71.1	85.3	89.8	61.8

* Chronic inflammation present in gastric antral biopsy specimens.
† Acute inflammation present in gastric antral biopsy specimens.
‡ Warthin-Starry stain of gastric antral biopsy specimen.
§ Urease test conducted on gastric antral biopsy specimen with results ascertained at 24 hours.
‖ Urea breath test (*UBT*) 60 minutes after administration of 150 mg of carbon-13–labeled urea.
¶ Serum antibodies to *H. pylori.*
(Courtesy of Cutler AF, Havstad S, Ma CK, et al: Accuracy of invasive and noninvasive tests to diagnose *Helicobacter pylori* infection. *Gastroenterology* 109:136–141, 1995.)

studied 315 patients referred to a gastroenterology unit by 65 British general practitioners and compared serology for *H. pylori* and symptom questionnaires before direct access endoscopy. In all age groups combined, serology was significantly better than the questionnaires at detecting peptic ulcers and gastric cancer. The authors concluded that serology is the method of choice in screening before direct access upper gastrointestinal endoscopy in those younger than 45 years of age. They feel that it best combines a high sensitivity for peptic ulcer disease with a large reduction in unnecessary negative endoscopies.

Blecker et al.[2] evaluated the significance of *H. pylori*–specific IgG antibodies in 542 apparently healthy women aged 20–40 years by determining the correlation between a positive enzyme-linked immunosorbent assay and the actual presence of an active *H. pylori* infection. Carbon 13–labeled UBTs performed in 85 seropositive and 65 randomly selected seronegative subjects were positive in 82 (96.5%) of 85 seropositive subjects and in none of the seronegative subjects, reflecting an actual presence of *H. pylori* in the gastric mucosa of the seropositive women. Although positive serologic findings were well correlated with an active infection in these patients, it is not clear whether such asymptomatic patients should be treated. Current guidelines do not call for treatment of such patients, but this could well change.

N.J. Greenberger, M.D.

References

1. Mendall MA, et al: Serology for *Helicobacter pylori* compared with symptom questionnaires in screening before direct access endoscopy. *Gut* 36:330, 1995.
2. Blecker U, et al: Serology as a valid screening test for *Helicobacter pylori* infection in asymptomatic subjects. *Arch Pathol Lab Med* 119:30–32, 1995.

Antibacterial Treatment of Gastric Ulcers Associated With *Helicobacter pylori*

Sung JJY, Chung SCS, Ling TKW, Yung MY, Leung VKS, Ng EKW, Li MKK, Cheng AFB, Li AKC (Prince of Wales Hosp, Hong Kong; Chinese Univ of Hong Kong)

N Engl J Med 332:139–142, 1995 119-96-42–2

Introduction.—A strong association between infection with *Helicobacter pylori* and gastric ulcers is unrelated to the use of nonsteroidal anti-inflammatory medications. The efficacy of antibacterial therapy without medication to suppress gastric acid for the treatment of patients with *H. pylori* infection and gastric ulcers unrelated to the use of nonsteroidal agents was studied.

Methods.—One hundred patients who had gastric ulcers seen on endoscopy and with *H. pylori* infection were randomly assigned to receive a 1-week course of antibacterial agents (500 mg of tetracycline, 120 mg of bismuth subcitrate, and 400 mg of metronidazole, each given 4 times per day orally) or a 4-week course of omeprazole (20 mg per day orally). After 5 and 9 weeks, follow-up endoscopies were performed. The endoscopists were not aware of the treatment assignments, but the patients and their physicians were. Eighty-five patients completed the trial.

Results.—At 5 weeks, *H. pylori* had been eradicated in 41 of 45 patients in the antibacterial treatment group (91.1%) and in 5 of the 40 in the omeprazole group (12.5%). The gastric ulcers were healed in 38 of the patients in the antibacterial group (84.5%) and in 29 of the omeprazole group (72.4%) (Table 2). At 9 weeks, the ulcers were healed in 43 of the patients in the antibacterial group and in 37 of the omeprazole group. The mean duration of pain during the first week of treatment was 1.9 days in the omeprazole group, compared with 3.6 days in the antibacterial treatment group. One year after treatment, recurrent gastric ulcers were found in 1 of 22 patients in the antibacterial treatment group (4.5%) and in 12 of 23 in the omeprazole group (52.2%). *Helicobacter pylori* was detected

TABLE 2.—Ulcer Healing and Duration of Pain, According to Treatment Group

Response to Treatment	Antibacterial Drugs	Omeprazole	*P* Value
Ulcer healing—no. of patients (%)			
Wk 5	38 (84.4)	29 (72.5)	0.28
Wk 9	43 (95.6)	37 (94.9)	1.00
Wk 13	45 (100)	38 (97.4)	0.46
Days with pain			
Wk 1	3.6 ± 3.0	1.9 ± 2.6	0.004
Wk 2–5	7.6 ± 9.5	4.4 ± 8.7	0.089

Notes: In the antibacterial treatment group, 45 patients completed the follow-up of 5, 9, and 13 weeks. In the omeprazole group, 40 patients completed the follow-up at 5 and 9 weeks, and 39 completed the follow-up at 13 weeks. Plus-minus values are means ± standard deviation.

in the 1 patient with a recurrent ulcer in the antibacterial treatment group and in 10 of the 12 patients with recurrent ulcers in the omeprazole group.

Conclusions.—Previous studies have found that *H. pylori* infection was the most important predictor of the recurrence of ulcers. One week of antibacterial therapy without acid suppression heals the ulcers as well as omeprazole and reduces the rate of their recurrence in patients with *H. pylori* infection and gastric ulcers unrelated to the use of nonsteroidal anti-inflammatory drugs.

► Although the results obtained with antibiotics alone are impressive, most authorities still recommend the use of both an antisecretory drug and antibiotics. The recurrence rate of gastric ulcer after antibiotic treatment alone is used for eradication of *H. pylori* has been 7%.[1] In the study by Seppala et al., the effect of *H. pylori* eradication on ulcer healing and the relapse rate were investigated in a multicenter trial of 239 gastric ulcer patients. Follow-up data were available for 205 patients after 1 year. Between 12 and 52 weeks, 2 (7%) ulcer relapses occurred in 29 *H. pylori*–negative patients and in 60 (47%) of 128 *H. pylori*–positive patients. The studies by Sung (summarized above) and Seppala indicate that healing of gastric ulcer is rapid and recurrence is *infrequent* after successful *H. pylori* eradication. Thus, *H. pylori* eradication changes the natural history of gastric ulcer disease much as it has for duodenal ulcer disease.

N.J. Greenberger, M.D.

Reference

1. Seppala K, et al: Cure of peptic gastric ulcer associated with eradication of *H. pylori*. *Gut* 36:834–837, 1995.

Effect of Acid Suppression on Efficacy of Treatment for *Helicobacter pylori* Infection

de Boer W, Driessen W, Jansz A, Tytgat G (Sint Joseph Ziekenhuis, The Netherlands; Academisch Medisch Centrum, Amsterdam)

Lancet 345:817–820, 1995 119-96-42-3

Purpose.—In patients with peptic ulcer disease, successful eradication of *Helicobacter pylori* infection leads to permanent cure. Triple therapy with bismuth, tetracycline, and metronidazole for 14 days yields the best cure rates; however, the side effects may limit compliance. Whether simultaneous acid inhibition with omeprazole could improve the results of 7-day triple therapy was investigated.

Methods.—A total of 108 consecutive patients with peptic ulcer disease and biopsy-proven *H. pylori* infection were studied. The patients were randomly assigned to receive 7 days of triple therapy with or without omeprazole, 20 mg given twice daily. Patients in the omeprazole group also received 3 days of pretreatment with omeprazole. Ten endoscopic biopsy specimens were obtained 4–6 weeks after treatment for urease testing, histologic examination, and culture to determine whether *H. pylori* had been eradicated.

Results.—The cure rate was 98% in the patients who received omeprazole vs. 83% in those who did not, for an efficacy difference of 15%. Omeprazole treatment led to a cure in 3 patients with metronidazole-resistant strains of *H. pylori.* The course of treatment was completed by 97% of patients; the side effects were generally mild. The omeprazole-treated patients had significantly fewer gastrointestinal side effects.

Conclusions.—For patients with peptic ulcer and *H. pylori* infection, the addition of omeprazole to triple therapy with bismuth, tetracycline, and metronidazole improves efficacy while reducing side effects. The efficacy of triple therapy plus omeprazole is high enough to obviate the need for diagnostic tests of cure in compliant patients. It is believed that this form of quadruple therapy is the best treatment approach for *H. pylori*–related ulcers.

► The authors have shown that a short 1-week course of quadruple therapy combines excellent efficacy independent of metronidazole resistance and a good tolerability, and they believe that this is the best treatment option for *H. pylori*–associated ulcers. They have also demonstrated that "pretreatment" with omeprazole for 3 days does not interfere with the efficacy of triple therapy; this is in contrast to omeprazole decreasing the efficacy of dual therapy. Single antimicrobial therapy with an antisecretory drug or double antimicrobial therapy alone does not result in high enough *H. pylori* eradication rates, i.e., rates greater than 90%. Although several current treatment regimens yield *H. pylori* eradication rates that are in this ballpark, additional studies are under way to determine whether drug regimens given for 7 days or less will prove equally efficacious with fewer side effects. For a comprehensive review of the treatment of *H. pylori* infection in the management of peptic ulcer disease, see the review article by Walsh and Peterson.[1]

N.J. Greenberger, M.D.

Reference

1. Walsh JH, Peterson WL: The treatment of *Helicobacter pylori* infection in the management of peptic ulcer disease. *N Engl J Med* 333:984–991, 1995.

Helicobacter pylori **Infection and Abnormalities of Acid Secretion in Patients With Duodenal Ulcer Disease**

El-Omar EM, Penman ID, Ardill JES, Chittajallu RS, Howie C, McColl KEL (Therapeutics Western Infirmary, Glasgow, Scotland; Queens Univ, Belfast, North Ireland)

Gastroenterology 109:681–691, 1995 119-96-42–4

Background.—The presence of *Helicobacter pylori* predisposes patients to duodenal ulcers (DUs). However, the manner in which this occurs is not well understood. Hypergastrinemia, which is induced by biologically active gastrin 17, is known to occur in the presence of *H. pylori* infection. Through the gastrin-releasing peptide (GRP) stimulation from the stomach antrum and body, it has been documented that production of acid can increase more dramatically in patients and in volunteers who are *H. pylori* positive. The effect of acid response after eradication of *H. pylori* was studied.

Methods.—The study participants included 36 patients with active DUs, of whom all were *H. pylori* positive, and 25 *H. pylori*–positive and 25 *H. pylori*–negative volunteers. Serum gastrin and gastric acid outputs were measured basally in all patients and volunteers, and also in response to administration of 10 and 40 pmol/kg/hr of GRP. The maximal acid response to exogenous gastrin administration was also determined. *Helicobacter pylori* eradication treatment was instituted in 29 DU patients and in 15 *H. pylori*–positive volunteers. The presence of *H. pylori* in patients and recruits was determined by carbon-14 urea breath tests.

Results.—Concentrations of basal acid secretion and basal gastrin secretion were higher in the *H. pylori*–positive volunteers and in patients with DUs than in *H. pylori*–negative volunteers, and the basal acid secre-

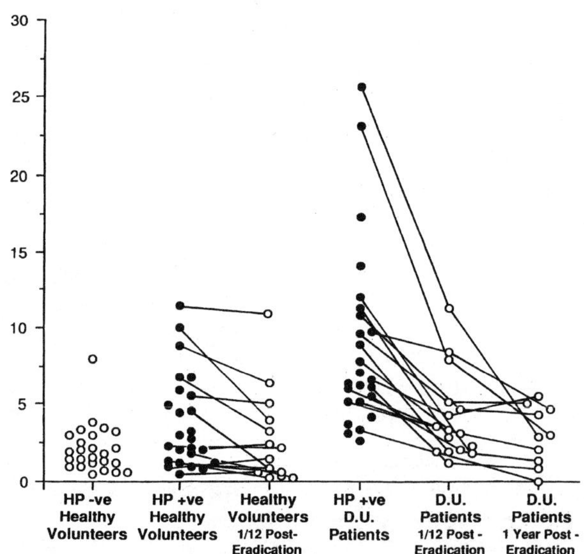

FIGURE 2.—Basal acid output in healthy volunteers and patients with duodenal ulcers (*DUs*) of varying *Helicobacter pylori* status (*solid circles, H. pylori* positive). Compared with that in *H. pylori*–negative healthy volunteers, basal acid output is increased in *H. pylori*–positive healthy volunteers ($P < 0.05$), *H. pylori*–positive patients with DUs ($P < 0.0001$), and patients with DUs 1 month after eradication ($P < 0.01$). (Courtesy of El-Omar EM, Penman ID, Ardill JES, et al: *Helicobacter pylori* infection and abnormalities of acid secretion in patients with duodenal ulcer disease. *Gastroenterology* 109:681–691, 1995.)

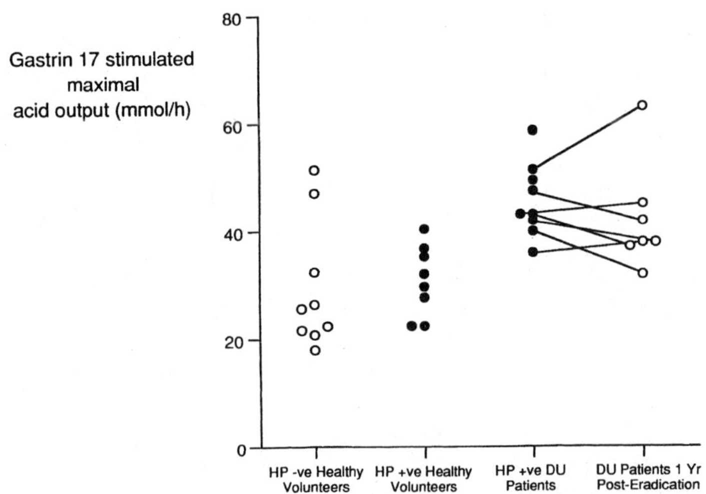

FIGURE 7.—Maximal acid output in response to gastrin 17 in individuals from the various groups in whom maximal response to gastrin-releasing peptide also was assessed (*solid circles, Helicobacter pylori* positive). Patients with duodenal ulcers (*DUs*) examined before and 1 year after *H. pylori* eradication are identified by *continuous lines*. Values in *H. pylori*–positive patients with DUs were higher than those in healthy volunteers with and without *H. pylori* ($P < 0.01$ for both) and were unchanged 1 year after eradication. (Courtesy of El-Omar EM, Penman ID, Ardill JES, et al: *Helicobacter pylori* infection and abnormalities of acid secretion in patients with duodenal ulcer disease. *Gastroenterology* 109:681–691, 1995.)

tions were still higher than in all normal volunteers 1 month after *H. pylori* eradication (Fig 2). However, the basal levels of gastrin secretion were comparable to those of *H. pylori*–negative controls. No correlation was found between the basal concentration of gastrin and basal acid output in *H. pylori*–positive individuals. *Helicobacter pylori*–positive individuals and patients with DUs showed an increase in both gastrin and acid response to a 40 pmol/kg/hr infusion of GRP compared with *H. pylori*–negative individuals. Both of these responses reached levels comparable to those found in *H. pylori*–negative individuals after eradication of *H. pylori*. In patients with DUs, there was a positive correlation between the GRP-stimulated gastrin concentration and the acid output. Maximal acid output in response to GRP infusion was found at a higher dosage for patients with infections compared with those without infections (100 pmol/kg/hr vs. 40 pmol/kg/hr). Maximal acid response to administration of gastrin in patients with DUs was still higher than that in either negative or positive volunteers 1 year after eradication therapy (Fig 7).

Discussion.—This study confirms previous reports indicating that basal acid output decreases after treatment for eradication of *H. pylori*. However, the increase in acid output observed in patients with DUs cannot be entirely attributed to gastrin release. The study results suggest that the increased output is associated with increased oxyntic mucosal as well as antral mucosal release of gastrin. Also, the presence of *H. pylori* alone could not completely explain the increased response in patients with DUs to GRP infusion. Patients with DUs had an increase in parietal cell mass, which accounted for the response to exogenous gastrin in *H. pylori*–positive patients. Even 12 months after eradication of *H. pylori,* the maximal acid output in response to gastrin in patients with DUs did not change. Therefore, the increase in cell mass in patients with DUs may have a hereditary component. The other abnormal responses seen in these individuals, including an increased basal and GRP-stimulated acid output, an increased ratio of basal acid output to maximal gastrin-stimulated acid output, and an increased ratio of maximal GRP-stimulated acid output to maximal gastrin-stimulated acid output, all resolve after appropriate treatment. The inability to decrease acid output in response to gastrin may result from a lack of inhibitory control of GRP in the antral and oxyntic mucosa. Therefore, the mechanism by which acid secretion in the duodenum is disrupted is probably related to the action of *H. pylori.*

► This elegant study confirms, extends, and clarifies the relationship between *H. pylori* infection and secretion of gastric acid in patients with DUs as well as healthy subjects. To recapitulate briefly, the data obtained indicate that in patients with DUs, *H. pylori* infection is associated with a markedly increased basal acid output and GRP-stimulated acid output; both fully resolve after eradication of the infection. The mechanism of the increased secretion of acid is unclear, but the findings are consistent with *impaired inhibitory control.* These disturbances in the regulation of acid secretion are likely to be relevant to the mechanism by which *H. pylori* infection predisposes to DU. Recent studies[1] argue against the hypothesis that degradation of gastric mucus by *H. pylori* is important in the pathogenesis of peptic ulcer.

It should be noted that intragastric acidity is a predictor of the success of *H. pylori* eradication.[2] Labenz et al. studied 50 patients with relapsing or complicated *H. pylori*–positive duodenal or gastric ulcer who were randomly treated with either omeprazole, 20 mg twice daily, plus amoxicillin, 1 g twice daily, or with omeprazole, 40 mg twice daily, plus amoxicillin, 1 g twice daily, over 2 weeks. A 24-hour gastric pH measurement was performed in all patients after treatment. The *H. pylori* cure rate was 67%, and patients who later turned out to have cures had higher pH values, both during nighttime and after meals. This study indicates that the success of eradication treatment with omeprazole and amoxicillin in patients with DUs who have *H. pylori* infection is clearly related to intragastric pH.

N.J. Greenberger, M.D.

References

1. Markisich DC, et al: *Helicobacter pylori* infection does not reduce the viscosity of human gastric mucus gel. *Gut* 36:327–329, 1995.
2. Labenz J, et al: Intragastric acidity as a predictor of the success of *Helicobacter pylori* eradication: A study in peptic ulcer patients with omeprazole and amoxicillin. *Gut* 37:39–43, 1995.

Regression of Primary Gastric Lymphoma of Mucosa-Associated Lymphoid Tissue Type After Cure of *Helicobacter pylori* Infection

Bayerdörffer E, for MALT Lymphoma Study Group (Univ of Munich; Free Univ of Berlin; Univ of Cologne, Germany; et al)

Lancet 345:1591–1594, 1995 119-96-42–5

Background.—Chronic *Helicobacter pylori* infection is present in most patients with mucosa-associated lymphatic tissue. *Helicobacter pylori* gastritis may be linked to lymphoma of mucosa-associated lymphoid tissue type (MALT). It has been suggested that primary gastric low-grade mucosa-associated lymphoma is linked to *H. pylori* infection. The effect of curing *H. pylori* infection on regression of these MALT lymphomas was investigated.

Methods.—A total of 33 patients aged 31–84 years with primary gastric low-grade MALT lymphoma were studied. Patients were treated with omeprazole, 120 mg/day, and amoxicillin, 2.25 g/day, for 14 days. Patients were examined every 4 weeks until tumors regressed completely.

Results.—All patients became negative for *H. pylori.* On histologic examination, 23 patients had complete tumor regression and 4 had partial tumor regression. In 6 patients, there was no change in tumor after cure of *H. pylori* infection (table). In these 6 patients, 1 was treated with chemotherapy and 5 were treated surgically; of these 5 patients, 4 had high-grade B-cell lymphoma and 1 had high-grade T-cell lymphoma. Of 16 of the 23 patients with complete tumor regression, polymerase chain reaction (PCR)

TABLE.—Relation Between Baseline Characteristics and Outcome

	Complete regression	Partial regression	No change
Number (%)	23 (70%)	4 (12%)	6 (18%)
Tumor stage (by histology)			
EI_1	23	4	2*
≥EII	0	0	4†
Endoscopic appearance			
Tumor	13	3	2
Ulcer	7	0	2
Erosions	1	0	0
Atypical mucosal relief	2	1	2
Tumor size (cm)‡	2 (1–10)	4 (3–8)	5 (2–8)
Time after eradication of *H. pylori* (months)	4·0 (0·5–8·5)	8·5 (4·0–12·0)	4·0 (3·5–6·0)
Age (years)	58·0 (31–74)	58·5 (32–84)	47·5 (35–78)
Male/female	12/11	2/2	4/2

Note: Data are number of patients or median (range).

* One patient also had a high-grade T-cell lymphoma, and 1 was primarily treated by chemotherapy so the exact tumor stage could not be determined.

† Pretreatment staging EI_1 found to be incorrect when resected stomach was examined by histology, when 5 of 6 patients in this group were given a diagnosis of high-grade lymphoma.

‡ Largest dimension measured on endoscopy with biopsy forceps.

(Courtesy of Bayerdörffer E, for MALT Lymphoma Study Group: Regression of primary gastric lymphoma of mucosa-associated lymphoid tissue type after cure of *Helicobacter pylori* infection. *Lancet* 345:1591–1594. Copyright by The Lancet Ltd., 1995.)

showed complete disappearance of monoclonal bands in 13 patients. There was no relapse of lymphoma during the 12-month follow-up.

Conclusions.—There may be a direct relation between primary gastric low-grade MALT lymphoma and lymphatic tissue in the gastric mucosa acquired from *H. pylori* infection. Complete tumor regression occurred in more than 80% of patients after cure of *H. pylori* infection associated with early-stage tumor, but no regression occurred in advanced tumor stages. Further studies should investigate whether complete remission lasts.

► These findings provide additional support for the concept that the development of primary gastric low-grade MALT lymphoma may be directly related to the lymphatic tissue in the gastric mucosa acquired through chronic *H. pylori* infection. In this fairly large series of 33 patients, it is impressive that complete tumor regression occurred in 23 patients after cure of *H. pylori* infection associated with early-stage tumor. Furthermore, there was no relapse during the follow-up of 12 months. However, only 13 of the 16 patients in this group studied by molecular biological techniques such as PCR showed complete loss of monoclonal bands. Whether patients with residual monoclonal bands will ultimately relapse remains to be determined by a longer follow-up. It is interesting to note that *all* patients became negative for *H. pylori* despite receiving treatment with only 2 drugs, i.e., amoxicillin and omeprazole, although the dosage of the latter drug was 120 mg/day.

N.J. Greenberger, M.D.

Misoprostol Reduces Serious Gastrointestinal Complications in Patients With Rheumatoid Arthritis Receiving Nonsteroidal Anti-Inflammatory Drugs: A Randomized, Double-Blind, Placebo-Controlled Trial

Silverstein FE, Graham DY, Senior JR, Davies HW, Struthers BJ, Bittman RM, Geis GS (Univ of Washington, Seattle; Baylor College of Medicine, Houston; Univ of Pennsylvania, Philadelphia; et al)

Ann Intern Med 123:241–249, 1995 119-96-42-6

Introduction.—The gastrointestinal side effects of nonsteroidal anti-inflammatory drugs (NSAIDs) have become a major health problem among patients receiving long-term therapy. In a randomized trial, it was determined whether concurrent administration of the synthetic prostaglandin misoprostol would reduce the incidence of serious upper gastrointestinal complications in patients with rheumatoid arthritis.

Patients and Methods.—The study participants were 8,843 men and women who were recruited from 664 family medicine, internal medicine, and rheumatology practices in the United States and Canada. All patients had chronic rheumatoid arthritis and were taking 1 of 10 NSAIDs at specified minimum doses. The patients were assigned in a double-blind manner to receive misoprostol (200 μg) or placebo tablets 4 times daily; they were then followed for 6 months for the development of definite upper gastrointestinal complications, as determined by clinical symptoms

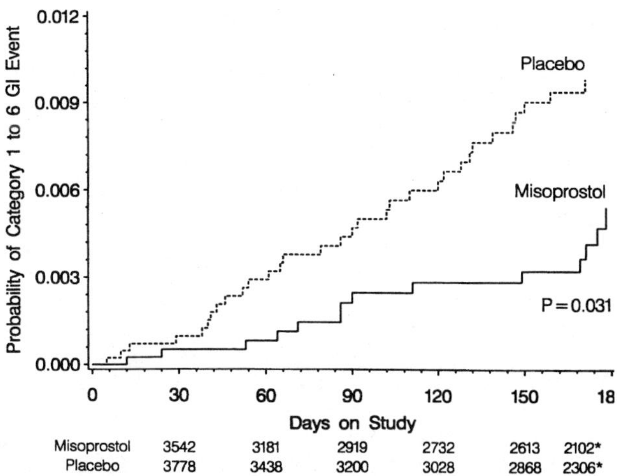

FIGURE 1.—Kaplan-Meier curves for gastrointestinal (*GI*) events in categories 1–6 for misoprostol and placebo groups. The difference between the curves is significant. The *numbers below the horizontal axis* are numbers of patients in the 2 groups remaining in the study at times shown. *Asterisks* indicate the number of patients in each group remaining in the study at 170 days. (Courtesy of Silverstein FE, Graham DY, Senior JR, et al: Misoprostol reduces serious gastrointestinal complications in patients with rheumatoid arthritis receiving nonsteroidal anti-inflammatory drugs: A randomized, double-blind, placebo-controlled trial. *Ann Intern Med* 123:241–249, 1995.)

or findings. The placebo group was expected to have an approximately 1% incidence of such complications during a 6-month period.

Results.—The overall rate of premature withdrawal from the study was 39%. Significantly more patients withdrew from the misoprostol group (42%) than from the placebo group (36%), a difference attributed to diarrheal symptoms associated with misoprostol. Of 242 suspicious gastrointestinal events reported by investigators, 49 patients were judged to have serious ulcer complications, 18 to have bleeding with no ulcer or erosion, and 28 to have possible previous but not active bleeding. Serious ulcer complications were reduced by 51% and all definite upper gastrointestinal complications by 44% in patients receiving misoprostol vs. placebo. The time-to-event analysis for serious events (categories 1–6) showed an advantage for misoprostol (Fig 1). Analysis of 18 potential risk factors for gastrointestinal complications showed significant indicators of increased risk to be age 75 years or older and a history of peptic ulcer, of gastrointestinal bleeding, or of cardiovascular disease. After adjusting for these factors, misoprostol continued to yield a significant reduction in serious upper gastrointestinal complications.

Conclusion.—In this group of mostly elderly, chronically ill patients with rheumatoid arthritis, misoprostol given concurrently with NSAID therapy significantly reduced the incidence of upper gastrointestinal complications. The drug more clearly reduced the risk for NSAID-induced ulceration than for gastrointestinal bleeding.

▶ This study by Silverstein and colleagues is the first randomized, double-blind, placebo-controlled trial using routine clinical criteria to determine the incidence of serious NSAID-induced upper gastrointestinal complications in arthritic patients, as detected under ordinary clinical practice conditions. Importantly, 4 factors identified patients at greatly increased risk of upper gastrointestinal complications; these factors were previous gastrointestinal bleeding, previous peptic ulcer, age 75 years or older, and a history of cardiac disease. Whereas patients with all 4 risk factors were found to have a 9% risk for a major complication in 6 months, the risk in patients who had none of these factors was only 0.4%. The reader is referred to 2 excellent editorials on NSAIDs and gastrointestinal side effects.[1, 2]

I agree with the recommendations of Levine.[2] He would first consider whether therapy with the NSAIDs could be stopped and replaced by therapy with other medications. If this was not possible, he would then prescribe low doses of NSAIDs such as ibuprofen and nabumetone. He would not use misoprostol in most patients requiring NSAIDs. However, for the small subgroup of patients with a history of peptic ulcer or gastrointestinal bleeding, especially elderly patients with concomitant cardiac disease, he would prescribe a dose of misoprostol that the patient could tolerate, such as 100–200 μg given 4 times per day.

N.J. Greenberger, M.D.

References

1. Hawkey CJ: Future treatments for arthritis: New NSAIDs, NO NSAIDs or No NSAIDs. *Gastroenterology* 109:614–616, 1995.
2. Levine JS: Misoprostol and nonsteroidal anti-inflammatory drugs: A tale of effects, outcomes, and costs (Editorial). *Ann Intern Med* 123:309–310, 1995.

43 Small Bowel

A Comparison of Symptoms After the Consumption of Milk or Lactose-Hydrolyzed Milk by People With Self-Reported Severe Lactose Intolerance

Suarez FL, Savaiano DA, Levitt MD (Univ of Minnesota, St Paul; Minneapolis Veterans Affairs Med Ctr)

N Engl J Med 333:1–4, 1995 119-96-43–1

Background.—Approximately 75% of adults worldwide have lactose malabsorption. After weaning, a reduction in lactase activity occurs in many individuals. Most individuals with lactose malabsorption have abdominal pain, bloating, flatulence, and diarrhea after consuming large doses of lactose, but their tolerance of smaller doses of lactose is controversial. Accordingly, the gastrointestinal symptoms of individuals who attributed their symptoms to severe lactose intolerance were investigated in a randomized, double-blind, crossover study.

Methods.—Thirty individuals who reported severe lactose intolerance were studied. Their ability to digest lactose was determined by measuring end-alveolar hydrogen concentrations after they drank 15 g of lactose in 250 mL of water. Then, the individuals drank 240 mL of milk each day for two periods of 1 week. Milk preparations were either a lactose-hydrolyzed milk with 2% fat, or milk with 2% fat and an artificial sweetener. Individuals rated their gastrointestinal symptoms.

Results.—Of the 30 individuals, 21 had lactose malabsorption and 9 were able to absorb lactose according to their breath hydrogen concentrations. The individuals' self-rated symptoms were between trivial and mild for abdominal pain, bloating, flatus, and diarrhea (Table 1). There were no significant differences in severity of symptoms between the 2 study periods.

Discussion.—Some individuals may incorrectly attribute abdominal distress to lactose malabsorption. These individuals were able to tolerate 240 mL of milk a day for 7 days with only mild gastrointestinal symptoms. Lactose-digestive aids may not be necessary when smaller doses of lactose are consumed.

▶ This important study involved patients who believed their gastrointestinal symptoms were due to lactose intolerance. However, when the subjects received either 240 mL of milk or lactose-hydrolyzed milk during the 1-week

TABLE 1.—Gastrointestinal Symptoms and Frequency of Flatus in 30 People With Self-Reported Severe Lactose Intolerance Who Drank 240 mL of Ordinary Milk or Lactose-Hydrolyzed Milk Daily for 1 Week*

Symptom	Ordinary Milk	Lactose-Hydrolyzed Milk	Difference	95% Confidence Interval†
Lactose-malabsorption group (n = 21)				
Bloating‡	0.6 ± 0.1	0.5 ± 0.1	0.1 ± 0.1	−0.2 to 0.4
Abdominal pain‡	0.4 ± 0.1	0.3 ± 0.1	0.1 ± 0.1	−0.1 to 0.3
Diarrhea (episodes/day)	0.1 ± 0.0	0.3 ± 0.1	−0.2 ± 0.1	−0.4 to 0.0
Flatus				
Perceived severity‡	1.1 ± 0.1	0.9 ± 0.1	0.2 ± 0.1	0.0 to 0.4
Frequency (episodes/day)	10.1 ± 1.5	7.6 ± 1.2	2.5 ± 1.1	0.2 to 4.8
Lactose-absorption group (n = 9)				
Bloating‡	0.6 ± 0.2	0.5 ± 0.2	0.2 ± 0.2	−0.3 to 0.7
Abdominal pain‡	0.6 ± 0.2	0.4 ± 0.2	0.2 ± 0.1	0.0 to 0.4
Diarrhea (episodes/day)	0.3 ± 0.2	0.2 ± 0.1	0.1 ± 0.2	−0.4 to 0.6
Flatus				
Perceived severity‡	0.9 ± 0.2	1.2 ± 0.2	0.3 ± 0.2	−0.2 to 0.8
Frequency (episodes/day)	11.8 ± 2.3	8.4 ± 1.9	3.4 ± 1.7	−0.53 to 7.3

* Data were analyzed by analysis of variance. Plus-minus values are means ± SEM.

† The 95% confidence intervals for the differences between the means for the severity or presence of symptoms include zero, indicating nonsignificance.

‡ Symptoms were ranked according to severity: *0* indicated no symptoms; *1*, trivial symptoms; *2*, mild symptoms; *3*, moderate symptoms; *4*, strong symptoms; and *5*, severe symptoms.

(Reprinted by permission of *The New England Journal of Medicine*. Suarez FL, Savaiano DA, Levitt MD: A comparison of symptoms after the consumption of milk or lactose-hydrolyzed milk by people with self-reported severe lactose intolerance. *N Engl J Med* 333:1–4, Copyright 1995, Massachusetts Medical Society.)

study periods, no significant differences were found in the severity of 4 symptoms, i.e., bloating, abdominal pain, flatus, and diarrhea. The authors conclude that individuals who believe they are lactose intolerant may mistakenly attribute a variety of symptoms to lactose intolerance.

Two points merit emphasis. First, there is considerable variation in the amount of milk that can be tolerated by individuals with a proven decrease in intestinal lactase activity. Although large amounts of lactose (50 g) cause symptoms in the majority of such patients, smaller amounts may not. For reference purposes, 8 oz of milk with 2% fat contains 12 g of lactose. Second, an important reason for the persistence of gastrointestinal symptoms in patients with lactose intolerance in diets containing variable amounts of lactose is the presence of a concurrent irritable bowel syndrome. Many such patients may erroneously attribute their recurrent symptoms, even while following a lactose-restricted diet, to sensitivity to small amounts of lactose. The study by Suarez et al. supports the concept. For a brief yet authoritative review of lactose intolerance, see Reference 1.

N.J. Greenberger, M.D.

Reference

1. Malagelada JR: Lactose intolerance (Editorial). *N Engl J Med* 333:53–54, 1995.

Stool Composition in Factitial Diarrhea: A 6-Year Experience With Stool Analysis

Phillips S, Donaldson L, Geisler K, Pera A, Kochar R (Mayo Clinic and Found, Rochester, Minn)
Ann Intern Med 123:97–100, 1995 119-96-43-2

Background.—Many patients with chronic diarrhea have no identifiable abnormalities and are classified as having "functional diarrhea." Analysis of stool water has been proposed as a way to obtain a more specific diagnosis in diarrhea of uncertain origin. The records of 325 patients referred for stool chemistry analysis during a 6-year period were reviewed to evaluate the diagnostic usefulness of this technique.

Methods.—Samples from 212 of the patients were adequate for analysis, and complete records were available in 202 cases. All of these patients had had diarrhea for at least 4 weeks. Although clinical evaluations were not uniform, most patients had endoscopy of the colon with biopsy, barium radiographs, stool microscopy and culture, investigations for malabsorption, and blood chemistry and hematologic screening tests performed. The final and most likely cause of diarrhea was recorded for each patient.

Results.—Factitial diarrhea was diagnosed in 35 patients including 30 in whom laxatives were identified and 5 whose stools showed evidence of having been diluted. Functional diarrhea, diagnosed when laboratory tests were negative, was found in 42 patients, and microscopic or collagenous colitis in 31. A diagnosis of malabsorption syndrome was made in 14 patients with sprue, pancreatic insufficiency, and diarrhea after gastrectomy and in whom fecal fat excretion was 7 g or more during 24 hours. The remaining 80 patients had various organic diseases (Table 1). The mean fecal concentration of sodium was significantly less in patients with osmotic diarrhea attributed to magnesium than in those taking secretory laxatives (Table 4). In patients with functional diarrhea of various origins, sodium concentrations were generally high and potassium concentrations

TABLE 1.—Final Diagnosis in 202 Patients

Diagnosis	Patients, *n*
Factitial diarrhea	
Laxative abuse	30
Stool dilution	5
Functional diarrhea	
Irritable bowel syndrome	22
After cholecystectomy	8
After infection	12
Microscopic or collagenous colitis	31
The malabsorption syndrome (sprue, diarrhea after gastrectomy, or chronic pancreatitis)	14
Miscellaneous	80

(Courtesy of Phillips S, Donaldson L, Geisler K, et al: Stool composition in factitial diarrhea: A 6-year experience with stool analysis. *Ann Intern Med* 123:97–100, 1995.)

TABLE 4.—Osmotic Gaps in Laxative Users*

Laxative	Patients	[NA]	[K]	Osmotic Gap Actual†	Osmotic Gap Calculated‡
		mM		*mOsm/kg*	
Osmotic	19	30 ± 5	44 ± 7	194 ± 15	143 ± 20
Secretory	11	104 ± 5	39 ± 4	39 ± 10	17 ± 7

* Values expressed as mean ± SE.
† Measured by subtracting 2([Na] + [K]) from the osmolality of fecal water.
‡ Calculated by subtracting 2([Na] + [K]) from 290 mOsm/kg.
(Courtesy of Phillips S, Donaldson L, Geisler K, et al: Stool composition in factitial diarrhea: A 6-year experience with stool analysis. *Ann Intern Med* 123:97–100, 1995.)

low. The osmotic gap of stool water was greater in patients with osmotic diarrhea than in those taking secretory laxatives (Fig 1).

Conclusion.—Fecal water analysis appears to have a definite but limited role in the diagnosis of chronic diarrhea. Because fecal hypotonicity indicates the addition of fluid to samples as might be done by patients with Munchausen syndrome, stool analysis does offer an inexpensive screening test for factitial diarrhea.

▶ This paper provides very useful information on the utility of stool composition in the assessment of patients with diarrheal disorders, and especially in patients with suspected factitial diarrhea. Not surprisingly, the latter group represented approximately 17% of the 202 patients studied in detail (Table 1). The osmotic gap of stool water has been 1 of 3 criteria generally used to differentiate between osmotic and secretory diarrhea, the other 2 being 24-hour stool volume and response to fasting. The data provided in this study indicate that values for osmotic gaps between 50 and 100

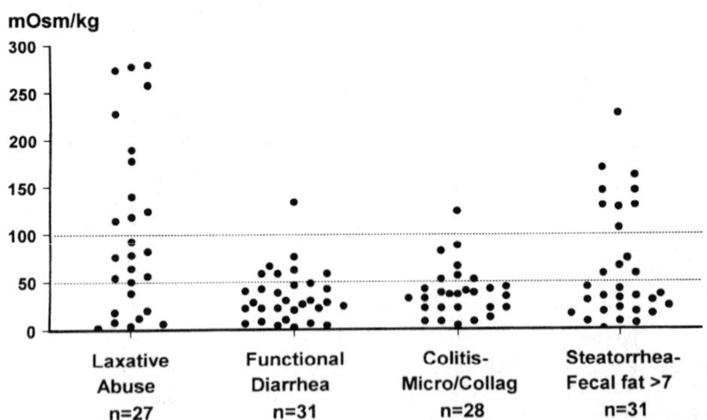

FIGURE 1.—The osmotic gap of stool water for subgroups of patients with diarrhea. The osmotic gap is derived from the following formula: 290 − [2(Na concentration + K concentration)]. Patients with negative values were not included, nor were patients with miscellaneous diagnoses. All patients with fecal fat excretion of more than 7 g/day were included, regardless of whether an underlying diagnosis was established. Values for osmotic gaps between 50 and 100 mOsm/kg (*dotted lines*) represent a "gray zone" between low (secretory diarrhea) and high (osmotic diarrhea) gaps. *Abbreviation: Micro/Collag,* microscopic and collagenous. (Courtesy of Phillips S, Donaldson L, Geisler K, et al: Stool composition in factitial diarrhea: A 6-year experience with stool analysis. *Ann Intern Med* 123:97–100, 1995.)

mOsm/kg represent a gray zone, whereas values greater than 100 mOsm/kg should suggest an osmotic diarrhea and in particular, laxative abuse. For a timely review of the evaluation of patients with chronic diarrhea, see the current concepts review article by Donowitz et al.[1]

N.J. Greenberger, M.D.

Reference

1. Donowitz M, Kokke FT, Saidi R: Current concepts: Evaluation of patients with chronic diarrhea. *N Engl J Med* 332:725–729, 1995.

The First Reported Outbreak of Diarrheal Illness Associated With *Cyclospora* in the United States

Huang P, Weber JT, Sosin DM, Griffin PM, Long EG, Murphy JJ, Kocka F, Peters C, Kallick C (Ctrs for Disease Control and Prevention, Atlanta, Ga)
Ann Intern Med 123:409–414, 1995 119-96-43–3

Background.—A weekend outbreak of diarrhea among housestaff physicians at a Chicago hospital was reported to the Division of Infectious Diseases in July 1990. The investigation of this diarrheal outbreak was described.

Methods and Findings.—Twenty-one case patients were identified among physicians and dormitory cohorts. All had had diarrhea lasting a median of 5 days. Symptoms included abdominal cramping, occurring in 76%; muscle aches in 52%; reduced appetite in 48%; fever in 48%; nausea in 43%; headache in 38%; constipation in 24%; vomiting in 24%; and chills in 19%. Typically, the symptoms occurred in a distinctive cycle of remissions and exacerbations that lasted for as long as several weeks. The results of investigations for known ova and parasites were negative. However, microscopic evaluation of stool specimens from 11 patients revealed many spherical bodies, 8–10 µm in diameter. These were identified as *Cyclospora* organisms. Follow-up specimens obtained from 7 patients showed that the organisms had disappeared by 8 weeks after onset of disease. Tap water in a physicians' dormitory was the most likely source of the outbreak. Stagnant water in a storage tank may have contaminated the water supply in that dormitory after a pump failed.

Conclusions.—This is the first report of a diarrheal outbreak associated with *Cyclospora* organisms in the United States. *Cyclospora* species may be a human enteric pathogen producing bouts of acute and relapsing diarrhea. Patients with unexplained, prolonged diarrhea should be tested for this pathogen.

► As the authors point out in their discussion, *Cyclospora* in this outbreak was fortuitously identified because the hospital served many patients with AIDS and because the hospital laboratory had implemented a monoclonal acid-fast staining procedure of all stool specimens to screen for *Cryptosporidium*. The data presented suggest that *Cyclospora* may be either a new or previously unrecognized pathogen that can cause acute or recurrent diarrhea. Accordingly, *Cyclospora* should be added to an ever-increasing list of pathogens in assessing patients with unexplained, prolonged diarrheal illness. Such considerations, obviously not complete, include amebiasis, giardiasis, *Campylobacter jejuni, Yersinia, Aeromonas, Plesiomonas,* cryptosporidia, microsporidia, *Mycobacterium avium intracellulare* (MAI) complex, *Clostridium difficile,* chlamydia, and cytomegalovirus.

N.J. Greenberger, M.D.

Current Use and Clinical Outcome of Home Parenteral and Enteral Nutrition Therapies in the United States

Howard L, Ament M, Fleming CR, Shike M, Steiger E (Albany Med College, NY; Univ of California, Los Angeles; Mayo Clinic Jacksonville, Fla; et al)
Gastroenterology 109:355–365, 1995 119-96-43–4

Background.—The use of home nutrition support has significantly increased in recent years. This type of therapy is expensive, particularly via the parenteral route. Use of Medicare home parenteral and enteral nutrition (HPEN) from 1989 to 1992 was analyzed to define the patterns, costs, and outcome of HPEN treatment.

Methods.—Data were derived from part B parenteral and enteral nutrition workload statistics compiled by the Health Care Financing Administration and by Blue Cross/Blue Shield of South Carolina, 1 of 2 national carriers responsible for determining HPEN eligibility of Medicare beneficiaries from 1986 to 1993. Disease distribution and therapy outcome were

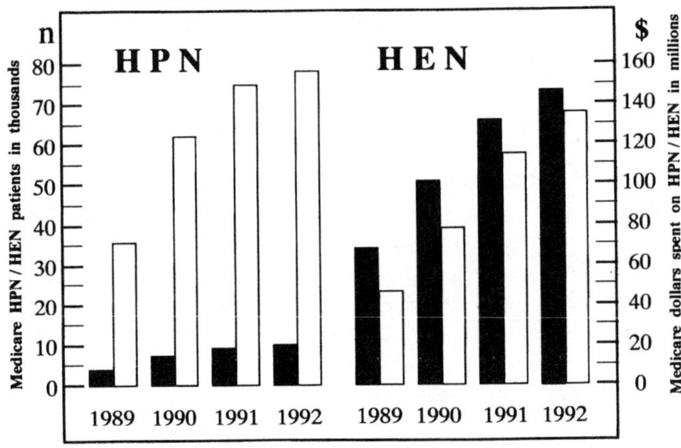

FIGURE 1.—An estimate of the number of Medicare patients receiving HPN and HEN in thousands (*solid bars*) and the dollars paid in millions (*open bars*) between 1989 and 1992. These estimates were derived from Medicare part B PEN workload statistics compiled by Blue Cross/Blue Shield of South Carolina (David Denny, personal communication, 2/93). This carrier processed approximately 75% of all Medicare PEN claims. Their workload statistics have been increased to provide an estimate of national Medicare activity. *Abbreviations: HPN,* home parenteral nutrition; *HEN,* home enteral nutrition; *PEN,* parenteral and enteral nutrition. (Courtesy of Howard L, Ament M, Fleming CR, et al: Current use and clinical outcome of home parenteral and enteral nutrition therapies in the United States. *Gastroenterology* 109:355–365, 1995.)

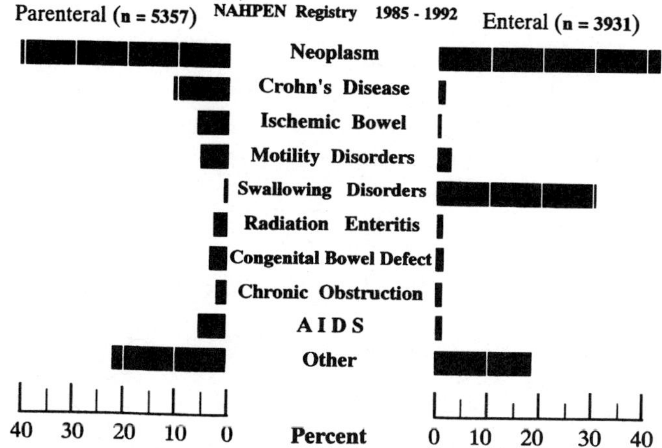

FIGURE 2.—Distribution of diagnoses in new patients receiving HPN and HEN reported to the North American HPEN (*NAHPEN*) Registry from 1985 to 1992. Values shown were percents of the total for each therapy category. *Abbreviations: HPN,* home parenteral nutrition; *HEN,* home enteral nutrition; *HPEN,* home parenteral and enteral nutrition. (Courtesy of Howard L, Ament M, Fleming CR, et al: Current use and clinical outcome of home parenteral and enteral nutrition therapies in the United States. *Gastroenterology* 109:355–365, 1995.)

assessed using National Registry information collected on 9,288 patients treated with HPEN from 1985 to 1992.

Results.—The use of HPEN doubled in the United States between 1989 and 1992, so that by 1992 there were approximately 40,000 parenteral nutrition and 152,000 enteral nutrition home patients. The money paid for Medicare beneficiaries receiving home enteral nutrition (HEN) and home parenteral nutrition (HPN) increased from $47 to $137 million and from $73 to $156 million, respectively, during the 4-year period (Fig 1). The average treatment time was calculated to be about 60 days for HPN and 70 days for HEN in 1992. A large proportion of the patients administered HPEN therapies had a short survival rate. The single most common diagnosis was cancer (Fig 2), and only 25% of patients with cancer were alive after 1 year. Outcome data showed that both HEN and HPN were safe and that the patient's primary disease strongly influenced rehabilitation and survival (Table 4).

Conclusion.—Data reviewed for this study suggest that Medicare HPEN prevalence rates are several times higher than the HPEN prevalence in the general population. A comparison with available data from other countries also suggests that there is a much higher use of HPEN therapies in the United States and that rapid expansion in these therapies has occurred in recent years. Furthermore, the costs reported for 1992 underestimate actual costs because nursing care, physician and laboratory fees, and hospitalization for therapy-related complications were not included. Examination of the risks and benefits of HPEN should consider the impact of primary diagnosis on expected long-term survival and rehabilitation. Age per se should not disqualify a patient from HPEN therapy.

TABLE 4.—Summary of Outcome on HPEN

Diagnosis/therapy	No. of patients	Age [yr (SD)]	Survival on therapy [% *(observed deaths/ expected deaths)*]*	Therapy status at 1 year [% (SEM)]†			Rehabilitation status in first year [% (SEM)]‡			Complications§ *(per patient yr)*	
				Full oral nutrition	Continued on HPEN therapy	Died	Complete	Partial	Minimal	HPEN	Non-HPEN
HPN											
Crohn's disease	562	36 (17)	96 (31/2.9)	70 (2)	25 (2)	2 (1)	60 (5)	38 (5)	2 (NA)	0.9	1.1
Ischemic bowel disease	331	49 (24)	87 (81/7.5)	27 (3)	48 (4)	19 (3)	53 (4)	41 (4)	6 (2)	1.4	1.1
Motility disorder	299	45 (22)	87 (81/3.1)	31 (3)	44 (4)	21 (3)	49 (4)	39 (4)	12 (3)	1.3	1.1
Congenital bowel defect	172	5 (14)	94 (20/1.6)	42 (6)	47 (6)	9 (3)	63 (6)	27 (5)	11 (4)	2.1	1.0
Hyperemesis gravidarum	112	28 (5)	100 (0/0.1)	100 (NA)	0 (NA)	0 (NA)	83 (4)	16 (4)	1 (NA)	1.5	3.5
Chronic pancreatitis	156	42 (17)	90 (9/0.6)	82 (3)	10 (3)	5 (2)	60 (5)	38 (5)	2 (NA)	1.2	2.5
Radiation enteritis	145	58 (15)	87 (47/3.2)	28 (5)	49 (5)	22 (4)	42 (6)	49 (6)	9 (3)	0.8	1.1
Chronic adhesive obstructions	120	53 (17)	83 (30/1.1)	47 (6)	34 (5)	13 (4)	23 (7)	68 (7)	10 (NA)	1.7	1.4
Cystic fibrosis	51	17 (10)	50 (254/0.05)	38 (7)	13 (5)	36 (7)	24 (6)	66 (7)	16 (5)	0.8	3.7
Cancer	2122	44 (24)	20 (1336/8.7)	26 (1)	8 (1)	63 (1)	29 (3)	57 (3)	14 (2)	1.1	3.3
AIDS	280	33 (12)	10 (182/0.8)	13 (3)	6 (2)	73 (4)	8 (NA)	63 (7)	29 (6)	1.6	3.3
HEN											
Neurological disorders of swallowing	1134	65 (26)	55 (447/31.5)	19 (2)	25 (2)	48 (2)	5 (1)	24 (2)	71 (3)	0.3	0.9
Cancer	1644	61 (17)	30 (885/13.6)	30 (2)	6 (1)	59 (2)	21 (3)	59 (3)	21 (3)	0.4	2.7

Note: Data from North American HPEN Patient Registry.

* Survival rates on therapy are values at 1 year calculated by life table method. This will differ from the percentage listed as "died" under therapy status because all patients with known end points are considered in this latter measure. Ratio of observed vs. expected deaths is equivalent to a standard mortality ratio.

† Not shown are those patients who were readmitted to the hospital or who had changed the type of therapy for 12 months.

‡ Rehabilitation is designated complete, partial, or minimal relative to the patient's ability to sustain normal age-related activity.

§ Complications refer only to those that resulted in rehospitalization.

Abbreviations: NA, not applicable (because the group was too small); *HPN*, home parenteral nutrition; *HEN*, home enteral nutrition; *HPEN*, home parenteral and enteral nutrition.

(Courtesy of Howard L, Ament M, Fleming CR, et al: Current use and clinical outcome of home parenteral and enteral nutrition therapies in the United States. *Gastroenterology* 109:355–365, 1995.)

► A recent report[1] provides further information on the prognosis of patients with nonmalignant chronic intestinal failure who are receiving long-term HPN. Two hundred seventeen adult patients with chronic intestinal failure who did not have cancer or AIDS were enrolled from 1980 to 1989 in approved HPN programs in Belgium and France. Prognostic factors were determined using multivariate analysis. Seventy-three patients died during the survey, and the mortality rate related to HPN complications accounted for 11% of deaths. Three independent variables were associated with a decreased risk of death: (1) patients younger than 40 years of age; (2) start of HPN after 1987; and (3) absence of chronic intestinal obstruction. The 2-year survival rate in patients younger than 60 years included after 1983 with a very short bowel was 90%.

N.J. Greenberger, M.D.

Reference

1. Messing B, et al: Prognosis of patients with nonmalignant chronic intestinal failure receiving long-term home parenteral nutrition. *Gastroenterology* 108:1005–1010, 1995.

Methotrexate for the Treatment of Crohn's Disease

Feagan BG, for the North American Crohn's Study Group Investigators (Univ of Calgary, Alta, Canada; Univ of Chicago; Univ of Alberta, Edmonton, Canada; et al)

N Engl J Med 332:292–297, 1995 119-96-43–5

Introduction.—Corticosteroids are effective in improving the symptoms of Crohn's disease. However, attempts to discontinue corticosteroid therapy fail in approximately 20% of patients, who continue to have both complications of the disease and chronic toxicity from the treatment. The efficacy of the anti-inflammatory drug methotrexate was assessed in patients who had chronically active Crohn's disease.

Methods.—A double-blind, placebo-controlled, multicenter study included 141 patients who had chronically active Crohn's disease despite having received at least 3 months of treatment with prednisone. The patients were randomly assigned to receive weekly injections with methotrexate, 25 mg IM, or placebo for 16 weeks. Randomization was done in a ratio of 2:1 favoring the active treatment: 94 patients received methotrexate and 47 received placebo. Prednisone was given in a starting dose of 20 mg/day and was tapered during a 10-week period if the patient's condition permitted. Clinical remission, defined as cessation of prednisone treatment and a Crohn's Disease Activity Index score of 150 points or less, was the main outcome measure.

Results.—At the end of the 16-week treatment, 39% of the methotrexate group vs. 19% of the placebo group were in clinical remission, for a relative risk of 1.95 (Fig 1). Overall, prednisone use was significantly less in the methotrexate group, particularly in the last 4 weeks of treatment. The mean Crohn's Disease Activity Index score was 162 points in the

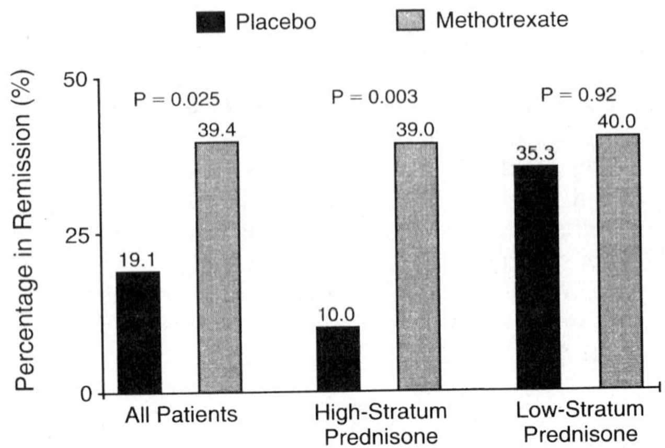

FIGURE 1.—Percentages of patients in remission at week 16, according to study group and stratum of daily dose of prednisone before study entry. The high-prednisone stratum was receiving a daily dose of more than 20 mg of prednisone and the low-prednisone stratum a daily dose of 20 mg or less, more than 2 weeks before randomization. The actual percentages are shown above the bars. The *P* values were derived by the Mantel-Haenszel chi-square test, with adjustment for study center. (Reprinted by permission of *The New England Journal of Medicine.* Feagan BG, for the North American Crohn's Study Group Investigators: Methotrexate for the treatment of Crohn's disease. *N Engl J Med* 332:292–297, Copyright 1995, Massachusetts Medical Society.)

methotrexate group vs. 204 points in the placebo group, although there were no significant differences in quality-of-life scores or serum concentrations of orosomucoid. Adverse events requiring cessation of treatment occurred in 17% of the methotrexate group vs. 2% of the placebo group. The most frequent events of this type in the methotrexate group were asymptomatically increased serum aminotransferase and nausea.

Conclusions.—Methotrexate is effective in improving symptoms and reducing prednisone requirements in patients with chronically active Crohn's disease. Methotrexate may be a useful alternative for patients who cannot tolerate prednisone or whose symptoms persist despite moderately high prednisone doses. A study using 15 mg of methotrexate once weekly to prevent relapse in patients with quiescent Crohn's disease is under way.

▶ This study provides data indicating that methotrexate was twice as likely as placebo to maintain patients with Crohn's disease in remission. After 16 weeks of treatment, however, many questions remain unanswered: Would such improvement be maintained over longer periods, i.e., years? Would oral therapy be effective? Is the site of Crohn's disease, i.e., small bowel or colon, a relevant factor? What is the long-term toxicity of methotrexate in Crohn's disease patients?

With regard to the last question, the reader is referred to a timely editorial by Weinblatt.[1] Weinblatt emphasizes that using methotrexate requires knowledge of the pharmacologic effects of the drug, awareness of its toxicity, and comprehensive understanding of the particular disease. Applying this to Crohn's disease, it would seem logical for the use of methotrexate to be considered *after* other treatments, such as sulfasalazine, 5-aminosalicylic (5-ASA) analogues, metronidazole, azathioprine, and 6-mercaptopurine (6-MP) have been tried.

Finally, the relatively short duration of the trial conducted by Feagan et al. brings to mind similar short-term trials with cyclosporine in Crohn's disease. Whereas short-term trials did indicate efficacy, more recent long-term trials[2] have failed to demonstrate sustained benefits.

N.J. Greenberger, M.D.

References

1. Weinblatt ME: Methotrexate for chronic diseases in adults. *N Engl J Med* 332:330–331, 1995.
2. Feagan BG, McDonald JWD, Rochon J, et al: Low-dose cyclosporine for the treatment of Crohn's disease. *N Engl J Med* 330:1846–1851, 1994.

►↓ It is estimated that Crohn's disease afflicts 500,000 Americans. Despite intensive research efforts, the pathogenesis of this disorder remains incompletely defined. In this setting, it is not surprising that treatment modalities are far from optimal. However, considerable progress has been made, and the following 6 articles highlight these advances.

Although medical therapy is the primary method of treatment, approximately 70% of patients will require surgery at some time. However, a particularly vexing problem is the high rate of recurrent disease, which in the literature is reported as ranging from 3% to 16% per year, depending in part on the criteria used to define recurrence.[1] Three of the following articles deal with this problem.

N.J. Greenberger, M.D.

Reference

1. McLeod RS, Wolff BG, Steinhart AH, et al: Prophylactic mesalamine treatment decreases postoperative recurrence of Crohn's disease. *Gastroenterology* 109:404–413, 1995.

Azathioprine and 6-Mercaptopurine in Crohn Disease: A Meta-Analysis

Pearson DC, May GR, Fick GH, Sutherland LR (Univ of Calgary, Alta, Canada)
Ann Intern Med 122:132–142, 1995 119-96-43-6

Purpose.—A meta-analysis of published, randomized, double-blind, placebo-controlled trials of azathioprine or 6-mercaptopurine for the treatment of Crohn's disease was performed to assess their effectiveness.

Study Design.—Relevant studies were chosen from the MEDLINE database (1966 to May 1994), abstracts from major gastrointestinal conferences, and references from published articles. Of the 222 studies reviewed, 9 met the inclusion criteria. Data were extracted by 3 independent observers on the basis of the intention-to-treat principle and were analyzed by regression analysis. Each study was rated for quality.

Findings.—Compared with placebo, treatment with either azathioprine or 6-mercaptopurine had an odds ratio of response of 3.09 in patients who had active Crohn's disease (Fig 1). The odds ratio of response to azathioprine in quiescent disease was 2.27 (Fig 2). For active disease, continuation of therapy for at least 17 weeks improved the response. For quiescent disease, a higher dose improved the response. In both cases, an increased cumulative dose improved the response. A steroid-sparing effect and improvement in fistulae were observed in both active and quiescent disease with these treatments. Increased antimetabolite therapy was also associated with increased adverse side effects, such as allergy, leukopenia, pancreatitis, and nausea.

Conclusions.—Azathioprine and 6-mercaptopurine are effective treatments for both active and quiescent Crohn's disease. Cumulative dose was an important factor in patient response, but adverse side effects also increased with increased dosage. Antimetabolite therapy should be initiated only after careful discussion of the risks and benefits with the affected patient.

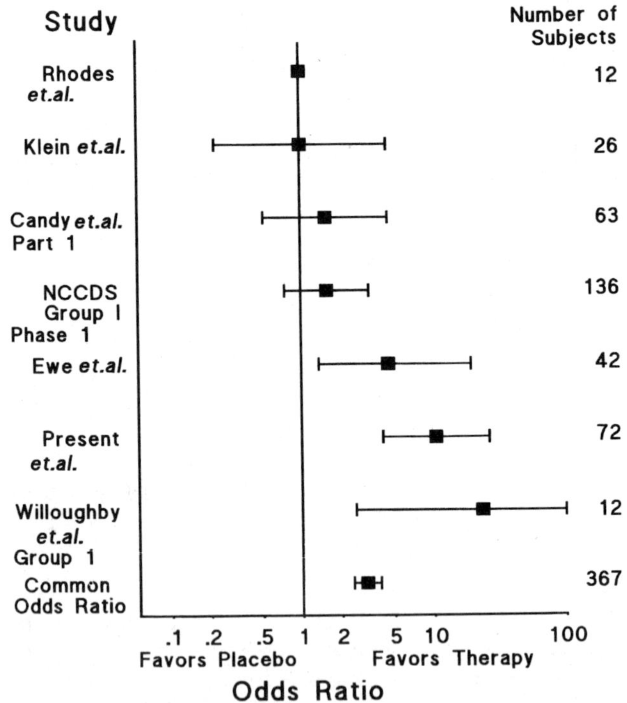

FIGURE 1.—Odds ratio of response in randomized controlled studies of azathioprine and 6-mercaptopurine for active disease. The odds ratio (log scale) for each study is represented by the *filled square,* and the 95% confidence intervals (*CIs*) are represented by *horizontal bars.* Values greater than 1 indicate a therapeutic benefit compared with placebo. The estimated common odds ratio for response was 3.09 (CI, 2.45–3.91). *Abbreviation: NCCDS,* National Cooperative Crohn's Disease Study. (Courtesy of Pearson DC, May GR, Fick GH, et al: Azathioprine and 6-mercaptopurine in Crohn disease: A meta-analysis. *Ann Intern Med* 122:132–142, 1995.)

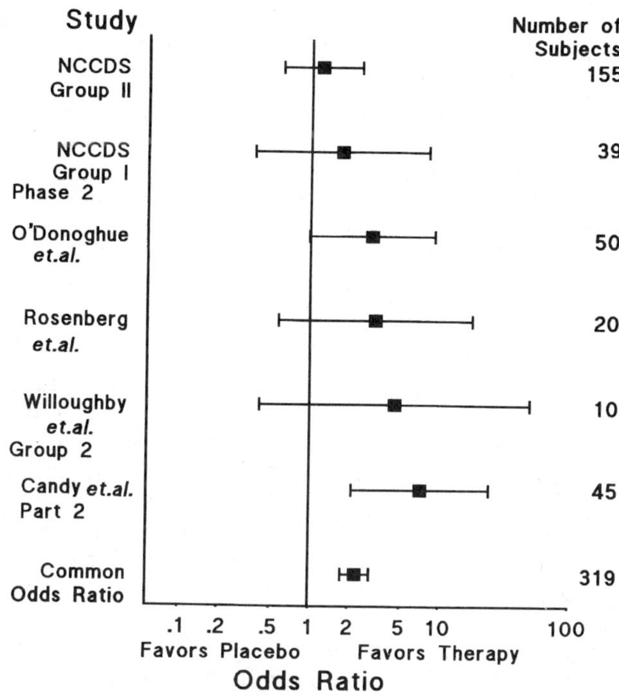

FIGURE 2.—Odds ratio of response in randomized controlled studies of azathioprine for maintenance therapy. The odds ratio (log scale) for each study is represented by the *filled square*, and the 95% confidence intervals (*CIs*) are represented by the *horizontal bars*. Values greater than 1 indicate a therapeutic benefit compared with placebo. The estimated common odds ratio for response was 2.27 (CI, 1.76–2.93). *Abbreviation: NCCDS,* National Cooperative Crohn's Disease Study. (Courtesy of Pearson DC, May GR, Fick GH, et al: Azathioprine and 6-mercaptopurine in Crohn disease: A meta-analysis. *Ann Intern Med* 122:132–142, 1995.)

► This study provides further support for the use of azathioprine and 6-mercaptopurine (6-MP) in the treatment of both active and quiescent Crohn's disease. The question arises as to when these drugs should be used. Clinicians now have several drugs and treatments that have been shown to be effective in the treatment of Crohn's disease; these include sulfasalazine, 5-aminosalicylic (5-ASA) preparations, corticosteroids (PO, enema, IV preparations), metronidazole, azathioprine and 6-MP, methotrexate, cyclosporine, and parenteral and enteral nutrition. Sulfasalazine or 5-ASA analogues and corticosteroids are the drugs usually used in patients with newly diagnosed Crohn's disease. Azathioprine and 6-MP are frequently used in several settings, including (1) to induce and/or maintain remission; (2) when there is failure to respond to initial therapy, as noted previously; (3) when there is a need to effect a reduction in steroid dosage, i.e., the steroid-sparing effect; and (4) to facilitate closure of enteroenteric, enterocutaneous, enterovesical, and rectovaginal fistulae. In this regard, corticosteroids are ineffective in the treatment of such fistulae, whereas azathioprine or 6-MP can be expected to effect fistula closure in approximately 40% to 50%

of cases, and this is more likely if intestinal obstruction is not present. The following article will address the use of metronidazole and 5-ASA analogues in the treatment of Crohn's disease.

N.J. Greenberger, M.D.

Controlled Trial of Metronidazole Treatment for Prevention of Crohn's Recurrence After Ileal Resection

Rutgeerts P, Hiele M, Geboes K, Peeters M, Penninckx F, Aerts R, Kerremans R (Univ Hosp Gasthuisberg, Belgium; Univ of Leuven, Belgium)

Gastroenterology 108:1617–1621, 1995 119-96-43-7

Objective.—A double-blind trial of metronidazole was done in 60 patients with Crohn's ileitis who underwent ileal resection and ileocolonic anastomosis with curative intent. The inflamed ileal segment was removed with 5–15 cm of uninvolved bowel, and the anastomosis was made with uninvolved colon.

Treatment.—Thirty patients received metronidazole, 20 mg/kg/day for 3 months, whereas 30 received a placebo. Seven actively treated patients and 2 placebo recipients withdrew from the study. The 2 groups were well matched clinically.

Results.—Severe recurrent disease developed in 43% of placebo patients and in 13% of those given metronidazole, for a significant difference. Only 4 actively treated patients compared with 15 placebo recipients had definite recurrent disease in the neoterminal ileum. Clinical recurrences were less frequent in metronidazole-treated patients for up to 3 years after surgery (Table 5), but the differences at 2 and 3 years were not significant.

Conclusion.—Administration of metronidazole for 3 months after curative resection of Crohn's ileitis reduces the severity of early recurrences and may delay symptomatic recurrences.

► This study provides further support for use of metronidazole to reduce both the frequency and severity of recurrent disease after ileal resection and ileocolic anastomosis, as well as delay such recurrences. Several additional studies cited by the authors also suggest efficacy of metronidazole in this setting. Although a significant difference in the rate of recurrence at 1 year

TABLE 5.—Metronidazole vs. Placebo for Prevention of Crohn's Recurrence After Ileal Resection: Clinical Outcome (Per Protocol Analysis)

	Clinical recurrence rates (%)		
	1 year	2 years	3 years
Placebo	7/28 (25)	12/28 (43)	14/28 (50)
Metronidazole	1/23 (4)	6/23 (28)	7/23 (30)
P	0.044	NS	NS

(Courtesy of Rutgeerts P, Hiele M, Geboes K, et al: Controlled trial of metronidazole treatment for prevention of Crohn's recurrence after ileal resection. *Gastroenterology* 108:1617–1621, 1995.)

was demonstrated in this study by Rutgeerts et al., the difference between patients given placebo and those given metronidazole failed to reach significance after the 2- and 3-year mark. However, this could be due to a type I error as a consequence of study groups that were too small.

The rationale for metronidazole use is as follows. Recurrence of new lesions after ileal resection is found almost exclusively in the neoterminal ileum, where anaerobic bacteria are present in very high concentrations, and metronidazole is an effective drug against gram-negative bacteria, both aerobic and anaerobic. The efficacy of metronidazole in this and similar studies provides additional evidence supporting the concept linking intestinal microflora and luminal contents to continued activity in Crohn's disease.

Finally, it should be noted that adverse effects occurred in 6 of 30 placebo-treated patients but in 17 of 30 metronidazole-treated patients. A high dose of metronidazole (20 mg/kg) was used by Rutgeerts et al., and lower doses, e.g., 10–15 mg/kg, should be studied in future investigations.

N.J. Greenberger, M.D.

Prophylactic Mesalamine Treatment Decreases Postoperative Recurrence of Crohn's Disease

McLeod RS, Wolff BG, Steinhart AH, Carryer PW, O'Rourke K, Andrews DF, Blair JE, Cangemi JR, Cohen Z, Cullen JB, Chaytor RG, Greenberg GR, Jaffer NM, Jeejeebhoy KN, MacCarty RL, Ready RL, Weiland LH (Univ of Toronto; Mayo Clinic, Rochester, Minn; Mayo Clinic, Jacksonville, Fla; et al)
Gastroenterology 109:404–413, 1995 119-96-43–8

Background.—About 80% of patients with Crohn's disease eventually need surgery. Unfortunately, the disease often recurs after such treatment. The value of mesalamine in reducing the risk of recurrent Crohn's disease after surgical resection was investigated.

Methods.—One hundred sixty-three patients with no evidence of residual disease after surgical resection were studied. By random assignment, patients received 1.5 g of mesalamine twice a day or placebo within 8 weeks of surgery. The maximum follow-up was 72 months.

Findings.—Symptomatic recurrence was documented in 31% of the patients in the active treatment group, compared with 41% of those in the control group. The relative risk of recurrence in the treatment group was 0.63 using an intention-to-treat analysis and 0.53 using an efficacy analysis. In addition, the endoscopic and radiologic rate of recurrence was significantly reduced, with relative risks of 0.65 and 0.64 in the 2 respective analyses. One serious side effect—pancreatitis—was documented in the mesalamine group.

Conclusions.—Mesalamine effectively reduces the symptomatic, endoscopic, and radiologic rate of recurrence after surgery for Crohn's disease. Additional research is needed to determine the best pharmacologic agents and dosage for prophylaxis and whether prophylaxis is of value in patients with residual disease after surgery.

► The report by McLeod et al. is one of several recent studies supporting the concept that mesalamine is effective in decreasing the risk of recurrence of Crohn's disease after surgical resection is performed.[1] It should be emphasized that higher doses of mesalamine, i.e., at least 3.0 g/day, have been required to demonstrate this effect. Other studies also demonstrate the effectiveness of mesalamine, 3.0 g/day, in decreasing the incidence of recurrent Crohn's disease.

Because metronidazole is also an effective drug in reducing the recurrence rate of Crohn's disease after surgery, it would seem desirable to design clinical trials comparing the use of a *combination* of metronidazole and mesalamine with the drugs given individually and with a placebo group.

N.J. Greenberger, M.D.

Reference

1. Greenberger NJ, Miner PB: Is maintenance therapy effective in Crohn's disease? *Lancet* 344:900–901, 1994.

Mesalamine in the Prevention of Endoscopic Recurrence After Intestinal Resection for Crohn's Disease

Brignola C, Cottone M, Pera A, Ardizzone S, Scribano ML, DeFranchis R, D'Arienzo A, D'Albasio G, Pennestri D, and the Italian Cooperative Study Group (Università di Bologna, Italy; Ospedale "Cervello," Palermo, Italy; Ospedale "Le Molinette," Torino, Italy; et al)

Gastroenterology 108:345–349, 1995 119-96-43-9

Introduction.—Trials using mesalamine as maintenance treatment for patients with Crohn's disease (CD) of the ileum have produced equivocal results. The efficacy of mesalamine in reducing endoscopic recurrence of CD after curative resection of the ileal or ileocecal lesion was evaluated in a double-blind, multicenter clinical trial.

Methods.—Within 1 month of surgery, patients were randomly assigned to receive either 2 tablets of mesalamine (Pentasa) 3 times daily for 12 months, or placebo tablets. Eighty-seven patients were recruited from 8 centers. After 1 year of treatment, a colonoscopy was performed and included 15 cm of anastomosed ileum. Overall endoscopic severity was expressed on a 5-point scale. If endoscopy was unable to reach the anastomosis, a double-contrast barium enema was performed.

Results.—Thirty-one of 44 patients receiving mesalamine were in clinical remission at 12 months. Of the 13 patients not in remission, 5 had side effects, 1 was lost to follow-up, and 7 had clinical relapse (Fig 1). Twenty-nine of 43 patients in the placebo group were in remission at 12 months. Of the 14 patients not in remission, 3 had side effects, 10 were in clinical relapse, and 1 dropped out because of protocol violation

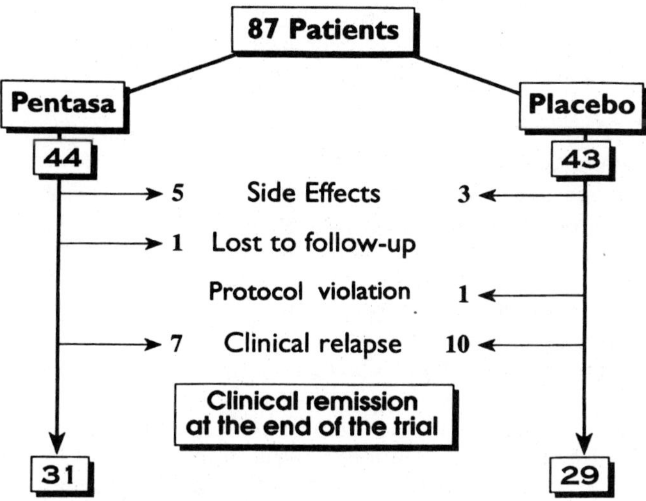

FIGURE 1.—Clinical outcome of patients divided according to the treatment received. (Courtesy of Brignola C, Cottone M, Pera A: Mesalamine in the prevention of endoscopic recurrence after intestinal resection for Crohn's disease. *Gastroenterology* 108:345–349, 1995.)

(Fig 1). The anastomosis was able to be reached in 51 patients by endoscopy. Nine patients underwent barium enema (Fig 2). Of the patients in remission, the endoscopic 5-point scores were significantly better in the treatment than placebo group. At 1 year, the rate of "overall severe recurrences" was 24% in the treatment group and 56% in the placebo group.

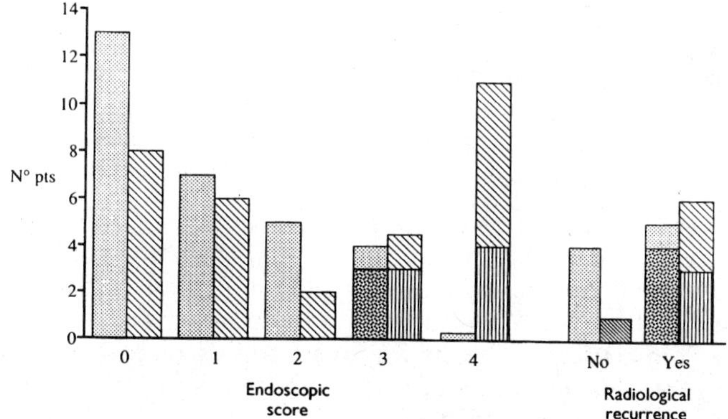

FIGURE 2.—Endoscopic score and radiologic recurrence divided according to the treatment received and to the clinical outcome within 12 months after surgery. Patients receiving Pentasa with clinical relapse (*solid bars*) or in remission (*dotted bar*); patients receiving placebo with clinical relapse (*striped bar*) or in remission (*slashed bar*). (Courtesy of Brignola C, Cottone M, Pera A, et al: Mesalamine in the prevention of endoscopic recurrence after intestinal resection for Crohn's disease. *Gastroenterology* 108:345–349, 1995.)

Conclusion.—The rate and severity of endoscopic recurrences after curative surgery for ileal CD is decreased with administration of mesalamine at 3 g/day. Results of long-term clinical outcome are pending.

▶ This study demonstrates that mesalamine is a useful drug to decrease both the frequency and severity of endoscopically proven recurrences after surgery in patients with ileal Crohn's disease. Endoscopically documented postoperative recurrent disease often occurs within a few months after surgery, even if resection margins are microscopically free of disease. Why the disease recurs primarily at the anastomotic site remains unknown. Nagel et al.[1] studied resection margins in Crohn's disease to clarify whether early lesions are relevant to the interpretation of postoperative recurrence. In Crohn's disease, a triad of early lesions occurring in *both* histopathologically unaffected and affected mucosa was recorded; the lesions noted were mucosal architectural alterations, epithelial bridge formation, and goblet-cell hyperplasia or hypertrophy or both. Importantly, these lesions were observed with histologically unaffected margins in *both* small and large bowel. These findings support the concept of diffuse involvement of the whole gastrointestinal tract by the disease process.

N.J. Greenberger, M.D.

Reference

1. Nagel E, et al: Scanning electron-microscopic lesion in Crohn's disease: Tolerance for the interpretation of postoperative recurrence. *Gastroenterology* 108:376–382, 1995.

Treatment of Crohn's Disease With Anti–Tumor Necrosis Factor Chimeric Monoclonal Antibody (cA2)

Van Dullemen HM, Van Deventer SJH, Hommes DW, Bijl HA, Jansen J, Tytgat GNJ, Woody J (Academic Med Ctr, Amsterdam; Centocor Inc, Malvern, Pa)

Gastroenterology 109:129–135, 1995 119-96-43–10

Background.—The mucosa of patients with active Crohn's disease exhibits increased concentrations of tumor necrosis factor (TNF). In several animal models, neutralization of this potent proinflammatory cytokine was shown to decrease recruitment of inflammatory cells and granuloma formation. Ten patients who had active Crohn's disease that was unresponsive to steroids were treated with an anti-TNF monoclonal antibody to evaluate its safety and efficacy.

Patients and Methods.—The 7 women and 3 men studied had a mean age of 33.6 years and a mean duration of Crohn's disease of 6.1 years. All had failed to respond to prednisone, 20 mg or more for at least 2 weeks. Patients who had started receiving azathioprine treatment within 3 months before enrollment were excluded, but concomitant treatment with prednisone and other immunosuppressive drugs was allowed. Treatment consisted of a single IV infusion of the anti-TNF chimeric

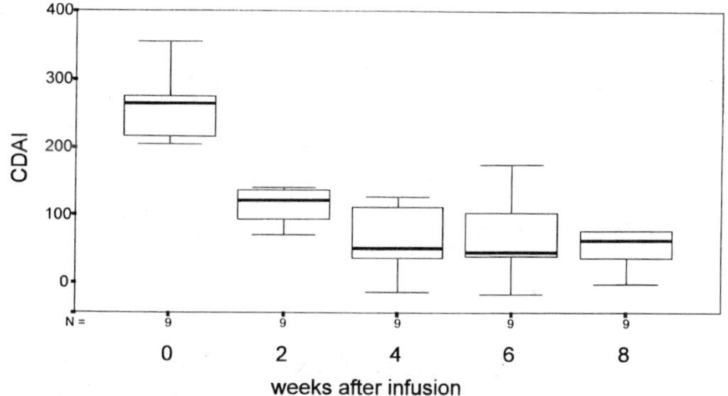

FIGURE 1.—Crohn's Disease Activity Index (*CDAI*) after infusion of cA2 (n = 9). Values represent means, *bars* represent the 25th and 75th percentiles, and *error bars* indicate the 5th and 95th percentiles ($P < 0.0001$). (Courtesy of Van Dullemen HM, Van Deventer SJH, Hommes DW, et al: Treatment of Crohn's disease with anti–tumor necrosis factor chimeric monoclonal antibody (cA2). *Gastroenterology* 109:129–135, 1995.)

monoclonal antibody (cA2) at a dose of 10 mg/kg, given over 2 hours. To evaluate the safety of a higher dose, the last 2 patients received 20 mg/kg of cA2.

Results.—One patient was excluded from efficacy evaluation because of incomplete data. Within 4 weeks after cA2 treatment, 8 of the remaining 9 patients showed normalization of Crohn's Disease Activity Index (CDAI) scores. Subjective symptoms improved after 1 week, and subjective scoring of response was good or excellent. The mean CDAI score decreased from 257 before treatment to 69 at week 8 (Fig 1). All previously observed ulcerations were found at videoendoscopy to have healed. Seven of the 8 responders were still in remission at week 8. In addition, extraintestinal manifestations of Crohn's disease, including arthritis, vanished with treatment. The infusion of cA2 was well tolerated and caused no adverse events. The single treatment failure was an elderly patient with persistent ulcers in the rectum.

Conclusion.—Treatment with cA2 was both safe and effective in these patients with Crohn's disease who had failed to respond to steroid treatment. A single infusion yielded an average response duration of 4 months. The success of cA2 supports the hypothesis that TNF plays a major role in the pathogenesis of the disease.

▶ This exciting report supports the hypothesis that TNF is of major importance in the pathogenesis of Crohn's disease. Although the number of patients treated with anti-TNF cA2 was small, the results were dramatic and suggest that cA2 may be useful in patients with Crohn's disease not responding to steroid treatment. This report also supports the concept that T-cell activation is quite important in the pathogenesis of Crohn's disease and that agents that interfere with T-cell activation might prove useful in the management of this disease.

N.J. Greenberger, M.D.

44 Colon

Incidence and Recurrence Rates of Colorectal Adenomas: A Prospective Study

Neugut AI, Jacobson JS, Ahsan H, Santos J, Garbowski GC, Forde KA, Treat MR, Waye J (Columbia Univ, New York; Mount Sinai School of Medicine, New York)

Gastroenterology 108:402–408, 1995 119-96-44–1

Introduction.—The frequency of adenomatous polyps (adenomas), the precursor lesions for most colorectal cancers, has been reported as prevalence rates based on autopsy or colonoscopy studies of symptomatic or high-risk patients. True incidence rates have been difficult to determine because most adenomas are asymptomatic. It has been assumed that the rate of recurrence is higher than the incidence rate of new adenomas, although there are no data on actual incidence or recurrence rates. Therefore, adenoma incidence and recurrence rates were prospectively determined in patients undergoing colonoscopy during a 2-year period.

Methods.—Clinical and demographic data were collected on all patients undergoing colonoscopy during the study. Of the 2,988 patients, 2,001 underwent colonoscopy extending at least to the splenic flexure and agreed to be interviewed regarding the colonoscopy findings. Of the 2,001 patients, 299 (case group) had at least 1 adenoma with no prior history of colon carcinoma, adenomas, or inflammatory bowel disease, and 508 (control group) had no colorectal neoplasia and no history of colorectal neoplasia or inflammatory bowel disease. Findings at subsequent colonoscopy, with a follow-up of up to 5 years, for patients in the 2 groups were analyzed to determine incidence and recurrence rates.

Results.—Repeat colonoscopies were performed on 19.4% of the control group and 59.5% of the case group during the follow-up. Among those who underwent follow-up studies, 24% of the control group and 46% of the case group had adenomas discovered at repeat colonoscopy. The risk of recurrence was highest in those with multiple adenomas on the initial colonoscopy (Fig 2).

Conclusions.—The first estimates of incidence rates for colorectal adenomas were reported, cumulatively approximating 16% for a 3-year period. The data support the assumption that the recurrence rate is significantly higher than the initial incidence rate, with the highest risk of recurrence occurring in patients with multiple adenomas at the initial

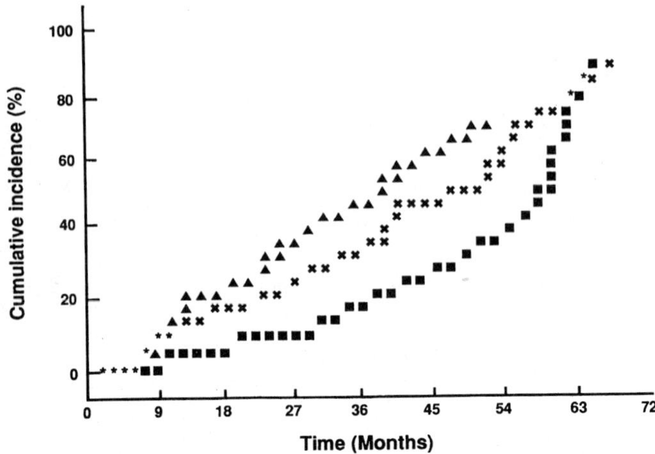

FIGURE 2.—Cumulative incidence rates of adenomatous polyps by time interval after initial colonoscopy. *Solid squares* indicate no adenomatous polyps; X, 1 adenomatous polyp; *solid triangles*, more than 1 adenomatous polyp. *Asterisk* indicates $P = 0.03$. (Courtesy of Neugut AI, Jacobson JS, Ahsan H, et al: Incidence and recurrence rates of colorectal adenomas: A prospective study. *Gastroenterology* 108:402–408, 1995.)

colonoscopy screening. These findings have significance for the design of chemoprevention trials and for recommendations for colorectal cancer screening.

▶ The following principal findings of this study bear emphasis:

- The recurrence rate was higher among patients with multiple adenomas at index colonoscopy
- The cumulative incidence rate for new adenomatous polyps after a normal colonoscopy was 16% at 3 years
- At a mean follow-up of 34 months, 46% of patients with adenoma detected at index colonoscopy had a recurrent adenoma
- The authors acknowledge that up to 10% of adenomas are missed on a single colonoscopy, and thus some of the incidence rate may represent missed adenomas.

N.J. Greenberger, M.D.

Aspirin and the Risk of Colorectal Cancer in Women

Giovannucci E, Egan KM, Hunter DJ, Stampfer MJ, Colditz GA, Willett WC, Speizer FE (Harvard Med School, Boston; Brigham and Women's Hosp, Boston; Harvard School of Public Health, Boston)

N Engl J Med 333:609–614, 1995 119-96-44–2

Introduction.—The results of research studies to determine the effect of aspirin use on the risk of colorectal cancer have been inconsistent. The possible correlation between colon and rectal cancers and aspirin usage was analyzed.

Methods.—Almost 90,000 women in the Nurses' Health Study with no diagnosis or any family history of colorectal cancer completed a baseline questionnaire on medication usage and diet. This was followed up every 2 years with another questionnaire on aspirin and other nonsteroidal anti-inflammatory drug usage. Cases of adenomatous polyps of both participants and their next of kin were documented. The association between aspirin use and the occurrence of a new colon or rectal cancer during a 12-year period was then analyzed.

Results.—During an 8-year period, 331 cases of not previously reported colorectal cancer were documented among women in the Nurses' Health Study. Individuals who in the initial questionnaire reported being regular aspirin users (those who took at least 2 aspirins per week) for 4 years did not have a lower risk of cancer development than did nonusers. A decrease in risk was observed for women who used aspirin regularly for at least 10 years, and this decrease became significant at 20 years of regular aspirin use. After controlling for other risk factors, women who on 3 consecutive questionnaires (which were filled out every 2 years) reported regular aspirin use were 38% less likely to have colorectal cancer develop. A significant inverse relationship was shown between the intake of 4–6 aspirins per week and the risk of development of colorectal cancer. These results are even more impressive because during the study, women who did take aspirin had a higher rate of endoscopy (Table 3).

Discussion.—In women, long-term use of aspirin (10 years or more) at a dosage of 4–6 tablets per week decreases the risk of colorectal cancer.

TABLE 3.—Frequency of Endoscopy and Detection of Adenomas According to the Level of Aspirin Use as Reported in 1980

Variable	Tablets per Week				
	0	1–3	4–6	7–14	>14
Endoscopy (% of cohort)*					
Before 1980	4.8	4.9	5.4	5.7	6.7
1980 or later					
Total	17.6	17.7	19.2	18.7	21.5
For fecal blood	4.7	4.6	5.2	5.3	6.6
Adenoma ≥ 1 cm (% of cohort)					
Total	0.40	0.37	0.42	0.35	0.38
Associated with fecal blood	0.19	0.15	0.19	0.19	0.21
Not associated with fecal blood	0.21	0.22	0.23	0.16	0.17
Adenoma ≥ 1 cm (% of those undergoing endoscopy)					
Total	2.3	2.1	2.2	1.8	1.8
Endoscopy for fecal blood	4.0	3.3	3.7	3.6	3.2
Endoscopy not for fecal blood	1.6	1.7	1.6	1.2	1.1

* Standardized for age according to the age distribution of the cohort.

(Reprinted by permission of *The New England Journal of Medicine*. Giovannucci E, Egan KM, Hunter DJ, et al: Aspirin and the risk of colorectal cancer in women. *N Engl J Med* 333:609–614, Copyright 1995, Massachusetts Medical Society.)

Endoscopy, which could lead to a possibly earlier detection of tumors, actually showed a decrease in the actual number of colorectal tumors among aspirin users. Possible mechanisms for the effect of aspirin in this instance include the inhibition of cyclooxygenase and subsequent inhibition of prostaglandin action, or the inhibition of phospholipase activity. Also, it has been documented that aspirin can modulate levels of prostaglandin levels in the rectal epithelium. Further research is needed, especially because low-dose aspirin has been shown to decrease the incidence of cardiovascular disease.

▶ This study showed a statistically significant reduction in the incidence of colorectal carcinoma in women who took 4–6 aspirin tablets per week for more than 10 years. As such, it mirrors similar findings reported in male aspirin users in whom a reduced incidence of colorectal carcinoma was also demonstrated.[1]

For an excellent brief review of the possible mechanisms whereby aspirin acts as a chemopreventive agent, see the editorial by Marcus.[2] Marcus postulates that it is possible that the effect of aspirin on neoplastic cells depends on its ability to change arachidonic acid metabolism, and perhaps also on interference with platelet function. He also makes the interesting recommendation that patients at risk for colorectal cancer (i.e., those with inflammatory bowel disease, previous adenoma, or large bowel cancer; a family history of colorectal cancer; or breast, ovarian, or endometrial cancer) should take a single 325-mg aspirin tablet every other day, assuming there are no contraindications to the use of aspirin. The ravages of colorectal cancer far exceed the possible complications of long-term treatment with aspirin.[2]

N.J. Greenberger, M.D.

References

1. Giovannuci E, Rim EB, Stampfer MJ, et al: Aspirin use and the risk for colorectal cancer and adenomas in male health professionals. *Ann Intern Med* 121:241–246, 1994.
2. Marcus AJ: Aspirin as prophylactic against colorectal cancer. *N Engl J Med* 333:656–657, 1995.

Fluorouracil Plus Levamisole as Effective Adjuvant Therapy After Resection of Stage III Colon Carcinoma: A Final Report

Moertel CG, Fleming TR, Macdonald JS, Haller DG, Laurie JA, Tangen CM, Ungerleider JS, Emerson WA, Tormey DC, Glick JH, Veeder MH, Mailliard JA (Mayo Clinic, Rochester, Minn; Fred Hutchinson Cancer Research Ctr, Seattle; Temple Univ, Philadelphia; et al)

Ann Intern Med 122:321–326, 1995 119-96-44–3

Introduction.—Most patients with carcinoma of the colon have completely grossly resectable disease. Adjuvant therapy may be used after potentially curative surgery to control any residual microscopic disease.

However, the most effective adjuvant regimen has not been established. The long-term effectiveness of a combination regimen of fluorouracil plus levamisole vs. levamisole alone was studied in patients who had surgically treated stage III disease.

Methods.—A total of 971 patients with stage III (Dukes stage C) colon cancer were randomly assigned to 1 of 3 treatment groups: observation only, levamisole alone, or levamisole plus fluorouracil. Treatment began after recovery from surgery. Patients in the group given levamisole only were given a 50-mg dose orally 3 times daily for 3 days; the regimen was repeated every 2 weeks for 1 year. Patients in the combination therapy group were given the same levamisole regimen plus 450 mg/m^2 body surface area of fluorouracil administered intravenously daily for 5 days, then weekly for 48 weeks.

Results.—All patients could be followed up for more than 5 years; the mean follow-up was 6.5 years. There have been recurrences in 177 of the 315 patients receiving no adjuvant treatment, in 172 of the 310 receiving levamisole alone, and in 119 of the 304 patients receiving fluorouracil plus levamisole. Patients receiving combination therapy had a strong recurrence-free interval benefit, whereas patients receiving levamisole had no increase in recurrence-free interval (Fig 1). Survival was similarly increased in the patients receiving combination therapy, who had a 33% reduction in mortality, whereas mortality was reduced by only 6% in patients treated with levamisole alone. Adverse reactions to levamisole were mild, infrequent, and reversible. Adverse reactions to combination therapy could be largely attributed to the use of fluorouracil and included nausea, infre-

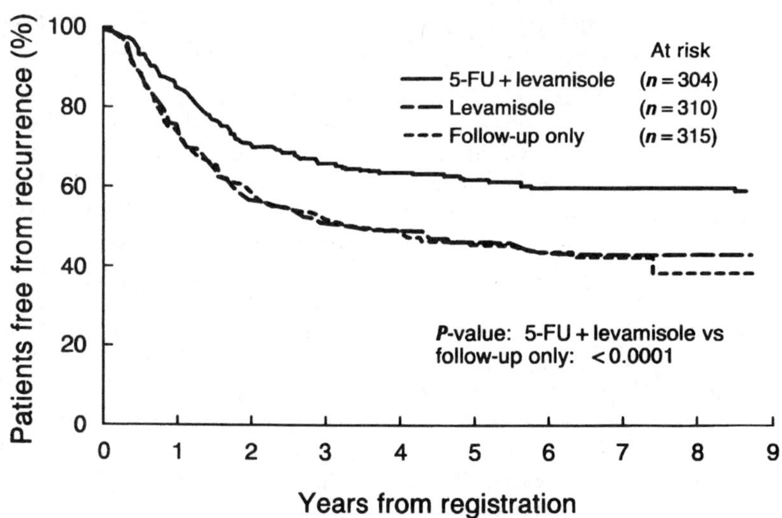

FIGURE 1.—Recurrence-free interval according to treatment arm. Patients who died without recurrence have been censored. *Abbreviation: 5-FU,* fluorouracil. (Courtesy of Moertel CG, Fleming TR, Macdonald JS: Fluorouracil plus levamisole as effective adjuvant therapy after resection of stage III colon carcinoma: A final report. *Ann Intern Med* 122:321–326, 1995.)

quent vomiting, stomatitis, diarrhea, dermatitis, fatigue, mild alopecia, and mild leukopenia. There was 1 drug-related death from profound leukopenia and sepsis in a patient given combination therapy. Mild, reversible abnormal liver function was observed in 40% of the patients receiving combination therapy.

Discussion.—The long-term follow-up clarifies that the 40% reduction in the recurrence rate seen in patients treated with a combination of levamisole and fluorouracil was not merely delayed; this treatment prevented recurrence. Similarly, the mortality rate is reduced by 33% with this adjuvant therapy regimen. Therefore, it is recommended that this regimen become standard management for postsurgical patients with stage III colon cancer.

► I would like to briefly recapitulate the major findings in this study. First, fluorouracil plus levamisole is tolerable adjuvant therapy to surgery. Second, this regimen has now been confirmed to substantially increase cure rates for patients with high-risk (stage III) colon cancer. Finally, the authors' recommendation that such a regimen should be considered standard treatment for all stage III patients not entered into clinical trials seems appropriate.

N.J. Greenberger, M.D.

Altered Rectal Perception Is a Biological Marker of Patients With Irritable Bowel Syndrome

Mertz H, Naliboff B, Munakata J, Niazi N, Mayer EA (Univ of California, Los Angeles; VA Sepulveda Med Ctr, Calif)

Gastroenterology 109:40–52, 1995 119-96-44–4

Objectives.—The usefulness of lowered visceral perception thresholds as a biological marker for irritable bowel syndrome (IBS) was studied. The prevalence and nature of altered rectal perception, the correlation of subjective symptoms with sensory thresholds for stool and discomfort, the existence of subgroups of IBS patients with different biological characteristics, the correlation between anal reflexes and physiology with rectal perception thresholds and symptoms, and the change with time in rectal sensory thresholds of patients with IBS were assessed.

Methods.—Fifteen normal controls and 100 patients with IBS completed a bowel symptom questionnaire regarding bowel habits, abdominal symptoms, and quality of life, and also completed the SCL-90 psychological symptom questionnaire to assess symptom severity. Fifteen patients who underwent both initial and 3-month follow-up rectal sensory testing completed a second questionnaire assessing retrospective changes in symptom severity. A computer-driven distention device and anorectal manometry were used to assess thresholds for the perception and intensity of sensations of stool (innocuous) and discomfort (aversive).

Results.—Altered perception of rapid-phase rectal distention appears to be a biological marker of IBS. Ninety-four percent of the patients with IBS

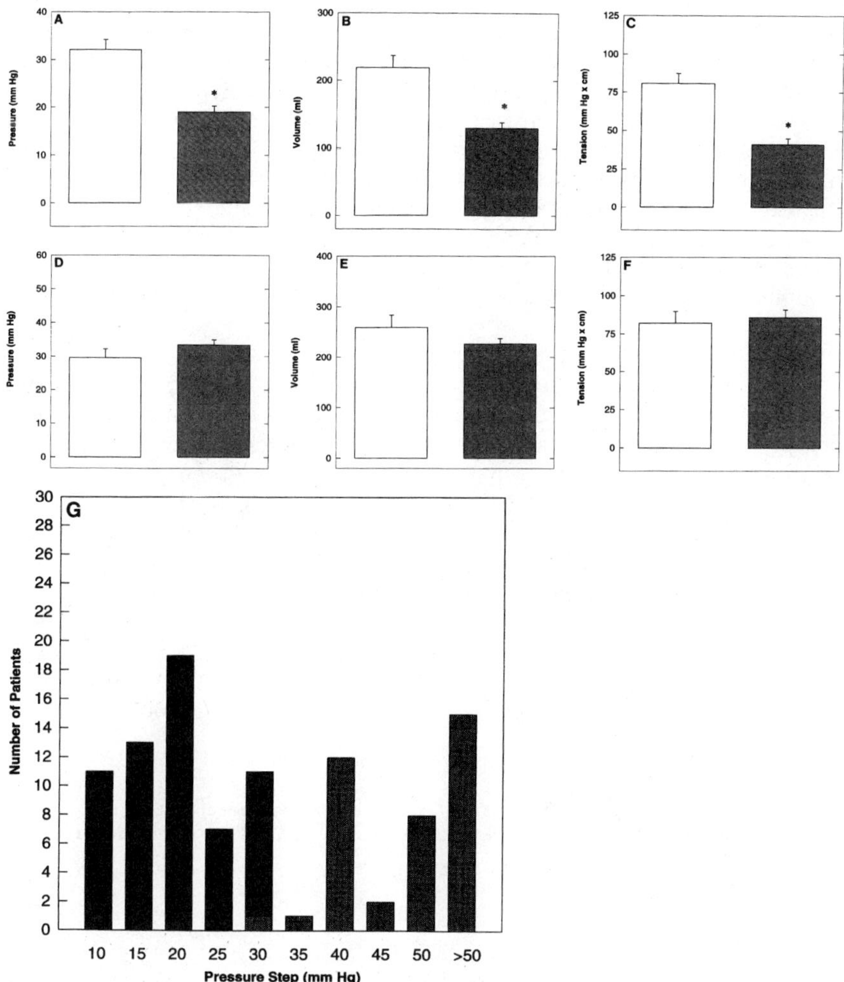

FIGURE 3.—Discomfort thresholds during rectal distention. **A–C**, during phasic distention, patients with irritable bowel syndrome (*IBS*) (*hatched bar*) have lower thresholds than normal controls (*open bar*) whether (**A**) pressure, (**B**) volume, or (**C**) tension is measured. Values are shown as mean ± SEM; $P < 0.001$. **D–F**, during slow ramp distention, patients with IBS and controls have similar thresholds. Values are shown as mean ± SEM. **G**, number of patients with low (*solid bar*) and normal (*crosshatched bar*) thresholds for discomfort at each pressure step during phasic distention. Normal threshold cutoff was based on 95% confidence interval for wall tension thresholds. There was overlap (1 patient) in threshold pressures between the 2 groups; median values for the 2 groups were separated by 6 pressure steps. Low threshold (n = 61): mean, 18 mm Hg; median, 20 mm Hg. Normal threshold (n = 39): mean, 47 mm Hg; median, 50 mm Hg. (Courtesy of Mertz H, Naliboff B, Munakata J, et al: Altered rectal perception is a biological marker of patients with irritable bowel syndrome. *Gastroenterology* 109:40–52, 1995.)

showed significantly lower thresholds for aversive sensations (intrarectal pressure, volume, or wall tension) than control subjects (Fig 3) , increased intensity ratings, or an altered viscerosomatic referral pattern. There were no differences between control and IBS patients with regard to thresholds for stool during rapid-phase rectal distention or for stool and discomfort during slow ramp distention (Fig 3). Viscerosomatic referral of sensation to the lower abdomen or suprapubic area was recorded by 79% of the IBS patients during rectal balloon distention, which often reproduced the patients' symptoms. In contrast, 93% of control subjects referred all sensations to the perianal area. Three IBS groups were identified by cluster analysis of physiologic parameters. The results of the 3-month follow-up indicate that an improvement in symptoms was associated with the development of normal thresholds in 36% of patients who were originally low-threshold individuals.

Conclusions.—Altered rectal perception is a reliable biological marker of IBS.

▶ These interesting observations indicate that altered rectal perception is present in almost all patients with IBS and that perception thresholds correlate with temporal changes in symptom severity, albeit determined retrospectively. Thus, visceral hyperalgesia may well represent a marker for IBS.

For an authoritative recent review on prognosis of IBS and the influence of the patient-physician interaction, see the article by Owens et al.[1] These investigators conclude that IBS is associated with a good prognosis, and the diagnosis is unlikely to be changed to that of an organic disease during follow-up. Furthermore, a positive physician-patient interaction may be related to reduced use of ambulatory health services by patients with IBS.

N.J. Greenberger, M.D.

Reference

1. Owens DM, Nelson DK, Talley NJ, et al: The irritable bowel syndrome: Long-term prognosis and the patient-physician interaction. *Ann Intern Med* 122:107–112, 1995.

45 Liver

Does the Healthy Hepatitis C Virus Carrier State Really Exist? An Analysis Using Polymerase Chain Reaction

Prieto M, Olaso V, Verdú C, Córdoba J, Gisbert C, Rayón M, Carrasco D, Berenguer M, Higón MD, Berenguer J (Hosp Universitario La Fe, Valencia, Spain)

Hepatology 22:413–417, 1995 119-96-45–1

Objectives.—Hepatitis C virus (HCV)–induced liver damage is not well understood. Reports exist of both HCV-associated hepatic damage and anti–HCV-positive individuals who appear healthy and have normal liver biopsy specimens. The relation between HCV viremia and the presence and severity of liver disease, and the prevalence of HCV RNA in the serum of anti–HCV-positive blood donors were studied.

Patients and Methods.—Ninety-eight blood donors who tested positive for anti-HCV antibodies and agreed to undergo a liver biopsy were studied. Anti-HCV antibodies were determined by enzyme-linked immunosorbent assay and confirmed by a second-generation recombinant immunoblot assay. Hepatitis C virus RNA was determined by a reverse transcription–polymerase chain reaction. Liver injury tests included aspartate transaminase (AST), alanine transaminase (ALT), alkaline phosphatase, and γ-glutamyl transpeptidase. Liver biopsy samples underwent histologic diagnosis.

Results.—Seventy-five percent of the asymptomatic anti–HCV-positive blood donors had histologic chronic hepatitis, and the amount of HCV RNA in serum from anti–HCV-positive blood donors correlated with the severity of liver injury (Fig 1). Only 3 blood donors had normal liver histology, 22 (22%) had minimal changes, and 73 (75%) had chronic hepatitis (1 with chronic lobular hepatitis, 40 with chronic persistent hepatitis [CPH], and 32 with chronic active hepatitis [CAH]). Hepatitis C virus RNA was detectable in 36% of the donors with minimal liver changes, 70% of those with CPH, and 87% of those with CAH, but it was not found in the 3 donors who had normal liver histology. Elevated serum levels of ALT were found in 4% of the donors with minimal liver changes, 45% of those with CPH, and 62% of those with CAH. There was no relationship between ALT levels and HCV RNA, but HCV RNA–positive donors had higher ALT levels than did HCV RNA–negative donors. Simi-

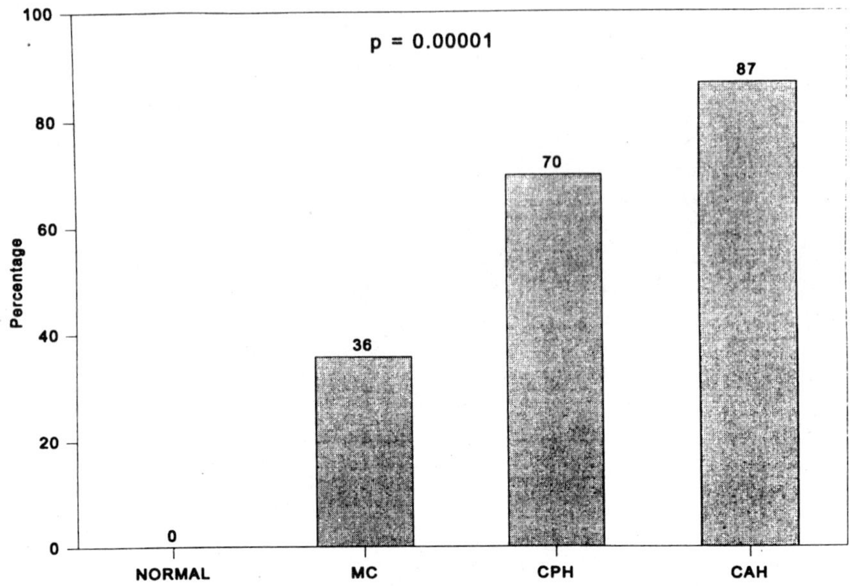

FIGURE 1.—Prevalence of hepatitis C virus (*HCV*) RNA in serum in anti–HCV-positive blood donors according to liver damage. *Abbreviations: MC,* minimal changes; *CPH,* chronic persistent hepatitis; *CAH,* chronic active hepatitis. (Courtesy of Prieto M, Olaso V, Verdú C, et al: Does the healthy hepatitis C virus carrier state really exist? An analysis using polymerase chain reaction. *Hepatology* 22:413–417, 1995.)

larly, HCV RNA–positive individuals had a significantly higher overall incidence of chronic hepatitis than HCV RNA–negative donors (88% vs. 50%).

Conclusions.—The prevalence of HCV RNA in anti–HCV-positive blood donors, but not serum ALT levels, correlates with the severity of liver injury. Also, a healthy HCV carrier state may exist as evidenced by the presence of HCV RNA in donors with minimal liver changes on biopsy specimens and normal serum ALT levels.

▶ Until recently, it was believed that asymptomatic HCV-positive patients who had a normal physical examination and normal liver tests, including serum aminotransferases, were unlikely to have significant changes in liver histology and did not need to be further evaluated. However, this paper by Prieto et al. and the following 2 abstracted articles (Abstracts 119-96-45–2 and 119-96-45–3) indicate that if such patients are viremic with positive tests for HCV RNA, there is a 50% to 75% likelihood of abnormal liver histology.

In a similar study by Shindo et al.,[1] 17 (89%) of 19 patients who were anti–HCV- and HCV RNA–positive with normal liver biochemical values showed histologic evidence of mild chronic hepatitis. Sookoian et al.[2] studied 58 HCV-positive blood donors. Of 26 patients with normal serum ALT values, liver biopsy specimens revealed normal findings or minimal lesions in 9, CPH in 13, CAH in 3, and cirrhosis in 1. Of 32 patients with raised ALT values, liver biopsy specimens showed CPH in 15 and CAH in 17. Several studies indicate that increased serum ALT values in HCV-positive patients correlate well with the presence of hepatic inflammation and fibrosis and indicate the need for liver biopsy.

N.J. Greenberger, M.D.

References

1. Shindo M, Arai K, Sokawa Y, et al: The virological and histological states of anti-hepatitis C virus-positive subjects with normal liver biochemical values (abstract). *Hepatology* 22:418–425, 1995.
2. Sookoian S, et al: Liver biopsy in anti-HCV(+) blood donors in Argentina. *Hepatology* 22:270A, 1995.

Liver Histology in Hepatitis C Infection: A Comparison Between Patients With Persistently Normal or Abnormal Transaminases

Healey CJ, Chapman RWG, Fleming KA (John Radcliffe Hosp, Oxford, England; Univ of Oxford, England)

Gut 37:274–278, 1995 119-96-45–2

Background.—Serologic tests have identified many individuals who are chronically infected by the hepatitis C virus (HCV) but who have minimal or no symptoms and normal liver biochemistry. Significant liver pathology may be demonstrated at biopsy, however, despite otherwise normal findings. To determine whether routine liver function tests can accurately reflect liver pathology, histologic findings were compared in 42 patients with HCV, 23 with abnormal liver function tests and 19 with persistently normal transaminases.

Patients and Methods.—All patients were positive for anti-HCV by second-generation enzyme-linked immunosorbent assay, had at least 3 serial estimations of serum aspartate transaminase (AST), and had undergone percutaneous liver biopsy. Abnormal liver function was defined as a transaminase activity greater than 45 IU/L at any testing occasion. Patients considered to have normal AST did not have transaminase activity above normal at any time. The risk factors present in each group included IV drug use, exposure to blood products, and sexual contact. Twenty-six of the 42 cases were detected at the time of blood donation, 8 had clinical disease, and 8 were referred because of known risk.

Results.—In the group of patients with normal AST activities, 2 (11%) had normal histologic examinations, 8 (43%) exhibited nonspecific reactive hepatitis, 6 (31%) had chronic persistent hepatitis, and 3 (16%) had chronic active hepatitis. Histologic examination in the group with abnormal liver biochemistry revealed chronic active hepatitis in 10 (43%), chronic persistent hepatitis in 6 (26%), reactive hepatitis in 5 (22%), and cirrhosis in 2 (9%). The group with abnormal liver function had a significantly higher average alcohol intake than the group with persistently normal AST.

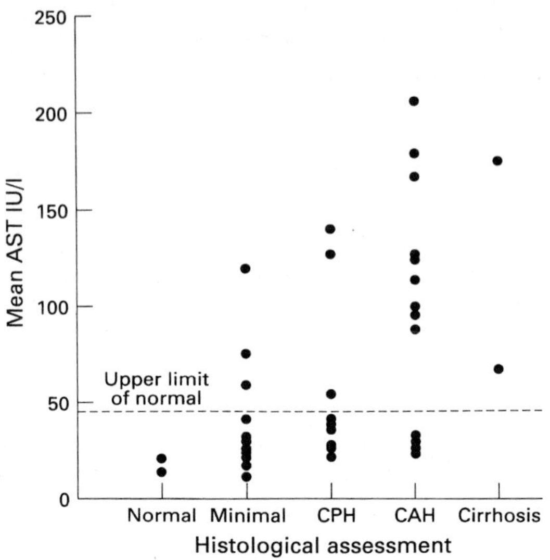

FIGURE 1.—Individual mean aspartate transaminase (*AST*) activities compared with histologic assessment in HCV infection. *Abbreviations: CPH,* chronic persistent hepatitis; *CAH,* chronic active hepatitis. (Courtesy of Healey CJ, Chapman RWG, Fleming KA: Liver histology in hepatitis C infection: A comparison between patients with persistently normal or abnormal transaminases. *Gut* 37:274–278, 1995.)

Conclusion.—Histologic findings showed significant liver pathology in patients with normal as well as abnormal liver biochemistry (Fig 1). Liver biopsy is therefore recommended in all cases of chronic HCV infection, even when liver transaminase values are persistently normal. Such a policy would help to identify those suitable for antiviral treatments and to inform patients of potentially beneficial changes in lifestyle.

▶ Recent studies indicate that 60% to 75% of hepatitis C–positive patients develop chronic hepatitis. This is more likely to occur in viremic individuals. Accordingly, HCV-positive patients should have a determination of HCV RNA. Until such assays become readily available at reasonable cost, one can obtain a confirmatory test, i.e., recombinant immunoblot assay (RIBA), with the inference that most RIBA-positive patients will be viremic. The question arises as to progression of liver disease in untreated asymptomatic individuals with normal serum aminotransferases. Ahmed et al.[1] addressed this question by carrying out serial liver biopsies 2 years apart in 29 such patients; 16 deteriorated, 4 improved, and 9 were unchanged. These and similar studies indicate that in asymptomatic RIBA-positive patients, initial histologic changes are mild. However, in many patients, there is a slow histologic progression over as short a period as 2 years. For additional information, as well as treatment recommendations, read the following article and comment.

N.J. Greenberger, M.D.

Reference

1. Ahmed MM: Histological progression of chronic hepatitis C virus (HCV), infection in untreated asymptomatic blood donors. *Hepatology* 22:2714, 1995.

Prevalence, Severity, and Risk Factors of Liver Disease in Blood Donors Positive in a Second-Generation Anti–Hepatitis C Virus Screening Test

Serfaty L, Nousbaum JB, Elghouzzi MH, Giral P, Legendre C, Poupon R (Hôpital Saint-Antoine, Paris; Hôpital Necker, Paris; Fondation Nationale de Transfusion Sanguine, Rungis, France)

Hepatology 21:725–729, 1995 119-96-45–3

Introduction.—The significance of anti–hepatitis C virus (HCV) enzyme-linked immunosorbent assay (ELISA) positivity in asymptomatic blood donors has not been established, particularly in regard to liver disease. The prevalence, severity, and risk factors of liver disease in a cohort of anti-HCV ELISA 2–positive donors were evaluated, according to the results of a confirmatory recombinant immunoblot assay (RIBA) 2 test.

Methods.—Of 132,769 consecutive blood donors, 483 tested positive for anti-HCV antibodies, using the HCV ELISA 2 test. Repeat and new donors accounted for 61% and 39% of reactivity, respectively. All HCV ELISA 2–positive donors were invited for a liver evaluation. Of 205 respondents, 98 were RIBA 2–positive, 35 were RIBA 2–indeterminate,

TABLE 2.—Epidemiologic, Serologic, and Histologic Characteristics of the 94 Anti-HCV ELISA 2–Positive Donors With Liver Biopsy, According to the RIBA 2 Test Results

	RIBA 2 Status		
Characteristics	Positive (n = 85)	Indeterminate (n = 6)	Negative (n = 3)
Age (yrs)*	39 ± 11	38 ± 7	46 ± 3
Sex ratio (M/F)	1.07	0.2	2
Transfusion (%)	30 (35)	4 (67)	0
IV drug abuse (%)	29 (34)	0	0
ALT† (IU/L, N < 35)*	49 ± 31	32 ± 28	18 ± 11
Anti-HBc + (%)	33 (39)	0	0
ELISA ratio*	5 ± 1.4	3.2 ± 1	1.9 ± 1.3
RIBA 2 Ab:			
5.1.1 + n (%)	55 (65)	0	0
C 100-3 + n (%)	58 (68)	1 (17)	0
C 33c + n (%)	79 (93)	1 (17)	0
C 22 3 + n (%)	85 (100)	4 (66)	0
Normal liver n (%)	4 (5)	3 (50)	3 (100)
CPH n (%)	30 (35)	2 (33)	0
CAH n (%)	45 (53)	1 (17)	0
Cirrhosis n (%)	6 (7)	0	0

* Mean ± standard deviation.

† At the time of donation.

Abbreviations: HCV, hepatitis C virus; *ELISA*, enzyme-linked immunosorbent assay; *RIBA*, recombinant immunoblot assay; *ALT*, alanine transaminase; *CPH*, chronic persistent hepatitis; *CAH*, chronic active hepatitis.

(Courtesy of Serfaty L, Nousbaum JB, Elghouzzi MH, et al: Prevalence, severity, and risk factors of liver disease in blood donors positive in a second-generation anti–hepatitis C virus screening test. *Hepatology* 21:725–729, 1995.)

TABLE 3.—Liver Disease According to ALT Activity in the RIBA 2–Positive Donors

	ALT Activity*		
	Elevated† (n = 72)	Normal (n = 13)	P*
Liver disease n (%)	71 (98.6)	10 (77)	.01
CPH n (%)	26 (36)	4 (30)	NS
CAH n (%)	39 (54)	6 (46)	NS
Cirrhosis n (%)	6 (9)	0 (0)	NS

* 3 consecutive assays, 2 months apart.
† At least once in the 3 assays.
‡ χ^2 test with Yates' correction.
Abbreviations: ALT, alanine transaminase; *RIBA*, recombinant immunoblot assay; *CPH*, chronic persistent hepatitis; *CAH*, chronic active hepatitis; *NS*, not significant.
(Courtesy of Serfaty L, Nousbaum JB, Elghouzzi MH, et al: Prevalence, severity, and risk factors of liver disease in blood donors positive in a second-generation anti–hepatitis C virus screening test. *Hepatology* 21:725–729, 1995.)

and 72 were RIBA 2–negative. Ninety-four of 107 donors to whom it was proposed underwent liver biopsy, and epidemiologic investigation, determination of alanine transaminase (ALT) activity, histologic investigation of liver biopsy specimens, and serum polymerase chain reaction (PCR) assay.

Results.—Eighty-five donors with liver biopsy were RIBA 2–positive. Of these, 81 had liver disease ranging from chronic persistent hepatitis to cirrhosis (Table 2). Three of 6 RIBA 2–indeterminant donors undergoing liver biopsy had liver disease (Table 2) compared with none of the 3 with negative RIBA 2 status (Table 2). Seventy-two (60%) RIBA 2–positive donors with liver biopsy had increased ALT activity, which increased to 85% after 2 supplemental assays (Table 3). The PCR indicated that 10 of 13 RIBA 2–positive donors with normal ALT activity had liver disease. Donors with cirrhosis were significantly different from other donors in age, sex ratio, alcohol consumption, and mean ALT activity in the 3 assays.

Conclusion.—Histologic examination of the liver is recommended when a RIBA 2 test is positive in a viremic donor. Serious liver disease can be present, despite normal ALT activity.

▶ Because asymptomatic anti-HCV–positive and HCV RNA–positive patients with normal aminotransferases often have significant hepatic histologic alterations, current recommendations call for such patients to undergo liver biopsy. However, interferon treatment is usually not recommended for those patients found to have minimal/mild hepatitis on liver biopsy. Such patients should be reviewed every 6 months and repeat liver biopsy done every 2–3 years.[1] If the biopsy specimens show worsening necroinflammatory disease or fibrosis or both, then treatment should be considered. These guidelines may well change within the next few years. In this regard, Booth et al.[1] point out that treatment in the early stages of HCV infection, when patients are asymptomatic with normal aminotransferases and minimal fibrosis on liver biopsy, offers the best opportunity for viral eradication. On the other hand, a reason for delaying treatment now stems from the rapid accumulation of data from numerous ongoing clinical trials and frequently changing recommendations. This is highlighted in Abstract 119-96-45–4.

N.J. Greenberger, M.D.

Reference

1. Booth JCL, et al: The management of chronic hepatitis C virus infection. *Gut* 37:440–454, 1995.

Clinical Outcomes After Transfusion-Associated Hepatitis C

Tong MJ, El-Farra NS, Reikes AR, Co RL (Huntington Mem Hosp, Pasadena, Calif)

N Engl J Med 332:1463–1466, 1995 119-96-45–4

Objective.—Because the natural course of chronic hepatitis C virus (HCV) infection acquired via blood transfusion remains uncertain, complications were examined in 131 such patients. Patients receiving multiple transfusions, intravenous drug users, those with HIV or hepatitis B infection, and those with alcoholic liver disease were excluded. The patients had an average age of 57 years when initially assessed and were an average of 35 years at the time they were transfused. The mean follow-up was nearly 4 years.

Observations.—Fatigue was by far the most common symptom. Only 2 of 67 patients with cirrhosis were jaundiced. Chronic hepatitis was present in 21% of patients, chronic active hepatitis in 23%, cirrhosis in 51%, and hepatocellular carcinoma in 5%. The interval between transfusion and histologic diagnosis was shortest for chronic hepatitis and longest for

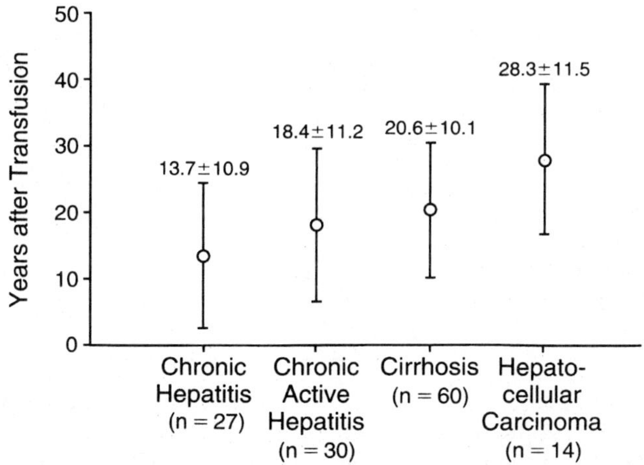

FIGURE 1.—Mean (± standard deviation) interval from blood transfusion to the diagnosis of diseases associated with hepatitis C in 131 patients. (Reprinted by permission of *The New England Journal of Medicine.* Tong MJ, El-Farra NS, Reikes AR, et al: Clinical outcomes after transfusion-associated hepatitis C. *N Engl J Med* 332:1463–1466, Copyright 1995, Massachusetts Medical Society).

hepatocellular carcinoma (Fig 1). Twenty patients died during follow-up, including 8 of complications of cirrhosis and 11 of hepatocellular carcinoma. Three patients with cirrhosis survived after undergoing orthotopic liver transplantation.

Implications.—Hepatitis C virus infection is a progressive disease that sometimes culminates in death from either liver failure or hepatocellular carcinoma. If blood products were screened for HCV, the risk of post-transfusion infection would be substantially reduced. Those already infected should receive antiviral treatment.

► In a group of patients seen at a referral hospital, chronic hepatitis C was a progressive disease and, in some patients, led to death from liver failure or hepatocellular carcinoma. Elimination of HCV would seem to be the most logical goal of therapy, not only to halt progression of the disease but also to reduce the likelihood of developing hepatocellular carcinoma. Evidence is accumulating in support of the concept that eradication of HCV, as documented by loss of HCV RNA, results in a decreased prevalence of hepatocellular carcinoma. Ishibashi et al.[1] followed 217 patients with chronic hepatitis C treated with interferon (INF); 44 patients had chronic persistent hepatitis and 173 patients had chronic active hepatitis. The patients were followed up 12 months after completion of INF therapy and were evaluated with ultrasound or CT. Diagnosis of hepatocellular carcinoma was confirmed by needle biopsy. Sixty-one patients were classified as responders and 156 as nonresponders to INF therapy. Four cases of hepatocellular carcinoma developed, all in nonresponders. These studies support the concept that INF therapy for chronic hepatitis C that results in eradication of HCV can retard the development of liver cirrhosis and hepatocellular carcinoma.

N.J. Greenberger, M.D.

Reference

1. Ishibashi K: Decreased prevalence of hepatocellular carcinoma in chronic hepatitis C after interferon therapy: Comparison between the responders and non-responders (abstract). *Hepatology* 22:173A, 1995.

Hepatic Hepatitis C Virus RNA as a Predictor of a Long-Term Response to Interferon-α Therapy

Shindo M, Arai K, Sokawa Y, Okuno T (Akashi Municipal Hosp, Japan; Kyoto Insts of Technology, Japan)

Ann Intern Med 122:586–591, 1995 119-96-45-5

Objective.—Factors predicting a long-term response were sought in 90 patients with chronic hepatitis C who were treated with interferon-α (INF-α). All the patients had a serum aminotransferase value at least 1.5 times the upper normal limit as well as histologically confirmed chronic hepatitis. All had antibody to hepatitis C virus (HCV) and HCV RNA in their sera, and they were negative for hepatitis B surface antigen.

TABLE 2.—Hepatitis C Virus (HCV) in Long-Term Responders to Interferon-α

Patient	Genotype	Serum HCV RNA*			Liver HCV RNA*			Liver Histologic Results		
		Before Therapy	After Therapy	1 Year After Therapy	Before Therapy	After Therapy	1 Year After Therapy	Before Therapy	After Therapy	1 Year After Therapy
1	III	3	Neg	Neg	3	Neg	Neg	CAH moderate	CPH	CPH
2	II	1	Neg	Neg	3	Neg	Neg	CAH moderate	NSRH	Normal
3	IV	3	Neg	Neg	2	Neg	Neg	CAH mild	CPH	NSRH
4	II	5	Neg	2	4	Neg	4	CAH mild	CPH	CPH
5	II	3	2	1	4	2	1	CPH	CPH	CPH
6	UC	3	Neg	Neg	4	Neg	Neg	CAH moderate	CPH	CPH
7	II	2	Neg	Neg	3	Neg	Neg	CAH severe	CAH mild	CPH
8	UC	1	Neg	Neg	3	Neg	Neg	CAH moderate	CPH	CPH
9	II	1	Neg	Neg	5	Neg	Neg	CPH	CPH	NSRH
10	II	3	Neg	Neg	3	Neg	Neg	CAH mild	NSRH	Normal
11	UC	2	Neg	Neg	3	Neg	Neg	CAH mild	NSRH	NSRH
12	II	3	Neg	Neg	3	Neg	2	CAH moderate	CPH	CPH
13	UC	1	Neg	Neg	3	Neg	Neg	CAH mild	NSRH	NSRH
14	III	2	Neg	Neg	6	Neg	Neg	CAH mild	CPH	NSRH
15	II	5	Neg	Neg	6	Neg	Neg	CAH mild	NSRH	Normal
16	III	2	Neg	Neg	3	Neg	Neg	CAH severe	CAH moderate	CPH
17	II	1	Neg	Neg	3	Neg	Neg	CAH severe	CPH	NSRH
18	III	3	Neg	Neg	4	Neg	Neg	CAH moderate	NSRH	NSRH
19	II	1	Neg	Neg	6	Neg	Neg	CAH moderate	NSRH	NSRH
20	UC	1	Neg	Neg	3	Neg	Neg	CAH moderate	NSRH	NSRH
21	IV	2	Neg	Neg	3	Neg	Neg	CPH	NSRH	Normal
22	II	1	Neg	Neg	2	Neg	Neg	CAH severe	CPH	CPH
Mean titer		2.1 ± 1.3			3.6 ± 1.2					

Note: Means are expressed ± standard deviation.
* Titers of HCV RNA in the serum and the liver are expressed as $\log_{10}$ per 50 μL of serum and as $\log_{10}$ per 1.5 μL of liver RNA, respectively.
Abbreviations: CAH, chronic acute hepatitis; *CPH*, chronic persistent hepatitis; *NSRH*, nonspecific reactive hepatitis; *neg*, negative; *UC*, unclassified type.
(Courtesy of Shindo M, Arai K, Sokawa Y, et al: Hepatic hepatitis C virus RNA as a predictor of a long-term response to interferon-α therapy. *Ann Intern Med* 122:586–591, 1995.)

Methods.—Human natural lymphoblastoid INF-α was given intramuscularly in a dosage of 6 MU 3 times weekly for 6 months. Viral titers were estimated in liver tissue and sera using the reverse transcriptase–polymerase chain reaction technique.

Results.—Twenty-two patients had normal serum levels of aminotransferase for more than 1 year after treatment. Twenty-five others responded transiently. Hepatitis C virus RNA was no longer detected in the liver or serum samples from 21 of the 22 long-term responders. It remained undetectable in the serum after 12 months in 91% of these patients and in the liver in 86% (Table 2). Liver histology was substantially less abnormal at 1 year, but a large majority of patients continued to have mild changes of chronic hepatitis. Hepatitis C virus RNA persisted in the liver of 76% of transient responders at the end of treatment, and in the serum of 36%. On multivariate analysis, the presence of HCV RNA in liver tissue at the end of treatment correlated with an increased risk of relapse.

Conclusion.—Hepatitis C virus infection is eradicated in most patients with chronic hepatitis C who are long-term responders to INF-α. Persistence of virus in the liver at the end of a course of treatment is a significant predictor of relapse.

▶ Several studies have demonstrated that several factors predict both an initial and a sustained response to INF-α treatment. These include viral level as evidenced by HCV RNA titer; HCV genotype; early clearance of HCV RNA; presence of cirrhosis; dose and duration of INF therapy; co-infection with multiple genotypes and/or hepatitis B; and presence or development of autoantibodies. Considerable attention has been devoted to HCV RNA titer and HCV genotype. Two key observations have been made:

- Persistence of HCV RNA negatively impacts outcome
- Certain genotypes, especially type 1B, are associated with significantly decreased response rates.

Three recent studies[1-3] highlight these findings.

N.J. Greenberger, M.D.

References

1. Carreno V, et al: Four year follow-up of patients with chronic hepatitis C treated with Interferon α (abstract). *Hepatology* 22:173A, 1995.
2. Takahashi M, et al: Long-term biochemical, virological and histological follow-up in patients with chronic hepatitis C treated with Interferon (abstract). *Hepatology* 22:174A, 1995.
3. Martinot M, et al: Predictors of response to alpha Interferon in chronic hepatitis: A multivariate analysis in 287 patients (abstract). *Hepatology* 22:174A, 1995.

Influence of the Genotypes of Hepatitis C Virus on the Severity of Recurrent Liver Disease After Liver Transplantation

Féray C, Gigou M, Samuel D, Paradis V, Mishiro S, Maertens G, Reynés M, Okamoto H, Bismuth H, Bréchot C (Paris South Univ, Villejuif, France; Hôpital Paul Brousse, Villejuif, France; Jinchi Med School, Tokyo; et al)

Gastroenterology 108:1088–1096, 1995 119-96-45–6

Introduction.—Hepatitis C virus (HCV) is now known to have at least 6 major genotypes, but the clinical relevance of these genotypes has yet to be determined. Orthotopic liver transplantation performed for HCV-related cirrhosis offers an opportunity for prospective investigation of the infection of normal livers by different types of HCV. The immunosuppressive regimen results in a high level of viral replication with infection of the allograft by HCV.

Patients and Methods.—From October 1985 to September 1991, 60 anti-HCV–positive patients underwent liver transplantation. The group included 51 men and 9 women with a mean age of 47 years. Forty-nine had end-stage cirrhosis and 11 had cirrhosis with hepatocellular carcinoma. Transfusions were the definite source of HCV infection in 4 patients and the possible source in 18. Precise surveillance of clinical, laboratory, and histologic parameters was available in all cases. Type-specific capsid primers and a line probe genotyping assay were used to determine HCV genotype.

Results.—Before transplantation, genotypes 1a, 1b, 2a, and 3a were detected in 12, 41, 5, and 1 of the 60 patients, respectively. One of the patients could not be classified. Forty-one patients had evidence of recurrent liver disease after transplantation. Acute hepatitis developed in 31 of the 40 patients infected by HCV type 1b after transplantation; 24 infected by type 1b had chronic active hepatitis. Among the 20 patients infected by other genotypes, acute hepatitis developed in 8 and chronic active hepatitis developed in 4. Three years after transplantation, the actuarial rates of acute and chronic active hepatitis were significantly higher in patients infected by type 1b than in those infected by other types (77% and 59% vs. 40% and 22%, respectively). The level of HCV viremia and HCV genotypes showed no statistical relation, either before or after transplantation. Patients in whom hepatitis developed after transplantation, however, had significantly increased serum HCV RNA values.

Conclusion.—Liver graft recipients infected by HCV type 1b were more likely than patients infected by other genotypes to have an aggressive course of recurrent infection after transplantation. Acute hepatitis resolved in only 1 of the 31 patients infected by type 1b; in contrast, 3 of 8 patients infected by other types had resolution of acute hepatitis. The marked differences observed in the relative pathogenicity of different HCV genotypes may have implications for the management of liver transplantation.

► Bravo and colleagues[1] have investigated the role of HCV genotypes in liver damage. Hepatitis C virus genotypes were determined and liver histology scored using the Knodell index in 78 patients. Thirty-two patients had co-infection with more than 1 genotype; this was most likely because 80% of the study population were former IV drug users. Patients carrying more than 1 HCV genotype had a higher probability of severe liver disease. When liver damage was stratified according to genotype 1b, a strong correlation was found between severe liver damage and this genotype. The authors conclude that both genotype 1b and co-infection with several HCV genotypes are associated with more severe liver histologic alterations in patients with chronic hepatitis C.

N.J. Greenberger, M.D.

Reference

1. Bravo R, et al: Coinfection with several HCV genotypes enhance liver damage in patients with chronic hepatitis C (abstract). *Hepatology* 22:273A, 1995.

A Comparison of Three Interferon Alfa-2b Regimens for the Long-Term Treatment of Chronic Non-A, Non-B Hepatitis

Poynard T, Bedossa P, Chevallier M, Mathurin P, Lemonnier C, Trepo C, Couzigou P, Payen JL, Sajus M, Costa JM, Vidaud M, Chaput JC, and the Multicenter Study Group (Hôpital de Bicêtre, Paris; Centre Natl de la Recherche Scientifique, Paris; Institut Pasteur, Lyons, France; et al)
N Engl J Med 332:1457–1462, 1995 119-96-45-7

Introduction.—Interferon-α (INF-α) reduces the serum levels of alanine aminotransferase in patients with chronic hepatitis C virus (HCV) infection, but it is not clear that these values accurately predict the state of the liver.

Objective.—One of 3 regimens of INF-α 2b treatment was administered for 18 months to consecutive patients with a histologic diagnosis of chronic non-A, non-B hepatitis and a serum alanine aminotransferase value more than 1.5 times normal. All patients received 3 million units subcutaneously 3 times weekly for 6 months. Subsequently, 103 patients (group 1) received the same treatment for 12 months longer; 101 (group 2) received 1 million units 3 times weekly for 1 year; and 99 (group 3) received no further treatment. Group 3 patients whose serum enzyme levels were increased for 3 consecutive months received the initial regimen.

Results.—Serum aminotransferase values at 18 months were normal in 45% of patients in group 1, 27% of those in group 2, and 30% of patients in group 3. Observation for up to 42 months showed that 22%, 10%, and 8% of these groups, respectively, continued to have normal serum enzyme values. Liver biopsy at 18 months demonstrated histologic improvement in 70% of patients in group 1, 48% of those in group 2, and 39% of patients in group 3 (Fig 1). Fully 61% of patients who had not responded at 6 months did have improved histology at 18 months. Similar responses were found in patients who did not respond at 3 months. Patients in group 1

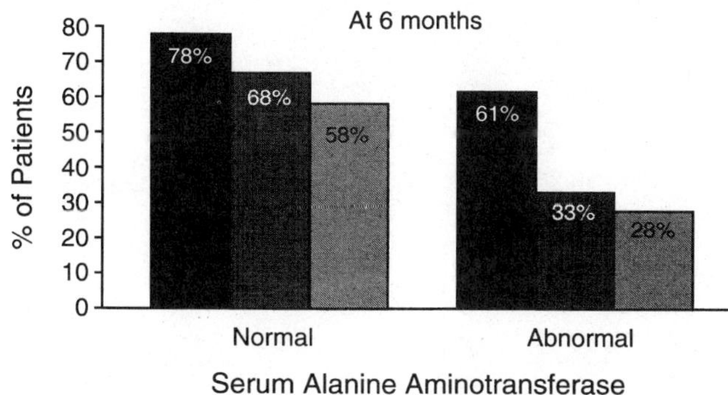

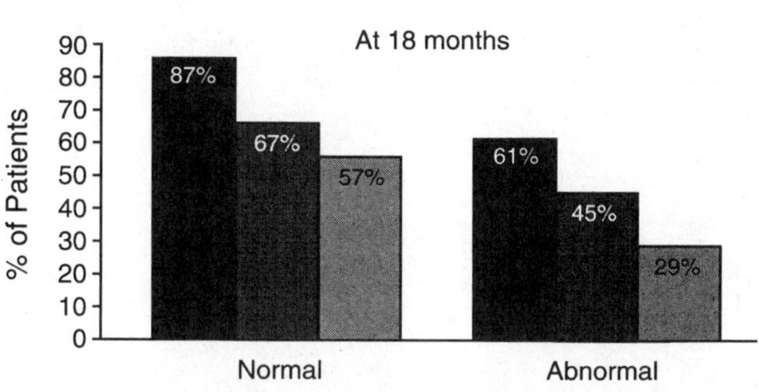

FIGURE 1.—Histologic improvement at 18 months in the 3 treatment groups, according to the serum alanine aminotransferase response at 6 months (**upper panel**) and 18 months (**lower panel**). (Reprinted by permission of *The New England Journal of Medicine.* Poynard T, Bedossa P, Chevallier M, et al: A comparison of three interferon alfa-2b regimens for the long-term treatment of chronic non-A, non-B hepatitis. *N Engl J Med* 332:1457–1462, Copyright 1995, Massachusetts Medical Society.)

had progressively better responses as time passed (Table 2). Significant adverse effects occurred in about one third of patients in all groups.

Conclusion.—The optimal regimen of INF-α 2b for patients with HCV infection consists of 3 million units 3 times a week for 18 months.

► A recent meta-analysis[1] of INF treatment of chronic hepatitis C indicates that the dose and duration of therapy clearly influence outcome. Niederau et al. analyzed 52 randomized trials of INF-α in chronic non-A, non-B, and C hepatitis, enrolling 3,749 patients. The key findings are as follows:

- Initial normalization of serum alanine aminotransferase (ALT) levels (1,499/2,927) (51.2%)
- Sustained normalization of ALT (482/2,218) (21.7%)
- Interferon treatment for more than 9 months (29.4%)
- Interferon treatment for less than 6 months (14.6%)

TABLE 2.—Normal Serum Alanine Aminotransferase Concentrations (Intention-to-Treat Analysis), Disappearance of Serum Hepatitis C Virus, and Residual Viremia

Group	Normal Serum Alanine Aminotransferase				No Serum Hepatitis C Virus	Residual Viremia (Branched DNA)*
	At 6 mo	At 18 mo	Between 7 and 18 mo	After treatment (19–42 mo)	After treatment	After treatment
	No. of patients (%)				No. of patients/total no. (%)	Mean ± SE
1 (n = 103)	51 (49.5)	46 (44.7)†	25 (24.3)‡	23 (22.3)§	17/26 (65.4)¶	18 ± 13 (n = 26)‖
2 (n = 101)	41 (40.6)	27 (26.7)	15 (14.9)	10 (9.9)	8/29 (27.6)	30 ± 9 (n = 29)
3 (n = 99)	38 (38.4)	30 (30.3)	7 (7.1)	8 (8.1)	9/29 (31.0)	32 ± 10 (n = 29)
Chi-square	2.8	8.2	11.4	10.5	10.5	
P value	0.23	0.02	0.003	0.005	0.005	0.008

* Expressed in multiples of 10^5 equivalent viral copies per milliliter.
† For group 1 vs. group 2, P = 0.008; for group 1 vs. group 3, P = 0.04.
‡ For group 1 vs. group 3, P < 0.001.
§ For group 1 vs. group 2, P = 0.02; for group 1 vs. group 3, P = 0.005.
¶ For group 1 vs. group 2, P = 0.005; for group 1 vs. group 3, P = 0.01.
‖ For group 1 vs. group 2, P = 0.003; for group 1 vs. group 3, P = 0.003.
(Reprinted by permission of *The New England Journal of Medicine*. Poynard T, Bedossa P, Chevaillier M, et al: A comparison of three interferon alfa-2b regimens for the long-term treatment of chronic non-A, non-B hepatitis. *N Engl J Med* 332:1457–1462, Copyright 1995, Massachusetts Medical Society.)

- Total INF dose greater than 240 million units (30.6%)
- Total INF dose less than 240 million units (10.8%)

Niederau et al. conclude that widely used therapy schedules, such as 3 million units of INF given thrice weekly for 6 months, result in insufficient long-term responses. This further affirms the conclusion drawn by Poynard et al. Future studies should focus on longer-term treatment and weekly doses exceeding 9 million units of INF.

N.J. Greenberger, M.D.

Reference

1. Niederau C, et al: Treatment of chronic non-A, non-B and C hepatitis with α interferon: A meta analysis of dose and duration. *Hepatology* 22:153A, 1995.

Hepatitis C Virus (HCV) Genotype, Tissue HCV Antigens, Hepatocellular Expression of HLA-A,B,C, and Intercellular Adhesion-1 Molecules: Clues to Pathogenesis of Hepatocellular Damage and Response to Interferon Treatment in Patients With Chronic Hepatitis C

Ballardini G, Groff P, Pontisso P, Giostra F, Francesconi R, Lenzi M, Zauli D, Alberti A, Bianchi FB (Univ of Bologna, Italy; Univ of Padova, Italy)

J Clin Invest 95:2067–2075, 1995 119-96-45–8

Background.—Recent studies of hepatocellular damage from hepatitis C virus (HCV) suggest that T cells have an important role in this process. Approximately half of the patients treated with α-interferon (α-INF), especially those infected by particular HCV genotypes and those with less intense viremia, have a primary response.

Objective and Methods.—The virologic and immunologic aspects of HCV infection were studied in 38 consecutive patients treated with either recombinant or lymphoblastoid α-INF, 24 of whom exhibited a primary response. These patients had normal transaminase levels and no serum HCV RNA 3 months after treatment. Twelve patients later relapsed. The HCV genotype was determined, and HCV-positive hepatocytes were quantified in liver tissue. In addition, the distribution of HLA-A,B,C and intercellular adhesion-1 molecules (ICAM-1) was studied, and CD8 T cells were counted.

Findings.—Patients infected by types 3, 1a, and 2 HCV were likelier than those with type 1b HCV to respond to INF treatment. Nonresponders had higher numbers of HCV-positive hepatocytes and expressed more HLA-A,B,C and ICAM-1 than did the patients who responded to treatment. Hepatitis C virus–related antigens were identified in liver tissue in 93% of nonresponders but also in 75% of responders. The presence of antigen could not be related to the clinical, histologic, or biochemical features of HCV infection. CD8-positive T cells were seen in contact with

TABLE 3.—CD8 T Cells in Relation to α-IFN Response, Tissue HCV Score, and HCV Genotype

		α-IFN response		Tissue HCV score				HCV genotype			
		NR	R	0	1	2	3	1b	1a	2	3
CD8, foci/10 mm^2	8.2	6.8	8.5	8.0	11.8	10.0	6.3	7.2	12.4	8.7	9.0
CD8, lobular/mm^2	84	84	98	72	121	93	76	80	75	80	129
ALT	105	105	102	83	168	97	86	86	174	142	139

Note: ALT, normal value, < 37 units/L. Data are reported as median values.

A significant correlation ($P < 0.03$) is found between ALT levels and the number of lobular CD8 T cells. Higher ALT levels (Wilcoxon rank sum test, $P < 0.001$) and higher numbers of lobular CD8 T cells (NS) were found in patients with tissue HCV score 1 vs. 3. Higher numbers of lobular CD8 T cells (Wilcoxon rank sum test, $P < 0.05$) and higher ALT levels (NS) were found in patients infected by genotype 3 vs. 1b.

Abbreviations: IFN, interferon; *HCV*, hepatitis C virus; *ALT*, alanine aminotransferase; *NS*, not significant.

(Courtesy of Ballardini G, Groff P, Pontisso P, et al: Hepatitis C virus (HCV) genotype, tissue HCV antigens, hepatocellular expression of HLA-A,B,C, and intercellular adhesion-1 molecules: Clues to pathogenesis of hepatocellular damage and response to interferon treatment in patients with chronic hepatitis C. *J Clin Invest* 95-2067–2075, 1995.)

infected hepatocytes, and the number of lobular cells of this type correlated with the level of alanine aminotransferase (Table 3).

Implications.—It appears that cytotoxicity mediated by T cells is a key aspect of liver cell damage in patients with HCV infection. A high level of viral replication in unresponsive patients infected by HCV type 1b may lead to a high level of expression of endogenous INF-inducible antigens such as HLA-A,B,C molecules. Exogenous INF may suppress viral replication when the endogenous INF system is not activated in this way.

▶ The data obtained in this study confirm previous observations indicating that patients infected with HCV genotype 1b display higher numbers of HCV-positive hepatocytes, which is probably linked to the lower response rate to INF treatment. The authors also emphasize that in patients with low activation of the endogenous INF system, *exogenous* INF might be successful in inhibiting viral replication, thereby moving the balance in favor of the immune system and facilitating the elimination of infected cells.

N.J. Greenberger, M.D.

High Prevalence of Serological Markers of Autoimmunity in Patients With Chronic Hepatitis C

Clifford BD, Donahue D, Smith L, Cable E, Luttig B, Manns M, Bonkovsky HL (Univ of Massachusetts Med Ctr, Worcester; Medizinische Hochschule Hannover, Germany)

Hepatology 21:613–619, 1995 119-96-45–9

Introduction.—Because treatment of hepatitis C (HCV) is so different from that of autoimmune hepatitis, it is important that they be diagnosed accurately. The pattern, prevalence, and clinical importance of serologic markers were defined in patients with chronic HCV, and these findings were compared with those of patients with liver diseases from other causes.

Methods.—The medical records of 244 unselected adult patients were retrospectively reviewed for HCV antibodies by second-generation enzyme immunoassay (EIA2) and/or 4-antigen recombinant immunoblot assay (RIBA). The age range of the 117 patients who met the criteria was 20–81 years. Laboratory data were reviewed for antimitochondrial antibodies (AMAs), antinuclear antibodies (ANAs), smooth-muscle antibodies (SMAs), cryoglobulins, and rheumatoid factor (RF). Sera from 41 patients had been tested for antibodies to antigens identified in microsomal preparations of liver and kidney (anti-LKM antibodies).

Results.—Forty-three of 65 patients tested for SMAs had a titer greater than or equal to 1:20. Thirty-five of 46 patients tested for RF had a titer greater than or equal to 1:160. Less frequently observed positive titers were as follows: ANAs, 13 of 92 patients with titers greater than or equal to 1:80; AMA, 1 of 48 patients with titers greater than or equal to 1:40; and cryoglobulins, 9 of 68 patients with titers greater than or equal to 5% (Fig 2). Forty of 41 patients tested for anti-LKM antibodies had negative

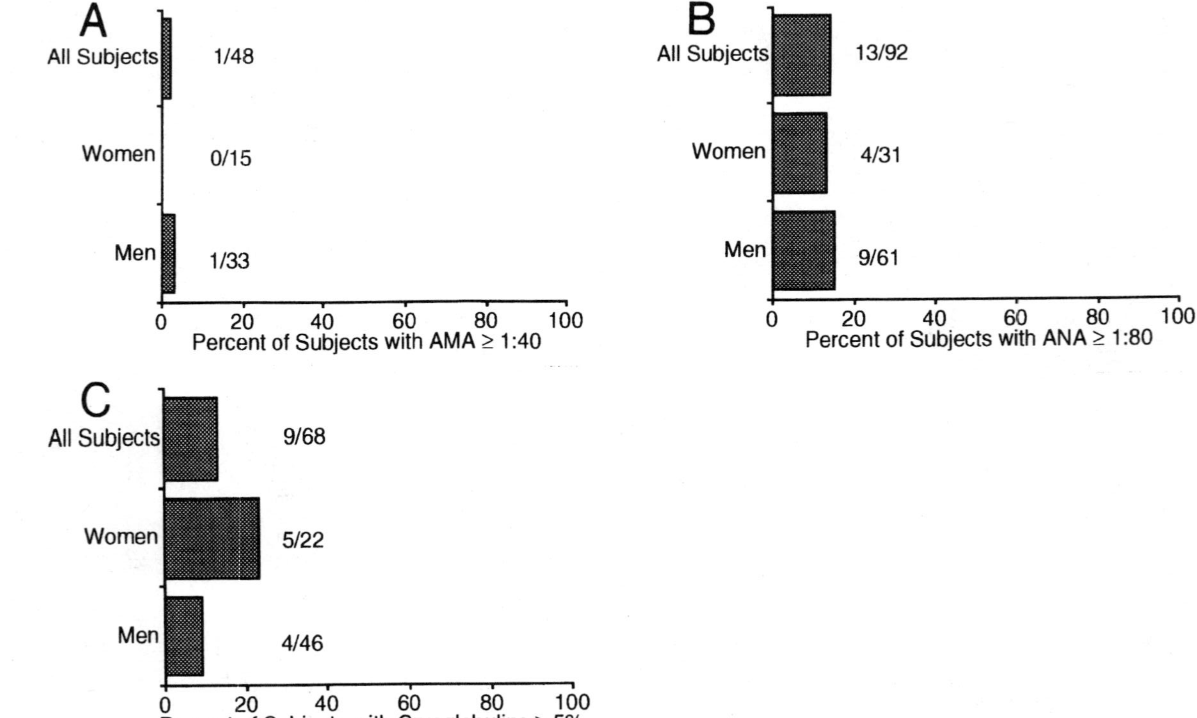

FIGURE 2.—Prevalence of antimicrobial antibodies (*AMAs*), antinuclear antibodies (*ANAs*), and cryoglobulins in patients with chronic hepatitis C virus (*HCV*). Blood samples were obtained from unselected patients with chronic HCV. The numbers to the right of the bars are the numbers of patients positive/total number tested. (Courtesy of Clifford BD, Donahue D, Smith L, et al: High prevalence of serological markers of autoimmunity in patients with chronic hepatitis C. *Hepatology* 21:613–619, 1995.)

results. When results of the prevalence of ANA, SMA, and AMA positivity for several liver diseases were combined with other series, it was found that the prevalence of SMA in chronic HCV was striking and also similar to that found in cryptogenic cirrhosis. No patients treated with interferon-α who had positive autoimmune markers had a worsening of disease.

Conclusion.—In patients with HCV, there was a high prevalence of autoimmune markers that were not specific for age or sex. The presence of these markers should not eliminate the use of interferon therapy. Patients should, however, be followed closely.

► That exacerbations of apparent autoimmune disease in patients with chronic viral hepatitis C can occur after initiation of treatment with interferon is described in the following article and the accompanying comment.

N.J. Greenberger, M.D.

Latent Autoimmune Hepatitis Triggered During Interferon Therapy in Patients With Chronic Hepatitis C

García-Buey L, García-Monzón C, Rodriguez S, Borque MJ, García-Sánchez A, Iglesias R, DeCastro M, Mateos FG, Vicario JL, Balas A, Moreno-Otero R (Universidad Autónoma de Madrid; Centro de Transfusiones de la CAM, Madrid)

Gastroenterology 108:1770–1777, 1995 119-96-45–10

Background.—Treatment with interferon (IFN) reduces serum levels of aminotransferase and improves liver histology in patients with chronic hepatitis C (CHC) infection; it also impedes viral replication. Prolonged treatment may, however, induce autoantibody formation and result in autoimmune disease, possibly directed against the liver. Hepatitis C virus (HCV) infection may be associated with autoimmunity.

Objective.—The findings were reviewed in 7 patients with autoimmune hepatitis (AIH) who initially received a diagnosis of true chronic active hepatitis C and who received IFN-α. Recombinant or lymphoblastoid IFN-α was given in a dose of 5–6 MU 3 times weekly for 2 months, followed by 3 MU 3 times a week for 10 months. The patients were among 144 with CHC who received IFN therapy.

Findings.—The 7 patients, all women, had a mean age of 42 years. Six had epidemiologic risk factors for HCV infection—4 received blood and 2 had major surgery. These patients had especially marked hepatitic activity and fibrosis. Most biopsy specimens revealed findings of both CHC and AIH. Constitutional symptoms increased before or at the time of an increase in serum alanine aminotransferase concentration. The mean enzyme level rose to 857 IU/L during IFN treatment, and IgG values also increased substantially (Fig 1). Two of the 3 patients with type 2 AIH were DR4-positive. All 4 patients with type 1 AIH were DR52-positive, and 2 of them were DR3-positive. Five of the 7 patients, including the 4 with

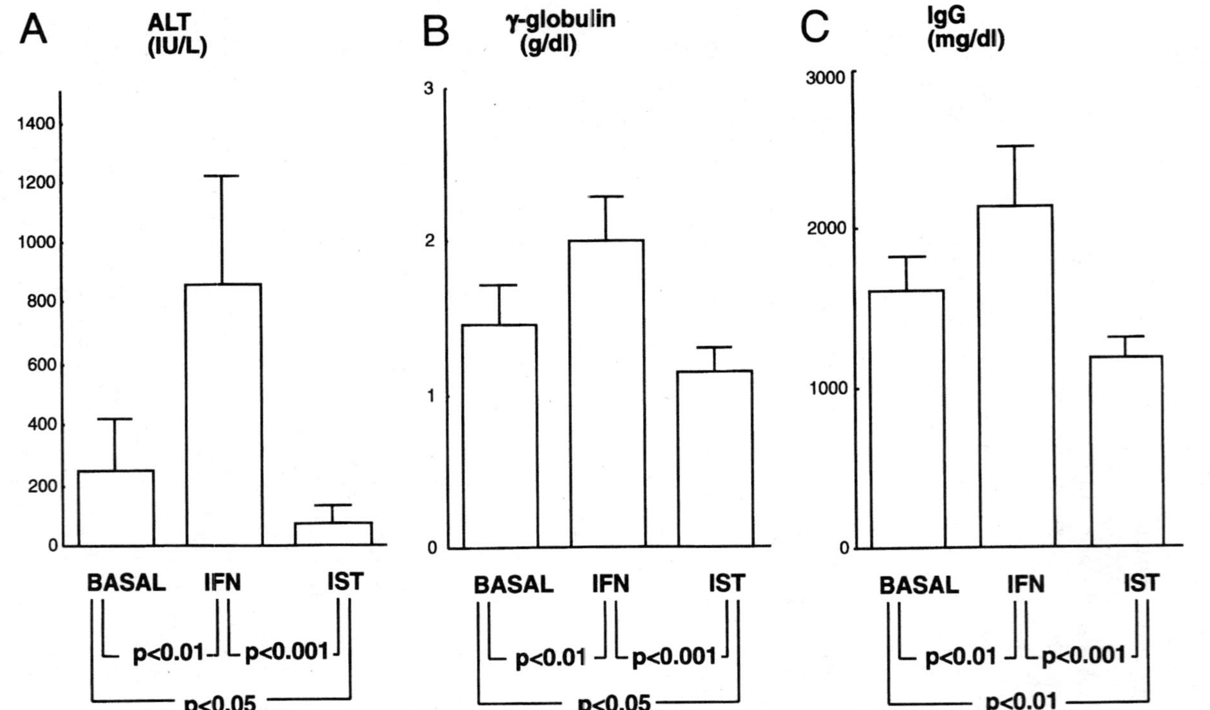

FIGURE 1.—(A) serum alanine aminotransferase (*ALT*); (B) γ-globulin; and (C) immunoglobulin G values on entry (*basal*) during interferon (*IFN*) treatment and with immunosuppressive therapy (*IST*). (Courtesy of García-Buey L, García-Monzón C, Rodriguez S, et al: Latent autoimmune hepatitis triggered during interferon therapy in patients with chronic hepatitis C. *Gastroenterology* 108:1770–1777, 1995.)

DR52, were positive for DQ2. All patients responded well to immunosuppressive treatment with steroid and azathioprine during follow-up of 8–16 months.

Conclusions.—Women with CHC may be genetically susceptible to AIH, which might be triggered by the immunostimulating effects of IFN. These patients appear to respond well to immunosuppressive therapy.

► This study clearly shows that the 7 patients had features of autoimmunity during IFN treatment for CHC, suggesting the presence of AIH along with authentic hepatitis C infection. The 7 patients were all women, had disproportionately increased serum alanine (ALT) levels, and all had (+) serologic markers of autoimmune liver disease (3 were positive for anti–liver and kidney microsomal [anti-LKM] antibodies and 4 were positive for antinuclear antibodies [ANAs]). All 7 patients responded to corticosteroids plus azathioprine therapy over 8–16 months.

Epstein-Barr virus (EBV) has also been described as a trigger for AIH in susceptible individuals.[1] Vento followed healthy relatives of 13 patients with chronic hepatitis, autoimmune type, and 7 cases of mononucleosis caused by the EBV. In 2 of the 7 patients, autoantibodies to the asialoglycoprotein autoantigen persisted and increased after infectious mononucleosis, and AIH developed within 4 months. These findings suggest that in susceptible individuals, EBV is a trigger for AIH.

Other reports[2] also indicate that the development of autoantibodies can interfere with the therapeutic response to IFN in CHC. García-Buey and colleagues studied 144 patients with CHC treated with IFN-α. The following autoantibodies were determined: ANA, antimitochondrial (AMA), smooth muscle (SMA), anti–LKM-1, antiparietal cell, antiplatelet, antithyroglobulin (TGA), antithyroid microsomal (TMA), and anti-ENA. Of the 144 patients treated with IFN, 7 had a paradoxical response aggravating their liver disease and triggering autoimmune phenomena. These patients received a diagnosis of AIH and were excluded from the study. Of the remaining 137 patients, 54 (39.4%) maintained a complete response with a negative HCV RNA determination in the vast majority. These patients with a sustained response had a significantly lower incidence of autoantibodies compared with nonresponders (5.6 vs. 19.3). The authors conclude that the presence of organ- and non–organ-specific autoantibodies is a factor predicting a poor response to IFN. Further, relapse was likely in patients with autoantibodies present before or developing after IFN treatment.

Billary et al.[3] describe 2 patients with combined features of autoimmune chronic hepatitis and hepatitis C who showed clinical, biochemical, and histologic responses to treatment with prednisone and azathioprine. They recommend that such patients be treated first with prednisone and azathioprine, and only if they do not respond should IFN therapy be considered.

N.J. Greenberger, M.D.

References

1. Vento SL: Epstein-Barr serves as a trigger for autoimmune hepatitis in susceptible individuals. *Lancet* 346:608–609, 1995.
2. García-Buey L, et al: The development of autoantibodies can interfere with the therapeutic response to interferon (IFN) in chronic hepatitis C (abstract). *Hepatology* 22:172A, 1995.
3. Billary S, et al: Chronic hepatitis with combined features of autoimmune chronic hepatitis and chronic hepatitis C: Favorable response to prednisone and azathioprine. *Ann Intern Med* 123:32–34, 1995.

Volunteer Blood Donors With Antibody to Hepatitis C Virus: Clinical, Biochemical, Virologic, and Histologic Features

Shakil AO, Conry-Cantilena C, Alter HJ, Hayashi P, Kleiner DE, Tedeschi V, Krawczynski K, Conjeevaram HS, Sallie R, Di Bisceglie AM, and the Hepatitis C Study Group (NIH, Bethesda, Md; Ctrs for Disease Control and Prevention, Atlanta, Ga)

Ann Intern Med 123:330–337, 1995 119-96-45–11

Background.—The clinical significance of antibody to hepatitis C virus (anti-HCV) in apparently healthy volunteer blood donors has not been established. The natural history of chronic hepatitis C in this population was further investigated.

Methods.—Sixty anti-HCV–positive blood donors were studied prospectively. Three groups of 20 donors each were formed. Group 1 had normal alanine aminotransferase (ALT) levels; group 2, ALT levels increased to values of less than twice the normal range; and group 3, ALT levels increased to values greater than twice the normal range.

Findings.—Donors with normal levels of ALT were older and more often female than were donors with abnormal levels. The 3 groups were comparable in their source of infection, disease duration, symptom score, and amount of alcohol intake. Hepatitis C virus RNA could be identified in 85% of the donors, more commonly in the groups with increased ALT levels (95% of patients) than in the group with normal levels (65% of patients). However, the groups had similar titers. An assessment of liver biopsy specimens revealed chronic hepatitis in 54 donors and cirrhosis in 1. There were only 3 normal liver biopsy specimens, all from HCV RNA–negative donors who had normal ALT levels.

Conclusions.—Chronic hepatitis C can be found in most blood donors with anti-HCV, irrespective of serum ALT levels. Donors with normal ALT concentrations and no HCV RNA in their serum usually have normal liver histologic findings or minimal changes. These donors have probably recovered from HCV infection.

► This important study indicates that asymptomatic patients with normal liver tests who are HCV-positive and HCV RNA–positive are likely to have histologic evidence of chronic hepatitis, which may range from chronic persistent to chronic active hepatitis and, in rare instances, to cirrhosis. The factors determining progression of the disease remain incompletely defined. Conversely, absence of HCV RNA in this setting indicates absence of both continuing infection and the potential for developing chronic liver disease.

N.J. Greenberger, M.D.

Molecular and Serologic Analysis in the Transmission of the GB Hepatitis Agents

Schlauder GG, Dawson GJ, Simons JN, Pilot-Matias TJ, Gutierrez RA, Heynen CA, Knigge MF, Kurpiewski GS, Buijk SL, Leary TP, Muerhoff AS, Desai SM, Mushahwar IK (Abbott Labs, North Chicago)

J Med Virol 46:81–90, 1995 119-96-45–12

Background.—Recently 2 flavivirus-like genomes have been cloned from tamarins infected with infectious serum derived from the human viral hepatitis GB strain, which induces hepatitis in these animals. The genomes may represent 2 independent viruses, GB virus-A (GBV-A) and GB virus-B (GBV-B).

Objective.—Further transmission studies have been performed in tamarins using newly developed reverse transcription–polymerase chain reaction and enzyme-linked immunosorbent assays to detect RNA and antibodies associated with GBV-A and GBV-B. The inocula included serum from a surgeon who had acute hepatitis—the original source of the GB agent.

Results.—The infectivity of both agents passed through a 0.1-μm filter. Sera from 8 infected tamarins contained 2 distinct genomes. In 4 other animals, the genomes were detected independently of one another. Specific antibody against GBV-B epitopes were present in sera of animals inoculated with both agents or with GBV-B alone. No animal had antibody against putative epitopes specific to GBV-A. All animals given serum containing GBV-B subsequently had increased liver enzymes, but inoculation of GBV-A had no such effect. Infection by the original infectious inoculum provided protection against reinfection by GBV-B but not GBV-A.

Conclusion.—The putative GB agent causing acute hepatitis actually consists of 2 independent viral agents.

► Two exciting reports[1, 2] have confirmed the identification of a new virus hepatitis agent, hepatitis G (HGV) and underscored its importance in posttransfusion acute and chronic hepatitis and in cirrhosis. The agent has a homology to hepatitis C and is most likely a member of the *Flaviviridiae* family. It has been absent in pretransfusion, and confirmed in posttransfusion blood specimens. This clearly implicates HGV as a cause of posttransfusion acute hepatitis. Not surprisingly, positive tests for GBV antibody and for GBV RNA have been confirmed in multiply transfused patients (hemophiliacs and thallasemics), patients with end-stage renal disease, and in patients with chronic hepatitis and cirrhosis. At this time, the GBV virus[1] and GBV-C[2] appear to be the same virus. Other members of the GBV virus family include GBV-A and GBV-B, but only GBV-C has been implicated in chronic liver disease. Infection with GBV virus may be more frequent as evidenced by the report[1] that 13 of 769 "normal" blood donors (1.7%) with negative tests for hepatitis B virus, HBC, and normal serum alanine aminotransferase values were positive for HGV antibodies.

N.J. Greenberger, M.D.

References

1. Kim JP, et al: Identification of a new hepatitis virus (HGV) and its implication in post transfusion hepatitis (abstract). *Hepatology* 22:218A, 1995.
2. Hadziyannis SJ: Infection with the Novel GBV-C virus in multiply transfused patients and in various forms of chronic liver disease (abstract). *Hepatology* 22:218A, 1995.

Acetaminophen (Paracetamol) Hepatotoxicity With Regular Intake of Alcohol: Analysis of Instances of Therapeutic Misadventure

Zimmerman HJ, Maddrey WC (George Washington Univ, Washington, DC; Armed Forces Inst of Pathology, Washington, DC; Univ of Texas Southwestern Med Ctr, Dallas)

Hepatology 22:767–773, 1995 119-96-45–13

Background.—Hepatic injury in alcoholics can result from the therapeutic use of acetaminophen (APAP). However, the extent of this phenomenon is unclear, and its importance is not widely appreciated. Sixty-seven alcoholics or regular drinkers sustaining hepatic injury after taking APAP with therapeutic intent were described.

Methods and Findings.—Sixty-four percent of the individuals were classified as alcoholic or drank more than 80 g of alcohol per day. Thirty-five percent drank 60 g/day or less, and the rest were vague in their descriptions of how much they drank. In 60% of the individuals, APAP doses were in the nontoxic range, being less than 6 g/day. In 40%, APAP doses were less than 4 g/day, and in 20%, between 4.1 and 6 g/day. A typical feature was the high level of aspartate transaminase (AST), ranging from 3,000 to 48,000 IU in more than 90% of the individuals. The mortality rate was nearly 20%.

Ninety-four cases of injury from therapeutic levels of APAP reported in the literature were similar to the current cases. Susceptibility appears to result from cytochrome P-4502EI induction by ethanol and glutathione depletion because of the effects of alcohol, the malnutrition often associated with alcoholism, and the depletion related to chronic APAP use and impaired glucuronidation from fasting (Table 1).

Conclusions.—These data add to the evidence that hepatic injury occurs in regular alcohol drinkers, especially chronic alcoholics, who take thera-

TABLE 1.—Characteristics of Cases of Hepatic Injury Associated With Therapeutic Use of Acetaminophen (*APAP*)

Characteristics	Registry	Literature
No. of cases	67	94
Male-female ratio	42/25 (1.7)	56/38 (1.5)
Age		
<30	7 (10%)	16 (17%)
30–50	39 (58%)	52 (54%)
>50	15 (24%)	24 (26%)
Unknown	6 (8%)	3 (3%)
Doses (g/d)		
<4	27 (40%)	22 (23%)
4.1–6	13 (20%)	25 (27%)
6.1–10	10 (15%)	17 (18%)
10.1–15	2 (3%)	1.3 (14%)
>15	5 (7%)	5 (5%)
Unclear	10 (15%)	13 (13%)
Duration of intake		
1 Day	7 (10%)	29 (30%)
1–7 Days	45 (67%)	38 (40%)
7–30 Days	4 (6%)	28 (30%)
>30 Days	8 (12%)	28 (30%)
Alcohol intake		
"Alcoholic" or "heavy"	17 (25%)	55 (60%)
Vague regular use	8 (12%)	
>80 g/d	18 (27%)	24 (34%)
~ 60 g/d	15 (22%)	5 (5%)
<60 g/d	9 (13%)	
Outcome		
Death	13* (18%)	19 (20%)
Recovered	52 (78%)	50 (53%)
Unknown	2 (3%)	26 (27%)
Zone 3 necrosis	14/16	23/26

* One of the surviving cases who was subjected to transplantation is included with the fatal cases.

(Courtesy of Zimmerman HJ, Maddrey WC: Acetaminophen (paracetamol) hepatotoxicity with regular intake of alcohol: Analysis of instances of therapeutic misadventure. *Hepatology* 22:767–773, 1995.)

peutic amounts of APAP. This distinctive syndrome is characterized by uniquely increased levels of AST. Because it poses a significant threat, a greater awareness of this syndrome is essential among the medical and lay community.

► In addition to alcohol, fasting has been shown to enhance the hepatotoxic effects of acetaminophen. Whitcomb and Block[1] found that recent fasting seemed more important than recent alcohol use among patients ingesting 4–10 g of acetaminophen per day. They suggest that fasting impairs glucuronidation and also depletes glutathione stores, thus enhancing conversion of acetaminophen to the toxic metabolite *N*-acetylbenzoquinonimine. Although the syndrome of liver injury related to acetaminophen plus alcohol use is distinctive and is marked by disproportionately increased serum levels of AST, it is disconcerting that it is not recognized as frequently as it should be. For an excellent recent review of acetaminophen poisoning, including methods to reduce acetaminophen absorption, use of antidotes, treatment recommendations, and prognostic factors, see the review article by Vale and Proudfoot.[2]

N.J. Greenberger, M.D.

References

1. Whitcomb DC, Block GD: Association of acetaminophen hepatotoxicity with fasting and ethanol use. *JAMA* 272:1845, 1994.
2. Vale JA, Proudfoot AT: Paracetamol (acetaminophen) poisoning. *Lancet* 346:547–552, 1995.

Diclofenac-Associated Hepatotoxicity: Analysis of 180 Cases Reported to the Food and Drug Administration as Adverse Reactions

Banks AT, Zimmerman HJ, Ishak KG, Harter JG (George Washington Univ, Washington, DC; Armed Forces Inst of Pathology, Washington, DC)

Hepatology 22:820–827, 1995 119-96-45–14

Introduction.—Nonsteroidal anti-inflammatory drugs (NSAIDs) appear to differ in terms of the character and severity of hepatic injury they may provoke. Diclofenac, approved in the United States in 1988 for treatment of osteoarthritis, rheumatoid arthritis, and ankylosing spondylitis, is reported in the medical literature to have caused approximately 60 cases of hepatic injury, primarily acute hepatocellular injury. The clinical, biochemical, and histologic features and possible mechanisms of diclofenac-associated hepatotoxicity were analyzed retrospectively in cases reported to the Food and Drug Administration (FDA) from November 1988 through June 1991.

Methods.—The FDA received 434 reports of diclofenac-associated hepatic injury during the review. After 254 cases were eliminated because of duplicate reporting, inadequate data, foreign sources, or other possible causes for liver enzyme abnormalities, 180 cases remained for study. The pattern of injury was classified as hepatocellular, cholestatic, mixed, or indeterminate, and the mechanism of injury as immunologic idiosyncrasy or metabolic idiosyncrasy.

Results.—The patient group included 142 women and 38 men, 68% of whom were older than 60 years. Osteoarthritis was the indication for diclofenac in 139 patients and rheumatoid arthritis in 22 patients. The ratio of females to males among cases of hepatic injury compared with the sex ratio of users of the NSAID yielded a relative risk of 2.0 for females. Two thirds of the patients had signs or symptoms, and one third were identified by increased levels of aspartate transaminase and alanine transaminase, noted incidentally or by monitoring. Jaundice was present in 50% of patients overall and in 75% of symptomatic patients. Seven of the 90 icteric patients died. In two thirds of the cases, the biochemical pattern of injury was hepatocellular or mixed hepatocellular. A pattern of cholestatic injury was present in 8% and an indeterminate pattern in 24%.

Sections of liver, available for 21 cases, showed hepatic injury 1 month after starting diclofenac in 24%, by 3 months in 63%, and by 6 months in 85%. No patient had evidence of hypersensitivity such as rash, fever, or eosinophilia, suggesting that metabolic idiosyncrasy was the probable mechanism.

Conclusion.—The hepatic injury induced by diclofenac is mainly hepatocellular, and the mechanism of injury appears to be metabolic idiosyncrasy. Most affected patients were women with osteoarthritis. Because half of all cases were detected in the first 2 months, physicians should consider possible hepatic toxicity when jaundice, nausea, or vomiting occur early after starting the drug.

▶ The data provided by this authoritative review suggest that diclofenac-related liver injury is especially likely to involve osteoarthritic females who have jaundice 1–6 months after starting diclofenac; injury is predominantly hepatocellular and is presumably caused by metabolic idiosyncrasy. For an excellent review of drug-induced hepatotoxicity, see the medical progress article on drug-induced hepatotoxicity.[1]

N.J. Greenberger, M.D.

Reference

1. Lee WM: Medical progress: Drug-induced hepatotoxicity. *N Engl J Med* 333:1118–1127, 1995.

Sclerotherapy With or Without Octreotide for Acute Variceal Bleeding

Besson I, Ingrand P, Person B, Boutroux D, Heresbach D, Bernard P, Hochain P, Larricq J, Gourlaouen A, Ribard D, Kara NM, Legoux J-L, Pillegand B, Becker M-C, Di Costanzo J, Metreau J-M, Silvain C, Beauchant M (Centre Hospitalier Universitaire de Poitiers, France)

N Engl J Med 333:555–560, 1995 119-96-45–15

Introduction.—Acute variceal bleeding is a major concern for patients with cirrhosis. Sclerotherapy is usually used to stop this bleeding, but rebleeding is common. Octreotide, a synthetic somatostatin analogue, is also effective in controlling this type of bleeding. The effectiveness of sclerotherapy alone, and in combination with octreotide therapy, in controlling acute variceal bleeding and preventing rebleeding in patients with cirrhosis was determined.

Methods.—A total of 199 patients with cirrhosis and either acute, active bleeding or evidence of recent bleeding were studied. After emergency sclerotherapy, the patients were randomly assigned to receive a continuous infusion of either octreotide, 25 μg/hr, or placebo for 5 days. The principal measures of outcome were survival for 5 days after sclerotherapy without rebleeding, and the amount of transfused blood that was required for these patients.

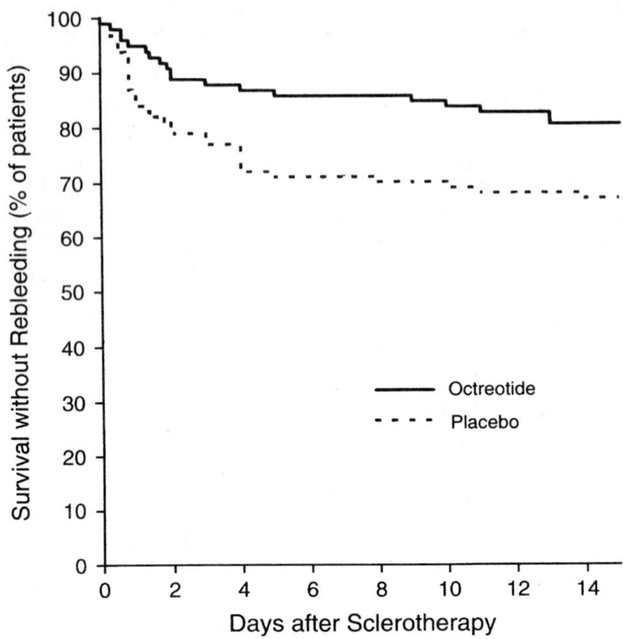

FIGURE 1.—Kaplan-Meier estimates of survival without rebleeding after sclerotherapy in the octreotide and placebo groups. Analysis was done on an intention-to-treat basis, and death was considered to be related to variceal bleeding, regardless of the precise cause (P = 0.02 by the adjusted Mantel-Haenszel test). (Reprinted by permission of *The New England Journal of Medicine.* Besson I, Ingrand P, Person B, et al: Sclerotherapy with or without octreotide for acute variceal bleeding. *N Engl J Med* 333:555–560, Copyright 1995, Massachusetts Medical Society.)

Results.—At 5 days, a significantly higher percentage of patients who received octreotide survived without rebleeding (87% vs. 71%). The number of units of blood transfused during the first 24 hours was also less in the octreotide group (1.2 units vs. 2.0 units). Among those who survived with no rebleeding at 5 days, 44% of patients who received octreotide did not require further blood transfusions after sclerotherapy, compared with 28% of patients who received placebo. Figure 1 shows the cumulative rates of survival without rebleeding at 15 days. Both groups had a mean cumulative survival rate at 15 days of 88%. Side effects were minimal.

Discussion.—At 5 days, a higher rate of survival without rebleeding was found for patients who received octreotide in addition to sclerotherapy, but the 15-day cumulative survival rate was unaffected by the mode of therapy. The rate of rebleeding documented in the placebo group was similar to the rate established in previous studies. Finally, 2 potential side effects of octreotide therapy—a decrease in glomerular filtration and encephalopathy—were not increased in those patients receiving octreotide.

► These findings indicate that the combination of sclerotherapy and octreotide is more effective than sclerotherapy alone in controlling variceal bleeding in patients with cirrhosis. However, it is important to note that there is no difference in the overall mortality rates with the 2 approaches to treatment. Octreotide, a synthetic somatostatin analogue, has a half-life of 1–2 hours, reduces collateral splanchnic blood flow, decreases the wedged:free hepatitic venous pressure gradient (WHVPG), and has been shown to be as effective as vasopressin without causing adverse systemic effects.[1]

N.J. Greenberger, M.D.

Reference

1. Hwong SJ, et al: A randomized controlled trial comparing octreotide and vasopressin in the control of acute esophageal variceal bleeding. *J Hepatol* 10:320–325, 1992.

Endoscopic Ligation Compared With Sclerotherapy for Treatment of Esophageal Variceal Bleeding: A Meta-Analysis

Laine L, Cook D (Univ of Southern California, Los Angeles; McMaster Univ, Hamilton, Ont, Canada)

Ann Intern Med 123:280–287, 1995 119-96-45–16

Introduction.—Endoscopic sclerotherapy decreases further bleeding in patients with esophageal variceal bleeding, but this treatment induces local and systemic complications and does not always prevent rebleeding. Endoscopic variceal ligation is based on the rubber-band ligation tech-

TABLE 4.—Results of Ligation Compared With Sclerotherapy for Treatment of Bleeding Esophageal Varices

Variable	Trials (Patients) *n*(*n*)	Odds Ratio (95% CI)*
Hemostasis for active bleeding	5 (106)	1.14 (0.44 to 2.90)
Variceal Obliteration	7 (547)	1.24 (0.87 to 1.76)
Rebleeding	7 (547)	0.52 (0.37 to 0.74)
Rebleeding caused by varices	5 (315)	0.47 (0.29 to 0.78)
Mortality	7 (547)	0.67 (0.46 to 0.98)
Mortality caused by bleeding	5 (368)	0.49 (0.24 to 0.996)
Complications†		
Esophageal stricture	7 (547)	0.10 (0.03 to 0.29)
Bleeding caused by treatment-induced ulcerations	7 (547)	0.56 (0.28 to 1.15)
Pulmonary infection	6 (524)	0.52 (0.21 to 1.34)
Bacterial peritonitis	5 (421)	0.74 (0.34 to 1.62)
Complications leading to death	5 (421)	0.47 (0.15 to 1.48)

* Odds ratios for ligation compared with sclerotherapy; all odds ratios favor ligation.
† Refers to number of patients with complications rather than to number of events.
Abbreviation: CI, confidence interval.
(Courtesy of Laine L, Cook D: Endoscopic ligation compared with sclerotherapy for treatment of esophageal variceal bleeding: A meta-analysis. *Ann Intern Med* 123:280–287, 1995.)

nique for hemorrhoids and has fewer complications than sclerotherapy. A meta-analysis of randomized clinical trials compared the 2 methods.

Methods.—MEDLINE was searched using the key words "varices and ligation" and "varices and band," and additional studies were sought through SCISEARCH and by scanning the reference lists of all articles obtained. Other sources were references for unpublished material, manufacturers of the ligation device, and researchers in the field of variceal hemorrhage. Eligible studies were randomized comparisons of endoscopic ligation and sclerotherapy in patients with esophageal variceal bleeding. Outcome measures were rebleeding, mortality, complications, or treatment sessions to obliteration.

Results.—Seven randomized trials involving 547 patients met inclusion criteria. The mean age of the study populations ranged from 46 to 56 years, and the mean follow-up ranged from 295 to 337 days. More than 99% of the patients had cirrhosis. The most common sclerosing agent used was sodium tetradecyl sulfate. When data for the studies were pooled, rebleeding was significantly less common with ligation than with sclerotherapy (Table 4). Both the mortality rate and the rate of death resulting from bleeding were reduced with ligation therapy compared with sclerotherapy. Ligation was also associated with a lower incidence of esophageal strictures and required fewer endoscopic treatment sessions to achieve variceal obliteration.

Conclusion.—Endoscopic sclerotherapy has been the standard treatment for patients with esophageal variceal bleeding. When data from 7 randomized trials were combined in meta-analysis, there was a 50% reduction in rebleeding with ligation compared with sclerotherapy. Because of lower rates of rebleeding, mortality, and complications, and the need for fewer endoscopic treatments, ligation should be considered the endoscopic therapy of choice in such cases.

► The authors conclude that on the basis of lower rates of rebleeding, mortality, and complications, and the need for fewer endoscopic treatments, ligation should be considered the endoscopic treatment of choice for patients with bleeding esophageal varices. However, they also point out that further large-scale studies with longer periods of follow-up will be helpful in more firmly establishing the utility of ligation therapy compared with sclerotherapy.

N.J. Greenberger, M.D.

The Transjugular Intrahepatic Portosystemic Stent-Shunt Procedure for Refractory Ascites

Ochs A, Rössle M, Haag K, Hauenstein K-H, Deibert P, Siegerstetter V, Huonker M, Langer M, Blum HE (Albert Ludwig Univ, Freiburg, Germany)

N Engl J Med 332:1192–1197, 1995 119-96-45–17

Objective.—The transjugular intrahepatic portosystemic stent shunt—a nonoperative side-to-side shunt between a main portal vein

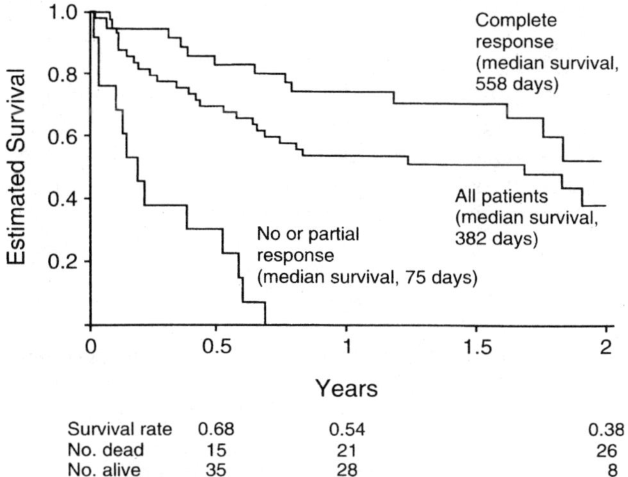

FIGURE 2.—Kaplan-Meier survival analysis of all patients and of patients according to their responses to treatment. (Reprinted by permission of *The New England Journal of Medicine*. Ochs A, Rössle M, Haag K, et al: The transjugular intrahepatic portosystemic stent-shunt procedure for refractory ascites. *N Engl J Med* 332:1192–1197, Copyright 1995, Massachusetts Medical Society.)

branch and a hepatic vein—has been effectively used to treat uncomplicated ascites in patients with variceal bleeding. It is an expandable metallic mesh device. This type of shunt was used in 50 of 62 consecutive patients with hepatic cirrhosis and treatment-resistant ascites. All patients had, besides ascites, other liver-related complications such as recent variceal bleeding or severe comorbidity.

Results.—The average follow-up was 426 days. A shunt was successfully established in all 50 patients, and the portal venous pressure gradient declined by 63% on average. Sixteen patients had 20 complications. Ascites lessened in 92% of patients and disappeared in 74%. Significant improvement took place within a week of stent placement. The serum creatinine level and creatinine clearance both had improved significantly at 6 months. Serum bilirubin levels increased initially but subsequently improved. Hepatic encephalopathy improved in 3 patients after stent placement but developed for the first time in 8 patients. Median survival was enhanced for patients whose ascites resolved (Fig 2).

Conclusion.—The transjugular intrahepatic portosystemic stent-shunt procedure is an effective treatment of refractory ascites in many patients with cirrhosis.

▶ The authors conclude that in this uncontrolled prospective study, the transjugular intrahepatic portosystemic shunt (TIPS) procedure was an effective treatment for many patients with liver cirrhosis and refractory ascites, but mortality from underlying diseases was substantial.

Hepatic encephalopathy after TIPS remains a significant problem. Somberg et al.[1] determined the incidence of new or worsened hepatic encephalopathy after TIPS in 108 adults, 77 of whom were followed for 1 year.

Post-TIPS encephalopathy was defined as new onset of clinical encephalopathy requiring treatment or worsening of preexisting encephalopathy within 1 year of TIPS. The overall incidence of new or worsened encephalopathy was 23% (18/77). *An increased risk of encephalopathy was associated with 3 factors, i.e., etiology of liver disease* other *than alcohol, female sex, and hypoalbuminemia.* Hepatic encephalopathy is a common complication of TIPS associated with specific risk factors, and these may be useful in the selection of appropriate candidates for this procedure.

N.J. Greenberger, M.D.

Reference

1. Somberg KA, et al: Hepatic encephalopathy after transjugular intrahepatic-portosystemic shunts: Incidence and risk factors. *Am J Gastroenterol* 90:549–555, 1995.

Trimethoprim-Sulfamethoxazole for the Prevention of Spontaneous Bacterial Peritonitis in Cirrhosis: A Randomized Trial

Singh N, Gayowski T, Yu VL, Wagener MM (Veterans Affairs Med Ctr, Pittsburgh, Pa; Univ of Pittsburgh, Pa)

Ann Intern Med 122:595–598, 1995 119-96-45–18

Background.—Spontaneous bacterial peritonitis can occur in 8% to 25% of patients with cirrhosis and ascites and is associated with a mortality rate of 30% to 50%. Attempts to prevent spontaneous bacterial peritonitis with antibiotic prophylaxis have been unsuccessful and have resulted in the emergence of highly resistant pathogens. However, trimethoprim-sulfamethoxazole (TMP-SMX) has shown in vitro activity against enteric gram-negative bacteria and streptococci. Its efficacy and safety in the prevention of spontaneous bacterial peritonitis in patients with cirrhosis and ascites were evaluated.

Methods.—Sixty consecutive patients with cirrhosis and ascites were stratified by the serum level of bilirubin, renal function, and the ascitic fluid protein level; they were then randomly assigned to either receive treatment with 1 double-strength tablet of TMP-SMX 5 times per week or no prophylaxis. Spontaneous bacteremia or spontaneous bacterial peritonitis was confirmed with ascitic fluid polymorphonuclear cell counts and/or ascitic fluid cultures.

Results.—Infectious complications occurred in 30% of the group not receiving prophylaxis and in 3% of the TMP-SMX group, with spontaneous bacterial peritonitis or spontaneous bacteremia occurring in 27% of the group not receiving prophylaxis and 3% of the TMP-SMX group. There were no adverse effects of treatment, including no hematologic toxicity.

Conclusions.—Trimethoprim-sulfamethoxazole is safe and effective for the prevention of spontaneous bacteremia or spontaneous bacterial peritonitis in patients with cirrhosis and ascites.

► These findings indicate that TMP-SMX was efficacious, safe, and cost-effective for the prevention of spontaneous bacterial peritonitis (SBP) in patients with cirrhosis. Sola et al.[1] performed a randomized controlled trial designed to compare whether therapeutic paracentesis is associated with a greater risk of SBP than diuretic therapy in patients with cirrhosis and ascites. They demonstrated that therapeutic paracentesis does not increase the short- and long-term risk of SBP in cirrhotics with tense ascites.

N.J. Greenberger, M.D.

Reference

1. Sola R, Andreu M, Coll S, et al: Spontaneous bacterial peritonitis in cirrhotic patients treated using paracentesis or diuretics: Results of a randomized study. *Hepatology* 21:340–344, 1995.

A Randomized, Double-Blind, Placebo-Controlled Trial of Ursodeoxycholic Acid in Primary Biliary Cirrhosis

Combes B, Carithers RL Jr, Maddrey WC, Lin D, McDonald MF, Wheeler DE, Eigenbrodt EH, Muñoz SJ, Rubin R, Garcia-Tsao G, Bonner GF, West AB, Boyer JL, Luketic VA, Shiffman ML, Mills AS, Peters MG, White HM, Zetterman RK, Rossi SS, Hoffmann AF, Markin RS (Univ of Texas, Dallas; Univ of Washington, Seattle; Thomas Jefferson Med College, Philadelphia; et al)

Hepatology 22:759–766, 1995 119-96-45–19

Objective.—The benefits of ursodeoxycholic acid (ursodiol) were evaluated in patients with primary biliary cirrhosis (PBC). Patients were stratified according to entry serum levels of bilirubin and liver histology (Ludwig criteria) to determine whether ursodiol was more effective in early or late stages of the disease.

Methods.—The multicenter, randomized, double-blind trial enrolled 151 patients, with 74 assigned to receive placebo and 77 to receive ursodiol. As is characteristic of PBC, most patients were women. The patients were grouped into 4 strata: (1) serum levels of bilirubin less than 2 mg/dL and stage I or II histology; (2) bilirubin less than 2 mg/dL and stage II or IV histology; (3) bilirubin ≥ 2 mg/dL and stage I or II histology; (4) bilirubin ≥ 2 mg/dL and stage III or IV histology. Ursodiol, 12 mg/kg/day, was administered as a single dose at bedtime. The effects of ursodiol and placebo were compared for symptoms, changes in biochemical parameters, liver histology, development of esophageal varices, ascites, or hepatic encephalopathy, liver transplantation, and death.

Results.—The 2 treatment arms were well matched at baseline for demographic and prognostic factors. Approximately 80% of patients completed the 2-year trial, and the dropout rate was comparable for placebo and ursodiol groups. Patients in strata 1 and 2 had major improvements in biochemical tests of the liver and in histology. In contrast, patients in strata 3 and 4 showed less improvement in laboratory tests and

TABLE 5.—Features of the 4 Major Randomized, Double-Blind, Controlled Trials of Ursodiol vs. Placebo in the Treatment of Primary Biliary Cirrhosis

	Poupon et al		Heathcote et al		Lindor et al		Combes et al	
	Placebo	Ursodiol	Placebo	Ursodiol	Placebo	Ursodiol	Placebo	Ursodiol
No. of patients	73	73	111	111	91	89	74	77
Percent women	89	95	95	91	87	91	92	86
Mean age (yrs)	52	54	55	57	52	54	49	49
Histological stage:								
I, II (%)	58	50	44	47	29	35	28	36
III, IV (%)	42	50	56	53	71	65	72	64
Mayo risk score	4.8	4.9	—	—	5.1	5.2	4.7	4.7
Duration of controlled trial	24 months		24 months		Up to 48 months Mean follow-up 24 months		24 months	
Daily dose (mg/kg)	13–15 in 2 doses		14 with evening meal		13–15 with meals and at bedtime		10–12 at bedtime	
Withdrawals	6 (8%)	5 (7%)	15 (14%)	10 (9%)	13 (14%)	5 (6%)	3 (4%)	2 (3%)
Completed 2-year trial	54 (74%)	62 (85%)	77 (69%)	89 (80%)	Uncertain		60 (80%)	63 (82%)
End point failures at 2 years:								
Death/transplantation	5* (7%)	5* (7%)	19 (17%)	12 (11%)	6† (7%)	6† (7%)	11 (15%)	12 (16%)
Developed cirrhosis	Not stated		Not stated		No difference		No difference	
Developed varices	Not stated		Not stated		No difference		No difference	
Ursodiol effects on:								
Symptoms	Not stated		No treatment effect		No treatment effect		No treatment effect on overall mean values, but significant decrease in development of severe fatigue/pruritus	

Laboratory tests	Improvements in bilirubin, alkaline phosphatase, GGT, AST, ALT, IgM, cholesterol	Improvements in bilirubin alkaline phosphatase, GGT, AST, ALT, IgM, cholesterol	Improvements in bilirubin, alkaline phosphatase, AST	Improvements in bilirubin, alkaline phosphatase, GGT, AST, ALT, IgM, albumin, particularly in patients with entry serum bilirubin <2 mg/dL
Histology	Better for piecemeal necrosis, parenchymal necrosis, portal and lobular inflammation, cholestasis, bile duct paucity and proliferation	Better for periportal ballooning and bile duct paucity	No effect on stage. Other features not yet reported.	Better for piecemeal necrosis, portal inflammation, and cholestasis in stratum 1; for fibrosis and cholestasis in stratum 2.

Abbreviations: GGT, γ-glutamyltransferase; *AST*, aspartate transaminase; *ALT*, alanine transaminase.

(Courtesy of Combes B, Carithers RL Jr, Maddrey WC, et al: A randomized, double-blind, placebo-controlled trial of ursodeoxycholic acid in primary biliary cirrhosis. *Hepatology* 22:759–766, 1995.)

no significant treatment effects in any histologic category. At the conclusion of the trial, ursodiol enrichment in fasting bile was approximately 40% and comparable in all strata, indicating that responses of patients in strata 1 and 2 were not attributable to greater ursodiol enrichment of the bile acid pool. Patients treated with ursodiol had a significant reduction in severe symptoms and in doubling of serum bilirubin levels. Major complications of liver disease occurred in 10.5% of patients with an entry serum bilirubin < 2 mg/dL and in 76.6% of those with ≥ 2 mg/dL, and the incidence of these complications did not differ between placebo and ursodiol groups. Treatment failure occurred at the same rate in placebo- and ursodiol-treated patients in strata 3 and 4.

Conclusions.—Patients with PBC who received ursodiol for 2 years benefited from the treatment when their disease was less advanced at entry (serum bilirubin, < 2 mg/dL). Findings in this series of patients were similar to those of previous trials (Table 5), demonstrating that ursodiol can improve test results, prevent certain features of histologic progression, and slow time to treatment failure in some patients with PBC.

► This and other studies provide data indicating that patients with advanced PBC are likely to benefit from receiving ursodiol (UDCA). In 65 PBC patients, Jorgensen and colleagues[1] compared UDCA-treated patients with complete normalization of biochemical functions to those without such improvement. Of 65 patients receiving UDCA, 12 (19%) showed normalization of liver biochemical tests at 2 years. The remaining 53 patients showed a less complete response. Mean alkaline phosphatase and total serum bilirubin values were significantly lower at entry in the patients whose liver biochemistry tests normalized, and percentage of UDCA in biliary bile acid was higher. Patients with biochemically and histologically less severe disease, and greater enrichment of biliary bile with UDCA, are more likely to respond favorably to the drug. The authors emphasize that the main objective of continued study will be to find out if normal liver biochemical functions can retard disease progression.

N.J. Greenberger, M.D.

Reference

1. Jorgensen RA, et al: Characterization of patients with a complete biochemical response to ursodeoxycholic acid. *Gut* 36:935–938, 1995.

The Hepatopulmonary Syndrome

Lange PA, Stoller JK (Cleveland Clinic Found, Ohio)

Ann Intern Med 122:521–529, 1995 119-96-45-20

Introduction.—Interactions between the lung and the liver have long been recognized. The current understanding of the hepatopulmonary syndrome (the association of severe hypoxemia and intrapulmonary vascular dilatations with hepatic dysfunction) was reviewed, using a literature search of all case reports, case series, and observational cohort studies published between 1986 and 1993.

Definition and Clinical Features.—Although patients may have other cardiopulmonary abnormalities, the triad of liver disease, an increased alveolar-arterial gradient while breathing room air, and evidence of intrapulmonary vascular dilatations defines the hepatopulmonary syndrome. The signs and symptoms include both liver disease features (gastrointestinal bleeding, esophageal varices, ascites, palmar erythema, splenomegaly) and pulmonary features (digital clubbing, cyanosis, dyspnea, platypnea, orthodeoxia). Other common cardiopulmonary features include alveolar hyperventilation with hypocapnia, systemic vasodilatation, elevated cardiac output, low pulmonary vascular resistance, low pulmonary artery pressures, pulmonary function abnormalities, and radiographic evidence of increased basilar interstitial and pulmonary vascular markings.

Mechanisms of Hypoxemia.—Intrapulmonary vascular dilatations are believed to be the primary cause of severe hypoxemia. Proposed mechanisms causing intrapulmonary vascular dilatations include failure of the liver to clear circulating pulmonary vasodilators, hepatic production of a circulating vasodilator, and hepatic inhibition of a circulating vasoconstrictor, with angiotensin II and nitric oxide among the substances probably involved. The vascular abnormalities are thought to produce diffusion-perfusion impairment, which refers to the inability of the oxygen molecules from the alveoli to diffuse to the center of the dilated capillary to oxygenate the hemoglobin, although supplemental oxygen can improve this impairment (Fig 1). Because cardiac output is typically increased in

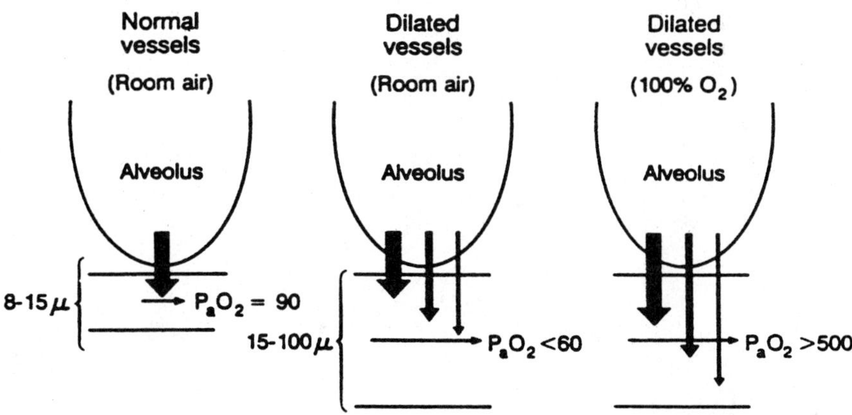

FIGURE 1.—Diffusion-perfusion impairment. Schematic diagram of the pulmonary vascular abnormality suspected in the hepatopulmonary syndrome. Driving pressure of alveolar arterial oxygen is depicted by *arrows*. (Reproduced with permission from Krowka MJ, Cortese DA: Severe hypoxemia associated with liver disease: Mayo Clinic experience and the experimental use of almitrine bismesylate. *Mayo Clin Proc* 62:164–173, 1987.)

patients with liver disease, reducing the transit time through pulmonary vessels, the opportunity for oxygen diffusion is reduced, further increasing the hypoxic potential.

The Diagnosis of Intrapulmonary Vascular Dilatations.—Contrast-enhanced echocardiography, technetium 99m–labeled macroaggregated albumin scanning, and pulmonary arteriography can detect these vascular abnormalities.

Treatment.—Medical therapy, including pharmacologic approaches, plasma exchange, and attempts at mechanical occlusion of intrapulmonary vascular dilatations, has been ineffective. Liver transplantation has resulted in reversal of the hepatopulmonary syndrome, indicating that hypoxemia is not a contraindication to liver transplantation.

Conclusions.—Although several characteristics of the hepatopulmonary syndrome have been elucidated, there is much need for further research in its diagnosis, pathophysiology, and treatment.

► In addition to intrapulmonic vascular dilatation, another factor contributing to the hepatopulmonary syndrome is portopulmonary hypertension. This can result in increased flow through the bronchial veins, causing arterial oxygen desaturation at rest and the development of bronchial varices. The latter can rupture, with the ensuing hemoptysis mistakenly diagnosed as pulmonary embolism, a not infrequent development in cirrhotic patients. Portopulmonary hypertension should be suspected if large azygos and hemizygous veins are visualized by chest films or CT scans of the lung.

N.J. Greenberger, M.D.

46 Biliary Tract

Prophylaxis Against Gallstone Formation With Ursodeoxycholic Acid in Patients Participating in a Very-Low-Calorie Diet Program

Shiffman ML, Kaplan GD, Brinkman-Kaplan V, Vickers FF (Med College of Virginia, Richmond; Health Management Resources, Boston; Ciba-Geigy Pharmaceutical Co, Summit, NJ)

Ann Intern Med 122:899–905, 1995 119-96-46–1

Objective.—Whether prophylactic treatment with ursodeoxycholic acid can prevent the formation of gallstones in patients participating in a very-low-calorie weight reduction program was investigated in a multicenter, double-blind, placebo-controlled trial.

Study Population.—The 1,004 patients enrolled in the 16-week study had a body mass index of at least 38 kg/m^2 and a normal ultrasonogram of the gallbladder. The age range was 18–70 years. No patient had an eating disorder or other problems that might compromise participation, and none were using oral bile salt preparations. The mean initial body weight was 128 kg, and the mean body mass index was 44 kg/m^2.

Methods.—The liquid protein diet that was used provided 520 kcal/day. Ursodeoxycholic acid was given in a daily dose of 300, 600, or 1,200 mg.

Results.—The active treatment was well tolerated. Gallstones developed in 28% of placebo recipients, in 8% of those given the lowest dose of ursodeoxycholic acid, and in only 2% of those given the highest daily dose (Fig 1). All actively treated groups were at significantly lower risk than patients given placebo. The proportion of ursodeoxycholic acid in the bile increased incrementally with the dose given. In women, but not in men, the rate of gallstone formation increased as the body mass index decreased.

Conclusions.—In patients on a strict weight-reducing diet, prophylaxis with 600 mg of ursodeoxycholic acid daily is effective in preventing the formation of gallstones. It may act by reducing cholesterol secretion into the bile, thereby lowering the cholesterol saturation index of bile.

► In their discussion, the authors point out that approximately 12% of the United States population and 18% of the women in the United States have gallstones. Well-defined risk factors for developing gallstones include obesity, pregnancy, family history, regional enteritis, and participation in weight-reduction dieting. The data obtained in this study show that prophylaxis against gallstone formation with ursodeoxycholic acid during well-defined,

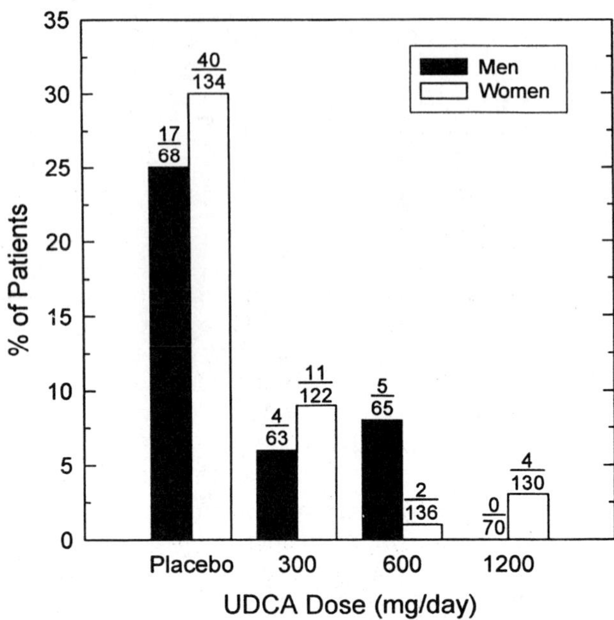

FIGURE 1.—Percentage of patients who had gallstones during the diet program. The *fractions above each bar* indicate the number of patients who had gallstones in each group over the total number of patients in each group. The values for all doses of ursodeoxycholic acid (*UDCA*) in both men and women were significantly lower than those for placebo. For women, the values for the 600-mg/day dose were significantly lower than those for the 300-mg/day dose. (Courtesy of Shiffman ML, Kaplan GD, Brinkman-Kaplan V, et al: Prophylaxis against gallstone formation with ursodeoxycholic acid in patients participating in a very-low-calorie diet program. *Ann Intern Med* 122:899–905, 1995.)

high-risk periods (such as after weight loss and after giving birth) has considerable potential to reduce health care costs associated with the treatment of gallstones and their complications.

N.J. Greenberger, M.D.

The Natural History of Gallstones: The GREPCO Experience

Attili AF, DeSantis A, Capri R, Repice AM, Maselli S, and the GREPCO Group
(Univ of L'Aquila, Italy; Univ of Rome)

Hepatology 21:656–660, 1995 119-96-46–2

Objective.—The natural course of gallstone disease was examined in 151 patients enrolled from 1981 to 1984 in the Group for Epidemiology and Prevention of Cholelithiasis study conducted in Rome. Thirty-three participants had symptoms at the outset. The patients were followed up clinically at intervals of 2 years or less.

Observations.—Biliary colic developed in 23.7% of the 118 initially asymptomatic patients. The cumulative probability of colic occurring within 10 years was 25.8%. Half of the initially symptomatic patients remained free of biliary colic during follow-up, although 3 of them had surgery shortly after entry to the study. Three asymptomatic and 2 symptomatic patients had acute cholecystitis develop. Cholecystectomy was performed in 23.7% of the initially asymptomatic patients and in 45.2% of those who were symptomatic initially (Fig 2). Surgery did not result in any deaths or complications. One patient died of gallbladder cancer.

Conclusion.—The natural course of gallstone disease is less benign than generally thought, even in patients who are initially asymptomatic.

▶ This study provides important information on the natural history of gallstones in 118 initially asymptomatic patients with cholelithiasis and 33 patients with symptoms. In contrast to the earlier report by Gracie and Ransohoff,[1] the results of the current study are less optimistic; biliary colic developed in approximately 25% of the asymptomatic patients followed for 10 years. Further, cholecystectomy was performed in 23.7% of the initially asymptomatic patients as compared with 45% of the symptomatic patients. The authors conclude by reaffirming that watchful waiting is the best course for patients with asymptomatic gallstones.

N.J. Greenberger, M.D.

Reference

1. Gracie WA, Ransohoff DF: The natural history of silent gallstones: The innocent gallstone is not a myth. *N Engl J Med* 307:798–800, 1982.

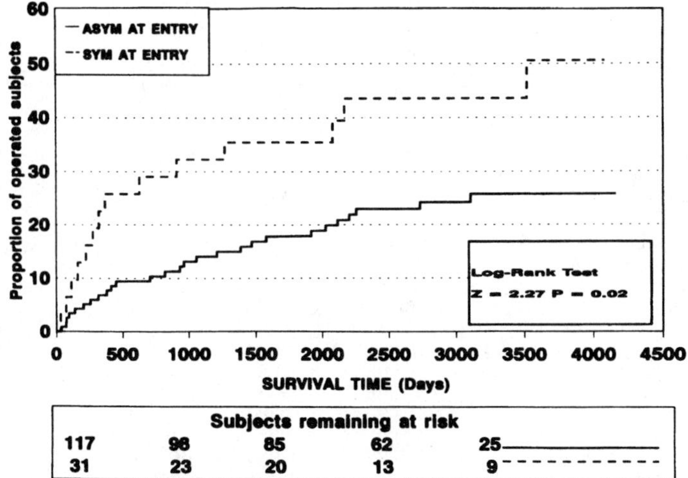

FIGURE 2.—Life-table analysis showing the cumulative probability of not being submitted to cholecystectomy in individuals who, at entry, were either asymptomatic (*ASYM*) or had already experienced at least 1 episode of biliary colic (*SYM*). (Courtesy of Attili AF, DeSantis A, Capri R, et al: The natural history of gallstones: The GREPCO experience. *Hepatology* 21:656–660, 1995.)

Intrahepatic Cholangiographic Appearance Simulating Primary Sclerosing Cholangitis in Several Hepatobiliary Diseases: A Postmortem Cholangiographic and Histopathological Study in 154 Livers at Autopsy

Terada T, Nakanuma Y (Kanazawa Univ, Japan)
Hepatology 22:75–81, 1995 119-96-46–3

Background.—Progressive fibrosing inflammation of the biliary tree without extrahepatic biliary obstruction or a history of biliary tract surgery characterizes primary sclerosing cholangitis (PSC). This fibrosis compresses the biliary tree and thus dilates the extrahepatic and intrahepatic bile ducts, which appear on cholangiography as a stricture with or without resultant dilatation of the biliary tree. This finding, along with histologic findings, confirms the diagnosis of PSC. However, PSC-like cholangiographic findings have been reported in patients with secondary sclerosing cholangitis. Therefore, the specificity of these cholangiographic findings

TABLE 1.—Postmortem Cholangiographic Findings in the Liver

	Cholangiographic Appearance			
Hepatobiliary Condition	Normal (%)	Stricture (%)	Stricture + Dilation (Beaded Appearance) (%)	Dilation (%)
APCD (n = 3)	0(0)	0(0)	2(67)	1(33)
Cirrhosis (n = 2)	0(0)	0(0)	1(50)	1(50)
Cirrhosis + HCC (n = 4)	0(0)	0(0)	3(75)	1(25)
HCC (n = 1)	0(0)	0(0)	1(100)	0(0)
Metastatic carcinoma (n = 13)	7(54)	2(15)	1(8)	3(25)
Involvement of leukemia or lymphoma (n = 12)	9(75)	1(8)	1(8)	1(8)
Submassive hepatic necrosis (n = 5)	3(60)	0(0)	2(40)	0(0)
Amyloidosis (n = 2)	1(50)	1(50)	0(0)	0(0)
Intrahepatic thrombosis (n = 1)	0(0)	1(100)	0(0)	0(0)
Extrahepatic obstruction (n = 2)	0(0)	0(0)	1(50)	1(50)
Gallstone (n = 7)	5(71)	0(0)	0(0)	2(29)
Hepatolithiasis (n = 1)	0(0)	0(0)	0(0)	1(100)
Chronic hepatitis (n = 4)	4(100)	0(0)	0(0)	0(0)
Fatty liver (n = 7)	7(100)	0(0)	0(0)	0(0)
Intrahepatic cholestasis (n = 5)	5(100)	0(0)	0(0)	0(0)
Hemosiderosis (n = 3)	3(100)	0(0)	0(0)	0(0)
Nodular transformation (n= 1)	1(100)	0(0)	0(0)	0(0)
Primary biliary cirrhosis (n = 1)	1(100)	0(0)	0(0)	0(0)
Miliary tuberculosis (n = 1)	1(100)	0(0)	0(0)	0(0)
Multiple nonparasitic cysts (n = 1)	1(100)	0(0)	0(0)	0(0)
Normal liver (n = 78)	76(97)	0(0)	0(0)	2(3)
Total (n = 154)	124(81)	6(4)	11(7)	13(8)

Note: All cases of cirrhosis were nonbiliary cirrhosis.

Abbreviations: APCD, adult-type polycystic disease of the liver and kidneys; *HCC*, hepatocellular carcinoma.

(Courtesy of Terada T, Nakanuma Y: Intrahepatic cholangiographic appearance simulating primary sclerosing cholangitis in several hepatobiliary diseases: A postmortem cholangiographic and histopathological study in 154 livers at autopsy. *Hepatology* 22:75–81, 1995.)

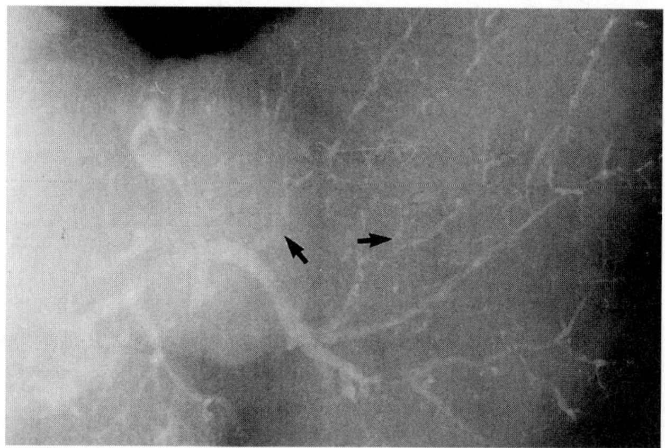

FIGURE 7.—Postmortem intrahepatic cholangiogram of a liver autopsy specimen (female, 47, with malignant lymphoma with diffuse liver involvement). The cholangiogram of the left lobe (posteroanterior direction) shows stenosis (*arrows*) and dilation, creating the "beaded appearance." (Courtesy of Terada T, Nakanuma Y: Intrahepatic cholangiographic appearance simulating primary sclerosing cholangitis in several hepatobiliary diseases: A postmortem cholangiographic and histopathological study in 154 livers at autopsy. *Hepatology* 22:75–81, 1995.)

was evaluated with postmortem intrahepatic cholangiography of liver autopsy specimens with a variety of liver diseases.

Methods.—Postmortem cholangiography was performed on 154 consecutive liver autopsy specimens. The intrahepatic cholangiograms were evaluated by a "blinded" examiner and categorized as stricture alone, stricture and dilatation, or dilatation alone. Liver sections were then obtained from 7 sites and examined histologically.

Results.—Cholangiographic PSC-like findings were found in patients with several hepatobiliary conditions (Table 1). They occurred frequently in patients with cirrhosis, hepatocellular carcinoma, adult-type polycystic disease of the liver and kidneys, submassive hepatic necrosis, amyloidosis, and intrahepatic thrombosis, and more rarely in patients with metastatic carcinomas and hepatic infiltration of leukemia or lymphoma cells (Fig 7). Histologic examination revealed that livers with a PSC-like cholangiographic appearance had intrahepatic bile ducts that were compressed by fibrosis, inflammatory infiltrates, liver and peribiliary cysts, infiltrating cancer cells, amyloid deposition, or portal thrombi. Histologic changes were more pronounced in livers with strictured than with dilated ducts and in livers with PSC-like cholangiographic findings than in those without this appearance.

Conclusions.—Because intrahepatic stricture with or without dilatation appears on the intrahepatic cholangiography in patients with several hepatobiliary diseases, all of these diseases, in addition to PSC, should be included in the differential diagnosis.

▶ This paper reminds us that a PSC-like cholangiographic appearance is frequently found in several disorders, including cirrhosis with or without hepatocellular carcinoma; adult polycystic disease of the liver and kidneys; submassive hepatic necrosis; amyloidosis; and intrahepatic extensive thrombosis. It was also found, albeit to a lesser extent, in patients with metastatic carcinoma and leukemic and lymphomatous infiltration of the liver. Clinicians should take such diseases into consideration when stricture, with or without dilatation, is found on intrahepatic cholangiography. For an excellent review on PSC, see the medical progress article by Lee and Kaplan.[1]

N.J. Greenberger, M.D.

Reference

1. Lee YM, Kaplan MM: Medical progress: Primary sclerosing cholangitis. *N Engl J Med* 332:924–933, 1995.

47 Pancreas

Interdigestive Cycling in Chronic Pancreatitis: Altered Coordination Among Pancreatic Secretion, Motility, and Hormones

Pieramico O, Dominguez-Muñoz JE, Nelson DK, Böck W, Büchler M, Malfertheiner P (Univ of Ulm, Germany; Gen Hosp, Meren, Italy; Univ of Magdeburg, Germany; et al)

Gastroenterology 109:224–230, 1995 119-96-47–1

Background.—Normally, pancreatic exocrine secretion cycles in concert with gastrointestinal motor activity and plasma concentration of pancreatic polypeptide (PP) during the interdigestive state. It has been hypothesized that pancreatobiliary secretion is an important modulator of gastrointestinal motility and that patients with chronic pancreatitis (CP) will also have motility abnormalities. However, animal studies have shown that canine pancreatectomy does not produce interdigestive gastrointestinal motility abnormalities. Therefore, the coordination of interdigestive cycling of exocrine and endocrine pancreatic secretion and gastrointestinal motor activity was studied in patients with and without CP.

Methods.—Gastrointestinal motility was monitored manometrically for at least 5 hours or until 2 interdigestive cycles were completed in 9 patients with CP and 13 healthy controls. Duodenal samples and blood samples were obtained every 15 minutes and analyzed for trypsin, chymotrypsin, amylase, and polyethylene glycol. Plasma concentrations of PP were assayed. The motility tracings were analyzed and correlated with enzyme secretion and PP release.

Results.—All the study patients demonstrated normal patterns of interdigestive motility, with no differences in any motility parameter. However, patients with CP demonstrated reduced PP release and shortened PP release cycles. Compared with controls, the patients with CP demonstrated substantially decreased peaks of trypsin, chymotrypsin, and amylase secretion and had shorter secretory cycles, although they cycled in synchrony. Two patients with severe CP had no fluctuations in their low PP plasma concentrations and enzyme secretion patterns. The cycles of motility, enzyme secretion, and PP release were closely correlated temporally in the control individuals. However, in the patients with CP, motility cycled in a temporal pattern similar to that of the controls but unrelated to the secretory and PP cycles, which correlated only with each other (Fig 3).

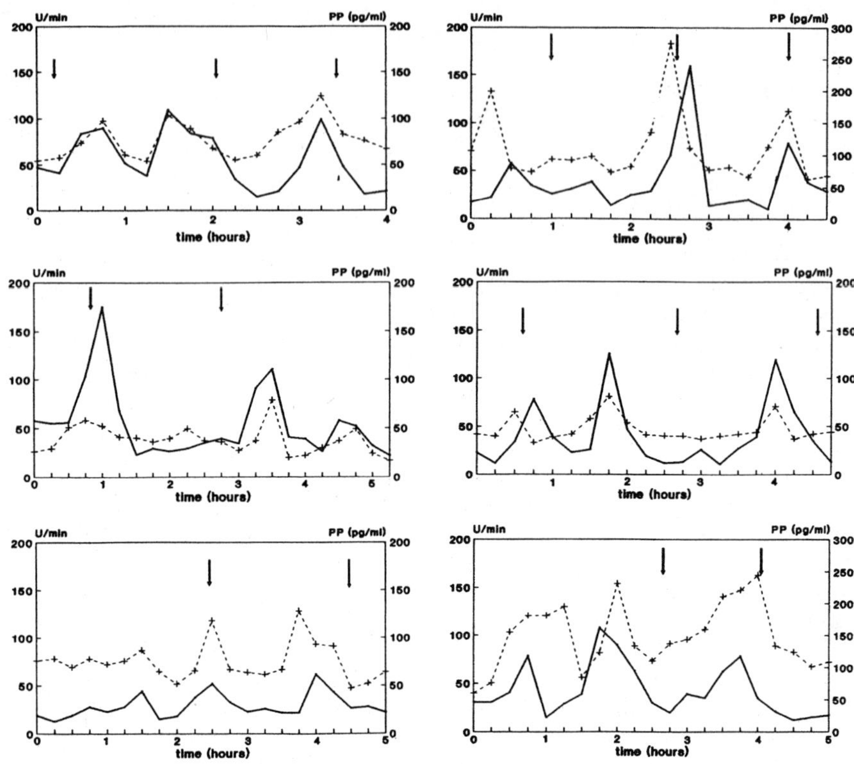

FIGURE 3.—Interdigestive trypsin output (*solid line*) and plasma concentrations of pancreatic polypeptide (*PP*) (*dashed line*) in 6 patients with chronic pancreatitis. *Arrows* indicate onset of duodenal phase III. Note the difference in the scale of vertical axes, which were expanded in comparison with those in the control example to allow visualization of cycling in chronic pancreatitis. (Courtesy of Pieramico O, Dominguez-Muñoz JE, Nelson DK, et al: Interdigestive cycling in chronic pancreatitis: Altered coordination among pancreatic secretion, motility, and hormones. *Gastroenterology* 109:224–230, 1995.)

Conclusions.—Although the cyclical pattern of interdigestive pancreatic secretion is altered in patients with CP, their interdigestive gastrointestinal motility pattern is not altered, suggesting that pancreatic secretion does not play a primary role in modulating motility.

Early Antibiotic Treatment in Acute Necrotising Pancreatitis

Sainio V, Kemppainen E, Puolakkainen P, Taavitsainen M, Kivisaari L, Valtonen V, Haapiainen R, Schröder T, Kivilaakso E (Helsinki Univ Central Hosp)
Lancet 346:663–667, 1995 119-96-47–2

Introduction.—Mortality from acute, severe pancreatitis remains high despite advances in treatment. Because infectious complications may indicate a poor outcome, prophylactic antibiotics are often recommended, even though the benefits of this therapy have not been confirmed in a controlled clinical study. The effects of cefuroxime therapy started early on admission were evaluated in 60 patients with alcohol-induced necrotizing pancreatitis.

Methods.—The patients studied had a C-reactive protein concentration greater than 120 mg/L within 48 hours of admission and low contrast enhancement of the pancreas on contrast-enhanced CT. Thirty of 60 consecutive patients were randomly assigned to receive cefuroxime, 4.5 g/day IV, at the time of admission. The remaining 30 patients were given no antibiotic treatment until infection was verified clinically or microbiologically, or after a secondary rise in C-reactive protein. Blood samples were cultured twice a week for each patient, and bacteriologic culture of urine samples was done twice a week. Infectious complications recorded were blood culture–positive sepsis, pneumonia and/or adult respiratory distress syndrome, urinary tract infection, and intra-abdominal abscess or infected necrosis.

Results.—The antibiotic and nonantibiotic groups were similar in mean age, sex distribution, duration of symptoms before admission, mean C-reactive protein concentrations within 48 hours of admission, and mean number of prognostic signs. Antibiotic treatment was subsequently started in all but 7 patients in the nonantibiotic group; 14 patients were treated because of suspected infection and 8 because of positive bacterial cultures. There were 84 infectious complications recorded, 30 in the antibiotic group and 54 in the nonantibiotic group. The mean number of infections per patient was significantly lower in the antibiotic group (1.8 vs. 1.0). Blood culture–positive sepsis occurred in 4 patients in the antibiotic group and 8 patients in the nonantibiotic group. Twice as many patients in the nonantibiotic group (14 vs. 7) needed operative intervention. Mortality was significantly higher in the nonantibiotic group (Table 5).

Conclusion.—Previous studies of prophylactic antibiotics were limited because the severity of pancreatitis was difficult to ascertain. All patients in this series, however, had extremely severe alcohol-induced pancreatitis verified by contrast-enhanced CT. Findings in these 2 groups of patients

TABLE 5.—Cause of Death and Mortality

	Antibiotic group	Nonantibiotic group
Fulminant course with irreversible shock	0	2
Verified *S. aureus* sepsis	0	1
Verified *E. faecalis* sepsis	0	1
Multiorgan failure and cultures of pancreatic necrosis positive for *S. epidermidis*	1	3
Total deaths	1	7*

*$P = 0.0284$, Fisher's exact test.

Abbreviations: S. aureus, *Staphylococcus aureus*; E. faecalis, *Enterococcus faecalis*; S. epidermidis, *Staphylococcus epidermidis*.

(Courtesy of Sainio V, Kemppainen E, Puolakkainen P, et al: Early antibiotic treatment in acute necrotising pancreatitis. *Lancet* 346:663–667. Copyright by The Lancet Ltd, 1995.)

with comparable disease severity indicate that prophylactic cefuroxime reduces mortality, probably by decreasing the frequency of sepsis.

► From July 1989 through November 1993, 820 patients with acute pancreatitis were treated at Helsinki University Central Hospital and 60 (7.3%) with severe necrotizing pancreatitis were randomized to placebo or antibiotic treatment groups. This incidence of severe pancreatitis in patients with alcohol-induced pancreatitis is similar to that in an earlier report by Gerzof et al.[1] in which the most common etiologic insult was also alcohol. In contrast to earlier studies in which a beneficial effect of antibiotics could not be demonstrated to influence the course of acute pancreatitis, the study by Saino et al. does suggest that an antibiotic (cefuroxime) given early in necrotizing pancreatitis is beneficial and may well reduce mortality, presumably by controlling sepsis. However, in patients with severe pancreatitis necrosis, it is important to document whether necrosis is, in fact, infected; in such cases, surgical drainage is usually indicated.

N.J. Greenberger, M.D.

Reference

1. Gerzof SG, et al: Early diagnosis of pancreatic infection by computed tomography–guided aspiration. *Gastroenterology* 93:1315–1320, 1987.

The Risk of Cancer Among Patients With Cystic Fibrosis

Neglia JP, FitzSimmons SC, Maisonneuve P, Schöni MH, Schöni-Affolter F, Corey M, Lowenfels AB, and the Cystic Fibrosis and Cancer Study Group (Univ of Minnesota, Minneapolis; Cystic Fibrosis Found, Bethesda, Md; European Inst of Oncology, Milan, Italy; et al)

N Engl J Med 332:494–499, 1995 119-96-47–3

Introduction.—Two to four percent of whites carry the cystic fibrosis gene, and approximately 25,000 Americans are affected with the disease. With advances in the care of cystic fibrosis, one third of all patients now reach adulthood, when the frequency of cancer increases. Some reports have suggested that the risk of cancer may be increased in patients with cystic fibrosis, especially digestive tract cancers and leukemia. The risk of cancer in patients with cystic fibrosis was analyzed.

Methods.—The occurrence of cancer was determined retrospectively in 28,511 United States and Canadian patients with cystic fibrosis from 1985 through 1992. Population-based data were used to calculate the expected cancer incidence, which was then compared with the number of observed cases. In addition, proportional incidence ratios were calculated to evaluate the association between specific cancers and cystic fibrosis in Europe.

Results.—During 164,764 person-years of follow-up in the North American cohort, a total of 37 cancers were observed. Because the expected number of cancers was 45.6, the ratio of observed to expected cancers was 0.8 (Table 3). There were 13 observed digestive tract cancers

TABLE 3.—Number of Cancers Observed and Number Expected Among North American Patients With Cystic Fibrosis

Type of Tumor* (ICD-9-CM Code)	Study Period	No. Observed/ No. Expected	Risk Ratio (95% CI)
Digestive tract (150–159)	1985–1992	13/2	6.5 (3.5–11.1)
	1988–1992	9/1.36	6.6 (3.0–12.6)
Hematopoietic (200–208)	1985–1988	8/11.85	0.7 (0.3–1.3)
	1988–1992	6/7.5	0.8 (0.3–1.7)
All other tumors	1985–1988	16/31.8	0.5 (0.3–0.8)
	1988–1992	14/20.1	0.7 (0.4–1.2)
Total	1985–1992	37/45.6	0.8 (0.6–1.1)
	1988–1992	29/29.8	1.0 (0.7–1.4)

* From 1985 to 1992, the specific tumors diagnosed consisted of 13 digestive tract cancers (esophagus, 1: stomach, 1; small intestine, 2; large intestine, 3; liver or biliary tract, 5; pancreas, 1), 8 hematopoietic cancers (lymphoma, 4; leukemia, 4), and 16 other types of tumors (tongue, 1; rhabdomyosarcoma, 1; malignant melanoma, 1; breast, 2; cervix, 2; testis, 4; brain, 5).

Abbreviations: ICD-9-CM, International Classification of Diseases, 9th Revision, Clinical Modification; CI, confidence interval.

(Reprinted by permission of *The New England Journal of Medicine.* Neglia JP, FitzSimmons SC, Maisonneuve P, et al: The risk of cancer among patients with cystic fibrosis. *N Engl J Med* 332:494–499, Copyright 1995, Massachusetts Medical Society.)

TABLE 4.—Association Between Cystic Fibrosis and Various Types of Cancer in European Patients

Type of Tumor (ICD-9-CM Code)	Case Patients	Controls*	Odds Ratio (95% CI)
Digestive tract (150–158)	11	28	6.4 (2.9–14.0)
Esophagus (150)	1	28	14.3 (1.4–148)
Bowel (152–154)	7	28	9.3 (3.5–25)
Pancreas (157)	2	28	31.5 (4.8–205)
Retroperitoneum (158)	1	28	3.4 (0.4–29)
Lymphatic or hematopoietic (200–208)	12	16	1.4 (0.6–3.2)
Lymphoma (200–202)	5	23	1.1 (0.4–3.0)
Myeloma (203)	1	27	17.2 (1.9–159)
Leukemia (204–208)	6	22	1.3 (0.5–3.4)
All other sites	16	12	0.7 (0.3–1.6)
Oral cavity (140–149)	1	27	2.4 (0.3–19.5)
Lung (162)	1	27	1.4 (0.1–16.8)
Bone or soft tissue (170–171)	2	26	0.7 (0.2–3.1)
Ovary (183)	1	27	0.9 (0.1–7.9)
Testis (186)	2	26	0.7 (0.1–3.3)
Eye (190)	1	27	2.0 (0.2–16.6)
Brain or nervous system (191–192)	3	25	0.7 (0.2–2.5)
Thyroid (193)	2	26	2.6 (0.5–21.1)
Endocrine (194)	3	25	5.4 (1.5–19.8)

* For digestive tract, bowel, and pancreatic tumors, the controls are patients with cystic fibrosis and all other types of cancer. For tumors at other sites, the controls are patients with cystic fibrosis and all other types of non–digestive tract cancer.

Abbreviations: ICD-9-CM, International Classification of Diseases, 9th Revision, Clinical Modification; CI, confidence interval.

(Reprinted by *The New England Journal of Medicine.* Neglia JP, FitzSimmons SC, Maisonneuve P, et al: The risk of cancer among patients with cystic fibrosis. *N Engl J Med* 332:494–499, Copyright 1995, Massacusetts Medical Society.)

compared with 2 expected, for a ratio of observed to expected cancers of 6.5. Of 39 cancers reported in the European study, 11 originated in the digestive tract. There was a positive association between digestive tract tumors and cystic fibrosis, with an odds ratio of 6.4 (Table 4).

Conclusions.—For patients with cystic fibrosis, the risk of cancer overall is similar to that of the general population. However, these patients have an elevated risk of digestive tract cancers, and more such cancers can be expected as patients live longer. Persistent or unexplained gastrointestinal symptoms in a patient with cystic fibrosis therefore warrant careful examination.

► These findings suggest that cystic fibrosis can be added to the growing list of genetic defects that are related to cancer. The authors emphasize that as the life span of cystic fibrosis patients increases, more digestive tract cancers will occur. Accordingly, unexplained gastrointestinal symptoms in such patients warrant careful evaluation.

N.J. Greenberger, M.D.

PART SIX

ENDOCRINOLOGY, DIABETES, AND METABOLISM

ROBERT D. UTIGER, M.D.

Introduction

The articles selected for this section encompass a broad spectrum of topics, like in previous years. They range from articles about the basic mechanisms of disease and new syndromes, seemingly rare but nevertheless biologically extremely instructive, to articles that address very practical aspects of the evaluation and management of many, even thousands, of patients. Some of the articles anticipated or accompanied the approval by the United States Food and Drug Administration of two new drugs—metformin and acarbose—for use in patients with non–insulin-dependent diabetes, which will probably have substantial impact on clinical practice. Other articles reported on the efficacy of established treatments, e.g., estrogen and radioactive iodine.

The chapter on the pituitary gland includes an article documenting the nonprogressive course of patients found to have a pituitary mass in the course of neuroradiologic studies done for some other purpose. The authors of another study suggest that some patients with pituitary apoplexy need not undergo surgery, contrary to usual practice, but may be managed conservatively. There are also two articles on hyponatremia, one describing a surprisingly high frequency after transsphenoidal surgery in patients with Cushing's disease and another describing the risk factors for hyponatremia among hospitalized patients with psychiatric disorders. While hyponatremia in patients in either group, or indeed in hospitalized patients in general, is not often severe and attributing symptoms to it is difficult, some water restriction will usually suffice to raise the serum sodium concentration, and clinical benefit may ensue.

Idiopathic adrenal insufficiency remains—according to a study from the United Kingdom—by far the most common cause of adrenal insufficiency. While probably also true in the United States, the proportion of patients in whom it is caused by infection is undoubtedly higher here, especially among those with HIV infection and AIDS. There is an article that describes the possible causes and diagnosis of adrenal insufficiency in patients with septic shock, in which the possibility of reversible cytokine-mediated pituitary-adrenal hypofunction is suggested. Maybe so, but whenever adrenal insufficiency is suspected in an acutely ill patient treatment should be initiated without delay (with minimal rapid testing); the question of the extent of adrenal insufficiency and its permanency can be considered later. I also included a report of a study of the effects of administration of the adrenal steroid dehydroepiandrosterone in middle-aged and older adults, primarily because there has been a good deal written—mostly in the lay press—about how its production declines with aging and how its administration may bolster immune responsiveness, prevent cancer, and do other wondrous things, and also because I have been asked about it by patients. The production of dehydroepiandrosterone does indeed decline with age, and when given exogenously under controlled conditions, it has some potentially beneficial hormonal effects and seems to make people feel better, but ....

The first article in the chapter on the thyroid gland describes the results of a 20-year follow-up study of subjects in the urban and rural community of Whickham (United Kingdom). The original survey provided the first extensive information about the frequency of thyroid disease in the community, and this new survey tells what happened to the same subjects in the next 20 years. The key finding is the very high risk of hypothyroidism in persons who had an elevated serum thyrotropin concentration and a positive test for thyroid antibodies at the first examination. Another important article in this chapter describes a 3-fold increase in the risk of atrial fibrillation in patients with low serum thyrotropin concentrations during a 10-year follow-up period, as compared with those with normal values; there was no increase in the risk of overt hyperthyroidism. Is this risk large enough to justify intervention routinely? I think not (see my comment on the article for more details). A third article contains a reminder that congestive heart failure can occur in patients with hyperthyroidism. I also included an article documenting that Graves' ophthalmopathy is not often progressive, justifying conservative management for most patients, and one on thyroxine therapy in patients with a solitary thyroid nodule. In the latter study, thyroxine was more effective than no therapy in reducing nodule size, but the benefit was limited to those patients with small nodules. The efficacy of thyroxine in patients with thyroid nodules has been studied previously, with conflicting results, and this new study by no means resolves the issue.

The topics of the articles in the chapter on parathyroid disorders range from studies on calcium absorption, to parathyroid disease, to skeletal disease in the elderly. One article describes parathyroid imaging with technetium-99m sestamibi. This seems the best procedure yet devised for imaging parathyroid tissue. I am not yet persuaded that it needs to be done routinely before parathyroid surgery, but it certainly is indicated before any reoperation. There are two articles about bone disease in patients with primary hyperparathyroidism. This is the complication of the disease about which we worry the most, particularly in those patients who have mild disease, for whom many physicians are reluctant to recommend neck exploration. The results of these two studies are reassuring in that they demonstrate that bone loss is not progressive in patients who are not treated and that it improves in those who are surgically treated. Finally, there are articles that reveal some of the risk factors for hip fracture and document the efficacy of estrogen in preventing these fractures.

The effects of estrogen deficiency in women are well known, but I doubt that anyone expected estrogen deficiency in men to affect primarily the skeleton, causing delayed epiphyseal closure and severe osteoporosis, as documented by Smith et al. in their report of a man who had no estrogen receptors and, therefore, complete estrogen resistance. Interestingly, this man had no hot flashes. Other articles in the chapter on reproduction indicate that men who are castrated as part of their treatment for carcinoma of the prostate may have hot flashes for years, and that in these men and also in women, hot flashes may be relieved by treatment with a progestin (megestrol acetate). I also included an article on the risks of carcinoma of the breast in postmenopausal women treated with estrogen, in which the authors found a small but significant time-dependent risk, especially with prolonged treatment and in older women, a risk not altered by concomitant progestin therapy.

The most important articles in the chapter on carbohydrate metabolism and diabetes mellitus are those that describe the efficacy of metformin and acarbose in patients with non–insulin-dependent diabetes. These are the first new treatments for diabetes to be introduced in the United States in many years. Both drugs effectively reduce blood glucose concentrations, although the best way to use either remains to be determined. Another question considered in this chapter is the extent to which blood glucose needs to be reduced to effect a reduction in risk of diabetic nephropathy and perhaps other complications of diabetes. The article on this topic suggests that reducing glycosylated hemoglobin values below a threshold (albeit elevated) value minimizes the risk of these complications; however, these (and other) data can also be interpreted to indicate that the risk is progressive and, therefore, treatment must be aimed at reducing glycosylated hemoglobin values to normal. This is not a theoretical debate, because if much of the advantage of lowering blood glucose concentrations can be achieved by moderately vigorous treatment, then many more patients will benefit, given that large reductions in blood glucose are more difficult to achieve and are accompanied by more frequent and severe hypoglycemia.

The problem of obesity is gradually being unraveled in terms of our understanding of both the metabolic abnormalities that make it so difficult for patients to maintain weight loss and the underlying mechanisms of obesity. The most striking advance made during the past year was the identification of the *ob* gene and its product in mice, which has already led to studies demonstrating that the product of the gene causes weight loss in obese animals, and that the gene seems to be normal in most obese humans. Some obese patients do have mutations in the gene for the β_3-adrenergic receptor, which might result in resistance to the lipolytic effects of catecholamines and could therefore contribute to obesity. This is an extremely active area of investigation, and new understanding of the pathophysiology of obesity and, probably, new treatments can be anticipated very soon.

Robert D. Utiger, M.D.

48 The Pituitary Gland

The Natural History of the Pituitary Incidentaloma

Donovan LE, Corenblum B (Univ of Calgary Health Sciences Centre, Alberta, Canada)

Arch Intern Med 155:181–183, 1995 119-96-48–1

Background.—With the wide availability of CT and MRI, unsuspected, endocrinologically silent pituitary masses, known as pituitary incidentalomas, have often been discovered. The most appropriate management for these patients is not known, but an aggressive approach seems unjustified because pituitary adenomas are discovered at autopsy in up to 27% of people. To develop a more rational approach to the management of pituitary incidentalomas, the natural course of untreated patients with these tumors was studied.

Methods.—In a prospective study, 31 adults with pituitary incidentalomas were followed for a mean of 6 years (range, 3–11 years). Fifteen patients had pituitary lesions less than 10 mm in diameter (mean, 5 mm), and 16 had lesions 10 mm or greater (mean, 15 mm). Clinical and biochemical assessment, CT or MRI of the pituitary, and visual field testing by Goldmann perimetry were performed at baseline, 6 months, and yearly thereafter.

Findings.—Tumor enlargement or complications occurred in 5 of the 16 patients with pituitary incidentalomas 10 mm or greater in diameter. The tumor enlarged by 2–5 mm in 4 patients, although 3 of these 4 patients remained asymptomatic during follow-up of 6–10 years. Two patients had complications. One had visual field impairment because of the enlarging mass, underwent transsphenoidal surgery, and then had permanent panhypopituitarism. The other had pituitary apoplexy during heparinzation for a coronary angiogram. In 4 patients with tumor diameters less than 10 mm, the size of the tumor decreased by 3–5 mm on the last CT; the other patients in this group had no change in the size of their pituitary mass.

Implications.—Pituitary incidentalomas usually follow a benign course for at least 6 years after discovery. Neurosurgical intervention is not necessary, particularly in patients with tumors less than 10 mm in diameter, but regular observation should be maintained.

► The occasional finding of a pituitary mass lesion in a patient in whom CT or MRI was done for another purpose raises several questions. What is the mass? Does it have any neurologic or endocrine effects? What should be done, both diagnostically and therapeutically?

Most of these masses are pituitary microadenomas (less than 10 mm in diameter), but some are macroadenomas and a few are cysts, metastatic lesions, granulomas, or infarcts.[1] The mass rarely causes headache, visual disturbance, or a clinically unrecognized syndrome of hormonal hypersecretion (acromegaly, Cushing's disease, etc.). With respect to hormonal evaluation, it is reasonable to measure serum cortisol (in the morning), thyroxine and thyrotropin, prolactin, testosterone (in men), and follicle-stimulating hormone (in men, any premenopausal woman who has amenorrhea or irregular cycles, and postmenopausal women). The results are nearly always normal, although a few patients have mild hyperprolactinemia.

What about therapy? In this study, in which the mean follow-up was quite long, few patients had an increase in the size of their mass, and all of them were in the macroadenoma group (the 1 patient who had surgery because his vision deteriorated proved to have a cystic craniopharyngioma). The increase in diameter varied from 2 to 5 mm and was not progressive in the 3 patients who had no clinical problems and did not undergo surgery. One might question the wisdom of this course, because there is no way to predict whether any increase will be progressive, but the results justify the procrastination. Others have reported similar results, although the duration of follow-up was shorter (mean, 22 months).[2]

Even if the incidental tumor is a macroadenoma, therefore, periodic clinical evaluation and imaging are all that are needed. With respect to imaging, it seems prudent to repeat it after 6 and 12 months and then yearly in patients with macroadenomas (I think yearly and then bi-yearly imaging is adequate for those with microadenomas). With respect to the type of imaging that should be done, to facilitate comparison I would do whatever had been done when the incidental mass was first detected.

R.D. Utiger, M.D.

References

1. Molitch ME: Evaluation and treatment of the patient with a pituitary incidentaloma. *J Clin Endocrinol Metab* 80:3–6, 1995.
2. Reincke M, Allolio B, Saeger W, et al: The 'incidentaloma' of the pituitary gland. *JAMA* 263:2772–2776, 1990. (1991 Year Book of Medicine, pp 501–503.)

Hypothalamic–Pituitary Dysfunction in Patients With Craniopharyngioma

Paja M, Lucas T, García-Uría J, Salamé F, Barceló B, Estrada J (Clínica Puerta de Hierro, Spain; Universidad Autónoma de Madrid, Spain)

Clin Endocrinol 42:467–473, 1995 119-96-48–2

Objective.—Endocrine function was evaluated before and after treatment in 35 patients (22 males and 13 females) who underwent surgery for craniopharyngioma in the years 1980–1992. The patient age range was 2–77 years, but most were adults in the third or fourth decade of life.

Preoperative Findings.—Sixteen of the 35 patients were seen with endocrine disorders, most often hypogonadism or diabetes insipidus. Nine patients had neurologic symptoms and 8 had a visual defect. Two children were seen with retarded growth. Six patients had symptoms of hypothyroidism and 4 of hypocortisolism. More than 80% of the patients had biochemical evidence of hypogonadotropic hypogonadism. Ten patients younger than 19 years of age had growth hormone deficiency. The serum thyroxine was low in 37% and serum cortisol was low in 35%. The incidence of diabetes insipidus was 38%. Seven patients had a high basal serum prolactin concentration.

Management and Outcome.—Thirty-one patients underwent craniotomy, and 4 a transsphenoidal operation. The craniopharyngioma was totally removed in 12 patients. There were no perioperative deaths. During an average follow-up of 50 months, tumor recurred in 4 patients after presumed total excision. Adults whose tumors were subtotally removed received radiotherapy 6–12 months after surgery; only one patient had a recurrence, which caused death a year after surgery. Ten younger patients who did not receive radiotherapy after subtotal tumor removal had recurrences. The visual fields of 9 eyes recovered postoperatively but decreased in 18 others, and 2 of these eyes became blind. Panhypopituitarism was documented in 80% of patients 2–3 months postoperatively (Fig 1), and most of the remainder had multiple deficiencies. Diabetes insipidus resolved in 2 patients but developed for the first time in 13 others.

Conclusions.—Hormonal disorders are very common in patients with craniopharyngioma both before and especially after treatment. Earlier diagnosis may limit the development of some of these problems as well as visual and neurologic problems.

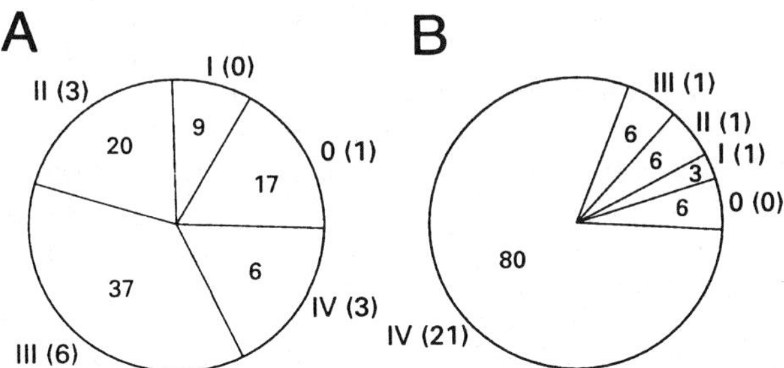

FIGURE 1.—Anterior pituitary deficits (**A**) before and (**B**) after surgery in 35 patients with craniopharyngioma. Roman numerals (I–IV) indicate the number of deficient hormones, including growth hormone, gonadotropins, adrenocorticotropic hormone, and thyroid-stimulating hormone. The percentage of patients in each group appears in the circle. *Arabic numbers within brackets* show the number of patients with diabetes insipidus in each group. (Courtesy of Paja M, Lucas T, García-Uría J, et al: Hypothalamic: Pituitary dysfunction in patients with crangiopharyngioma. *Clin Endocrinol* 42:467–473, 1995. Reproduced by permission of Blackwell Science, Ltd.)

Peripartum Hypopituitarism and Lymphocytic Hypophysitis

Patel MC, Guneratne N, Haq N, West TET, Weetman AP, Clayton RN (Keele Univ, Stoke on Trent, England; Princess Royal Hosp, Telford, England; Northern Gen Hosp, Sheffield, England)

Q J Med 88:571–580, 1995 119-96-48–3

Background.—When associated with pregnancy, hypopituitarism is mainly the result of Sheehan's syndrome and lymphocytic hypophysitis. The former is associated with hypotension during parturition, whereas the latter is associated with pituitary mass effects and pituitary hormone deficiencies, and ultimately requires pituitary biopsy for proof.

Objective.—The clinical course of 5 women in whom pregnancy-associated hypopituitarism was believed to be caused by lymphocytic hypophysitis was evaluated.

Findings.—The symptoms occurred during or immediately after pregnancy. Two women had visual field defects, and 3 had nonspecific illness related to deficiencies of anterior pituitary hormones. Four of the women were unable to lactate, and 4 were initially amenorrheic. Four had secondary hypothyroidism; another had painless thyroiditis 6 months post partum. Four women had hypocortisolemia, and 1 had normal cortisol secretion. Four had undetectable plasma prolactin concentrations, and 1 had hyperprolactinemia. All the women had abnormal short corticotropin stimulation tests, although 1 had only marginally abnormal results with a normal plasma cortisol response to hypoglycemia. Initially, 4 women had enlarged pituitary glands on MRI, but follow-up scans showed a return of the gland size to normal. Tests of serum for antipituitary and other organ-specific autoantibodies were negative. None of the women had complicated pregnancies, and the 2 who underwent cesarean section had no episodes of hypotension.

Implications.—Lymphocytic hypophysitis is more common than previously thought, but the variable and nonspecific symptoms and tendency to recovery make the diagnosis difficult. The diagnosis should be considered in postpartum women with persistent malaise who have concomitant hypothyroidism, hypocortisolemia, or both. The condition tends to be detected earlier in women with amenorrhea and those with visual impairment developing in the last trimester of pregnancy without antecedent pituitary disease. It should be treated conservatively, as the pituitary enlargement frequently regresses with time.

► These two papers (Abstracts 119-96-48–2 and 119-96-48–3) deal with interesting, albeit unusual, causes of hypopituitarism: craniopharyngioma and lymphocytic hypophysitis. The former is an "old" disorder, usually thought of as a disorder of children and adolescents, so a reminder that it can occur in adults seemed worthwhile. The latter is a "new" disorder, first described about 30 years ago, and is now probably a more important cause of hypopituitarism in the postpartum period than pituitary infarction (Sheehan's syndrome).

Craniopharyngiomas are most common in children, but they can occur at any age. The majority are located above the sella turcica (54% in the paper of Paja et al.); however, some are both suprasellar and intrasellar (40%), and a few are entirely intrasellar (6%). They are often calcified, cystic, or both, especially in children. Most patients (83% in this series) have 1 or more anterior pituitary hormone deficiencies, and some (20% in this series) have modest hyperprolactinemia, as, of course, do patients with large pituitary adenomas. Diabetes insipidus is a strong clue to the presence of a craniopharyngioma, because of the suprasellar location of many of the tumors. This study nicely documents the high likelihood of additional hormonal abnormalities after treatment (see Figure 1 in the original article). This is because the tumors tend to be large and are located in an area where it is difficult to remove them without further disturbing the hypothalamus and the hypothalamic-pituitary portal circulation. Furthermore, the tumor must usually be approached by a craniotomy, which is more hazardous and from which most patients recover more slowly than if they had undergone transsphenoidal surgery.

Lymphocytic hypophysitis is an ill-defined inflammatory disease of the anterior pituitary that has been diagnosed most often during the first year post partum (all the patients in this study, 15 of 38 in a summary study[1]) or during pregnancy (usually the third trimester), but it can occur distant from pregnancy and rarely in men. The symptoms may be those of a pituitary mass lesion (headache and visual abnormalities); adrenal, thyroid, or gonadal insufficiency; or both. Imaging studies characteristically show a homogeneously enlarged pituitary gland, sometimes extending above the sella turcica with enhancement after administration of a contrast agent. The diagnosis can only be proven by biopsy (or excision), which reveals lymphocytic infiltration, a few plasma cells, and some residual pituitary cells. Biopsy is justifiable if there is a pituitary mass that is causing visual impairment (meaning that in many patients, including the 5 women described in this article, the diagnosis is presumed). Some patients have had spontaneous improvement in some or all manifestations of the disorder after weeks or months, making reports of benefit during glucocorticoid therapy difficult to interpret, whereas others have gradually developed panhypopituitarism.

This disorder is presumed to be an autoimmune disease, mostly on the basis of the pathological findings, the presence of antipituitary antibodies or other autoantibodies in a few patients, and the induction of hypophysitis in animals by injecting various foreign antigens. However, autoimmune diseases characteristically remit during the latter part of pregnancy and do not usually worsen during the first few months post partum, both of which are times when lymphocytic hypophysitis often becomes clinically evident. Whatever its cause, it should certainly be considered in any woman who develops symptoms of pituitary disease either during or fairly soon after pregnancy. When the onset is during the postpartum period, it can be distinguished from postpartum pituitary infarction by the absence of a history of postpartum hemorrhage, the presence of symptoms of a pituitary mass, and the radiologic finding of an enlarged pituitary gland.

R.D. Utiger, M.D.

Reference

1. Powrie JK, Powell M, Ayers AB, et al: Lymphocytic adenohypophysitis: Magnetic resonance imaging features of two new cases and a review of the literature. *Clin Endocrinol (Oxf)* 42:315–322, 1995.

Conservative Management of Pituitary Apoplexy: A Prospective Study

MacCagnan P, Macedo CLD, Kayath MJ, Nogueira RG, Abucham J (Escola Paulista de Medicina, Sao Paulo, Brazil)
J Clin Endocrinol Metab 80:2190–2197, 1995 119-96-48–4

Background.—Pituitary apoplexy as a complication of a pituitary tumor necessitating immediate neurosurgical intervention has been thought to be rare. However, recent reports suggest that pituitary apoplexy is more common than was believed and that surgery is not always the best treatment. This prospective study examined the efficacy of conservative treatment.

Methods.—Twelve patients with the diagnosis of pituitary apoplexy established by CT imaging were studied. The patients' initial symptoms included headache, visual impairment, or ophthalmoplegia. Eleven patients received dexamethasone, 2 to 16 mg/day, intravenously. Surgery was undertaken when there was no improvement in vision or consciousness after dexamethasone was given.

Findings.—Of the 7 patients treated conservatively, 6 completely recovered from ophthalmoplegia, and 1 improved. On follow-up CT scans, 4 patients had resolution of their tumor and 3 patients had residual pituitary masses. Five patients had surgery, with improvement in vision and consciousness; all 5 patients had residual masses on follow-up imaging studies. One patient in each group had a recurrence. The frequencies of pituitary deficiencies in the surgical and conservative treatment groups were comparable. However, when the analysis included only patients with tumors that disappeared after the apoplexy, the prevalence of pituitary deficiencies was higher in the conservative treatment group. An anaylsis of the clinical and CT results showed that visual impairment did not improve during dexamethasone treatment, whereas the presence of a large hypodense region in the tumor predicted complete tumor resolution.

Conclusions.—Patients with pituitary apoplexy but no visual loss or impairment in consciousness may be conservatively treated.

▶ Pituitary apoplexy is characterized by sudden onset of headache, nausea and vomiting, hypotension, blurring or loss of vision, diplopia, and impaired consciousness and is generally considered a surgical emergency. This study indicates that some patients, in particular those who do not have loss of vision, impaired consciousness, or a large pituitary tumor or evidence of multiple hemorrhages, do well when treated with a high dose of glucocorticoid and subsequently do not need surgery. I doubt that these results will dissuade most physicians from recommending surgery in nearly all these patients, but at the least they indicate that there is an alternative.

Most patients with pituitary apoplexy have previously unrecognized pituitary macroadenomas (greater than 1 cm in diameter), and many have evidence of hypopituitarism at the time of hospitalization.[1] They should be treated immediately with a high dose of dexamethasone or hydrocortisone and probably also with thyroxine, regardless of whether surgery is planned. Extensive hormonal studies need not be done immediately (and were not done in this study), because the results are likely to change even if the patient is not operated on; however, they are mandatory several weeks or so later. The tendency is to assume that pituitary function will decline if the patient is operated on and an attempt is made to remove all of the tumor. However, pituitary hormone deficiencies may disappear after surgery, presumably because of relief of compression of the pituitary stalk or pituitary tissue itself.[1]

Computed tomography or MRI (and surgery) reveals regions of hemorrhage, necrosis, or both, or cysts (probably reflecting old hemorrhage) in 15% to 20% of pituitary macroadenomas. These superimposed abnormalities are usually small, and few patients recall having a severe or unusual headache, much less the nausea and vomiting, blurring or loss of vision or diplopia, or altered consciousness that characterize pituitary apoplexy. It is, therefore, likely that pituitary apoplexy is a good deal more common than we recognize clinically, and, indeed, spontaneous subclinical infarction of a pituitary macroadenoma can occur.[2]

R.D. Utiger, M.D.

References

1. Arafah BM, Harrington JF, Madhoun ZT, et al: Improvement of pituitary function after surgical decompression for pituitary tumor apoplexy. *J Clin Endocrinol Metab* 71:323–328, 1990. (1991 Year Book of Medicine, pp 510–512.)
2. Onesti ST, Nisniewski T, Post KD: Clinical versus subclinical pituitary apoplexy: Presentation, surgical management, and outcome in 21 patients. *Neurosurgery* 26:980–986, 1990.

Isolated Hyponatremia After Transsphenoidal Pituitary Surgery

Olson BR, Rubino D, Gumowski J, Oldfield EH (Natl Inst of Child Health and Human Development, Bethesda, Md; Natl Inst of Neurological Disorders and Stroke, Bethesda, Md)

J Clin Endocrinol Metab 80:85–91, 1995 119-96-48–5

Background.—In patients undergoing transsphenoidal pituitary surgery, hyponatremia may occur in isolation or before the onset of postoperative diabetes insipidus. This hyponatremia is believed to result from nonosmotic release of arginine vasopressin from damaged nerve terminals in the posterior pituitary. Hyponatremia occurring after transsphenoidal surgery differs from acute postoperative hyponatremia in general surgical patients in that it is not iatrogenic, it occurs later after surgery, and no specific morbidity and mortality have been described. Fifty-eight patients undergoing transsphenoidal pituitary adenomectomy were examined to determine the incidence and time course and incidence of hyponatremia after the operation.

Methods.—The study subjects were 58 patients with Cushing's disease operated on during 1992. Thirty-five were women, 12 were men, and 11 were children. Six patients had postoperative diabetes insipidus or volume depletion. In the remaining 52 patients, the incidence of hyponatremia, its time of onset and duration, and the factors associated with it were evaluated.

Findings.—Twelve of the 52 patients (23%) had isolated hyponatremia, defined as a plasma sodium concentration of less than 135 mmol/L, during their postoperative course. Isolated hyponatremia occurred in 33% of the women, 17% of the men, and none of the children. Seven percent had symptomatic hyponatremia, defined as a plasma sodium concentration of 125 mmol/L or less, with a new onset of headache, nausea, and vomiting.

Hyponatremia began early in the postoperative period and worsened slowly for 7 days; antidiuresis peaked on postoperative day 7. Plasma vasopressin concentrations measured during hyponatremia in 2 patients were inappropriately high, suggesting that unregulated vasopressin release played a role in the hyponatremia. Patients with and without hyponatremia were comparable in terms of their plasma cortisol concentrations, glucocorticoid replacement regimen, and pituitary adenoma size. The nadir plasma sodium concentrations were lower in the women recently exposed to estrogen combined with documented posterior pituitary trauma during surgery. When hyponatremia developed, the patients were treated with fluid restriction. None had progressive neurologic symptoms or other morbidity, and none died.

Conclusions.—Isolated hyponatremia is common after transsphenoidal surgery for Cushing's disease and is probably caused by inappropriate vasopressin release. The outcome is good, most likely because of the mild degree and slow rate of development of hyponatremia. All patients undergoing transsphenoidal surgery should have daily monitoring of plasma sodium concentrations for at least 1 week. Mild fluid restriction should be instituted for patients with a trend toward hyponatremia 5–7 days postoperatively, especially menstruating women with posterior pituitary trauma during surgery.

► Hyponatremia has not traditionally been considered a complication of transsphenoidal pituitary surgery, although a few isolated cases have been reported. However, it is clear from this study of 52 patients with corticotropic adenomas (Cushing's disease) and another study of 86 patients with a variety of pituitary tumors (19 of whom had corticotropic adenomas)[1] that hyponatremia is a common complication of this operation. In the latter series, hyponatremia was more common (58%) in the patients with corticotropic adenomas compared with other pituitary tumors (31%). The frequency of hyponatremia, defined as a plasma (or serum) sodium concentration less than 135 mmol/L in both studies, was 23% and 37%, respectively, and the mean nadir values were between 125 and 130 mmol/L. More women were affected in both series, as is true for hyponatremia after any operation.[2] The nadir values were 7–9 days after surgery. About half the patients had symptoms like headache, nausea, and vomiting, which might be attributed to hyponatremia, but some of the nonhyponatremic patients had similar symptoms.

The associated biochemical findings in the hyponatremic patients were those of excess vasopressin action—low plasma and high urine osmolality; plasma vasopressin concentrations, when measured, were usually inappropriately elevated. What might cause abnormal vasopressin release after pituitary surgery? One possibility is operative trauma. Recorded posterior pituitary trauma was associated with hyponatremia in the study of Olson et al.; on the other hand, there was no association between hyponatremia and either tumor size or the occurrence of diabetes insipidus either 1–2 days or several weeks or months after surgery (2 patients in the combined series developed permanent diabetes insipidus). Another possibility is that the hyponatremia was a result of corticotropin (ACTH) and cortisol deficiency, a well-known cause of excess vasopressin secretion.[3] All the patients received perioperative glucocorticoid therapy, making that possibility unlikely, although it is possible that a decrease in plasma cortisol concentrations from high to normal might contribute to the excess vasopressin secretion in patients with Cushing's syndrome. Finally, fluid intake may be excessive. Excess vasopressin secretion does not cause much hyponatremia if oral or parenteral fluid intake is not excessive also. I suspect many of these patients are overhydrated immediately after surgery, in anticipation that they may develop diabetes insipidus (which, in fact, is rare after transsphenoidal surgery), and they probably drink more, too, either because they are encouraged to do so or because of a transient, unphysiologic increase in thirst.

Today, many patients who undergo transsphenoidal surgery leave the hospital in 3–4 days. It is prudent to determine the plasma sodium concentration at that time, advise the patient to restrict fluids if it is low, and warn the patient about the possibility of symptomatic hyponatremia. More aggressive testing is not warranted, in view of the limited degree and short duration of hyponatremia in nearly all patients.

R.D. Utiger, M.D.

References

1. Sane T, Rantakari K, Poranen A, et al: Hyponatremia after transsphenoidal surgery for pituitary tumors. *J Clin Endocrinol Metab* 79:1395–1398, 1994.
2. Ayus JC, Wheeler JM, Arieff AI: Postoperative hyponatremic encephalopathy in menstruant women. *Ann Intern Med* 117:891–897, 1992. (1994 YEAR BOOK OF MEDICINE, pp 563–565.)

3. Oelkers W: Hyponatremia and inappropriate secretion of vasopressin (antidiuretic hormone) in patients with hypopituitarism. *N Engl J Med* 321:492–496, 1989.

Risk Factors for the Development of Hyponatremia in Psychiatric Inpatients

Siegler EL, Tamres D, Berlin JA, Allen-Taylor L, Strom BL (Univ of Pennsylvania, Philadelphia; Philadelphia Veterans Affairs Med Ctr, Pa; Mount Sinai School of Medicine, New York)

Arch Intern Med 155:953–957, 1995 119-96-48–6

Background.—Hyponatremia occurs in about 2.5% of all hospitalized patients, but its prevalence among patients in a long-term psychiatric institution was reported as 6.4% in 1 study. Hyponatremia can cause lethargy, headache, confusion, or coma, and psychiatric treatment often must be altered or interrupted pending medical treatment of the hyponatremia. To determine the risk factors for the development of hyponatremia in psychiatric inpatients, the records of 1,905 patients residing at a tertiary psychiatric care facility (over a 3-year period) were reviewed.

Methods & Findings.—Sixty-four patients (3.4%) had serum sodium concentrations less than 130 mmol/L. None of these patients had psychogenic polydipsia. The medical history of each of these patients was compared with that of 3 control patients. Univariate (Table 1) and multivariate analyses revealed significant associations of hyponatremia with female sex, systolic blood pressure, elevated serum creatinine, abnormal serum potassium, diabetes mellitus, hypertension, chronic obstructive pulmonary disease, and administration of diuretics, tricyclic antidepressants, calcium antagonists, and fluoxetine. The strongest associations with hyponatremia were for abnormal serum potassium concentrations, diuretic therapy, and fluoxetine therapy.

Discussion.—Among psychiatric inpatients, hyponatremia is associated with therapy with several drugs and several co-morbid conditions that either have an impact on, or reflect impairment of, the handling of free water by the kidney. Serum sodium concentrations should be monitored in patients hospitalized for psychiatric treatment who have multiple risk factors for hyponatremia. If hyponatremia develops, early initiation of free-water restriction or discontinuation of responsible medications is indicated.

▶ The frequency of hyponatremia in any clinical study is inevitably based on a numerical value for the serum sodium concentration, usually chosen arbitrarily and without regard for the occurrence of symptoms (it was 130 mmol/L in this study). That is not surprising, because identification on clinical grounds would be very difficult. The symptoms of mild hyponatremia—lethargy, anorexia, nausea, headache, and confusion—are vague, and even if present, they may be due to the underlying cause of hyponatremia or

TABLE 1.—Risk Factors for Hyponatremia: Univariate Data

Risk Factor	No. (%) of Cases (n = 54)	No. (%) of Control Subjects (n = 192)	Odds Ratio (95% Confidence Interval)
Demographics			
Female	51(80)	126 (65)	2.1 (1.04–4.1)
Elderly (≥ 65) y	37(58)	45 (23)	4.5 (2.5–8.1)
Comorbidities			
Affective disorder	33 (52)	100 (52)	0.97 (0.6–1.7)
Diabetes mellitus	17 (27)	5 (3)	13.5 (4.8–38.6)
Hypertension	36 (56)	22 (11)	9.9 (5.1–19.3)
Congestive heart failure	15 (23)	7 (4)	8.1 (3.1–20.8)
Chronic obstructive pulmonary disease	6 (9)	1 (0.5)	19.8 (2.3–167.5)
Coronary artery disease	14 (22)	11 (5)	4.6 (2.0–10.8)
Abnormal potassium	17 (26)	5 (3)	13.5 (4.7–38.5)
Smoking			
Nonsmoker	37 (63)	104 (56)	1.0 (referent)
Current smoker	12 (20)	75 (40)	0.4 (0.2–0.8)
Quit within past 6 mo	10 (17)	8 (4)	3.5 (1.3–9.5)
Drugs			
Diuretic	19 (30)	6 (3)	13.1 (4.9–34.7)
Neuroleptic	15 (23)	51 (26)	0.8 (0.4–1.6)
Benzodiazepine	23 (36)	54 (28)	1.4 (0.8–2.6)
Monoamine oxidase inhibitor	3 (4)	6 (3)	1.5 (0.4–6.3)
Tricyclic antidepressant	15 (23)	27 (14)	1.9 (0.9–3.8)
β-Blocker	8 (13)	11 (6)	2.4 (0.9–6.1)
Calcium antagonist	16 (25)	8 (4)	7.7 (3.1–1.19)
Angiotensin-converting enzyme inhibitor	15 (23)	3 (2)	19.3 (5.4–69.3)
Nitrates	8 (13)	5 (3)	5.3 (1.7–17)
Fluoxetine	12 (18.7)	7 (4)	6.1 (2.3–16.3)

(Courtesy of Siegler EL, Tamres D, Berlin JA, et al: Risk factors for the development of hyponatremia in psychiatric inpatients. *Arch Intern Med* 155:953–957, 1995. Copyright 1995, American Medical Association.)

entirely unrelated to either the hyponatremia or its cause(s). Besides, it is better to identify hyponatremia before important symptoms occur and when it may be readily corrected by simple maneuvers like changes in medication and modest restriction of fluid intake.

Like in patients hospitalized on medical services,[1] hyponatremia among patients hospitalized for treatment of acute psychiatric disorders is multifactorial, being associated with multiple drugs and disorders. The immediate causes are undoubtedly a combination of impaired inhibition of vasopressin secretion (inappropriate vasopressin secretion) and increased fluid intake, because of increased thirst or excess parenteral administration, and increased sodium excretion, although the mechanisms responsible for these changes usually remain undefined.[2] Plasma vasopressin is hard to measure, and so we rely on measurements of plasma and urine osmolality to make inferences about vasopressin secretion. Thirst also is hard to measure, and we tend not to think much about it; however, I suspect that it is not normally inhibited by hypo-osmolality in many sick patients. I am not aware that fluoxetine or tricyclic antidepressant or calcium channel antagonist drugs stimulate vasopressin secretion or thirst, but I suspect that any drug or illness that affects central neurotransmitter function could do so.

A few patients with major psychiatric disease, especially those with schizophrenia, have severe polydipsia, and some of them have hyponatremia.[3] They, too, have impaired inhibition of vasopressin secretion, and they may also have increased renal sensitivity to vasopressin.[4] These patients differ from those described in this study mostly in degree, and they should also be treated primarily with fluid restriction.

R.D. Utiger, M.D.

References

1. Anderson RJ: Hospital-associated hyponatremia. *Kidney Int* 29:1237–1247, 1986.
2. Goldman MB, Luchins DJ, Robertson GL: Mechanisms of altered water metabolism in psychotic patients with polydipsia and polyuria. *N Engl J Med* 318:397–403, 1988.
3. Illowsky BP, Kirch DG: Polydipsia and hyponatremia in psychiatric patients. *Am J Psychiatry* 145:675–683, 1988.
4. Riggs AT, Dysken MW, Kim SW, et al: A review of disorders of water homeostasis in psychiatric patients. *Psychosomatics* 32:132–148, 1991.

49 The Adrenal Glands

Eighty-Six Cases of Addison's Disease

Kong M-F, Jeffcoate W (City Hosp, Nottingham, England)

Clin Endocrinol 41:757–761, 1994 119-96-49–1

Purpose.—Addison's disease is a rare condition. Affected patients tend to present in crisis to general medical teams and are not necessarily referred to specialist units. The goals of this study were to define the prevalence, incidence, and causes of Addison's disease. In addition, the criteria for diagnostic interpretation of the short corticotropin (ACTH) test were studied.

Methods.—All patients having Addison's disease who had been admitted to the hospitals in Nottingham, England, from 1987 to 1993 were reviewed.

Findings.—Eighty-six cases of Addison's disease were identified; 66 patients were still alive and in the city. The prevalence of the disease was calculated as 110 per million population. In 93% of the patients, the presumed cause was autoimmune destruction of the adrenal cortex. Two patients had metastatic cancer, and 3 unrelated patients had late-onset adrenoleukodystrophy. None of the cases were attributed to tuberculosis, however. During the study, 21 new cases of Addison's disease were diagnosed, for a calculated incidence of 5.6 per million per year. Based on an examination of the biochemical basis of the diagnosis in the 21 new cases, the authors suggest criteria for interpretation of the short ACTH test: a baseline serum cortisol of 250 nmol/L (9.0 µg/dL) or less and a value of 600 nmol/L (22 µg/dL) or less 30 minutes after ACTH injection indicate the presence of Addison's disease.

Discussion.—Nearly all the patients had autoimmune adrenal insufficiency and, surprisingly, not a single case was attributed to tuberculosis.

► A number of "new" causes of primary adrenal insufficiency have been identified in recent years, including cytomegalovirus, atypical mycobacterial, and other infections in patients with HIV infection (and maybe the HIV-1 virus itself); ketoconazole therapy; hypercoagulable and hypocoagulable states; and adrenoleukodystrophy (or adrenomyeloneuropathy); of course, its causation by metastatic carcinoma and tuberculosis (though not in this series) should not be forgotten either. (Acute adrenal insufficiency in patients with septic shock is considered in the Abstract 119-96-49–2). Nevertheless, easily the most common cause is what the authors of this study call autoimmune destruction of the adrenal cortex, but which is perhaps more often still called idiopathic adrenal insufficiency, or autoimmune adrenalitis.

The key clinical manifestations of chronic adrenal insufficiency, which are independent of its cause, are anorexia, weight loss, fatigue, weakness, hyperpigmentation, salt-craving, and symptoms of postural hypotension. Two types of findings lead to the presumptive diagnosis of autoimmune adrenalitis: (1) the absence of symptoms and signs of any disorder known to cause adrenal insufficiency, and (2) the presence of other autoimmune endocrinopathies, e.g., hypothyroidism or goiter caused by chronic autoimmune thyroiditis, Graves' hyperthyroidism, or premature ovarian failure. In this series, of the 81 patients presumed to have autoimmune adrenalitis, 25%, 11%, and 13%, respectively, had these disorders.

From 50% to 80% (55% in this study) of patients with autoimmune adrenalitis have antiadrenal antibodies, as detected by immunofluorescence. What these antibodies do is uncertain, but in some patients, the antibodies are directed against steroid 21-hydroxylase activity or, less often, other adrenal enzymes;[1] antibodies that block the action of ACTH also have been detected in a few patients.[2] I know of no study in which tests for all these different antibodies were done in a group of patients, so their overall frequency is uncertain; also, there is no compelling evidence that they do, in fact, cause adrenal dysfunction in vivo. The absence of these antibodies in a substantial proportion of patients means that testing for them is not a useful clinical test to determine the cause of adrenal insufficiency in an individual patient.

Patients suspected of having primary adrenal insufficiency should have measurements of serum electrolytes, creatinine, cortisol, and ACTH. The latter 2 tests are preferably done early in the morning, when both should be abnormal (low cortisol, high ACTH) in a patient with primary adrenal insufficiency; later in the day, when the serum cortisol is rather low in normal subjects, only the serum ACTH may be abnormal in a patient with primary adrenal insufficiency.[3, 4] A normal serum ACTH concentration is strong evidence against primary adrenal insufficiency but does not exclude ACTH deficiency. I think that the diagnosis of primary adrenal insufficiency should then be confirmed by measurements of serum cortisol and aldosterone before and 60 minutes after administration of cosyntropin (synthetic ACTH).

R.D. Utiger, M.D.

References

1. Rees Smith B, Furmaniak J: Adrenal and gonadal autoimmune disease. *J Clin Endocrinol Metab* 80:1502–1505, 1995.
2. Wulffraat NM, Drexhage HA, Bottazzo G-F, et al: Immunoglobulins of patients with idiopathic Addison's disease block the in vitro action of adrenocorticotrophin. *J Clin Endocrinol Metab* 69:231–238, 1989.
3. Oelkers W, Diederich S, Bahr V: Diagnosis and therapy surveillance in Addison's disease: Rapid adrenocorticotropin (ACTH) test and measurement of plasma ACTH, renin activity and aldosterone. *J Clin Endocrinol Metab* 75:259–264, 1992. (1993 Year Book of Medicine, pp 522–526.)

4. Grinspoon SK, Biller BMK: Laboratory assessment of adrenal insufficiency. *J Clin Endocrinol Metab* 79:923–931, 1994.

Adrenal Insufficiency Occurring During Septic Shock: Incidence, Outcome, and Relationship to Peripheral Cytokine Levels

Soni A, Pepper GM, Wyrwinski PM, Ramirez NE, Simon R, Pina T, Gruenspan H, Vaca CE (Lincoln Med and Mental Health Ctr, Bronx, NY; New York Med College, Valhalla)

Am J Med 98:266–271, 1995 119-96-49–2

Objectives.—Adrenal insufficiency has been reported in association with septic shock. The incidence of adrenal insufficiency during septic shock, and the effects of steroid supplementation on outcome in patients with impaired adrenal function were determined, and a possible correlation between adrenal function and peripheral blood cytokine concentrations was investigated.

Methods.—The study included 21 consecutive patients who were admitted to a medical and surgical ICU with septic shock and 11 normal subjects. Cortisol, tumor necrosis factor-α (TNF-α), and interleukin-6 (IL-6) concentrations were measured before and after infusion of low (1 μg) and standard (250 μg) doses of corticotropin (ACTH) given intravenously within 24 hours of the diagnosis of septic shock. Patients with an insufficient adrenal response to ACTH, which was defined as a serum cortisol concentration of less than 18 μg/dL (500 nmol/L) after the standard ACTH test, were treated with high doses of glucocorticoids. Plasma hormone and cytokine concentrations and survival data were compared between the patients with an adequate adrenal response and those with adrenal insufficiency.

Results.—Five (23.8%) patients had adrenal insufficiency, as defined above, and the other 16 patients had adequate adrenal reserve. The mean plasma TNF-α concentrations did not differ significantly between the patients in the 2 groups. The TNF-α concentrations correlated inversely with mean arterial pressure in the patients with adequate adrenal reserve but not those with adrenal insufficiency. The plasma IL-6 concentrations tended to be lower in patients with adrenal insufficiency, suggesting that a deficient IL-6 response to sepsis may contribute to understimulation of the pituitary-adrenal axis. Three patients with adrenal insufficiency received glucocorticoid therapy, with rapid improvement in hemodynamic parameters. Despite this recovery from the acute crisis, the mortality rate in patients with adrenal insufficiency was 80% at 4 weeks, as compared with 44% in patients with adequate adrenal reserve. At autopsy, 2 patients with adrenal insufficiency had intact adrenal cortices.

Discussion.—Adrenal insufficiency can occur in patients with septic shock and should be suspected in those patients who do not respond to conventional treatment. The standard-dose ACTH infusion test is adequate for detecting adrenal insufficiency. Pending the availability of the results, a trial of high doses of glucocorticoids is reasonable and may improve short-term survival in patients with adrenal insufficiency, but their overall mortality is worse than that of patients with septic shock and adequate adrenal reserve.

► The possibility of acute adrenal insufficiency is often raised in patients with septic shock who are responding poorly to antimicrobial drug and supportive therapy. How often these patients do, in fact, have acute adrenal insufficiency and its mechanism are uncertain. In this study, the diagnosis was based on a serum cortisol concentration less than 18 μg/dL (500 nmol/L) 30 minutes after administration of ACTH, a fairly standard definition.[1] The mean basal serum cortisol concentration in this group was about 9 μg/dL (248 nmol/L); the other patients had a mean basal serum cortisol concentration of about 26 μg/dL (717 nmol/L). The increment in serum cortisol after ACTH was about 5 μg/dL (138 nmol/L) in both groups of patients, as compared with 14 μg/dL (386 nmol/L) in the normal subjects. The smaller than normal response in the patients with septic shock who had normal adrenal responsiveness is in keeping with the general rule that the serum cortisol response to ACTH varies inversely with the basal serum cortisol concentration. The mean basal plasma ACTH concentration in the patients with adrenal insufficiency was slightly lower than that in the normal subjects [17 vs. 21 pg/mL (3.0 vs. 4.7 pmol/L)], and it was 41 pg/mL (9.0 pmol/L) in the other patients. The overall results are not unique; in another study of 32 patients with septic shock, 13 had poor cortisol responses to ACTH; all 32 died, as compared with 6 deaths among the other 19 patients.[2]

These results suggest that adrenal insufficiency in patients with septic shock is a result of both decreased ACTH secretion and decreased adrenal responsiveness to ACTH. Certainly, sepsis, hypotension, or associated coagulation disturbances could affect ACTH or adrenal secretion. While there is little direct evidence in support for a role for these factors, it seems very likely that they cause increased production of many cytokines, and that cytokines are important mediators of the pituitary-adrenal response to acute illness, which would surely include septic shock.[3] Exogenously administered interleukin-6 stimulates ACTH secretion,[4] as do other inflammatory cytokines; they also may have direct effects on the adrenal. The authors' studies of plasma IL-6 (supranormal in the patients with adequate adrenal function and subnormal in those with adrenal insufficiency) and tumor necrosis factor-α (supranormal in both patient groups) are compatible with, but hardly prove, a role for the former in reducing ACTH secretion and for the latter in reducing adrenal responses to stimulation. The actions of these substances could be transient, so that surviving patients might not have permanent adrenal insufficiency; the substances are more likely to be paracrine than endocrine, making unraveling their actions even more difficult.

There is no doubt that the occurrence of adrenal insufficiency, whatever its causes, contributes to the mortality of septic shock and related disorders. Because it may result from impaired ACTH secretion as well as impaired adrenal secretion, simultaneous measurements of ACTH and cortisol cannot be relied on for diagnosis, unlike in healthier outpatients.[5] Instead, an

ACTH stimulation test should be done, with measurements of serum cortisol before and 60 minutes after ACTH administration (some normal subjects have higher values at 60 than at 30 minutes). As a general rule, if the diagnosis is considered serious enough to warrant testing, the patient should be treated immediately; the treatment can always be stopped if the test results are normal.

R.D. Utiger, M.D.

References

1. Grinspoon SK, Biller BMK: Laboratory assessment of adrenal insufficiency. *J Clin Endocrinol Metab* 79:923–931, 1994.
2. Rothwell P, Udwadia ZF, Lawler PD: Cortisol response to corticotropin and survival in septic shock. *Lancet* 337:582–583, 1991.
3. Chrousos GP: The hypothalamic-pituitary-adrenal axis and immune-mediated inflammation. *N Engl J Med* 332:1351–1362, 1995.
4. Mastorakos G, Chrousos GP, Weber JS: Recombinant interleukin-6 activates the hypothalamic-pituitary-adrenal axis in humans. *J Clin Endocrinol Metab* 77:1690–1694, 1993.
5. Oelkers W, Diederich S, Bahr V: Diagnosis and therapy surveillance in Addison's disease: Rapid adrenocorticotropin (ACTH) test and measurement of plasma ACTH, renin activity, and aldosterone. *J Clin Endocrinol Metab* 75:259–264, 1992. (1993 YEAR BOOK OF MEDICINE, pp 522–525.)

Assessing the Hypothalamo-Pituitary-Adrenal Axis in Patients on Long-Term Glucocorticoid Therapy: The Short Synacthen Versus the Insulin Tolerance Test

Kane KF, Emery P, Sheppard MC, Stewart PM (Univ of Birmingham, England)
Q J Med 88:263–267, 1995 119-96-49–3

Introduction.—Long-term glucocorticoid treatment suppresses hypothalamo-pituitary-adrenal (HPA) function and may lead to adrenocortical atrophy. The insulin tolerance test is traditionally used to assess the HPA axis, but the short synacthen (corticotropin) test is a reliable alternative procedure in patients having pituitary disease. It is safer than the insulin tolerance test, and may be done on an outpatient basis. Some reports suggest, however, that it is less sensitive in evaluating the HPA axis in glucocorticoid-treated patients.

Objective and Methods.—The 2 tests were compared in 22 patients (17 women and 5 men; mean age, 50 years) who had received prednisolone in single daily doses of 3 to 10 mg for an average of 5.3 years (range, 0.75 to 15 years). The most common indications were rheumatoid arthritis and systemic lupus erythematosis. The tests were administered in random order at a 1-week interval, with glucocorticoid therapy being withheld on the morning of each test. The insulin test was considered positive if the peak plasma cortisol concentration 30 to 120 minutes after 0.15 IU/kg of insulin exceeded 500 nmol/L (18 μg/dL). The corticotropin test, done by injecting 250 μg of synthetic corticotropin ($ACTH_{1-24}$) intramuscularly, was considered positive if the 30-minute plasma cortisol concentration exceeded 550 nmol/L (20 μg/dL).

Results.—Five of the 22 patients had normal responses in both tests, 9 failed both tests, and the results were discordant in 8 patients. All the latter patients failed the corticotropin test but passed the insulin tolerance test. There was very close correlation between the peak cortisol concentration after insulin and the 30-minute value after corticotropin (Fig 1). The dose of prednisolone and the duration of treatment were inversely correlated with the plasma cortisol response in both tests. Patients failing both tests tended to have taken a higher dose of prednisolone for longer than those who passed.

Conclusions.—The corticotropin-stimulation test is a reliable and safe means of evaluating the HPA axis in patients receiving long-term glucocorticoid therapy. The more time-consuming and less safe insulin tolerance test may be reserved for patients who have poor responses to corticotropin.

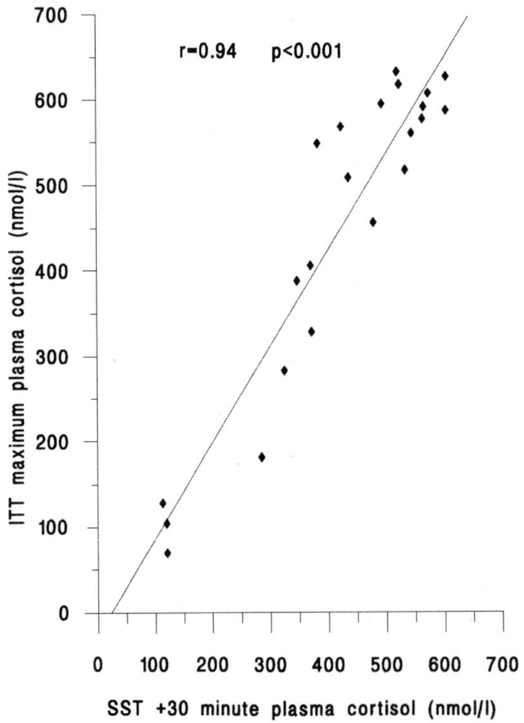

FIGURE 1.—Correlation between the peak plasma level of cortisol after insulin-induced hypoglycemia and the plasma level of cortisol after the administration of 250 μg of IM synacthen in 22 patients receiving long-term corticosteroid therapy. (Courtesy of Kane KF, Emery P, Sheppard MC, et al: Assessing the hypothalamo-pituitary-adrenal axis in patients on long-term glucocorticoid therapy: The short synacthen versus the insulin tolerance test. *Q J Med* 88:263–267, 1995. Reprinted by permission of Oxford University Press.)

▶ The patients in this study were taking daily doses of prednisolone in the range of what would be given to a patient with Addison's disease and which, therefore, in a person with normal pituitary-adrenal function would be expected to reduce but not abolish endogenous ACTH and adrenal secretion. In fact, their basal plasma cortisol concentrations on the 2 study days (about 24 hours after a dose of prednisolone) averaged 218 nmol/L (7.9 µg/dL), so that they must have been secreting some ACTH. Their responses to ACTH and insulin hypoglycemia, therefore, should not have been so discordant. One reason for the discordance is that the authors measured plasma cortisol 5 times after the administration of insulin but only once (30 minutes) after the administration of ACTH, and the values are nearly always a little higher 60 minutes after ACTH injection.[1] Another reason is that the threshold value for a normal plasma cortisol response to ACTH was set 50 nmol/L (1.8 µg/dL) higher than the response to insulin, for no physiologic reason that I can think of. Lowering the plasma cortisol response to ACTH considered normal by that amount reduces by half the discordance between the 2 tests, and Figure 1 shows that the correlation between the responses is very good.

As a practical matter, there is rarely any need to do any type of stimulation test in patients taking a small dose of glucocorticoid. If the patient becomes acutely ill, additional glucocorticoid will be given, without waiting for any tests. If elective surgery is planned, a test could be done, but it is easier to give more glucocorticoid then, too. If glucocorticoid therapy is to be discontinued, I recommend measuring plasma cortisol in the morning, 18–24 hours after the last dose. If the value is 220 to 280 nmol/L (8 to 10 µg/dL) or more, therapy can be discontinued. If not, the dose can be reduced slightly, and the patient can be retested in a month or so. If a test is to be done, I prefer the ACTH test. It is simpler, safer, and quicker, and both the results shown in Figure 1 and those in the literature suggest it is a reliable test of ACTH deficiency as well as of primary adrenal insufficiency.[2]

R.D. Utiger, M.D.

References

1. Dickstein G, Shechner C, Nicholson WE, et al: Adrenocorticotrophin stimulation test: Effects of basal cortisol level, time of day, and suggested new sensitive low dose test. *J Clin Endocrinol Metab* 72:773–778, 1991.
2. Lindholm J, Kehlet H: Re-evaluation of the clinical value of the 30-minute ACTH test in evaluating the hypothalamic-pituitary-adrenal function. *Clin Endocrinol (Oxf)* 26:53–59, 1987.

Effects of Replacement Dose of Dehydroepiandrosterone in Men and Women of Advancing Age

Morales AJ, Nolan JJ, Nelson JC, Yen SSC (Univ of California, La Jolla; Nichols Inst Reference Labs, San Juan Capistrano, Calif)

J Clin Endocrinol Metab 78:1360–1367, 1994 119-96-49–4

Introduction.—Aging is accompanied by a progressive decline of adrenal secretion of dehydroepiandrosterone (DHEA) and its sulfate ester (DHEAS), paralleling that of the growth hormone/insulin-like growth factor–I (GH-IGF-I) axis. Epidemiological data support beneficial effects of DHEA and DHEAS, but their biological role in humans remains elusive. The hypothesis that the decline in DHEA secretion contributes to the shift from anabolism to catabolism associated with aging was tested.

Methods.—A dose of 50 mg of DHEA or placebo was administered orally at bedtime each day to 17 women and 13 men ranging in age from 40 to 70 years. All the subjects in the double-blind, placebo crossover trial were nonobese nonsmokers, had stable dietary and exercise regimens, and were taking no medications. Fifteen of the women were menopausal, and 8 were receiving estrogen replacement therapy. Each subject received DHEA and placebo for 3 months in random order. Serum concentrations of androgens, lipids, apolipoproteins, IGF-I, IGF-binding protein-1 (IGFBP-1) and IGFBP-3; insulin sensitivity; percent body fat; libido; and sense of well being were measured during each treatment period.

Results.—After initiation of DHEA, serum DHEA and DHEAS concentrations increased in both men and women, reaching values typically found in young adults. These concentrations were maintained throughout the 3-month treatment period and then declined to baseline values within 2 weeks after DHEA was discontinued. Serum concentrations of androgens increased 2-fold in women; men had only a small rise in serum androstenedione and no change in testosterone. Neither men nor women had changes in serum sex hormone–binding globulin, estrone, or estradiol concentrations. There was a slight decline in serum high-density lipoprotein concentrations in women, but there were no other lipid changes. Percent body fat and insulin sensitivity did not change. Serum IGF-I concentrations increased and IGFBP-1 decreased significantly in both sexes, despite a lack of change in the mean 24-hour serum GH and IGFBP-3 concentrations, suggesting increased availability of IGF-I to target tissues. No change in libido was reported. The majority of both men (67%) and women (82%) noted an improved sense of well-being while receiving DHEA, whereas less than 10% reported any change after placebo administration.

Conclusion.—A replacement dose of DHEA raised serum DHEA and DHEAS concentrations in men and women over age 40 years to values found in younger persons and induced an increase in bioavailable IGF-I, supporting the hypothesis that DHEA has a biological function in humans. Physical and psychological well-being may be enhanced with DHEA replacement.

► Both the cause and the consequences, if any, of the progressive 80% decline in both serum DHEA and DHEAS concentrations from about age 25 years to age 80 years are unexplained.[1] Virtually all the DHEA and most of the DHEAS come from the adrenal, although sulfation of DHEA can occur in many tissues. With respect to the decline in DHEA and DHEAS production, all one can say is that the activity of the adrenal enzyme (17-20-lyase) that removes the steroid side chain declines, but why it declines is not known.

Little is known about the consequences of the age-related decline in serum DHEA (and DHEAS) concentrations; indeed, little is known about the biological activity of DHEA. It may have either androgenic or estrogenic effects, depending on the sex and age of the person.[2] Its androgenic activity probably results from its peripheral conversion to androstenedione and then testosterone, whereas its estrogenic activity results from androgen-to-estrogen conversion. Some data suggest that persons with lower serum DHEA and DHEAS concentrations have more cardiovascular disease and cancer, and less immunocompetence than those with higher concentrations, and that among patients with HIV infection, those with lower serum DHEAS concentrations have lower CD4 cell counts.[3] Morales et al. attempted to get at some of these questions from a mechanistic point of view. The subjects given DHEA had some potentially beneficial effects (small increases in serum androstenedione, testosterone, and insulin-like growth factor–I concentrations) that were not consistent among the sexes, in addition to the rather substantial increases in psychological and physical well-being.

I don't know what these results mean, but it is safe to say that they will lead to more studies of DHEA, in search for a simple solution to the ravages of aging and the disorders that accompany it. I wouldn't bet on its efficacy.

R.D. Utiger, M.D.

References

1. Orentreich N, Brind JL, Rizer RL, et al: Age changes and sex differences in serum dehydroepiandrosterone sulfate concentrations throughout adulthood. *J Clin Endocrinol Metab* 59:551–555, 1984.
2. Ebeling P, Koivisto VA: Physiological importance of dehydroepiandrosterone. *Lancet* 343:1479–1481, 1994.
3. Wisniewski TL, Hilton CW, Morse EV, et al: The relationship of serum DHEA-S and cortisol levels to measures of immune function in human immunodeficiency virus-related illness. *Am J Med Sci* 305:79–83, 1995.

Diagnosis and Treatment of Primary Hyperaldosteronism

Blumenfeld JD, Sealey JE, Schlussel Y, Vaughan ED Jr, Sos TA, Atlas SA, Müller FB, Acevedo R, Ulick S, Laragh JH (New York Hosp–Cornell Med Ctr, New York; Veterans Affairs Med Ctr, Bronx, NY)

Ann Intern Med 121:877–885, 1994 119-96-49–5

Background.—Primary hyperaldosteronism is characterized by hypertension, hypokalemia, and low plasma renin activity. It is most often caused by an adrenal adenoma. The clinical and laboratory features of primary hyperaldosteronism were evaluated, and diagnostic test results were assessed to determine which feature(s) test results might differentiate surgically curable forms of this disorder.

Patients and Methods.—Eighty-two patients with primary aldosteronism were retrospectively reviewed. Blood pressure, serum electrolytes, urinary aldosterone and electrolytes, CT scans, plasma renin and aldosterone before and during upright posture, plasma atrial natriuretic peptide, and adrenal venous plasma aldosterone and cortisol values were evaluated. Blood pressure, serum electrolytes, and plasma renin activity after treatment were also assessed.

Results.—Plasma aldosterone/renin ratios were higher in the patients with primary aldosteronism—independent of its cause—as compared with patients with other types of hypertension (Fig 2). The patients with adrenal adenomas had higher systolic and diastolic blood pressures, lower serum potassium concentrations, and higher urinary 18-methyl oxygenated cortisol-metabolite excretion than did the patients with bilateral adrenal

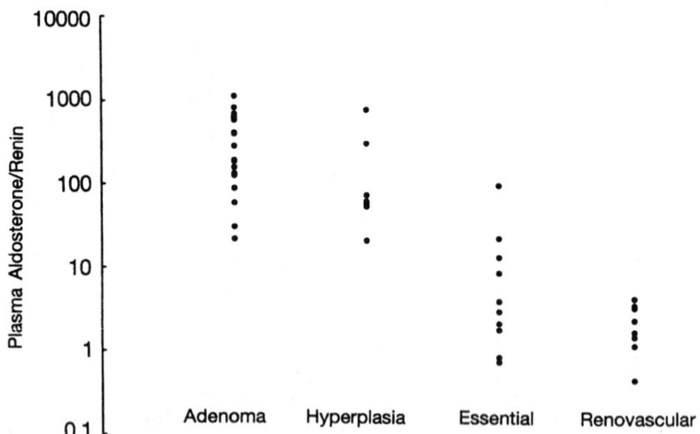

FIGURE 2.—Comparison of the ratio of plasma aldosterone to plasma renin activity for primary aldosteronism (aldosterone-producing adenoma and nonadenomatous adrenal hyperplasia) and renovascular and essential hypertension. A ratio of greater than 50 helped identify patients with primary aldosteronism. (Courtesy of Blumenfeld JD, Sealey JE, Schlussel Y, et al: Diagnosis and treatment of primary hyperaldosteronism. *Ann Intern Med* 121:877–885, 1994.)

hyperplasia. Aldosterone secretion lateralized to 1 adrenal gland and did not increase during the postural stimulation test in the patients with adenomas. Urinary aldosterone excretion before surgery also correlated with diastolic blood pressures in these patients. In the patients with adenomas, hypertension was cured by surgery in 35% and was improved in another 56%, as compared with 38% and 12%, respectively, of the patients with bilateral adrenal hyperplasia; however, most of the patients with hyperplasia were not operated on. In most of the nonoperated patients, hypertension could be controlled with drugs.

Conclusions.—Among patients with primary hyperaldosteronism, tests that can differentiate adrenal adenomas from adrenal hyperplasia include the postural stimulation test, urinary excretion rates of 18-oxocortisol and 18-hydroxycortisol, and adrenal vein sampling.

▶ The key finding that should lead to consideration of primary aldosteronism in a hypertensive patient is unexplained hypokalemia. Once this is confirmed, urinary potassium excretion should be measured. If inappropriately high, indicating renal potassium wasting, then plasma renin activity and plasma aldosterone should be measured simultaneously.[1] If the plasma aldosterone/renin ratio is high, indicative of an increase in the former and the appropriate compensatory decrease in the latter, then hyperaldosteronism is likely, and detailed studies to determine its cause are indicated. It is best to discontinue all antihypertensive drugs (indeed, all drugs) before undertaking even screening tests; this is because so many of them interfere with potassium metabolism (thiazides) or the renin-angiotensin-aldosterone system itself (β-adrenergic antagonists, calcium-channel antagonists).

The traditional causes of primary aldosteronism are an adrenal adenoma and bilateral adrenal hyperplasia, but a few patients have multiple adenomas or unilateral adrenal hyperplasia (or at least have no tumor and are cured by unilateral adrenalectomy). Patients with tumors tend to be younger, and their hypertension and hypokalemia tend to be more severe; however, that knowledge is not of much value in evaluating individual patients, and as shown in Figure 2, baseline plasma aldosterone/renin ratios are similar in the 2 groups. The possibility of glucocorticoid-remediable aldosteronism should not be forgotten.[2]

The importance of distinguishing between an adrenal adenoma and bilateral adrenal hyperplasia in patients with primary aldosteronism is that patients who have a tumor are more often—but by no means invariably—cured by surgery. Many biochemical and radiological tests have been proposed for differential diagnosis. Among them, the most reliable seem to be the postural stimulation test, some measurement of 18-hydroxylation of adrenal steroids, and either CT or MRI of the adrenal glands. The postural test consists of measurements of plasma aldosterone soon after arising in the morning and after upright posture and ambulation for 4 hours. Plasma aldosterone concentrations characteristically decline slightly in patients with an adrenal tumor, as a result of the lack of postural rise in plasma renin and the dependence of plasma aldosterone on plasma corticotropin (ACTH), which declines during the morning. In contrast, plasma renin and aldosterone both rise in patients with bilateral adrenal hyperplasia. With respect to measurements of 18-hydroxylated steroids, these investigators measured them in urine, but measuring plasma 18-hydroxycorticosterone is easier.[3] Nearly all patients with an adrenal adenoma have concentrations greater than 100 ng/dL (2.7 nmol/L), whereas the values are lower in patients with adrenal hyperplasia. Finally, while the sensitivity of adrenal CT or MRI for detection of an aldosterone-secreting adenoma is only about 80%, no one would undertake an operation for one of these tumors without doing one of these tests. Indeed, a major dilemma is what to do if the biochemical data suggest an adenoma but none is detected by imaging. Adrenal radionuclide imaging or adrenal vein catheterization studies may still uncover an adenoma, but neither procedure is simple, inexpensive, and completely reliable.

Primary aldosteronism, whatever the cause, can be treated effectively nonsurgically with spironolactone, potassium-sparing antihypertensive drugs (triamterene or amiloride), or more conventional antihypertensive drugs and potassium supplementation.[4] Furthermore, as documented in this study, hypertension is not always cured by excision of an aldosterone-secreting adrenal adenoma, and bilateral adrenalectomy is not recommended for patients with bilateral adrenal hyperplasia (recall that half the patients in this series who had this operation were not improved). These facts make it inappropriate to carry out costly and cumbersome diagnostic tests that are not highly reliable to prove the existence of an aldosterone-secreting adenoma in patients in whom the results of simpler tests are confusing or contradictory.

R.D. Utiger, M.D.

References

1. McKenna TJ, Sequeira SJ, Heffernan A, et al: Diagnosis under random conditions of all disorders of the renin-angiotensin-aldosterone axis, including primary hyperaldosteronism. *J Clin Endocrinol Metab* 73:952–957, 1991. (1993 Year Book of Medicine, pp 525–526.)
2. Rich GM, Ulick S, Cook S, et al: Glucocorticoid-remediable hyperaldosteronism in a large kindred: Clinical spectrum and diagnosis using a characteristic biochemical phenotype. *Ann Intern Med* 116:813–820, 1992. (1993 Year Book of Medicine, pp 527–529.)
3. Kem DC, Tang K, Hanson CS, et al: The prediction of anatomical morphology of primary aldosteronism using serum 18-hydroxycorticosterone levels. *J Clin Endocrinol Metab* 60:67–73, 1985.
4. Levi M: Primary hyperaldosteronism. *Am J Med Sci* 300:189–202, 1990.

50 The Thyroid Gland

The Incidence of Thyroid Disorders in the Community: A Twenty-Year Follow-Up of the Whickham Survey

Vanderpump MPJ, Tunbridge WMG, French JM, Appleton D, Bates D, Clark F, Evans JG, Hasan DM, Rodgers H, Tunbridge F, Young ET (Univ of Oxford, England)

Clin Endocrinol 43:55–68, 1995 119-96-50–1

Background.—Cross-sectional studies have provided some data on the prevalence of thyroid disease in the community, but data on incidence are few. The Whickham Survey provided thyroid disorder prevalence data from a representative cross-section of a British community (2,779 adults) from 1972 to 1974. A 20-year follow-up to this survey was completed to examine the incidence and natural history of thyroid disorders in the community.

Findings.—Thirty percent of the 2,779 subjects in the original survey had died. Of the 1,877 known survivors, 96% were available to participate in the follow-up, and 91% underwent clinical, biochemical, and immunologic testing for thyroid disease. Outcome information (morbidity and mortality) was available for 97% of the original cohort. The mean incidence of hypothyroidism was 4.1 per 1,000 survivors per year among women and 0.6 per 1,000 survivors per year among men. The mean incidence of hyperthyroidism was negligible among men but was 0.8 per 1,000 survivors per year among women. The incidence rates were similar when data from the deceased participants were included. The risk of hypothyroidism, but not hyperthyroidism, increased with age. The frequency of goiter decreased during the 20-year period. Thyroid antibody status was associated with goiter only in women and only at follow-up. Odds ratios for developing hypothyroidism, given the presence of a particular risk factor at the initial survey, were calculated. Raised serum thyrotropin (TSH) concentrations yielded an odds ratio of 8 for women and 44 for men (Table 7). Positive antithyroid antibodies were associated with an odds ratio of 8 for women and 25 for men. The odds ratios were 38 for women and 173 for men who had both of these risk factors. Family history of thyroid disease was not associated with occurrence of hypothyroidism, nor were fasting serum cholesterol and triglyceride concentrations.

TABLE 7.—Development of Spontaneous Hypothyroidism at Follow-Up in Female Survivors: Odds Ratios (With 95% Confidence Intervals)

TSH raised, regardless of THY AB status	14 (9–24)
THY AB−, regardless of TSH status	13 (8–19)
If THY AB−, effect of raised TSH alone	8 (3–20)
If THY AB−, additional effect of raised TSH	5 (2–11)
If TSH normal−, effect of THY AB− alone	8 (5–15)
If TSH raised, additional effect of THY AB−	5 (1–15)
TSH raised and THY AB−, combined	38 (22–65)

Abbreviations: TSH, thyroid-stimulating hormone; *THY AB+,* thyroid antibody positive; *THY AB−,* thyroid antibody negative.

(Courtesy of Vanderpump MPJ, Tunbridge WMG, French JM, et al: The incidence of thyroid disorders in the community: A twenty-year follow-up of the Whickham survey. *Clin Endocrinol* 43:55–68, 1995. Reprinted by permission of Blackwell Science, Ltd.)

Comments.—For women with both antithyroid antibodies and elevated serum TSH concentrations, the annual risk of hypothyroidism developing is 4.3%. The presence of either factor alone also increases the risk of hypothyroidism, and the higher the serum TSH concentration is above 2 mU/L, the greater the risk. For women with a raised serum TSH value alone, the theoretical risk of lifelong thyroxine therapy must be balanced against the need for follow-up care, because approximately one third of these women will become hypothyroid within 20 years.

▶ This is the only study I know of in which the frequency of hypothyroidism, hyperthyroidism, and goiter were looked at twice in a random sample of the adult population in a period of many years. That some subjects developed hypothyroidism, hyperthyroidism, or goiter is not surprising, but the disappearance of goiter in 182 women and 35 men, with no change in thyroid function in most of them, is surprising. I would have thought that most of the goiters were caused by chronic autoimmune thyroiditis and would not disappear during follow-up.

Among the 1,051 women and 826 men in the cohort, 81 and 10, respectively, developed hypothyroidism at some time during the follow-up period. In the new survey, 91 of 1,704 subjects had high serum TSH concentrations; 29 of the 91 had newly detected hypothyroidism, and 15 were taking thyroxine. The study is particularly useful in providing a lot of data about the extent to which the presence of thyroid antibodies and subclinical hypothyroidism (elevated serum TSH concentrations but normal serum thyroxine concentrations) are risk factors for the occurrence of overt hypothyroidism. Restating the risk factor results given in the abstract, the annual risk of developing overt hypothyroidism was 4.3% per year among the women with high serum TSH concentrations and antithyroid antibodies 20 years earlier, 2.6% per year in those with high serum TSH concentrations, and 2.1% per year in those with antithyroid antibodies, as compared with 0.4% per year for all women; the risk increased progressively as the serum TSH increased. These same factors also greatly increased the risk of hypothyroidism in men, notwithstanding its much lower frequency in them. These results lend substance to the view that individuals with both abnormalities should be treated with thyroxine, even if one doesn't want to treat subjects with either abnormality alone. I confess to having been reluctant even to measure antithyroid antibodies in subjects with subclinical hypothyroidism, much less to treat them merely on the grounds that they might become hypothyroid, but I may need to change that policy.

Many fewer subjects developed hyperthyroidism (only 16 women, or 0.08% per year, and no men) during the 20-year period. In the new survey, 73 of 1,704 subjects had low serum TSH concentrations; of these, 26 were taking thyroxine and 5 had newly identified hyperthyroidism. Unfortunately, the first survey was done before sensitive TSH assays were introduced,[1] so we do not know what proportion of the subjects had low serum TSH concentrations (subclinical hyperthyroidism) then or the extent to which a low value was a risk factor for subsequent hyperthyroidism.

R.D. Utiger, M.D.

Reference

1. Tunbridge WMG, Evered DC, Hall R, et al: The spectrum of thyroid disease in a community: The Whickham survey. *Clin Endocrinol (Oxf)* 7:481–493, 1977.

Thyroid Function and Thyroid Size in Normal Pregnant Women Living in an Iodine Replete Area

Berghout A, Endert E, Ross A, Hogereil HV, Smits NJ, Wiersinga WM (Univ of Amsterdam, The Netherlands; Univ of Nijmegen, The Netherlands)

Clin Endocrinol 41:375–379, 1994 119-96-50–2

Background.—There are numerous changes in thyroid function during pregnancy. In general, thyroid activity increases in early pregnancy and slightly declines thereafter. In areas of even mild iodine deficiency, thyroid size increases during pregnancy.

Study Design.—In a prospective study, thyroid size and function were monitored serially in 10 normal iodine-replete women who completed pregnancy after artificial insemination.

Results.—Thyroid volume, measured by ultrasonography, did not change during pregnancy, being 10.3 mL at baseline and 10.6, 9.6, and 9.4 mL during the first, second, and third trimesters, respectively. Plasma free thyroxine and free triiodothyronine concentrations tended to decline during pregnancy, whereas serum thyrotropin (TSH) concentrations decreased and then increased slightly, all values being within the normal (nonpregnant) range. Plasma thyroglobulin concentrations did not change significantly during pregnancy, confirming the lack of substantial change in plasma TSH concentrations.

Conclusions.—Thyroid volume and secretion do not change during pregnancy in areas where iodine intake is adequate.

► Thyroid secretion increases during early pregnancy, even though serum thyroid hormone concentrations increase very little, for several reasons. The large amount of chorionic gonadotropin secreted during early pregnancy has some thyroid-stimulating activity. The estrogen-induced increase in serum thyroxine-binding globulin means that more thyroxine must be produced just to occupy the increased number of binding sites (which accounts for the well-known increase in serum total thyroxine concentrations that occurs during pregnancy) and maintain a normal serum free thyroxine concentration. Finally, there is an increase in thyroxine clearance, some being deiodinated by the placenta and some transferred to the fetus. The magnitude of the increase in thyroxine secretion is modest (about 40%) based on the increase in thyroxine dosage needed to maintain normal TSH secretion in hypothyroid women during pregnancy.[1, 2]

This need for increased thyroid hormone synthesis and secretion could result in goiter, and the notion that thyroid enlargement is common (and "physiological") in pregnant women persists. When iodine intake is adequate (greater than 150 μg/day), as in The Netherlands (where this study was done) and in the United States, goiter does not occur.[3, 4] When iodine intake is marginal, however, thyroid size does increase, and the increase can be minimized by iodine supplementation.[5]

In the United States, thyroid enlargement in a pregnant women is not often caused by inadequate dietary iodine intake but by the same things that cause goiter in nonpregnant women. These include chronic autoimmune thyroiditis, lithium carbonate therapy, and Graves' disease. Clinical manifestations of thyroid dysfunction need not be present. The disorders unique to pregnancy that are associated with hyperthyroidism—hyperemesis gravidarum and trophoblastic tumors—rarely cause goiter.

R.D. Utiger, M.D.

References

1. Mandel SJ, Larsen PR, Seely EW, et al: Increased need for thyroxine during pregnancy in women with primary hypothyroidism. *N Engl J Med* 323:91–96, 1990. (1991 YEAR BOOK OF MEDICINE, pp 532–533.)
2. Kaplan MM: Monitoring thyroxine treatment during pregnancy. *Thyroid* 2:147–152, 1992.
3. Levy RP, Newman DM, Rejall LS, et al: The myth of goiter in pregnancy. *Am J Obstet Gynecol* 137:701–703, 1980.
4. Nelson M, Wickus GG, Caplan RH, et al: Thyroid gland size in pregnancy: An ultrasound and clinical study. *J Reprod Med* 32:888–890, 1987.
5. Glinoer D, De Nayer P, Delange F, et al: A randomized trial for the treatment of mild iodine deficiency during pregnancy: Maternal and neonatal effects. *J Clin Endocrinol Metab* 80:258–269, 1995.

Autoimmunity and Thyroid Function in Patients With Chronic Active Hepatitis Treated With Recombinant Interferon Alpha-2a

Preziati D, La Rosa L, Covini G, Marcelli R, Rescalli S, Persani L, Del Ninno E, Meroni PL, Colombo M, Beck-Peccoz P (Istituti di Scienze Endocrine, Milan, Italy; Medicina Interna Centro Migliavacca, Milan, Italy; Ospedale Maggiore IRCCS, Milan, Italy; et al)

Eur J Endocrinol 132:587–593, 1995 119-96-50–3

Background.—The occurrence of overt autoimmune disease has been reported in patients with both malignant disease and chronic viral infections during long-term therapy with recombinant interferon-α-2a (IFN-α). This study evaluated the prevalence of organ- and non–organ specific autoantibodies and the risk of developing autoimmune diseases in patients with chronic hepatitis C (CAH-HCV) and hepatitis-B (CAH-HBV) infections during IFN-α therapy.

Patients.—Eighty-six patients with CAH-HCV and 51 patients with CAH-HBV were studied. Most patients had longstanding community-acquired hepatitis. The patients with CAH-HCV were given IFN-α, 6 mega (million) units (MU) 3 times a week until serum alanine aminotransferase concentrations became normal, followed by 2-3 MU 3 times a week for the remainder of the year. The patients with CAH-HBV received a similar regimen, but for only 6 months.

Results.—At baseline, 9% of the patients with CAH-HCV and 4% of those with CAH-HBV had clinical or biochemical signs of thyroid disorders. The remaining patients were euthyroid, but 42% of the CAH-HCV patients and 10% of the CAH-HBV patients had antithyroid autoantibodies. During IFN-α therapy, 40% of the CAH-HCV and 10% of the CAH-HBV patients without antithyroid antibodies initially had positive antithyroid antibody tests, irrespective of the cumulative IFN-α dosage. Among the 35 patients with CAH-HCV treated for 12 months, 12 (34%) had thyroid disorders develop, including 8 who had antithyroid antibodies before treatment. Seven patients had permanent primary hypothyroidism; 1, transient hypothyroidism; and 4, hyperthyroidism. Most of the thyroid disorders occurred within 6 months of treatment, although one developed at 12 months and another 6 months after IFN-α withdrawal. In contrast, only 1 patient with CAH-HBV had hyperthyroidism during IFN-α therapy.

At baseline, 5 (14%) of the CAH-HCV and 3 (19%) of the CAH-HBV patients had elevated titers of antinuclear autoantibodies. During IFN-α treatment, antinuclear autoantibodies were found in 10 (36%) of the CAH-HCV patients but in none of the patients with CAH-HBV. None of the patients had any manifestations of systemic autoimmune diseases.

Conclusions.—In patients with CAH-HCV and CAH-HBV, long-term IFN-α therapy is associated with appearance or increased titer of antithyroid antibodies and with the development of hypothyroidism and hyperthyroidism, irrespective of the cumulative dosage of IFN-α. Thyroid disorders develop more often in patients with CAH-HCV than in CAH-HBV patients, presumably because of their high prevalence of thyroid autoantibodies before treatment. The risk of development of organ-specific autoimmunity should be assessed carefully in patients with long-standing hepatitis who are candidates for IFN-α treatment.

▶ Thyroid disease is a well-recognized side effect of interferon-α, which has become standard therapy for patients with chronic hepatitis B and C infections and is also being used in patients with various tumors. The thyroid disease takes several forms: permanent hyperthyroidism (Graves' disease), permanent hypothyroidism (usually with no goiter), and painless or silent thyroiditis (transient hyperthyroidism followed by transient hypothyroidism, transient hyperthyroidism alone, or transient hypothyroidism alone). The frequency of these disturbances has varied from 5% to about 50% in different studies, for no obvious reasons discernible to me. As in this study, it has tended to be higher in patients with chronic hepatitis C than in those with chronic hepatitis B, and it is definitely higher in patients who have antithyroid antibodies before therapy.[1, 2] The effects are drug- but not disease-specific in that the same thyroid disorders occur in patients with tumors treated with IFN-α.[3] Interferon-α has a variety of immunomodulatory effects, but how it activates thyroid autoimmune disease (and other autoimmune diseases) is not known. It also has direct thyroid inhibitory actions in vitro. In contrast, interferon-γ has no effects on thyroid antibody formation or thyroid function.[4]

As a practical matter, patients who are to receive IFN-α should have a serum thyrotropin (TSH) determination, and they should be clinically evaluated for both hyperthyroidism and hypothyroidism periodically during therapy. Obviously, one could also measure serum TSH during therapy, but I see no particular reason to do so unless some symptoms or signs of thyroid disease are present. Should the patient have evidence of hyperthyroidism, then thyroid radioiodine uptake should be measured to distinguish transient (low uptake) from more permanent (high uptake) hyperthyroidism. Should hypothyroidism occur, the patient should be treated unless the hypothyroidism is very mild, in which case therapy can be delayed to determine whether it will subside. A test for antithyroid peroxidase antibodies could also be done before interferon therapy is begun, but the absence of antibodies does not mean there is no risk of thyroid disease during therapy.

R.D. Utiger, M.D.

References

1. Lisker-Melman M, Di Bisceglie AM, Usala SJ, et al: Development of thyroid disease during therapy of chronic viral hepatitis with interferon alfa. *Gastroenterology* 102:2155–2160, 1993.
2. Watanabe U, Hashimoto E, Hisamitsu T, et al: The risk factor for development of thyroid disease during interferon-α therapy for chronic hepatitis C. *Am J Gastroenterol* 89:399–402, 1994.
3. Ronnblom L, Alm GV, Oberg KE: Autoimmunity after alpha-interferon therapy for malignant carcinoid tumors. *Ann Intern Med* 115:178–183, 1991.
4. Kung AWC, Jones BM, Lai CL: Effects of interferon-γ therapy on thyroid function, T-lymphocyte subpopulations and induction of autoantibodies. *J Clin Endocrinol Metab* 71:1230–1234, 1990.

Low Serum Thyrotropin Concentrations as a Risk Factor for Atrial Fibrillation in Older Persons

Sawin CT, Geller A, Wolf PA, Belanger AJ, Baker E, Bacharach P, Wilson PWF, Benjamin EJ, D'Agostino RB (Boston Veterans Affairs Med Ctr; Boston Univ; Framingham Heart Study, Mass)

N Engl J Med 331:1249–1252, 1994 119-96-50–4

Background.—Atrial fibrillation is a well-recognized manifestation of hyperthyroidism. Although low serum thyrotropin concentrations are an established indicator of hyperthyroidism, they may also be found in persons with no clinical evidence of this disorder. Clinically euthyroid elderly persons were investigated to determine whether low serum thyrotropin concentrations are a risk factor for subsequent atrial fibrillation.

Participants and Methods.—Serum thyrotropin concentrations were measured in 2,007 persons, 814 men and 1,193 women, aged 60 years or older, who were living at home. None of the participants had atrial fibrillation. Sixty-one had low values defined as ≤ 0.1 mU/L; 187 had slightly low values, defined as > 0.1–0.4 mU/L; 1,576 had normal values, defined as > 0.4–5.0 mU/L, and 183 had high values, defined as > 5.0 mU/L. The frequency of atrial fibrillation was determined during a 10-year follow-up period.

Results.—Thirteen persons with low serum thyrotropin values, 23 with slightly low values, 133 with normal values, and 23 with high values experienced atrial fibrillation during the follow-up period. At 10 years, the cumulative incidence of atrial fibrillation was 28% among those with low values, as compared with 11% among those with normal values. The age-adjusted incidence of atrial fibrillation was 28 and 10 per 1,000 person-years among the persons with low and normal values, respectively. After adjusting for other established risk factors, the persons with low values had a 3.1 relative risk of atrial fibrillation compared with those with normal values. The 10-year incidence of atrial fibrillation did not differ significantly between persons with slightly low and high values and those with normal values. Only one person who developed atrial fibrillation had overt hyperthyroidism at the same time.

Conclusions.—Low serum thyrotropin concentrations are associated with an increased risk for atrial fibrillation among persons aged 60 years and older.

► The proven risks of subclinical hyperthyroidism are atrial fibrillation (or other cardiovascular problems, e.g., tachycardia and diastolic dysfunction),[1] accelerated bone loss[2, 3] and overt hyperthyroidism. According to this large study, the risk of atrial fibrillation during the 10-year follow-up period was increased about 3 times among euthyroid persons with unequivocally low serum thyrotropin concentrations (≤ 0.1 mU/L) but only slightly decreased in those with slightly low values. The low serum thyrotropin concentrations were most likely caused by small increases in serum thyroid hormone concentrations rather than by the other common causes of low serum thyrotropin values—nonthyroidal illness and secondary (central) hypothyroidism—for several reasons. The study subjects were all outpatients, and among those in the low serum thyrotropin group, the mean serum thyroxine concentration was higher (but not above the upper limit of normal in any subject) than that in the patients with normal serum thyrotropin concentrations; about 60% were taking thyroid hormone. Most, although not all,[4] patients with nonthyroid illness who have low serum thyrotropin concentrations are quite sick, often so sick they are in an ICU; secondary hypothyroidism is rare; and patients with either usually have low serum thyroxine concentrations.

What should be done if the serum thyrotropin concentration is persistently low in a seemingly euthyroid patient who has a normal serum free thyroxine value? If the patient is taking thyroid hormone, the dose should be reduced. If not, then a cause for the subclinical hyperthyroidism should be sought. The known causes are a hyperfunctioning thyroid adenoma, a multinodular goiter, and Graves' disease; the former 2 disorders should be detectable by palpation, but the latter certainly may not be. Sawin et al. did not report the results of thyroid palpation in their patients, and I know of no large series of patients with subclinical hyperthyroidism in which the cause was carefully sought. A possible next step is to measure thyroid radioiodine uptake and perhaps do a thyroid radionuclide scan, but I would do these tests only if I intended to treat the patient.

Which patients with subclinical hyperthyroidism should be treated? I do not recommend treatment simply because the serum thyrotropin concentration is low. The risk of atrial fibrillation, while increased, is not high, and the risk of overt hyperthyroidism is very low. In the 10-year study by Sawin et al., it occurred in 2 of the 192 persons who developed atrial fibrillation (one at the same time and one later) and in 4 of 1,815 who did not; in a 1-year study in the United Kingdom, it occurred in 1 of 66 patients with low serum thyrotropin concentrations.[5] Furthermore, among patients with low serum thyrotropin concentrations, a substantial proportion have normal values 1 or more years later; this was the case in 19 of the 36 persons who were restudied in the study of Sawin et al. and in 40 of 61 in the British study.[5]

I do recommend therapy if the patient has atrial fibrillation, some other cardiac problem, accelerated bone loss, or any other condition that might be ameliorated by a small reduction in thyroid secretion. Because of its simplicity and safety, the best treatment is radioiodine; antithyroid drug therapy is less attractive because of its side effects and the need for lifelong therapy, at least in those patients with nodular thyroid disease.

R.D. Utiger, M.D.

References

1. Biondi B, Fazio S, Carella S, et al: Cardiac effects of long term thyrotropin suppressive therapy with levothyroxine. *J Clin Endocrinol Metab* 77:334–338, 1993.
2. Faber J, Galloe AM: Changes in bone mass during prolonged subclinical hyperthyroidism due to L-thyroxine treatment: A meta-analysis. *Eur J Endocrinol* 130:350–356, 1994. (1995 Year Book of Medicine, p 610.)

3. Schneider DL, Barrett-Connor EL, Morton DJ: Thyroid hormone use and bone mineral density in elderly women: Effects of estrogen. *JAMA* 271:1245–1249, 1994. (1995 YEAR BOOK OF MEDICINE, pp 610–612.)
4. Eggertsen R, Petersen K, Lundberg P-A, et al: Screening for thyroid disease in a primary care unit with a thyroid stimulating hormone assay with a low detection limit. *BMJ* 297:1586–1592, 1988.
5. Parle JV, Franklyn JA, Cross KW, et al: Prevalence and follow-up of abnormal thyrotropin (TSH) concentrations in the elderly in the United Kingdom. *Clin Endocrinol (Oxf)* 34:77–83, 1991.

Thyrotoxicosis-Induced Congestive Heart Failure in an Urban Hospital

Wilson BE, Newmark SR (Univ of Nevada, Las Vegas)
Am J Med Sci 308:344–348, 1994 119-96-50–5

Background.—Previous reports have linked thyrotoxicosis to a number of different cardiac complications, including atrial fibrillation, functional cardiomyopathy, and congestive heart failure. The latter has been reported to be an unusual complication of thyrotoxicosis, occurring mainly in older patients. A review was performed to determine the frequency of thyrotoxicosis-associated congestive heart failure among hospitalized adults.

Methods.—The review included all admissions to a 535-bed urban public hospital over a 14-month period. Those admitted with a diagnosis of atrial fibrillation or congestive heart failure of unclear cause were screened for thyrotoxicosis by biochemical tests.

Findings.—One hundred seventy-seven patients with a principal diagnosis of atrial fibrillation and 21 with a principal diagnosis of thyrotoxicosis were admitted during the study. Concomitant atrial fibrillation and thyrotoxicosis were present in 11 patients, representing 6% of the atrial fibrillation group. Five of these 11 patients had clinically apparent congestive heart failure with no signs of other organic heart disease and were designated group A. The other 6 had only atrial fibrillation and were designated group B. The average age was 36 years in group A, as compared with 49 years in group B. On echocardiographic examination, the mean number of enlarged cardiac chambers was 2.8 in group A, as compared with 1.0 in group B. Left ventricular function was normal in 4 of the 5 patients in group A. The 2 groups had similar mean serum thyroxine, albumin, and hematocrit values, left ventricular percent shortening, and left atrial diameters. All group A patients had reversal of their arrhythmia and heart failure with antithyroid therapy.

Conclusions.—Thyrotoxicosis-induced congestive heart failure may not be as rare in young patients as previous reports have suggested. Patients with this complication of thyrotoxicosis usually have dilated cardiomyopathy and high-output failure. Thyrotoxicosis should remain high on the list of differential diagnoses in young adults with cardiomyopathy.

► The finding of overt hyperthyroidism in 6% of patients with atrial fibrillation in this study is not surprising, in view of data indicating that subclinical hyperthyroidism can be found in between 4% and 15% of patients with atrial fibrillation (reviewed in Reference 1). I am surprised that about half the patients with hyperthyroidism and atrial fibrillation had congestive heart failure, and that they were younger than those who did not have heart failure. They also had more cardiac chamber enlargement, although they did not have thicker ventricular walls; however, their hyperthyroidism was not more severe biochemically than that in patients with no heart failure. Whether they had a more rapid ventricular rate, more weight loss, or more skeletal muscle weakness than the patients with no heart failure is not stated. Since cardiac function became normal after antithyroid treatment, they can be considered to have had hyperthyroid cardiomyopathy, whatever that is. I assume that the hyperthyroid patients who did not have atrial fibrillation did not have heart failure either, but no information about this group is provided. Most of the patients with heart failure in this study had a normal ejection fraction, but in other studies it was low,[2] which seems to me to provide more evidence of muscle dysfunction.

The average age of the 11 hyperthyroid patients with atrial fibrillation in this study must have been about 43 years, an unusually young age, and the incidence of atrial fibrillation among them (11 of 21 patients, 52%) was unusually high, almost surely because all the patients were hospitalized. In a study of 880 hyperthyroid patients, the proportions with atrial fibrillation who were in the third through eighth decades were, respectively, 1%, 1%, 1%, 8%, 17%, and 0%, and the overall incidence was 3%.[3] Other reported rates range from 9% to 22% (summarized in Reference 1).

This study serves as a reminder that both atrial fibrillation and heart failure occur in young patients with hyperthyroidism. The appropriate treatment, whatever the age of the patient, is methimazole (radioactive iodine acts too slowly), control of the ventricular rate with digoxin or a β-adrenergic antagonist drug if the heart failure is considered mainly rate-related, and a diuretic drug. Whether to initiate anticoagulant therapy is a much more difficult question. I do not think it is indicated in patients who have uncomplicated atrial fibrillation, because about 65% revert to sinus rhythm with antithyroid drug or radioiodine treatment,[4] but I would advise it if the patient also has other risk factors for thromboembolism, such as heart failure, left atrial enlargement, or a history of thromboembolic disease.

R.D. Utiger M.D.

References

1. Woeber KA: Thyrotoxicosis and the heart. *N Engl J Med* 327:94–98, 1992.
2. Umpierrez GE, Challapalli S, Patterson C: Congestive heart failure due to reversible cardiomyopathy in patients with hyperthyroidism. *Am J Med Sci* 310:99–102, 1995.
3. Nordyke RA, Gilbert FI Jr, Harada ASM: Graves' disease: Influence of age on clinical findings. *Arch Intern Med* 148:626–631, 1988.
4. Nakazawa HK, Sakurai K, Hamada N, et al: Management of atrial fibrillation in the post-thyrotoxic state. *Am J Med* 72:903–906, 1982.

Natural History of Thyroid Associated Ophthalmopathy

Perros P, Crombie AL, Kendall-Taylor P (Western Gen Hosp, Edinburgh, Scotland)

Clin Endocrinol 42:45–50, 1995 119-96-50–6

Introduction.—As many as half of patients with Graves' disease have ophthalmopathy. Although little is known about the natural course of thyroid-related ophthalmopathy, many believe that most patients improve spontaneously over time.

Objective.—The course of mild-to-moderate thyroid-associated ophthalmopathy was examined in 59 patients referred to a thyroid-eye clinic. None had undergone surgery or received glucocorticoid or other drug therapy for their eye disease. Patients who were hyperthyroid received carbimazole until they became euthyroid, and thyroxine then was added. The patients were followed every 3 to 6 months for a median time of 1 year.

Observations.—Ophthalmopathy improved spontaneously in 64% of patients, remained stable in 22%, and progressed in 14%. At the time of initial evaluation, patients who later improved could not be distinguished from those who remained stable or deteriorated with respect to sex, age, the duration of ocular disease, type of antithyroid therapy, or thyroid function, but those who deteriorated and later required glucocorticoid or surgical treatment had more severe eye involvement. The changes in ophthalmopathy index—a composite score based on grading of soft tissue inflammation, exophthalmos and other eye findings (maximum score, 26)—distinguished the patients who improved or remained stable on the one hand and those who deteriorated progressively on the other (Fig 1).

Conclusions.—More than 80% of patients in this series with mild to moderate thyroid-associated ophthalmopathy improved spontaneously or remained stable over time.

► In patients with Graves' hyperthyroidism, ophthalmopathy is most likely to occur within the year before or after they become hyperthyroid. Its occurrence afterward has led to suggestions that it can be induced by antithyroid treatment, and there is some evidence that it is somewhat more likely to occur after radioactive iodine therapy than after subtotal thyroidectomy or during antithyroid drug therapy.[1] More important inciting factors than the type of antithyroid therapy are hypothyroidism and persistent hyperthyroidism.[2, 3] Thus, the way to minimize the risk of the development or worsening of Graves' ophthalmopathy is effective antithyroid treatment, with care being taken to avoid even transient hypothyroidism. Since smoking is a strong risk factor for ophthalmopathy,[4] I wouldn't hesitate to suggest that cessation of smoking would minimize the risk of development or worsening of ophthalmopathy, although evidence that cessation at this time in the course of Graves' disease is beneficial is lacking.

What we learn from this study is that ophthalmopathy, once present in sufficient severity to warrant referral of the patient to a specialized thyroid-eye clinic, but not so severe that immediate aggressive treatment is deemed necessary, usually improves or at least does not worsen. Grading systems for ophthalmopathy don't convey a very clear picture of the problem, but suffice it to say that the patients entering this study probably had some combination of moderate eyelid retraction, moderate periorbital edema, mild diplopia, and moderate proptosis. About 20% of the patients were not euthyroid and were treated to correct their thyroid dysfunction; all were advised to use methylcellulose eye drops and to sleep with the head of the bed raised.

These results confirm my long-held views that Graves' ophthalmopathy is not usually progressive and may gradually subside, and that major interventions are best avoided in the absence of compelling indications. These are, broadly speaking, severe persistent periorbital and conjunctival inflammation, visual impairment from optic neuropathy, and corneal ulceration. Another argument for a conservative approach is that the major interventions,

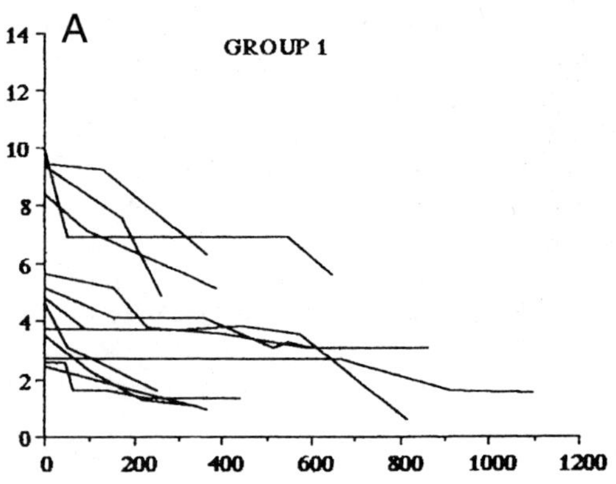

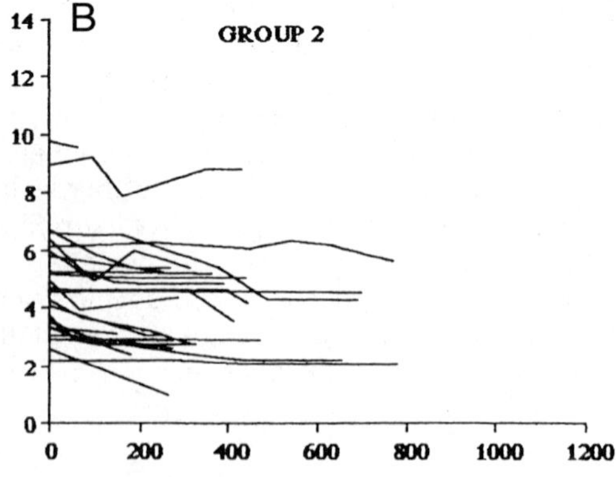

(Continued)

Fig 1 (cont.)

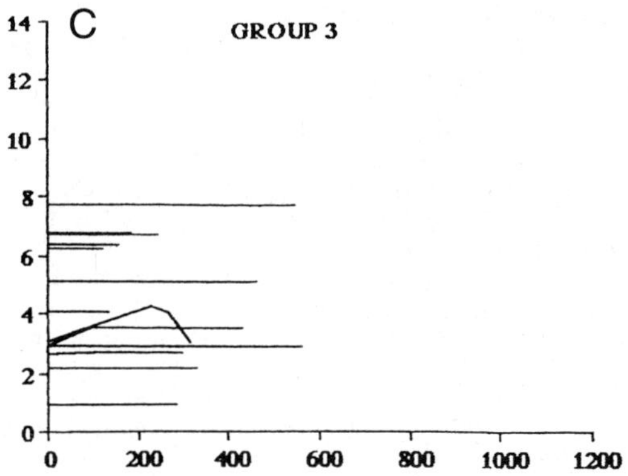

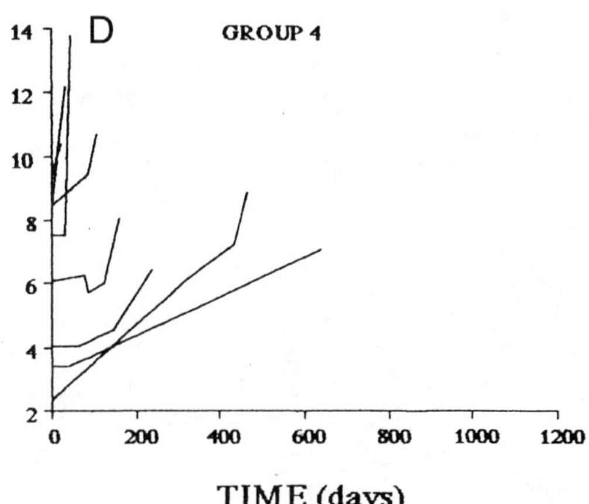

FIGURE 1.—Serial ophthalmopathy index measurements of patients with thyroid-associated ophthalmopathy. **A,** group 1 (improvement in ophthalmopathy index of 2 points or greater); **B,** group 2 (improvement in ophthalmopathy index of less than 2 points); **C,** group 3 (stable eye disease); and **D,** group 4 (progressive deterioration). The mean values for the 2 eyes of each patient are shown. (Courtesy of Perros P, Crombie AL, Kendall-Taylor P, et al: Natural history of thyroid associated ophthalmopathy. *Clin Endocrinol* 42:45–50, 1995. Reprinted by permission of Blackwell Science, Ltd.)

i.e., glucocorticoid therapy, orbital radiotherapy, and orbital decompression, are not uniformly effective, safe, or simple, nor are the reasons to choose among them well-defined. My preference is to use glucocorticoid therapy for patients whose main problem is periorbital and conjunctival inflammation and orbital decompression for those with optic nerve or corneal disease; however, radiotherapy has its advocates (see Reference 5 for a series of papers discussing all aspects of this problem). My real preference, as I said above, is to procrastinate as long as vision is not impaired; as documented by Perros et al., more often than not the need for aggressive therapy subsides.

R.D. Utiger, M.D.

References

1. Tallstedt L, Lundell G, Torring O, et al: Occurrence of ophthalmopathy after treatment for Graves' hyperthyroidism. *N Engl J Med* 326:1733–1738, 1992. (1993 Year Book of Medicine, pp 534–535.)
2. Tallstedt L, Lundell G, Blomgren H, et al: Does early administration of thyroxine reduce the development of Graves' ophthalmopathy after radioiodine treatment? *Eur J Endocrinol* 130:494–497, 1994. (1995 Year Book of Medicine, pp 620–622.)
3. Prummel MF, Wiersinga WM, Mourits MPh, et al: Effect of abnormal thyroid function on the severity of Graves' ophthalmopathy. *Arch Intern Med* 150:1098–1101, 1990. (1991 Year Book of Medicine, pp 526–527.)
4. Prummel MF, Wiersinga WM: Smoking and risk of Graves' disease. *JAMA* 269:479–482, 1993.
5. DeGroot LJ, Gorman CA, Pinchera A, et al: Therapeutic controversies: Radiation and Graves' ophthalmopathy. *J Clin Endocrinol Metab* 80:339–349, 1995.

Radioiodine Therapy Compared in Patients With Toxic Nodular or Graves' Hyperthyroidism

Franklyn JA, Daykin J, Holder R, Sheppard MC (Univ of Birmingham, England)

Q J Med 88:175–180, 1995 119-96-50–7

Introduction.—The optimum dose of radioiodine for patients with hyperthyroidism has yet to be determined, and many physicians simply administer a single fixed dose instead of determining an individualized dose based on thyroid size or radioiodine uptake. Whether a standardized dose would be appropriate for patients with both toxic nodular and Graves' hyperthyroidism was determined.

Patients and Methods.—The study participants were 103 patients with hyperthyroidism who were receiving their first radioiodine dose. Fifty-nine had Graves' disease, and 44 had a toxic multinodular goiter. Disease severity was judged by serum free thyroxine (T_4) and free triiodothyronine (T_3) concentrations before any therapy. All patients received a single 5-mCi (185 MBq) dose of radioiodine. Those who remained hyperthyroid at 6 months were given a second dose of 10 mCi (370 MBq) and were reassessed at 12 months.

Results.—As expected, the patients with Graves' disease were younger than those with toxic multinodular goiter and had a higher prevalence of antithyroid antibodies. At 6 months, 34.1% of the patients with toxic multinodular goiter had persistent hyperthyroidism, as compared with 55.9% of those with Graves' disease, and the cure rate (euthyroidism or hypothyroidism) was greater in the former group (65.9% vs. 44.1%) (Table 2). At 12 months, 80.6% of the patients with toxic multinodular goiter and 74.5% with Graves' disease were cured of their hyperthyroid-

TABLE 2.—Thyroid Status in Patients With Toxic Nodular Hyperthyroidism (n=44) or Graves' Hyperthyroidism (n=59) 6 Months After Treatment With a Single 5-mCi Dose of Radioiodine

	Hyperthyroid	Euthyroid	Hypothyroid	Euthyroid + hypothyroid
Toxic nodular hyperthyroidism	15 (34.1%)	24 (54.5%)	5 (11.4%)	29 (65.9%)
Graves' disease	33 (55.9%)	10 (16.9%)	16 (27.1%)	26 (44.1%)

(Courtesy of Franklyn JA, Daykin J, Holder R, et al: Radioiodine therapy compared in patients with toxic nodular or Graves' hyperthyroidism. *Q J Med* 88:175–180, 1995. Reprinted by permission of the Oxford University Press.)

ism. The probability of achieving euthyroidism or hypothyroidism at 6 months was related inversely to the baseline serum T_4 concentration—indicative of disease severity—and to the administration of carbimazole before or after radioiodine therapy, but it was unrelated to the cause of the hyperthyroidism.

Conclusion.—The 6-month cure rate was higher in patients with hyperthyroidism caused by toxic multinodular goiter than in those with Graves' disease, but the differences in outcome between the 2 groups reflected the severity of hyperthyroidism and the administration of carbimazole rather than an effect of the diagnostic category. These results, in opposition to a widely held view, indicate that patients with toxic multinodular goiter should not routinely receive a higher dose of radioiodine than those with Graves' disease.

► The 5-mCi (185-MBq) dose of radioiodine given to these patients in the United Kingdom is considerably smaller than what would be given in the United States, regardless of whether their hyperthyroidism was caused by Graves' disease or by a toxic multinodular goiter. In this country, most patients with Graves' hyperthyroidism are treated with 10–15 mCi (370–555 MBq), whether as a fixed or a calculated dose, and most patients with a toxic multinodular goiter are treated with 15–25 mCi (555–926 MBq). The difference in administered doses cannot be explained by differences in 24-hour radioiodine uptake in the 2 countries, but it is at least in part due to the reluctance of physicians in the United Kingdom to use radioiodine at all. As an aside, I know of no data indicating that any method of dose calculation, no matter how complicated, is any better than giving a fixed dose, as Franklyn et al. did.

The results of this study, however, as shown in Table 2, clearly indicate that 5 mCi (185 MBq) is too little, because too many patients remained hyperthyroid. I would not, unlike the authors, attribute this largely to the concomitant antithyroid drug therapy given before or after radioiodine administration to about half of all patients. Antithyroid drug therapy given either before or after radioiodine treatment certainly may, but does not uniformly, reduce the efficacy of radioiodine.

The main reason to give larger doses of radioiodine to patients with Graves' hyperthyroidism is that, destructive therapy having been agreed upon, it is more sensible to give enough radioiodine to do the job right so that the patient does not have persistent hyperthyroidism. The invariable trade-off, of course, is that more patients become hypothyroid; there is no scheme by which one can estimate dosage so most patients become euthyroid and only a few either remain hyperthyroid or become hypothyroid. In a large United States study in which patients received a variety of fixed doses, 70% of those treated with 5 mCi (185 MBq) were either euthyroid or hypothyroid 1 year later, as compared with 87% of those treated with 10 mCi (370 MBq).[1] No distinction was made between hypothyroidism and euthyroidism in this study, but hypothyroidism undoubtedly was more common in the latter group. The difference in hypothyroidism at 1 year, however, is of little importance, because so-called late hypothyroidism (more than 1 year post treatment) occurs at a rate of about 2% per year, whatever the initial dose of radioactive iodine. Indeed, some argue that the thing to do is administer enough radioiodine, say 15–20 mCi (555–740 MBq), to make nearly everyone hypothyroid within the first year after treatment, so that there is no need to worry about the patient becoming hypothyroid at some later time (Of course, one then has to worry that the patient will stop taking thyroxine!).

The rationale for the use of even larger doses in patients with a toxic multinodular goiter is that most of them have only a small increase in radioiodine uptake and the therapeutic dose will not be evenly distributed throughout the thyroid. Notwithstanding the results of Franklyn et al., most studies in both the United States and elsewhere have confirmed the need for larger doses in these patients.

I subscribe to the view that radioiodine should be given in sufficient dosage to do it right the first time. For patients with Graves' hyperthyroidism, that means 10–12 mCi (370–444 MBq), and for those with toxic multinodular goiter, 15–20 mCi (555–740 MBq), with upward adjustments if the patient has a large goiter.[1] I do not usually recommend either pre- or post-treatment antithyroid drug therapy, except for severely hyperthyroid patients and some older patients who I think will benefit from the more rapid action of the drug.

Another issue is whether 24-hour thyroid radioiodine uptake should be measured before radioactive iodine therapy. In the United States, most do this test to be sure that thyroid uptake is high and the treatment dose is not wasted, either because the patient had received stable iodine or has thyroiditis. Six-hour uptake measurements are just as good for this purpose and are more convenient for the patient; their use should be encouraged.[2]

R.D. Utiger, M.D.

References

1. Nordyke RA, Gilbert FI Jr: Optimal iodine-131 dose for eliminating hyperthyroidism in Graves' disease. *J Nucl Med* 32:411–416, 1991.
2. Hennessey JV, Berg LA, Ibrahim MA, et al: Evaluation of early (5 to 6 hours) iodine 123 uptake for diagnosis and treatment planning in Graves' disease. *Arch Intern Med* 155:621–624, 1995.

Levothyroxine and Potassim Iodide Are Both Effective in Treating Benign Solitary Solid Cold Nodules of the Thyroid

La Rosa GL, Lupo L, Giuffrida D, Gullo D, Vigneri R, Belfiore A (Univ of Catania, Italy)

Ann Intern Med 122:1–8, 1995 119-96-50-8

Objective.—Most patients with hypofunctioning (cold) nodules of the thyroid are managed medically. The effectiveness of levothyroxine and potassium iodide in the treatment of benign solitary cold thyroid nodules was studied.

Study Design.—In a randomized, controlled study, 80 patients (77 women and 3 men) with solitary cold thyroid nodules proven to be benign by fine-needle aspiration biopsy were assigned to receive no treatment, thyroxine at an initial dose of 1.0 µg/kg daily that then was adjusted so that serum thyrotropin concentrations were ≤ 0.3 mU/L (average dose, 1.94 µg/kg), or potassium iodide, 1.5 mg orally every 2 weeks. After 1 year of treatment, the thyroxine or iodide was discontinued and the patients were reevaluated 4 months later; the initially untreated patients received thyroxine and were followed up for another year.

Outcome.—Seventy patients completed the 1-year study. Both thyroxine and potassium iodide effectively reduced nodule volume, as measured by ultrasonography, as compared with no treatment. The mean nodule volume decreased by 40% in the 23 patients receiving thyroxine and by 23% in the 25 patients receiving potassium iodide but increased by 11% in the 22 untreated patients. A "clinically relevant" decrease in nodule volume (≥ 50%) was noted in 39% of patients receiving thyroxine and 20% of patients receiving potassium iodide but none of the untreated patients. There was no difference in the decrease in nodule volume between the thyroxine and potassium iodide groups. Only nodules with a volume of 10 mL or less decreased in size, and most nodules in which the decrease was clinically relevant had an initial volume of 5 mL or less (Table 5). Nodule volume did not increase in any of the treated patients but did increase in 14% of untreated patients. When therapy was discontinued, 25% of patients treated with either thyroxine or potassium iodide had an increase in nodule volume, and 2 of 11 untreated patients who were treated subsequently with thyroxine had a ≥ 50% decrease in nodule volume.

Conclusion.—Thyroxine and, to a lesser extent, potassium iodide effectively arrests the growth or reduces the volume of benign solitary cold thyroid nodules, especially small nodules, in some patients.

► I believe that this is the sixth randomized trial of thyroxine therapy in patients with a solitary, solid, hypofunctioning, benign thyroid nodule. In these studies, nodule size was determined by ultrasonography, palpation, and occasionally both; when both were used, the response as measured by palpation was less. I agree with the authors that the most important or, as they say, "clinically relevant" result is the proportion of patients in whom the size of the nodule decreased by 50% or more. By this criterion, thyroxine

TABLE 5.—Nodule Volume Changes During the 12-Month Study

Treatment Group	Class of Nodule Volume	Decrease	Volume Change No Change *n*	Increase
Levothyroxine		9	14	0
(*n* = 23)	<5 mL (*n* = 12)	8	4	0
	5.1–10 mL (*n* = 7)	1	6	0
	>10 mL (*n* = 4)	0	4	0
Potassium iodide		5	20	0
(*n* = 25)	<5 mL (*n* = 15)	5	10	0
	5.1–10 mL (*n* = 6)	0	6	0
	>10 mL (*n* = 4)	0	4	0
No treatment		0	19	3
(*n* = 22)	<5 mL (*n* = 15)	0	13	2
	5.1–10 mL (*n* = 3)	0	3	0
	>10 mL (*n* = 4)	0	3	1

* Variations (decrease or increase) indicate changes of 50% or more of initial volume.

(Courtesy of La Rosa GL, Lupo L, Giuffrida D, et al: Levothyroxine and potassium iodide are both effective in treating benign solitary solid cold nodules of the thyroid. *Ann Intern Med* 122:1–8, 1995.)

therapy was effective in 39% of the patients, and no untreated patient had any decrease during the 1-year study. Note, however, that only 1 of the 11 patients whose nodule was greater than 5 mL in volume (assuming a sphere, this works out to a nodule 2.2 cm in diameter) had a response to thyroxine (Table 5). In the other studies, the proportion of treated patients who responded was similar or lower (9% to 39% as assessed by palpation and 0% to 14% by ultrasonography), and a few patients who received either no treatment or placebo also had decreases.[1] One reason for the varying results is that solitary nodules, even as described above, are heterogeneous; some are hyperplastic nodules and others are true benign tumors.

These results do not persuade me that patients with solitary thyroid nodules should be treated. The efficacy of thyronine is obviously limited, and in some patients the nodule eventually disappears without treatment.[2] Besides, thyroxine-treated patients must have periodic serum thyrotropin measurements to be sure that the dose of thyroxine is not too high. Therefore, I prefer periodic physical examination and either rebiopsy or excision if the nodule enlarges. If treatment is given because the patient desires it or because the reader is more impressed than I that thyroxine is effective, it should be given for at least 1 year; in this study, mean nodule volume decreased progressively during that interval.

I do not know how to explain the benefit of potassium iodide in this study. The patients were not markedly iodine-deficient (anyone whose urinary iodine excretion was less than 8 µg/dL [about 80 µg/day] was excluded), and their serum thyrotropin concentrations did not decline during therapy. One can only speculate that the increase in iodide intake somehow reduced growth or replication of the cells of the nodule.

R.D. Utiger, M.D.

References

1. Cooper DS: Thyroxine suppression therapy for benign nodular disease. *J Clin Endocrinol Metab* 80:331–334, 1995.
2. Kuma K, Matsuzuka F, Kobayashi A, et al: Outcome of long standing solitary thyroid nodules. *World J Surg* 16:583–588, 1992.

51 The Parathyroid Glands and Bone

An Investigation of Sources of Variation in Calcium Absorption Efficiency

Barger-Lux MJ, Heaney RP, Lanspa SJ, Healy JC, DeLuca HF (Creighton Univ, Omaha, Neb; Univ of Wisconsin, Madison)

J Clin Endocrinol Metab 80:406–411, 1995 119-96-51–1

Introduction.—The measurement of the efficiency of calcium absorption under standard conditions yields wide variations, even among healthy subjects of similar age and estrogen status. Forty-one healthy premenopausal women were evaluated in an investigation of possible sources of interindividual variation in calcium absorption efficiency.

Methods.—The women's mean age was 36 years, they were of normal weight for their height, and none were taking medications that affect calcium metabolism or skeletal physiology. None were pregnant or likely to become pregnant soon. Variables measured included dietary factors, humoral regulators, intestinal motility, mucosal histology, mucosal vitamin D receptor levels, and calcium absorption efficiency. Half the women were taking 25-hydroxyvitamin D (25OHD), 20 µg/day. Vitamin D status was compared for summer test dates (May through November) and winter test dates (December through April).

Results.—In winter tests only, the calcium absorption fraction was significantly higher in the 25OHD-treated group. There were significant positive correlations between the efficiency of calcium absorption and serum 25OHD concentrations (Fig 1), intestinal transit time, and urinary calcium-creatinine ratio. No correlations were found, however, between the level of 1,25-dihydroxyvitamin D receptors in duodenal mucosa or serum 1,25-dihydroxyvitamin D and calcium absorption efficiency, nor were any dietary variables correlated with the calcium absorption fraction.

Conclusion.—Factors identified as playing a role in the interindividual variation in calcium absorption among healthy premenopausal women included serum 25OHD, mouth-to-cecum transit time, and fasting urinary calcium-creatinine ratio. Taken together, these factors explained 44% of

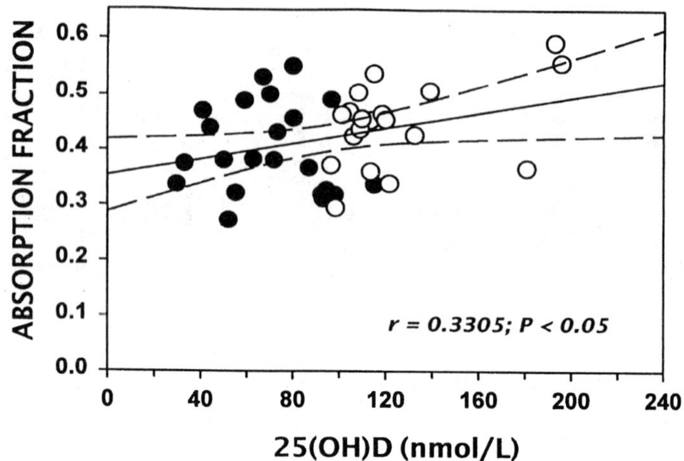

FIGURE 1.—Relationship between 25-hydroxyvitamin D (*25OHD*) and the calcium absorption fraction in healthy premenopausal women, some of whom (*open circle*) were pretreated with 25OHD before testing. (Courtesy of Barger-Lux MJ, Heaney RP, Lanspa SJ, et al: An investigation of sources of variation in calcium absorption efficiency. *J Clin Endocrinol Metab* 80:406–411, 1995. Copyright, The Endocrine Society.)

the observed variation in calcium absorption efficiency. Most of the biological vitamin D activity in human serum appeared to be explained by 25OHD.

► The best-known facts about calcium absorption are that it is largely dependent on vitamin D and that the efficiency of absorption decreases as intake increases. For example, in a large study of calcium absorption in normal middle-aged women, calcium absorption decreased from an average of 46% when the intake was 200 mg daily to 22% when the intake was 1,000 mg daily.[1] Another fact is that the between-individual variation in absorption is very large, being approximately threefold. Absorption decreases slightly with age (0.2%/year) after age 40 years, and it decreases further after menopause independent of age. Data of this sort led an NIH Consensus panel to recommend that 25- to 50-year-old women should consume 1,000 mg of calcium daily and women older than 50 years of age should consume 1,500 mg daily.[2]

This new study provides additional information about the factors that affect calcium absorption and therefore might explain some of the large interindividual and age-related variations in absorption. That vitamin D is important is not surprising, but the finding of a positive correlation between serum concentrations of 25-hydroxyvitamin D, but not serum 1,25-dihydroxyvitamin D, and fractional calcium absorption is surprising. The latter is generally considered the active form of vitamin D, but 25-hydroxyvitamin D does react to some extent with vitamin D receptors. Furthermore, it is worth remembering that the serum concentration of 25-hydroxyvitamin D is about 1,000-fold higher than that of 1,25-dihydroxyvitamin D; therefore, the notion that the former is itself an important determinant of calcium absorption is plausible. The correlation between calcium absorption and the urinary calcium/creatinine ratio could not be explained by hormonal factors, and its slope was shallow, meaning that urinary calcium excretion was not much lower when absorption was low than when it was high.

These results thus explain some of the variables affecting calcium absorption, and they reinforce the need for adequate amounts of vitamin D, regardless of which form of the hormone is most important. They in no way minimize the importance of dietary intake of calcium. Indeed, they reinforce that need. Measurements of calcium absorption are not practical in clinical practice, which means that the worst should be assumed and, therefore, calcium intake should be generous for all. Indeed, the recommended intake for older women should probably be higher.

R.D. Utiger, M.D.

References

1. Heaney RP, Recker RR, Stegman MR, et al: Calcium absorption in women: Relationships to calcium intake, estrogen status, and age. *J Bone Miner Res* 4:469–475, 1989.
2. NIH Consensus Development Panel: Optimal calcium intake. *JAMA* 272:1942–1948, 1994.

Primary Hyperparathyroidism: Is Technetium ^{99m}-Sestamibi/Iodine-123 Subtraction Scanning the Best Procedure to Locate Enlarged Glands Before Surgery?

Hindié E, Melliere D, Simon D, Perlemuter L, Galle P (Henri Mondor Univ Hosp, Creteil, France)

J Clin Endocrinol Metab 80:302–307, 1995 119-96-51–2

Background.—Surgery for primary hyperparathyroidism can fail because of nonrecognition of multiglandular disease or parathyroid adenomas in aberrant positions. Several current imaging techniques have not proven to be as sensitive or specific for locating abnormal glands in patients who have not undergone surgery as are experienced surgeons. Technetium-99m–sestamibi scanning has recently been found to be very sensitive in locating enlarged parathyroid glands. The sensitivity, false positive rate, and impact on surgery of ^{99m}Tc-sestamibi/iodine-123 (^{123}I) subtraction scanning were evaluated.

Methods.—In 30 patients with primary hyperparathyroidism, ^{99m}Tc-sestamibi/^{123}I subtraction imaging was performed before first surgery. The results were compared with the surgical findings.

Results.—Imaging detected 26 solitary adenomas, and 27 were found at the time of surgery. Three patients had multiglandular parathyroid hyperplasia; imaging predicted multiglandular involvement in 2 of these patients, and a solitary image was seen in the third. The smallest gland detected by imaging weighed 125 mg. Two mediastinal adenomas were detected before surgery and were excised via a median sternotomy. Image analysis was hindered in 10 patients because of concomitant nodular thyroid disease and led to 1 false positive imaging result.

Conclusion.—Technetium-99m–sestamibi/iodine-123 subtraction imaging is excellent for locating enlarged parathyroid glands, although image interpretation can be difficult in patients with thyroid nodules and multiglandular disease cannot always be identified.

► Using ^{99m}Tc-sestamibi/^{123}I subtraction imaging to identify abnormal parathyroid glands looks very promising, as documented in this study and several others (summarized in Reference 1). Parathyroid adenomas weighing as little as 125 mg can be detected, as can adenomas located in the mediastinum. At this relatively early stage, this technique seems to be more sensitive and specific than other parathyroid imaging methods, including thallium-technetium subtraction imaging, ultrasonography, CT, and MRI. Biologically, the basis for the high uptake of ^{99m}Tc-sestamibi seems to be the mitochondria-rich nature of hyperfunctioning parathyroid tissue. Practically, false positive results may occur in patients with thyroid nodules, particularly those that do not take up iodine well. The results may be falsely negative not only in a few patients with parathyroid adenomas but also in some with parathyroid hyperplasia.

This is a localization, not a diagnostic, procedure. Even as a localization procedure, I do not think it should be done routinely in previously untreated patients with primary hyperparathyroidism (see Reference 2 for a dissenting view). In these patients, a good surgeon finds abnormal parathyroid tissue more often than any imaging procedure. This is especially likely to occur in those patients who have primary parathyroid hyperplasia, and in them, the finding of a single abnormal parathyroid gland (using this or any other imaging procedure) may lead to less care being taken to search for multiple abnormal parathyroid glands. This imaging procedure is indicated, probably as the first choice, in a patient in whom neck exploration was unsuccessful, but it is difficult to resist doing multiple procedures in these particular patients in a quest for certainty because reexploration of the neck is so difficult.

R.D. Utiger, M.D.

References

1. Mitchell BK, Kinder BK, Cornelius E, et al: Primary hyperparathyroidism: Preoperative localization using technetium-sestamibi scanning. *J Clin Endocrinol Metab* 80:7–10, 1995.
2. Caixas A, Berna L, Piera J, et al: Utility of ^{99m}Tc-sestamibi as a first-line imaging procedure in the preoperative evaluation of hyperparathyroidism. *Clin Endocrinol* 43:525–530, 1995.

Biochemical Hyperparathyroidism and Bone Mineral Status in Patients Treated Long-Term With Lithium

Nordenström J, Elvius M, Bågedahl-Strindlund M, Zhao B, Törring O
(Huddinge Univ Hosp, Sweden; Karolinska Hosp, Stockholm)

Metabolism 43:1563–1567, 1994 119-96-51–3

Introduction.—Calcium homeostasis is affected by lithium carbonate, which is widely used in the treatment of patients with manic-depressive psychoses. The high intracellular calcium concentrations typical of patients with bipolar affective disorders are reduced with lithium treatment, suggesting a mechanism for its beneficial effect. However, patients taking lithium may develop parathyroid hyperplasia and hypercalcemia.

Methods.—Parathyroid function was studied in 23 normal subjects and 26 patients with bipolar or unipolar affective disorder who had been treated with lithium for a minimum of 10 years. For comparison, parathyroid function was also determined in 50 patients with primary hyperparathyroidism, and 21 patients with parathyroid hormone–dependent hypercalcemia after renal transplantation (tertiary hyperparathyroidism). Serum calcium, ionized calcium, phosphate, osteocalcin and parathyroid hormone were measured. All lithium-treated patients had normal kidney function and no musculoskeletal pain or kidney stones. Bone mineral density (BMD) of the whole body, femoral neck and lumbar spine was determined by dual-energy x-ray absorptiometry.

Findings.—As compared with the normal subjects, the lithium-treated patients had higher serum ionized calcium concentrations, but serum parathyroid hormone concentrations were similar in the two groups. Fifty-four percent had an elevated serum calcium or parathyroid hormone concentration. These changes were in the same direction, but not as prominent as those in the groups with primary or tertiary hyperparathyroidism. The values for bone density were slightly higher in the lithium-treated patients than in the normal subjects. Serum parathyroid hormone and osteocalcin concentrations were positively correlated in the lithium group, possibly explaining their higher bone density values.

Conclusion.—Patients receiving long-term lithium therapy have biochemical findings of mild primary hyperparathyroidism but no decrease in bone density.

► Lithium carbonate increases parathyroid hormone secretion to some extent in everyone who receives it, and it causes hypercalcemia in a few patients because it diminishes the sensitivity of parathyroid secretion to inhibition by calcium. In this study of patients treated for 10 years or longer, the majority had mild hypercalcemia and inappropriate—if not overtly elevated—serum parathyroid hormone concentrations. The basic observation that chronic lithium carbonate therapy causes hypercalcemia is not new, but the bone density results are; they indicate that lithium-induced hyperparathyroidism does not cause bone disease.

The effect of lithium carbonate therapy on parathyroid secretion is gradual. In one study, treatment for less than 6 months had no effect, whereas patients treated for 36–300 months (mean, 103 months) had slightly higher serum ionized calcium concentrations (although few had hypercalcemia), higher serum parathyroid hormone concentrations, and bigger parathyroid glands (measured by ultrasonography) than did normal subjects.[1] The biochemical findings were similar in a group of patients treated for an average of 6.6 years[2] and in another study of patients treated for more than 10 years.[3] Despite the chronic but minimal hypercalcemia, nephrolithiasis is not a problem, because urinary calcium tends to be low (the hypercalcemia is very modest and renal calcium reabsorption is increased by parathyroid hormone).

Any patient with hypercalcemia, especially if the cause is not obvious, should be asked about lithium. First, lithium alone can cause hypercalcemia. Second, it probably also worsens hypercalcemia in patients with primary hyperparathyroidism. Whether to discontinue lithium, of course, depends on the degree of hypercalcemia, the need for lithium, and whether something else can be substituted for it, but nothing need be done if the hypercalcemia is mild and uncomplicated.

R.D. Utiger, M.D.

References

1. Mallette LE, Khouri K, Zengotita H, et al: Lithium treatment increases intact and midregion and intact parathyroid hormone and parathyroid volume. *J Clin Endocrinol Metab* 68:654–660, 1989.
2. Christiansen C, Baastrup PC, Lindgreen P, et al: Endocrine effects of lithium: II. Primary hyperparathyroidism. *Acta Endocrinol* 88:528–534, 1978.
3. Stancer HC, Forbath N: Hyperparathyroidism, hypothyroidism, and impaired renal function after 10 to 20 years of lithium treatment. *Arch Intern Med* 149:1042–1045, 1989.

Longitudinal Measurements of Bone Density and Biochemical Indices in Untreated Primary Hyperparathyroidism

Silverberg SJ, Gartenberg F, Jacobs TP, Shane E, Siris E, Staron RB, Bilezikian JP (Columbia Univ, New York)

J Clin Endocrinol Metab 80:723–728, 1995 119-96-51–4

Introduction.—Surgery is not indicated for many patients with asymptomatic primary hyperparathyroidism. However, there is concern that untreated primary hyperparathyroidism may have deleterious effects on the skeleton. The effect of untreated hyperparathyroidism on biochemical and bone densitometric indexes was prospectively evaluated in 66 patients.

Methods.—The patients were enrolled in a longitudinal study of primary hyperparathyroidism. For most patients, medical follow-up, rather than parathyroidectomy, was recommended according to the guidelines of the Consensus Development Conference on the Management of Asymptomatic Primary Hyperparathyroidism; others declined or had contra-

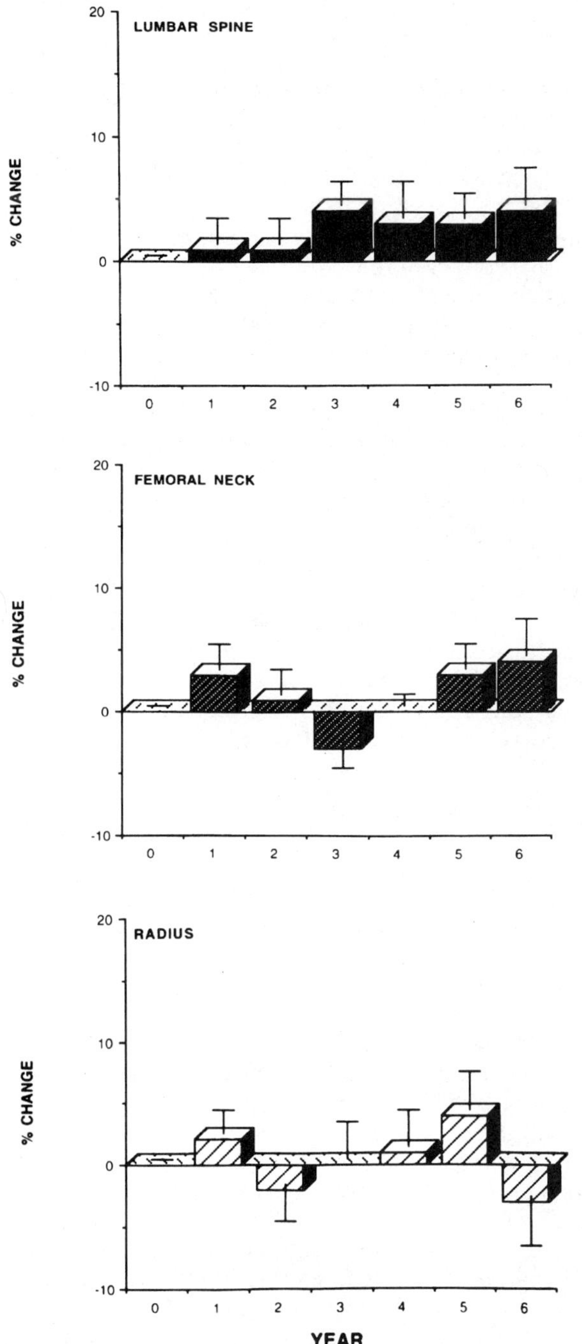

FIGURE 3.—Course of bone mineral density over 7 annual measurements. Cumulative percent change (from 0 year baseline) in bone mineral density by site. (Courtesy of Silverberg SJ, Gartenberg F, Jacobs TP, et al: Longitudinal measurements of bone density and biochemical indices in untreated primary hyperparathyroidism. *J Clin Endocrinol Metab* 80:723–728, 1995. Copyright, The Endocrine Society.)

indications to operation. During follow-up the patients underwent routine clinical evaluation and had serum and urine biochemical tests performed every 4 months. Bone mineral densitometry was performed at study entry and then yearly at the lumbar spine, femoral neck, and radius.

Results.—The study group included 11 men with a mean age of 58 years, 11 premenopausal women with a mean age of 43 years, and 44 postmenopausal women with a mean age of 63 years. None of the women were taking estrogen. For both the group as a whole and the subgroup of postmenopausal women, there was no change in serum calcium, phosphorus, parathyroid hormone, vitamin D, or alkaline phosphatase during the 6-year follow-up. Similarly, there were no changes in urinary calcium, hydroxyproline and hydroxypyridinium cross-link excretion, nor in lumbar spine, femoral neck, and radial bone mineral density (Fig 3). The patients enrolled in the study who initially met guidelines for surgery but were not operated on were younger than the others (mean age, 50 years vs. 62 years) and had higher urinary calcium excretion. Their biochemical and bone mineral density values also did not change during follow-up.

Conclusion.—Because primary hyperparathyroidism often occurs without symptoms or signs, the need for routine surgery has been questioned. However, the disease often affects postmenopausal women, leading to concern about accelerated bone loss and increased risk of fracture. The results of this study, however, suggest that mild primary hyperparathyroidism is not associated with progressive biochemical or skeletal abnormalities.

▶ Most patients with primary hyperparathyroidism are asymptomatic, and they remain so for prolonged periods, as was true of the 66 patients in this study. These facts have led to much debate about who should be treated—meaning neck exploration—and also to the development of the criteria for surgery used in this study (serum calcium greater than 12 mg/dL [3.0 mmol/L], urinary calcium excretion greater than 400 mg/day [10 mmol/day], presence of any manifestations of the disease [stones, overt bone disease, etc.], abnormal renal function, and age younger than 50 years).[1] These are reasonable criteria, but they should not be followed slavishly—nor were they by Silverberg et al. Twenty-four of their patients met the criteria but were not operated on (or they refused operation). The wisdom of these criteria is confirmed by the results of this study, in which no patient had clinical manifestations or biochemical progression of their disease during the 6-year follow-up.

Note that low bone density is not a criterion for surgery, but there is little doubt that hyperparathyroidism causes bone loss, especially of cortical bone. In this study, the patients' initial radial, femoral neck, and lumbar spine bone density values were, respectively, −1.3, −0.8, and −0.3 standard deviations below the mean for age- and sex-matched normal subjects. The follow-up results are remarkable in that there was no loss of bone density at any site (Fig 3), even though some age- and menopause-related loss would have been expected. These results add substantially to already published work that progressive bone loss does not occur in primary hyperparathyroidism,[2] and there is evidence that it is not a risk factor for vertebral or hip fractures.[3, 4]

That bone density is, on average, low in these patients when first studied means that accelerated bone resorption must occur very early in the course of hyperparathyroidism and that there is a lag period before bone formation increases to balance and even exceed the increase in resorption. The alternate possibility—that although bone resorption is not persistently increased and even declines to less than normal, bone formation is not increased—is unlikely, because the patients had biochemical evidence of increased bone resorption and formation both when they were first studied and during follow-up.

Might a subgroup of these patients, e.g., postmenopausal women, be at more risk for bone loss? They were not in this study. I should note that in cross-sectional studies in postmenopausal women with primary hyperparathyroidism, the bone density of the radius, femoral neck, and lumbar spine was higher in those who had taken estrogen for at least 2 years than in those who had not taken any estrogen after the menopause.[5] So excess parathyroid hormone does not block the ability of estrogen to inhibit bone resorption.

Should bone density be measured in everyone with mild primary hyperparathyroidism and, if so, how should the information be used? If surgery is planned anyway, there is no need for the measurement. If it is not, the finding of reasonably normal bone density would not change the recommendation. If bone density is low, particularly in the femoral neck, then surgery ought to be recommended, not so much because of what might happen without it but, rather, because bone density will increase after the hyperparathyroidism is cured (see Abstract 119-96-51–5).

R.D. Utiger, M.D.

References

1. National Institutes of Health: Consensus development conference statement on primary hyperparathyroidism. *J Bone Miner Res* 6:9S–13S, 1991.
2. Rao DS, Wilson RJ, Kleerekoper M, et al: Lack of biochemical progression or continuation of accelerated bone loss in mild asymptomatic primary hyperparathyroidism: Evidence for biphasic disease course. *J Clin Endocrinol Metab* 67:1294–1298, 1988.
3. Wilson RJ, Rao DS, Ellis B, et al: Mild asymptomatic primary hyperparathyroidism is not a risk factor for vertebral fractures. *Ann Intern Med* 109:959–962, 1988.
4. Larsson K, Ljunghall S, Krusemo UB, et al: The risk of hip fracture in patients with primary hyperparathyroidism: A population-based cohort study with a follow-up of 19 years. *J Intern Med* 234:585–593, 1993.
5. McDermott MT, Perloff JJ, Kidd GS: Effects of mild asymptomatic primary hyperparathyroidism on bone mass in women with and without estrogen replacement therapy. *J Bone Miner Res* 9:509–514, 1994.

Increased Bone Mineral Density After Parathyroidectomy in Primary Hyperparathyroidism

Silverberg SJ, Gartenberg F, Jacobs TP, Shane E, Siris E, Staron RB, McMahon DJ, Bilezikian JP (Irving Ctr for Clinical Research, New York; Columbia Univ, New York)

J Clin Endocrinol Metab 80:729–734, 1995 119-96-51–5

Background.—Patients with primary hyperparathyroidism tend to lose mainly cortical bone, with cancellous (trabecular) bone being relatively spared. Little is known about the changes in bone density after successful parathyroidectomy, especially at sites of cancellous bone. It is conceivable that the operation, which often is done to prevent osteoporosis in postmenopausal women, might have adverse effects on cancellous bone density.

Objective.—Thirty-four patients meeting accepted criteria for parathyroidectomy successfully underwent the operation and were followed for up to 4 years afterward. Eleven were men and 23 were women, 17 of whom were postmenopausal. The criteria for surgery included age 50 years or younger; a serum calcium concentration greater than 12 mg/dL (3.0 mmol/L); a history of kidney stones or hypercalcuria; reduced radial bone mineral density; and neuromuscular signs of primary hyperparathyroidism.

Initial Status.—Twenty-seven patients had a parathyroid adenoma, 5 had parathyroid hyperplasia, and 2 had both. Bone turnover was slightly increased.

Postoperative Status.—All patients had normal biochemical values a year after parathyroid surgery. Bone mineral density was significantly increased in the lumbar spine at this time (Fig 1), and it increased by 13% at this site during the 4-year follow-up period. Bone density also increased in the femoral neck and to a lesser extent in the distal radius—which contains more cortical bone than the other sites.

Implications.—Bone mineral density increases significantly at sites of cancellous bone in patients with primary hyperparathyroidism who successfully undergo parathyroid surgery. Cortical bone density sometimes substantially increases as well.

► These results demonstrate quite clearly that both cortical and cancellous (trabecular) bone density increase after successful surgical treatment of primary hyperparathyroidism and that much of the improvement occurs in the first year after surgery. Although these patients met standard criteria for surgery (see comment after Abstract 119-96-51–4), their baseline values for bone density were no different than those in the patients described in Abstract 119-96-55–4 who were not operated on.

As shown in Figure 1, the pattern of increase in bone density after cure varied, with the improvement being somewhat greater and continuing longer in regions rich in cancellous bone (lumbar spine) and cancellous and cortical bone (femoral neck), where bone remodeling is more rapid than in cortical

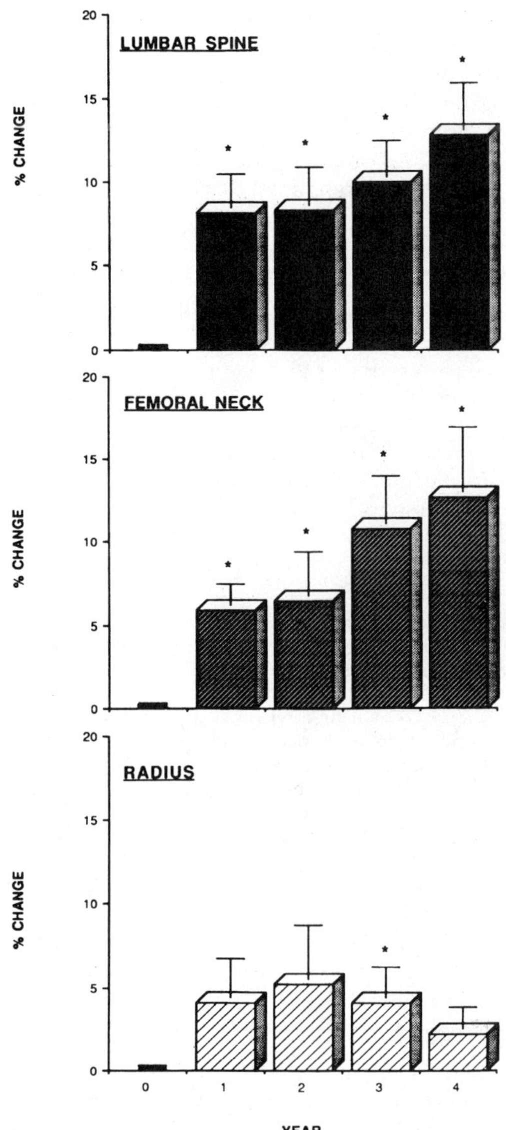

FIGURE 1.—Bone mineral density after parathyroidectomy, cumulative percentage change in bone mineral density after parathyroidectomy by site. *Asterisk* represents change from year 0 baseline at $P < 0.05$. (Courtesy of Silverberg SJ, Gartenberg F, Jacobs TP, et al: Increased bone mineral density after parathyroidectomy in primary hyperparathyroidism. *J Clin Endocrinol Metab* 80:729–734, 1995. Copyright, The Endocrine Society.)

bone (radius). This pattern was unexpected, because both the density and histology of cortical bone are more abnormal in unoperated patients (see Abstract 119-96-51–4 and Reference 1). Recovery tended to be greater in those patients with lower initial bone density values, and it was as great in postmenopausal women as in other patients. I should note that only 13 patients were studied 4 years after surgery, and I cannot tell whether bone density at the different sites reached mean values for age- and sex-matched normal subjects in any of the patients during follow-up. Nevertheless, the improvement is impressive; for example, it is greater than that which occurs in postmenopausal women treated with estrogen. In other studies, bone density increased in the femoral neck but not in the lumbar spine during the first year after surgery,[2] and it increased substantially (but not to normal) in the radius (the only site measured) within the first 10 months, after which it increased very little.[3] I don't know the reason for these discrepancies, but of these 3 studies, that of Silverberg et al. was considerably larger and more comprehensive than the others.

It is reassuring to know that bone may be regained after cure of hyperparathyroidism. I think that this finding puts measurement of bone density in patients with primary hyperparathyroidism on firmer footing. That bone density increases, rather than simply stabilizes, makes me more inclined to recommend surgery for patients with asymptomatic hyperparathyroidism in whom bone density is low.

R.D. Utiger, M.D.

References

1. Parisien M, Silverberg SJ, Shane E, et al: The histomorphometry of bone in primary hyperparathyrodism: Preservation of cancellous bone structure. *J Clin Endocrinol Metab* 70:930–938, 1990.
2. Clyde JW, Wittert GA, Gilchrist NL, et al: The effect of parathyroidectomy on bone mineral density in primary hyperparathyroidism. *N Z Med J* 105:71–72, 1992.
3. Martin P, Bergmann P, Gillet C, et al: Long-term irreversibility of bone loss after surgery for primary hyperparathyroidism. *Arch Intern Med* 150:1495–1497, 1990.

Prevention of Bone Loss by Vitamin D Supplementation in Elderly Women: A Randomized Double-Blind Trial

Ooms ME, Roos JC, Bezemer PD, van der Vijgh WJF, Bouter LM, Lips P (Vrije Universiteit, Amsterdam; Free Univ Hosp, Amsterdam)
J Clin Endocrinol Metab 80:1052–1057, 1995 119-96-51–6

Introduction.—The elderly population is at risk for vitamin D deficiency, which may be an important risk factor for hip fractures. Vitamin D supplementation for the elderly has few or no side effects, and by reducing bone turnover and bone loss, it may reduce the incidence of fractures. However, there are few data from randomized, double-blind trials. The effects of vitamin D supplementation on bone turnover and bone loss in elderly women were evaluated.

Methods.—The double-blind, placebo-controlled trial included 348 women aged 70 years or older (mean age, 80 years), who were randomly assigned to receive either vitamin D_3 supplementation, 400 IU/day, or placebo for 2 years. Bone mineral density was measured at the femoral neck and trochanter of both hips and at the distal radius. These measurements were made at baseline in all women, after 1 year in 283, and after 2 years in 248. Biochemical measurements were made as well.

Results.—After 1 year, the women in the vitamin D group had a 35 nmol/L (14 ng/mL) increase in serum 25-hydroxyvitamin D, a 7 pmol/L (3 pg/mL) increase in serum 1,25-dihydroxyvitamin D, and a 0.5% increase in the urinary calcium-creatinine ratio. They also had a small but significant decrease in serum parathyroid hormone. Vitamin D supplementation had no effect on measures of bone turnover. In the left femoral neck, bone mineral density increased by 1.8% in the first year, 0.2% in the second year, and 1.9% overall, expressed as the difference in mean change compared with the placebo group. Bone mineral density in the right femoral neck increased by 1.5%, 1.1%, and 2.6%, respectively. There were no significant changes in bone mineral density of the femoral trochanter or distal radius.

Conclusions.—Vitamin D_3 supplementation, 400 IU/day, prevents bone loss in elderly women. It improves vitamin D status to the young adult range while slightly decreasing parathyroid hormone secretion and increasing bone mineral density at the femoral neck. The increase in bone mineral density would be expected to reduce the risk of hip fracture, although a reduction will be difficult to detect and may differ for femoral neck and trochanteric fractures.

▶ This article provides more evidence—if more is needed—that vitamin D supplementation is beneficial in elderly persons. As compared with younger persons, older persons eat less vitamin D,[1] go outdoors less, and wear more clothes when they do go outside; the capacity of their skin to produce vitamin D is also decreased. As a result, they have lower serum 25-hydroxyvitamin D concentrations. There is also some evidence that aging is associated with decreased conversion of 25-hydroxyvitamin D to 1,25-dihydroxyvitamin D and, possibly, decreased vitamin D stimulation of intestinal calcium absorption. Vitamin D is also important for normal bone metabolism and muscle function. In older women, bone density and serum 25-hydroxyvitamin D concentrations are correlated.[2]

This Dutch study of elderly women confirms that vitamin D supplementation not only has beneficial effects on vitamin D and parathyroid function but also increases femoral neck bone density. Dietary calcium intake, estimated by recall, ranged from about 600 to 1,200 mg daily in the 2 groups and was not supplemented. The mean serum 25-hydroxyvitamin D concentration doubled, but many women still had concentrations in the low-normal range, suggesting that a larger dose might be more beneficial. Note that although femoral bone density did not increase during the second year, the initial increase was sustained. Whether bone loss eventually resumes despite continued supplementation is not known but seems likely; nevertheless any increase in bone density will lower fracture risk somewhat. The occurrence of fractures is not mentioned, but few would be expected in a study of this size. In a French study of 3,270 elderly women given 800 IU of vitamin D and 1,200 mg of calcium daily,[3] the risk of hip and other nonvertebral fractures was reduced significantly.

The new results—even in the absence of fracture data—strengthen the evidence that vitamin D and calcium intake should be supplemented in older persons. I think that the intake of vitamin D should be 800 IU daily, or 5,000 IU once weekly; that of calcium should be 1,500 mg daily. In view of the evidence indicating that changes in overall vitamin D economy begin much earlier, we should consider increasing vitamin D intake at a considerably earlier age.

R.D. Utiger, M.D.

References

1. O'Dowd KJ, Clemens TL, Kelsey JL, et al: Exogenous calciferol (vitamin D) and vitamin D endocrine status among elderly nursing home residents in the New York city area. *J Am Geriatr Soc* 41:414–421, 1993. (1994 YEAR BOOK OF MEDICINE, pp 597–598.)
2. Villareal DT, Civitelli R, Chines A, et al: Subclinical vitamin D deficiency in postmenopausal women with low vertebral bone mass. *J Clin Endocrinol Metab* 72:628–634, 1991. (1992 YEAR BOOK OF MEDICINE, pp 493–495.)
3. Chapuy MC, Arlot ME, Duboeuf F, et al: Vitamin D_3 and calcium to prevent hip fractures in elderly women. *N Engl J Med* 327:1637–1642, 1992. (1994 YEAR BOOK OF MEDICINE, pp 607–609.)

Risk Factors for Hip Fracture in White Women

Cummings SR, for the Study of Osteoporotic Fractures Research Group
(Prevention Sciences Group, San Francisco)
N Engl J Med 332:767–773, 1995 119-96-51–7

Objective.—White women have a 1 in 6 risk of hip fracture during their lifetime. However, no comprehensive prospective studies have assessed the risk factors for hip fracture. In a cohort of older women, many potential risk factors were identified, bone mass was measured, and the group was followed up for hip fractures.

Methods.—A total of 9,516 white women aged 65 years and older with no previous hip fracture received a questionnaire, interview, physical examination, and measurement of calcaneal (trabecular) bone density. The women were followed by telephone every 4 months for an average of 4.1 years to ascertain the incidence of hip fracture.

Results.—During the follow-up, there were 192 non–motor vehicle accident–related hip fractures and 565 deaths; 92 women were lost to follow up. Sixteen independent risk factors for hip fracture were identified in multivariate age-adjusted analyses, including a history of maternal hip fracture (double the risk), weight loss since age 25 years, being tall at age 25 years, poor self-rated health, previous hyperthyroidism, therapy with benzodiazepines or anticonvulsant drugs, increased caffeine intake, and spending 4 hours a day or less on their feet. Examination findings associated with increased risk were the inability to rise from a chair without using the arms, poor depth perception, poor contrast sensitivity, and

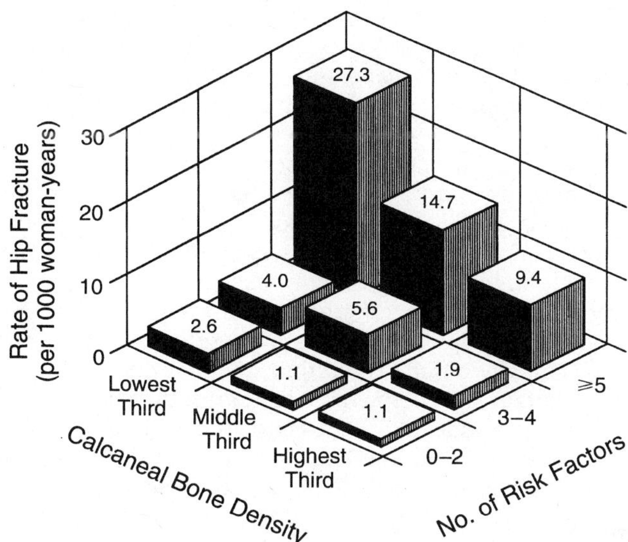

FIGURE 2.—The annual risk of hip fracture according to the number of risk factors and the age-specific calcaneal bone density. The risk factors are as follows: age 80 years or older; maternal history of hip fracture; any fracture (except hip fracture) since the age of 50 years; fair, poor or very poor health; previous hyperthyroidism; anticonvulsant therapy; current long-acting benzodiazepine therapy, current weight less than at the age of 25 years; height at the age of 25 years greater than or equal to 168 cm; caffeine intake more than the equivalent of 2 cups of coffee per day, on feet 4 hours or less per day; no walking for exercise; inability to rise from chair without using arms; lowest quartile (standard deviation greater than 2.44) of depth perception; lowest quartile (≤ 0.70 unit) of contrast sensitivity; and pulse rate greater than 80 beats per minute). (Reprinted by permission of *The New England Journal of Medicine.* Cummings SR, for the Study of Osteoporotic Fractures Research Group: Risk factors for hip fracture in white women. *N Engl J Med* 332:767–773, 1995. Copyright 1995, Massachusetts Medical Society.)

tachycardia at rest. Low calcaneal bone density was an independent risk factor. The annual risk of hip fracture was related to the number of risk factors (Fig 2).

Conclusions.—Multiple risk factors are associated with hip fractures in older white women, especially in those women with low bone density.

► The original article on which this abstract is based has a table (Table 3) listing 17 factors that were associated with later hip fracture in this prospective cohort study of nearly 10,000 women. Only a maternal history of hip fracture, an inability to rise from a chair without using one's arms, and anticonvulsant drug therapy were associated with a relative risk of 2.0 or more; factors of lesser importance were related to thinness, muscular or visual impairment, physical inactivity (less than 4 hours/day on feet), caffeine ingestion, or benzodiazepine therapy, previous hyperthyroidism, previous fracture, and bone density. Many of these factors remained important after correction for bone density, suggesting that their effect was mediated via falling or changes in bone quality rather than density.

Factors not associated with hip fracture included age of menopause, alcohol consumption in past year, history of breast-feeding or oophorectomy, thyroid hormone therapy, antacid therapy, thiazide therapy, dietary calcium intake, and self-reported osteoarthritis. The relative risk of hip fracture in the 13.9% of women who were taking estrogen at baseline and had no history of osteoporosis or fracture was 0.3 (95% confidence interval, 0.1 to 1.1), indicative of a protective effect.

It is easy to be skeptical about the importance of risk factors that increase risk very little, particularly when many factors (probably about 50) are evaluated; much of the information is obtained from the study subject, and many of the questions concern rather distant events. The cumulative effect of the many risk factors, however, is rather impressive (Fig 2), even in the women with higher bone density. Furthermore, many of these factors—or ones very similar to them—were identified as being important in a case-control study of hip fracture in black women.[1] Notwithstanding evidence from case-control (and, in some instances, prospective randomized) studies that estrogen, calcium, vitamin D compounds, and calcitonin protect against hip fracture,[2] much of the risk can be related to factors that have nothing to do with bone density. These factors, e.g., alertness, vision, strength, and coordination, relate to the likelihood of falling and are often amenable to relatively simple interventions.

R.D. Utiger, M.D.

References

1. Grisso JA, Kelsey JA, Strom BL, et al: Risk factors for hip fracture in black women. *N Engl J Med* 330:1555–1559, 1994. (1995 Year Book of Medicine, pp 655–657).
2. Kanis JA, Johnell O, Gullberg GB, et al: Evidence for efficacy of drugs affecting bone metabolism in preventing hip fracture. *BMJ* 305:1124–1128, 1992. (1994 Year Book of Medicine, pp 602–604.)

Effect of Age on Bone Density and Bone Turnover in Men

Wishart JM, Need AG, Horowitz M, Morris HA, Nordin BEC (Royal Adelaide Hosp, South Australia; Inst of Med and Veterinary Science, Adelaide, South Australia; Univ of Adelaide, South Australia)

Clin Endocrinol 42:141–146, 1995 119-96-51–8

Introduction.—There are few data on the patterns and causes of age-related bone loss in men. Men need androgen to achieve optimal bone mass and androgen production declines with age, but it is unclear whether the age-associated declines in bone mass and serum androgen concentrations in men are related. Associations between age, bone status, plasma androgens, and indicators of bone resorption and formation were studied in normal men.

Methods.—The cross-sectional study included 147 normal men, aged 20–83 years. Bone density was measured in the forearm, lumbar spine, femoral neck, Ward's triangle, and trochanter by dual-energy x-ray absorptiometry. Markers of bone resorption and formation were determined as well, including serum procollagen I C-terminal peptide (PICP), osteocalcin, bone alkaline phosphatase, and procollagen I C-terminal telopeptide; fasting urine hydroxyproline/creatinine, pyridinoline/creatinine, and deoxypyridinoline/creatinine ratios; and a serum free androgen index (FAI) calculated as serum testosterone/sex hormone–binding globulin.

Results.—There was a significant relationship between body mass index and age and a negative correlation between dietary calcium intake and age. There was an age-related decline in serum free androgen index values, because serum testosterone declined and sex hormone-binding globulin increased. The serum free androgen index decreased by 26% between the third and fourth decades and then by 16% between the fourth and fifth decades. The decline continued at a slower rate into the eighth decade. The markers of bone formation all declined with age, though the associations with age were not linear and the patterns of decline varied. The markers of bone resorption fell in comparable ways, with the greatest decreases between the third and fourth decades. Strong associations were noted between the markers of bone resorption and the markers of bone formation. The best marker of bone formation was serum procollagen I C-terminal peptide, which was correlated with serum free androgen values after adjustment for age and body mass index. Bone density decreased significantly after age 50 years at most sites (Fig 3). For example, between ages 50 and 80 years, the rates of bone loss in the forearm, Ward's triangle and the femoral neck were 0.6%, 0.7%, and 0.5%/year, respectively. After correction for age, there were no significant correlations between bone

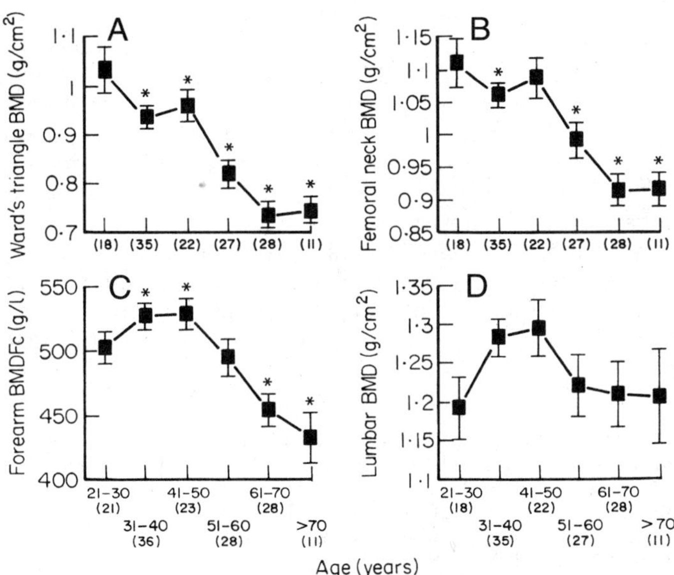

FIGURE 3.—Effects of age on bone density in (**A**) Ward's angle; (**B**) femoral neck; (**C**) forearm; and (**D**) lumbar spine in 141 normal men. The numbers in each group are given in parentheses. Data are mean values ± SEM. $*P < 0.05$. *Abbreviation: BMD,* bone mineral density. (Courtesy of Wishart JM, Need AG, Horowitz M, et al: Effect of age on bone density and bone turnover in men. *Clin Endocrinol* 42:141–146, 1995. Reproduced by permission of Blackwell Science, Ltd.)

density and serum free androgen index values or any of the biochemical markers of bone formation or resorption.

Conclusions.—Normal men lose little bone before the age of 50 years, but bone loss increases thereafter. No biochemical changes occurred at that age that might reflect or cause the onset of bone loss.

► Like women, men lose both cortical and trabecular bone with age; of course, they also have hip, radial, and vertebral fractures, albeit considerably less often. However, the pattern and the mechanism of bone loss differ among men and women. In men, the initiation of bone loss is age-related, and it continues at the same rate for several decades, after which it may cease (although note the small number of men in the group older than 70 years of age in Figure 3), whereas in women the initiation of bone loss is primarily menopause-related and the rate of bone loss is greatest during the first 5–10 years after the menopause, after which it slows appreciably (but does not cease). In men, the values for the tests of bone formation (serum procollagen I C-terminal peptide, osteocalcin, and bone alkaline phosphatase) and bone resorption both declined, suggesting that the primary cause of the declining bone density in older men is decreased bone formation. In women, the primary cause of bone loss in the early postmenopausal years is increased bone resorption, with a secondary but necessarily inadequate increase in bone formation.

The calculated yearly rates of bone loss in men from 50 to 80 years of age in this and other cross-sectional studies were low,[1, 2] as compared with the rates calculated from repeated measurements in one of the earlier studies.[1] The risk factors for bone loss in men include smoking, obesity, physical inactivity, alcohol consumption, glucocorticoid therapy, and declining testosterone (and perhaps growth hormone) secretion.[3] Dietary calcium and vitamin D intake might also be expected to be important, but in one 3-year study of well-nourished men (estimated dietary calcium intake of 1,159 mg/day) in the United States (Portland, Oregon), calcium and vitamin D supplementation did not slow bone loss.[1]

No one recommends measurements of bone density in older men. However, the fact that they lose bone and that some reversible factors are known to be associated with increased bone loss should be kept in mind.

R.D. Utiger, M.D.

References

1. Orwoll ES, Oviatt SK, McClung MR, et al: The rate of bone mineral loss in normal men and the effects of calcium and cholecalciferol supplementation. *Ann Intern Med* 112:29–34, 1990.
2. Burger H, van Daele PLA, Algra D, et al: The association between age and bone mineral density in men and women aged 55 years and over: The Rotterdam study. *Bone Miner* 25:1–13, 1994.
3. Kelepouris N, Harper KD, Gannon F, et al: Severe osteoporosis in men. *Ann Intern Med* 123:452–460, 1995.

52 The Reproductive System

Estrogen Resistance Caused by a Mutation in the Estrogen-Receptor Gene in a Man

Smith EP, Boyd J, Frank GR, Takahashi H, Cohen RM, Specker B, Williams TC, Lubahn DB, Korach KS (Univ of Cincinnati, Ohio; Univ of North Carolina, Chapel Hill; Natl Inst of Environmental Health Sciences, Research Triangle Park, NC)

N Engl J Med 331:1056–1061, 1994 119-96-52–1

Background.—Although mutation of the estrogen-receptor gene was previously thought to be lethal, recent case reports and experiments in mice appear to contradict that belief. Mice of both sexes with disrupted estrogen-receptor genes were found to be viable, and 2 female patients—1 with a placental aromatase deficiency and 1 with a full mutation in the aromatase cytochrome *P-450* gene—were reported to survive as pseudohermaphrodites. A unique case of estrogen resistance in a man was described.

Case Report.—Man, 28, had tall stature and progressive genu valgum. His birth weight and early growth and development were normal, but he continued to grow slowly after adolescence despite normal development of secondary sex characteristics. Radiographic evaluation revealed unfused epiphyses. The patient reported strong heterosexual interest and no history of sex-identity disorder. His height and span were above the 95th percentile, and his proportions were eununchoid. Physical examination revealed bilateral axillary acanthosis nigricans and a skin tag in the left axilla. The patient's bone age was 15 years. Comparison of radiographs with others taken 10 years earlier revealed bone demineralization with minimal epiphyseal maturation. The patient's karyotype was 46,XY; his sperm showed subnormal viability. His glucose tolerance was impaired and he had hyperinsulinemia. His serum testosterone concentration was normal, but concentrations of estradiol, estrone, follicle-stimulating hormone, and luteinizing hormone were high. The patient was treated with high-dose transdermal ethinyl estradiol for 6 months, but he had no increase in serum concentration of any estrogen-dependent protein. Conformation analysis of the estrogen-receptor gene of peripheral blood lymphocyte DNA revealed that exon 2 had a variant banding pattern suggestive of a homozygous mutation, and sequencing indicated the mutation introduced a stop codon. The translated protein would therefore be truncated and functionally inactive. The patient's parents were second cousins and were heterozygous carriers of the mutation.

Discussion.—Disruptive mutation of the estrogen receptor gene is not necessarily lethal, but in a male it may cause tall stature, continued slow linear growth, markedly delayed skeletal maturation, and osteoporosis. Estrogen therefore appears to be important for both men and women to promote normal bone development and mineralization.

▶ The clinical abnormalities (delayed epiphyseal maturation, continued slow linear growth, and osteoporosis) in this man with no estrogen receptors attest to the importance of estrogen in skeletal maturation and bone mineralization. These same abnormalities are known to occur in men with hypogonadism,[1] in whom they have usually been attributed to androgen, not estrogen, deficiency. That they can occur in a man with normal serum testosterone (and dihydrotestosterone) concentrations (and do not occur in patients with complete androgen resistance[2]) demonstrates the primacy of estrogen as the gonadal hormone responsible for normal skeletal maturation and maintenance of normal bone mass.

In men, estrogen is also thought to have a role in sexual behavior and in regulating gonadotropin secretion, and possibly in spermatogenesis and carbohydrate metabolism. In this respect, the results in this man are somewhat conflicting. He had normal sexual function and a normal sperm count, but decreased sperm viability. His serum follicle-stimulating hormone (FSH) and luteinizing hormone (LH) concentrations were high, in spite of normal serum testosterone concentrations and high serum estrogen concentrations. Given the high serum LH concentrations, I would have expected his serum testosterone concentrations to be higher, but perhaps conversion of testosterone to estradiol (and other unmeasured steroids) in the testes was sufficiently stimulated to prevent an increased amount of testosterone from reaching the circulation. In any event, these hormonal values support the notion that estrogen is a regulator of FSH and LH secretion in men, even in the face of substantial amounts of testosterone. The patient's glucose intolerance and hyperinsulinemia could be aggravated by, if not attributed to, deficient estrogen action.

The mutation of the gene for the estrogen receptor in this man would be expected to lead to synthesis of a protein that lacked both the DNA- and estrogen-binding regions of the normal receptor. In other words, estrogen should be totally inactive, unless there are nonnuclear actions of estrogen. The absence of any response to a large transdermal dose of estrogen indicates there are no such actions, nor do I know of any evidence for their existence. I also know of no counterpart to this syndrome in women. A woman with severe estrogen deficiency caused by a genetic defect in aromatase has been reported;[3] she had normal female internal genitalia, some virilization of external genitalia, and additional virilization at puberty, but she had no pubertal breast development or growth spurt and no menarche.

That estrogen deficiency has similar skeletal effects in men and women was unexpected. Presumably, treatment (excluding estrogen) should be similar, e.g., calcium, vitamin D, and a diphosphonate. As with any new syndrome, one may ask "Has it been missed?" I think it could have been—for instance, in a man with delayed pubertal growth or osteoporosis if only serum testosterone were measured. We will learn how much the phenotype varies and more about the importance of estrogen in men as more patients with this disorder are identified.

R.D. Utiger, M.D.

References

1. Orwoll ES, Klein RF: Osteoporosis in men. *Endocr Rev* 16:87–116, 1995.
2. Zachmann M, Prader A, Sobel EH, et al: Pubertal growth in patients with androgen insensitivity: Indirect evidence for the importance of estrogen in pubertal growth in girls. *J Pediatr* 108:694–697, 1986.
3. Conte FA, Grumbach MM, Ito Y, et al: A syndrome of female pseudohermaphrodism, hypergonadotropic hypogonadism, and multicystic ovaries associated with missense mutations in the gene encoding aromatase (P450arom). *J Clin Endocrinol Metab* 78:1287–1292, 1994.

Effect of Digital Rectal Examination on Serum Prostate-Specific Antigen in a Primary Care Setting

The Internal Medicine Clinic Research Consortium

Arch Intern Med 155:389–392, 1995 119-96-52–2

Objective.—Prostate cancer screening commonly includes serum prostate-specific antigen (PSA) measurement and digital rectal examination. Rectal examination could spuriously elevate the serum PSA concentration, although no such change has been documented in normal subjects. The possibility that rectal examination affects serum PSA was assessed among men in a primary care clinic.

Methods.—The study included 202 men aged 50 years or older (mean age, 67 years) attending a Veterans Affairs internal medicine clinic. All men underwent rectal examination for assessment of prostate size and nodularity. Blood for serum PSA measurement was taken immediately before and 30 minutes after the examination. All of the men also provided information about voiding in a questionnaire.

Results.—After the rectal examination, the mean serum PSA concentration increased by a mean of 0.26 μg/L. In 2.9% of the men, PSA increased from less than 4 μg/L before to more than 4 μg/L afterward. Voiding score was significantly but weakly associated with the serum PSA value, with a correlation coefficient of 0.17. Compared with the men with normal or borderline results on rectal examination, serum PSA concentrations were higher in men with an enlarged prostate. However, serum PSA concentrations were not higher in the men with prostatic nodularity.

Conclusions.—An internist performing digital rectal examination in elderly men may cause a statistically significant but not clinically important increase in the serum PSA concentration. For men with clinical indications for serum PSA measurement, previous rectal examination should not preclude blood sampling for PSA determination at that visit. The symptoms and findings on rectal examination are not helpful in selecting a patient population for whom serum PSA screening would likely be useful.

▶ The extent to which the serum PSA concentration might rise after rectal examination is of obvious practical importance in interpreting the results of the test. While the mean serum PSA concentration increased after the examination in this study by a statistically significant amount (mean, 0.26 μg/L; range, −2.37 to +4.44 μg/L), the increase is surely biologically unimportant, and 22% of the men had no increase (or a decrease). Since absolute threshold values—usually 4.0 μg/L—are used to decide who should be evaluated further, it is no surprise that there were a few men in whom the value before the rectal examination was below and the postexamination value was above the threshold. Whether any of the men had a preexamination value above and a postexamination value below this threshold—and, therefore, would have been spared further evaluation had only the second test been done—is not mentioned in the paper; however, there must have been a few. Also not mentioned is a more important result needed to interpret the importance of the small increase, namely the reproducibility of the assay.

These results confirm most other work on this subject in normal men, regardless of whether the postexamination serum PSA determinations were done a few minutes or several hours after the examination;[1, 2] rectal examination does not result in an increase in serum PSA concentration, whether the examination is done by internists or urologists. (The few men with prostate nodules had no increase in serum PSA, but I don't know what happens in men with prostate cancer.) This lack of increase simplifies the interpretation of an abnormal postrectal examination value. What it does not do, of course, is say anything about the value of serum PSA measurement as a test for prostatic disease that is not otherwise detectable. While the test has been recommended by several national organizations for the early detection of prostatic cancer, serum PSA values are elevated in men with other prostatic disorders and there is no evidence for improved survival in men whose tumors were detected by screening serum PSA measurements.[3] Serum PSA measurements may have value as a tumor marker in men with proven prostatic cancer, but as a diagnostic test its time has not yet come.

R.D. Utiger, M.D.

References

1. Yuan JJ, Coplen DE, Petros JA, et al: Effects of rectal examination, prostatic massage, ultrasonography and needle biopsy on serum prostate specific antigen levels. *J Urol* 147:810–814, 1992.
2. Crawford ED, Schutz MJ, Clejan S, et al: The effect of digital rectal examination on prostate-specific antigen levels. *JAMA* 267:2227–2228, 1992.
3. Kramer BS, Brown ML, Prorok PC, et al: Prostate cancer screening: What we know and what we need to know. *Ann Intern Med* 119:914–923, 1993.

Prevalence and Duration of Hot Flashes After Surgical or Medical Castration in Men With Prostatic Carcinoma

Karling P, Hammar M, Varenhorst E (Univ of Health Sciences, Linköping, Sweden)

J Urol 152:1170–1173, 1994 119-96-52-3

Introduction.—Hot flashes are a natural occurrence in menopausal women, a result of declining serum estrogen concentrations. They also may occur in men with advanced prostatic cancer who undergo bilateral

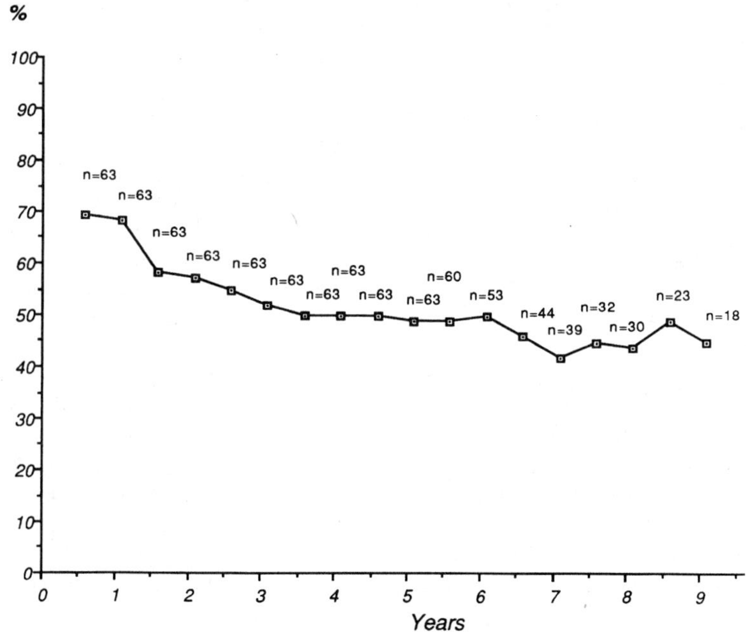

FIGURE p 1,171.—Prevalence of hot flashes among patients treated with surgical or pharmacologic castration in long-term perspective (1–9 years). (Courtesy of Karling P, Hammar M, Varenhorst E: Prevalence and duration of hot flushes after surgical or medical castration in men with prostatic carcinoma. *J Urol* 152:1170–1173, 1994.)

orchiectomy or "medical castration." In women, the flashes often cease 2–5 years after menopause, but whether they also resolve spontaneously in men is not clear.

Methods.—Seventy-seven men with prostatic cancer diagnosed 6–11 years earlier, who had either undergone bilateral orchiectomy or received gonadotropin-releasing hormone analogue therapy, were questioned about vasomotor symptoms. Sixty-three men, aged 65–91 years, completed the questionnaire. Fifty-three men had had orchiectomy as their only treatment.

Findings.—More than two thirds of the men (68%) reported having hot flashes, which continued for 5 years in 48% and for 8 years in 43% (Fig). More than a third of the men who were affected reported having 4 to 10 hot flashes a day. Most flashes began with a feeling of heat in the face. Thirteen men were bothered much or all of the time by their symptoms, in that they had to change clothes often, felt insecure when with others, and had problems sleeping.

Conclusions.—Most men rendered severely hypogonadal by surgery or medical treatment have hot flashes. The hot flashes tend to persist and may be very distressing. They should be treated at an early stage.

► The induction of androgen deficiency by either orchiectomy or gonadotropin-releasing hormone therapy is standard treatment for men with disseminated prostatic carcinoma. The major adverse consequences are impotence and hot flashes. I was surprised that so many of the men reported having had hot flashes and that they continued to have them for so many years. The accuracy of the men's memory for the sequelae of treatment 5 or more years earlier may be questioned, but very similar results were recently reported elsewhere.[1] These figures for the proportion of men affected and the frequency and persistence of hot flashes are very similar to those in postmenopausal women.[2] Hot flashes are much less common in men with spontaneously occurring hypogonadism, presumably because their androgen (and estrogen) deficiency develops more slowly and is rarely as severe.

Hot flashes are caused by sympathetic activation of hypothalamic thermoregulatory centers, which leads to peripheral vasodilatation, elevation in skin temperature, and perspiration. They may be ameliorated by estrogen, androgen (although I do not know whether they are ameliorated by androgens that, unlike testosterone, cannot be converted to estrogens), clonidine, and progestational steroids (see Abstract 119-96-52–4). For men with prostatic carcinoma who had an orchiectomy or who are receiving antiandrogen therapy, of course, only the latter 2 (and estrogen) are appropriate therapy.

R.D. Utiger, M.D.

References

1. Bucholz N-P, Mattarelli G, Bucholz M-MH: Post-orchiectomy hot flushes. *Eur Urol* 26:120–122, 1994.

2. Berg G, Gottwall T, Hammar M, et al: Climacteric symptoms among women aged 60–62 in Linkoping, Sweden, in 1986. *Maturitas* 10:193–199, 1988.

Megestrol Acetate for the Prevention of Hot Flashes

Loprinzi CL, Michalak JC, Quella SK, O'Fallon JR, Hatfield AK, Nelimark RA, Dose AM, Fischer T, Johnson C, Klatt NE, Bate WW, Rospond RM, Oesterling JE (Mayo Clinic and Mayo Found, Rochester, Minn; Siouxland Hematology Oncology Assocs, Sioux City; Carle Cancer Ctr Community Clinical Oncology Program, Urbana, Ill; et al)

N Engl J Med 331:347–352, 1994 119-96-52–4

Objective.—Because estrogen replacement therapy may stimulate the growth of breast cancer, the effectiveness of low-dose megestrol acetate in eliminating hot flashes and its safety were examined in 97 women with a history of breast cancer who had had hot flashes at least 7 times per week for 1 month or longer. Sixty-six men with prostatic cancer who had received androgen deprivation treatment (surgical or medical orchiectomy) and had hot flashes also were studied.

Treatment.—After 1 week of observation, the patients received either megestrol acetate in a dose of 20 mg twice daily or placebo for 4 weeks, followed by a 4-week crossover. Treatment was given on a double-blind basis. The patients kept a record of their symptoms.

Results.—Treatment with megestrol acetate significantly reduced the frequency of hot flashes in both men and women (Table 2). In general, 2–3 weeks of megestrol therapy were needed to achieve the maximal effect. About one third of women had vaginal bleeding while receiving megestrol acetate. There was no indication that appetite was stimulated by 4 weeks of treatment.

TABLE 2.—Frequency and Severity of Hot Flashes During the Fourth Week of the First Treatment Period

	Megestrol Acetate	Placebo	*P* Value
	% of baseline daily average		
Frequency of hot flashes (median)			
Women (n = 80)	26	73	< 0.001
Men (n = 60)	20	81	< 0.001
Both (n = 140)	23	79	< 0.001
Hot-flash score (median)			
Women (n = 80)	17	73	< 0.001
Men (n = 60)	13	84	< 0.001
Both (n = 140)	15	79	< 0.001

Conclusion.—Megestrol acetate markedly reduces the frequency of hot flashes in women who have had breast cancer and men receiving androgen deprivation therapy for prostatic cancer.

▶ This study documents that progestational steroids are effective treatment for hot flashes in both women and men. In women, the obvious first choice is estrogen, but for some women, notably those with carcinoma of the breast, estrogen is generally thought to be contraindicated (a view recently challenged[1]). In men who have metastatic prostatic carcinoma treated to make them hypogonadal, in whom hot flashes are common (see Abstract 119-96-52–3), megestrol acetate is probably the first choice; one alternative is clonidine, which has more side effects. Megestrol acetate did not eliminate hot flashes in these patients (Table 2), and a higher dose has proven more effective.[2]

Megestrol acetate (Megace) has other actions, some of which are beneficial. It has antitumor effects in women with carcinoma of the breast and endometrium. In patients with wasting disorders, notably cancer and AIDS, larger doses, 80–240 mg/day, stimulate appetite and cause weight gain—mostly an increase in body fat.[3, 4] These latter effects *may* be due to its glucocorticoid properties. In a study of 4 patients with AIDS, a dose of 240 mg/day inhibited corticotropin and cortisol secretion substantially (mean 8 AM plasma cortisol concentration, 11.0 µg/dL [303 nmol/L] before and 1.5 µg/dL [41 nmol/L] after 1 month).[5] One patient who had symptoms of adrenal insufficiency and low plasma corticotropin and cortisol concentrations after discontinuation of this dose was described in the same report. (I think even lower doses will inhibit pituitary-adrenal function; I recently saw a man with AIDS taking 80 mg/day who had a very low basal plasma cortisol concentration that increased only modestly to 11 µg/dL [303 nmol/L] after corticotropin stimulation). Also, overt Cushing's syndrome was reported in a woman with endometrial carcinoma taking higher doses.[6]

R.D. Utiger, M.D.

References

1. Cobleigh MA, Berris RF, Bush T, et al: Estrogen replacement therapy in breast cancer survivors: A time for change. *JAMA* 272:540–545, 1994.
2. Erlik Y, Meldrum DR, Lagasse LD, et al: Effect of megestrol acetate on flushing and bone metabolism in post-menopausal women. *Maturitas* 3:167–172, 1981.
3. Von Roenn JH, Armstrong D, Kotler DP, et al: Megestrol acetate in patients with AIDS-related cachexia. *Ann Intern Med* 121:393–399, 1984.
4. Oster MH, Enders SR, Samuels SJ, et al: Megestrol acetate in patients with AIDS and cachexia. *Ann Intern Med* 121:400–408, 1994.
5. Leinung MC, Liporace R, Miller CH: Induction of adrenal suppression by megestrol acetate in patients with AIDS. *Ann Intern Med* 122:843–845, 1995.
6. Steer KA, Kurtz AS, Honour JW: Megestrol-induced Cushing's syndrome. *Clin Endocrinol* 42:91–93, 1995.

Circulating Hormone Levels in Menopausal Women Receiving Different Hormone Replacement Therapy Regimens: A Comparison

Castelo-Branco C, Martínez de Osaba M, Fortuny A, Iglesias X, González-Merlo J (Univ of Barcelona, Spain)

J Reprod Med 40:556–560, 1995 119-96-52–5

Objective.—A study was conducted to compare plasma concentrations of sex hormones in menopausal women after the administration of different hormone replacement therapy regimens.

Treatment.—Ninety women aged 43–57 years, 1–3 years postmenopausal, were studied in a randomized, comparative study; 85 completed one year of follow-up. Fifteen women received conjugated equine estrogen (CEE), 0.6 mg/day, cyclically; 17 received transdermal estradiol (E_2), 50 µg/day, cyclically; and 17 received CEE, 0.6 mg/day, continuously; all these women also received 2.5 mg of medroxyprogesterone acetate (MPA) for the last 12 days of each cycle. A fourth group of 19 women received CEE, 0.625 mg/day, and MPA, 2.5 mg/day, continuously. Twenty-two women served as treatment-free control subjects. Plasma hormone concentrations were measured before and during the 6th and 12th months of hormone replacement therapy, between days 21 and 24 of estrogen administration. Endometrial biopsy was performed between 5 and 7 days after the addition of the progestin.

Results.—During hormone replacement therapy, plasma follicle-stimulating hormone (FSH), luteinizing hormone (LH), and prolactin (PRL) concentrations decreased; estradiol (E_2), estrone (E_1), and sex hormone–binding globulin (SHBG) concentrations increased; and testosterone (T), androstenedione (A_4), and dehydroepiandrosterone sulfate (DHEAS) concentrations did not change. There were no significant differences between treatment groups in plasma FSH, LH, PRL, E_2, T, A_4, or DHEAS values, whereas E_1 and SHBG values were higher in the women who received oral than those who received transdermal hormone replacement therapy. None of the regimens lowered plasma FSH and LH concentrations to within the range found in normal premenopausal women. Endometrial biopsies showed that only continuous estrogen/progesterone administration effectively protected the endometrium from hyperplastic changes.

Conclusions.—In postmenopausal women, usual doses of estrogen reduce plasma gonadotropin concentrations modestly, and also lower (unexpectedly) plasma prolactin concentrations. Although MPA dosage was not the focus of this study, MPA, 2.5 mg/day, was inadequate to prevent endometrial hyperplasia unless given continuously.

► Increasing numbers of postmenopausal women are receiving estrogen replacement therapy, not only to treat menopausal symptoms but also to prevent cardiovascular disease and osteoporosis. Furthermore, although the number of regimens being used has increased, there is little information about their comparative effects. The 4 regimens used in this study are probably the most popular, with the trend in the past few years being toward continuous administration of both estrogen and progesterone. The advantage of continuous therapy is that there is no cyclic vaginal bleeding, although about 40% of women have some irregular breakthrough bleeding during the first several months of treatment. The dose of progesterone (nearly always given as medroxyprogesterone, as in this study) needed to prevent endometrial hyperplasia is lower (2.5 mg daily) when it is given continuously than when it is given intermittently (5 mg/day). Continuous progestin administration does not interfere with the beneficial effects of estrogen on serum cholesterol concentrations, and it may enhance the effect of estrogen on bone.[1]

The results of this study indicate that these several regimens have very similar effects on plasma estrogen and gonadotropin concentrations. Although the plasma estrone and estradiol concentrations during treatment were similar to those in young women, plasma gonadotropin concentrations decreased very little (5% to 15%). At least in the case of follicle-stimulating hormone, the lack of substantial decrease is probably because of the absence of ovarian inhibin. Nothing is said about efficacy with respect to amelioration of menopausal symptoms, but no differences would be expected.

R.D. Utiger, M.D.

Reference

1. Munk-Jensen N, Nielsen SP, Obel EB, et al: Reversal of postmenopausal vertebral bone loss by oestrogen and progestogen: A double blind placebo controlled study. *BMJ* 296:1151–1152, 1988.

The Use of Estrogens and Progestins and the Risk of Breast Cancer in Postmenopausal Women

Colditz GA, Hankinson SE, Hunter DJ, Willett WC, Manson JE, Stampfer MJ, Hennekens C, Rosner B, Speizer FE (Brigham and Women's Hosp, Boston; Harvard Med School, Boston; Harvard School Public Health, Boston)

N Engl J Med 332:1589–1593, 1995 119-96-52–6

Background.—Although several studies and meta-analyses have examined the relationship between postmenopausal estrogen therapy and risk of breast cancer, the findings have been inconclusive. Particularly in question is the effect of combining a progestin with estrogen therapy and the influence of age on the risk. These questions were examined in analysis of 1992 data from the Nurses' Health Study.

Methods.—The Nurses' Health Study, established in 1976, collected prospective data periodically on known or suspected risk factors for cardiovascular disease and cancer. Data from the 1992 follow-up questionnaire were examined with regard to the diagnosis of breast cancer and postmenopausal hormone therapy, and the association was analyzed. There were 1,935 cases of breast cancer during 725,550 person-years of follow-up, and 69,586 women were postmenopausal in 1990.

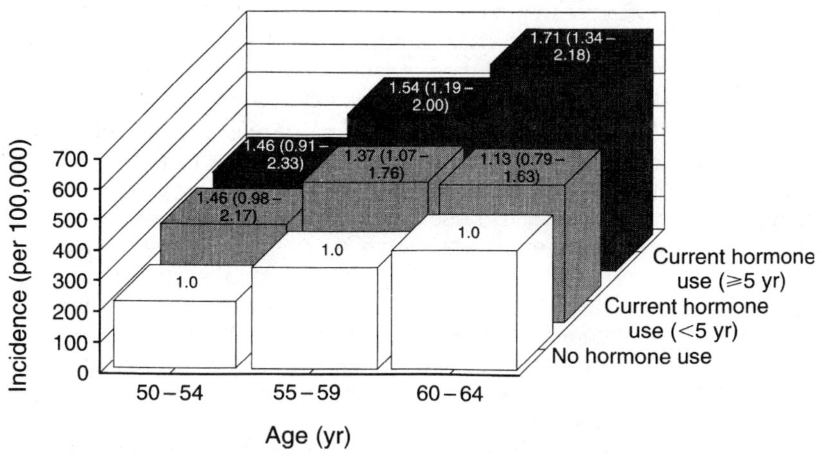

FIGURE 1.—Incidence and relative risk of breast cancer according to age and the duration of current postmenopausal hormone therapy. Relative risks and 95% confidence intervals are shown on the top of the bars; relative risks are expressed in comparison with the risk among women in each age group who never received hormone therapy. Data have been adjusted for age at menopause, type of menopause, and family history of breast cancer in a proportional hazards analysis. (Reprinted by permission of *The New England Journal of Medicine.* Colditz GA, Hankinson SE, Hunter DJ, et al: The use of estrogens and progestins and the risk of breast cancer in postmenopausal women. *N Engl J Med* 332:1589–1593, 1995.)

Results.—Between 1978 and 1992, the relative risk of breast cancer rose to 1.32 among women treated with estrogen alone, 1.41 among women treated with estrogen plus progestin, and 2.24 among women treated with progestin alone, as compared with women who had never received either treatment. There were no significant differences in relative risk of breast cancer between the 3 groups. The risk of breast cancer also increased with age. After adjustment for age, risk increased significantly only among women who had received hormone therapy for 5 years or more (Fig 1).

Conclusions.—The risk of breast cancer is increased among postmenopausal women currently treated with estrogen alone or estrogen and progestin in combination. Therefore, the addition of progestin does not reduce the risk of breast cancer associated with estrogen treatment, suggesting that ductal cells in the breast do not respond to progestin in the same way as does the endometrium, where progestin has a protective effect. Postmenopausal hormone therapy may be a particularly strong risk factor with advancing age.

► This report adds substantially to the already voluminous literature concerning whether the risk of breast cancer is increased in postmenopausal women who take estrogen replacement therapy. The strengths of the study include the large number of case and control women, the repeated questioning of the women (undoubtedly a highly motivated group), and the meticulous documentation of the tumors. The key findings are the similar, albeit small, increase in risk among women taking estrogen alone and those taking estrogen and progestin, and the increased risk in older women who had taken estrogen for many years. These results both support and conflict with those of approximately 40 previous cohort or case-control studies, and they conflict with those of a case-control study from northwestern Washington State, published a month later, that evaluated 537 women with breast cancer.[1] The results of several meta-analyses suggest there is little or no risk among women taking moderate doses of estrogen for less than 8 or 10 years, but there is a small risk (relative risk, rarely greater than 1.5) when therapy is prolonged or the dose is higher.[2, 3]

One reason not to dismiss these small risks is that they have biological plausibility. Among women treated with estrogen, the risk is dose- and time-dependent. Women who have greater lifelong estrogen production (e.g., women who have early menarche and late menopause, and obese postmenopausal women) have an increased risk of breast cancer. Another reason not to dismiss these risks is that women are now being advised to take estrogen for many years, even throughout their life, so as not to lose the skeletal and perhaps cardiovascular benefits of estrogen.

A component part of the recently launched Women's Health Study is a prospective randomized trial of cyclic estrogen-progestin therapy in postmenopausal women; in time, it will provide more information about all the effects of this treatment. However, methods of estrogen-progestin therapy are changing, and this fact may alter both the risk of breast cancer and the beneficial effects of estrogen. More women now receive transdermal estrogen, and continuous estrogen-progestin therapy is becoming the norm. These differences could change the risk of breast cancer in either direction. Furthermore, new synthetic progestins and estrogens are being developed, e.g., estrogens with more skeletal and fewer uterine and mammary effects than naturally occurring estrogen.

I do not believe that the possible small risk of breast cancer outweighs the benefits of estrogen-progestin therapy in postmenopausal women or estrogen therapy alone in women who have had a hysterectomy. However, the problem should be mentioned in any discussion of estrogen therapy, and no doubt some women will prefer not to be treated because of this risk.

R.D. Utiger, M.D.

References

1. Stanford JL, Weiss NS, Voigt LF, et al: Combined estrogen and progestin hormone replacement therapy in relation to risk of breast cancer in middle-aged women. *JAMA* 274:137–142, 1995.
2. Dupont WD, Page DL: Menopausal estrogen replacement therapy and breast cancer. *Arch Intern Med* 151:67–72, 1991. (1992 Year Book of Medicine, pp 505–506.)
3. Colditz GA, Egan KM, Stampfer MJ: Hormone replacement therapy and the risk of breast cancer: Results from epidemiologic studies. *Am J Obstet Gynecol* 168:1473–1480, 1993.

Fluoxetine in the Treatment of Premenstrual Dysphoria

Steiner M, for the Canadian Fluoxetine/Premenstrual Dysphoria Collaborative Study Group (McMaster Univ, Hamilton, Ont, Canada; Univ of Toronto, Canada; Univ of British Columbia, Vancouver; et al)

N Engl J Med 332:1529–1534, 1995 119-96-52–7

Objective.—Premenstrual dysphoria, which affects 3% to 8% of North American women, results in tension, irritability, and dysphoria and has negative health consequences. Although the disorder has characteristics similar to depression and anxiety states that are known to result from serotonergic dysfunction, no satisfactory treatment for premenstrual dysphoria has been found. The results of a multicenter, double-blind, placebo-controlled study to assess the efficacy and safety of fluoxetine, a serotonergic drug, in women with premenstrual dysphoria are presented.

Methods.—After a 2-cycle washout period, 313 women, aged 20 to 45 years, received either placebo, 20 mg/day of fluoxetine, or 60 mg/day of fluoxetine for 6 menstrual cycles. Late luteal-phase visual analogue-scale (0 to 100 mm) scores for tension, irritability, and dysphoria were measured during each cycle.

Results.—A total of 180 women completed the study, and 277 women were included in the efficacy study. Women receiving either 20 or 60 mg/day of fluoxetine had a significant reduction in symptoms, as compared with placebo (Fig 1). Marked improvement, defined as a 75% improvement in symptoms, occurred in 32% of the cycles in which the women

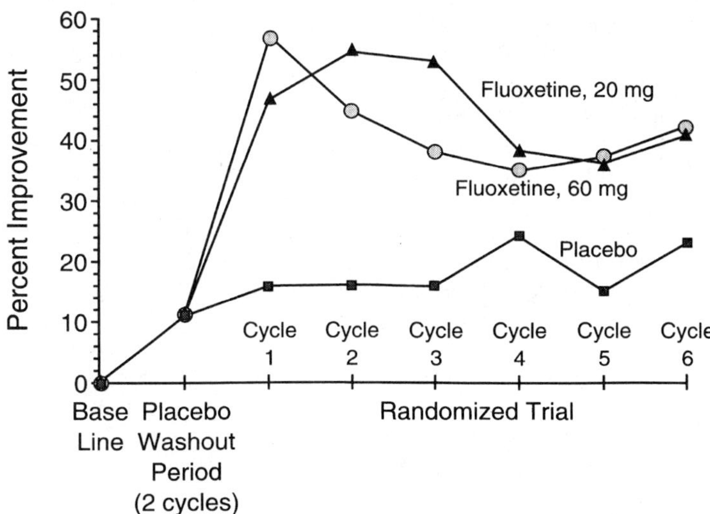

FIGURE 1.—Percent improvement in the total luteal-phase scores of the visual analogue scale for the 180 women who completed the protocol ($P < 0.001$). The degree of improvement recorded during the placebo washout period did not differ between groups (mean improvement, 11.2%). (Reprinted by permission of *The New England Journal of Medicine*. Steiner M, for the Canadian Fluoxetine/Premenstrual Dysphoria Collaborative Study Group: Fluoxetine in the treatment of premenstrual dysphoria. *N Engl J Med* 332:1529–1534, 1995. Copyright 1995, Massachusetts Medical Society.)

received fluoxetine but only 14% of cycles involving placebo. The women in the 60-mg fluoxetine group had more side effects, including insomnia, nausea, fatigue or lethargy, and anorexia, and 33% dropped out of the study because of side effects. The total dropout rate for all causes (side effects, lack of efficacy, other reasons) was 42%. When the medication was discontinued, symptoms returned.

Conclusion.—Fluoxetine at a dose of 20 mg/day may be useful in treatment premenstrual dysphoria.

► Premenstrual dysphoria (formerly called premenstrual syndrome and late luteal phase dysphoric disorder) is a symptom complex of psychological or behavioral symptoms, such as irritability, dysphoria, tension, anxiety, insomnia and headache, sufficient to interfere with daily activities and interpersonal relationships during the luteal phase of the menstrual cycle. It is the timing and periodicity of the symptoms, not the symptoms per se, that define the syndrome. That the symptoms are related in some way to cyclic pituitary-gonadal function is clear, because they are largely abolished by oophorectomy, whether done surgically or by treatment with a gonadotropin-releasing hormone agonist drug. However, women with this syndrome have no abnormalities in pituitary-gonadal function during their cycles, and induction of luteolysis and menses very soon after ovulation does not prevent the appearance of the symptoms at the expected time. Postovulatory surges in estrogen and progesterone secretion, even if for only a few days, seem to be necessary but are not sufficient for the disorder. Many of these women also have somatic symptoms, such as anorexia, changes in appetite, bloating, edema, and breast engorgement, but these alone occur in many other women and are not an integral part of the syndrome.

The results of this study suggest a beneficial effect of fluoxetine, but one wonders about the generalizability of the results. The women were very carefully selected, in that they had symptoms sufficiently severe to impair their activities for at least 1 year and then for 2 more months after entering the study. The dropout rates in all 3 groups were about 40%, mostly due to a lack of efficacy in the placebo group and side effects in the fluoxetine groups. The results shown in Figure 1 are the mean of the scores for tension, irritability, and dysphoria. Note that the improvement in late luteal phase symptoms was prompt, but there was no further improvement with time. Note also that these results are from only the 180 women who completed the 6-cycle trial; from the actual scores given in a table in the original article, the symptoms disappeared in few women. Nevertheless, there was substantial improvement in these three symptoms during many cycles, and the results of scoring of other symptoms were similar. The lower dose of fluoxetine was the better dose, having fewer side effects and as much efficacy as the larger dose.

It seems reasonable to treat women whose lives are disrupted by this disorder, but the decision is theirs; whether less severely affected women should be treated is not clear. How to treat is another question. Treatment with fluoxetine only during the luteal phase might be as effective as continuous therapy, and there is a report of efficacy of a single dose given during the early luteal phase.[1] Alprazolam also was found to be beneficial in a recent study,[2] although the change in symptom scores seems to have been less than occurred in this study of fluoxetine. What will prove most effective is not known, but at least effective, albeit incompletely effective, therapy for this disorder is now available.

R.D. Utiger, M.D.

References

1. Daamen MJ, Brown WA: Single-dose fluoxetine in management of premenstrual syndrome. *J Clin Psychiatry* 53:210–211, 1992.
2. Freeman EW, Rickels K, Sondheimer SJ, et al: A double-blind trial of oral progesterone, alprazolam, and placebo in treatment of severe premenstrual syndrome. *JAMA* 274:51–57, 1995.

53 Carbohydrate Metabolism and Diabetes Mellitus

Efficacy of Metformin in Patients With Non-Insulin-Dependent Diabetes Mellitus

DeFronzo RA, Goodman AM, and the Multicenter Metformin Study Group
(Univ of Texas, San Antonio; Lipha Pharmaceuticals, New York)
N Engl J Med 333:541–549, 1995 119-96-53–1

Purpose.—Until early 1995, sulfonylurea drugs were the only oral therapy available for patients with non–insulin-dependent diabetes mellitus (NIDDM) in the United States. At that time, metformin was approved for use in the treatment of NIDDM. Two randomized, placebo-controlled studies were performed to assess the results of metformin treatment in moderately obese patients with NIDDM whose disease was poorly controlled with diet alone or diet plus a sulfonylurea drug.

Methods.—Both studies evaluated the effects of 29 weeks of metformin treatment. In protocol 1, 289 patients whose diabetes was poorly controlled by diet alone were assigned to either metformin or placebo. In protocol 2, 632 patients whose diabetes was poorly controlled by diet plus glyburide were assigned to receive metformin, glyburide, or both. Efficacy was assessed by measurements of plasma glucose, both while the patients were fasting and after oral glucose administration; plasma lactate, lipid, and insulin concentrations; and glycosylated hemoglobin.

Results.—In protocol 1, the mean fasting plasma glucose concentration at the end of the study was 189 mg/dL (10.6 mmol/L) in the metformin group and 244 mg/dL (13.7 mmol/L) in the placebo group, and the respective glycosylated hemoglobin values were 7.1% and 8.6%. In protocol 2, mean fasting plasma glucose concentration was 187 mg/dL (10.5 mmol/L) in the metformin plus glyburide group, as compared with 261 mg/dL (14.6 mmol/L) in the glyburide-only group (Fig 2); the respective glycosylated hemoglobin values were 7.1% and 8.7%. The results in the metformin-only group were similar to those of the glyburide-only group. Symptoms consistent with hypoglycemia occurred in 18% of patients

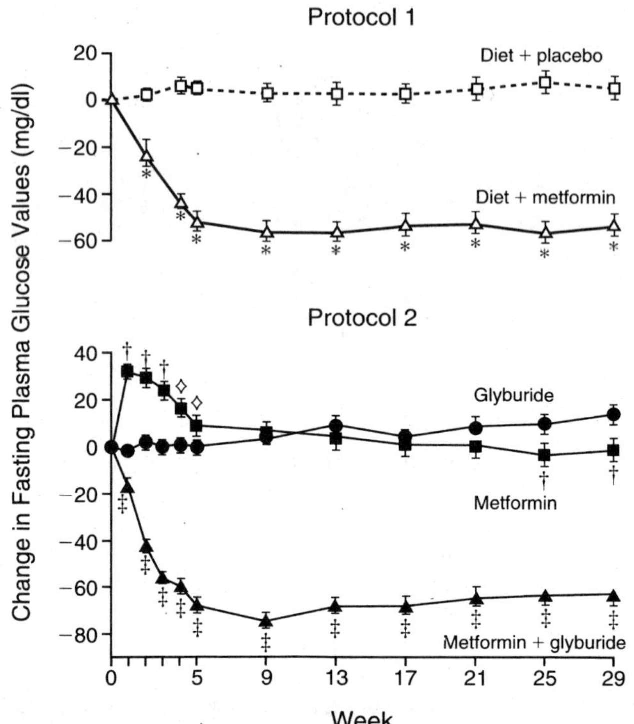

FIGURE 2.—Mean (± SE) changes in fasting plasma glucose concentrations in patients with non–insulin-dependent diabetes mellitus who were enrolled in protocol 1 or 2. The *asterisks* indicate significant differences ($P < 0.001$) between the groups in protocol 1; the *daggers*, significant differences ($P < 0.001$) between the metformin and glyburide groups; the *diamonds*, significant differences ($P < 0.01$) between the metformin and glyburide groups; and the *double daggers*, significant differences between the combination-therapy and glyburide groups. To convert values for glucose to millimoles per liter, multiply by 0.056. (Reprinted by permisison of *The New England Journal of Medicine*. DeFronzo RA, Goodman AM, and the Multicenter Metformin Study Group: Efficacy of metformin in patients with non-insulin-dependent diabetes mellitus. *N Engl J Med* 333:541–549, 1995. Copyright 1995, Massachusetts Medical Society.)

receiving metformin and glyburide, as compared with 3% of those in the glyburide-only group and 2% of those in the metformin-only group.

The patients in both protocols who received metformin had significant declines in plasma total and low-density lipoprotein cholesterol and triglyceride concentrations. None of the treatments was associated with a significant change in fasting plasma lactate concentration.

Conclusions.—For patients with NIDDM whose disease is poorly controlled with diet or sulfonylurea therapy, metformin, given alone or combined with a sulfonylurea drug, is well tolerated and can improve not only glycemic control but also plasma lipid concentrations.

► The 2 studies described in this paper indicate the efficacy and safety of metformin in patients with NIDDM, either as sole therapy in patients unresponsive to diet or combined with glyburide in patients who are unresponsive to the latter (all initially had fasting plasma glucose values greater than 140 mg/dL [7.8 mmol/L], but patients with symptomatic hyperglycemia were excluded). While the baseline fasting and postprandial plasma glucose concentrations and the glycosylated hemoglobin values were slightly higher in the patients already receiving glyburide, the declines in fasting (and postprandial) plasma glucose concentrations and glycosylated hemoglobin values were substantial and similar in magnitude in both studies.

The maximal dose of metformin allowed was 2,550 mg (three 850-mg tablets), and about 85% of patients were taking this dose at the end of the study. The major side effects of metformin were nausea and diarrhea. Anorexia and weight loss, often mentioned in earlier studies of metformin, were not prominent. In fact, anorexia was not listed among the side effects of metformin, and weight loss in the metformin groups varied from 0.3 to 3.8 kg. Metformin alone does not cause hypoglycemia, because it acts primarily by inhibiting hepatic glucose output;[1] as plasma glucose concentrations decline, so does insulin secretion. The occurrence of symptoms of hypoglycemia in 18% of the patients treated with metformin and glyburide might argue against wide use of the combination, but hypoglycemia was never documented. A curious finding was a 20% to 30% decrease in serum vitamin B_{12} concentrations in the metformin-treated patients, probably caused by interference with absorption of vitamin B_{12}-intrinsic factor complexes. No patient became anemic during the 29-week study, and in Europe and Canada, where metformin has been available for years, megaloblastic anemia in metformin-treated patients is very rare. Detailed studies of lactate metabolism during metformin therapy in small numbers of patients have revealed no abnormalities in plasma lactate concentrations and lactate turnover,[1] but the drug can cause lactic acidosis. The incidence seems to be about 4 cases per 100,000 patient-years, about 5% of that of its long-withdrawn predecessor phenformin. It nearly always occurs in patients with renal, cardiovascular, or hepatic disease, and no one with any of these diseases should be given metformin.

Metformin is available as 500-mg tablets, with recommendations that the initial dose be 500 mg given twice daily with meals and that the maximal dose not exceed 2,500 mg. Who should receive it? The most obvious candidates are patients with NIDDM being treated with a sulfonylurea drug who are poorly controlled[2] in whom addition of or change to insulin has been the alternative until now. With respect to patients with newly diagnosed or diet-resistant NIDDM, metformin may be as appropriate as a sulfonylurea drug, and it is probably the treatment of choice for more obese patients and those who have high plasma lipid concentrations. It has also been effective in improving glycemic control and plasma lipid concentrations in insulin-treated patients with NIDDM.[3]

R.D. Utiger, M.D.

References

1. Stumvoll M, Nurjhan N, Perriello G, et al: Metabolic effects of metformin in non–insulin-dependent diabetes mellitus. *N Engl J Med* 333:550–554, 1995.
2. Crofford OB: Metformin. *N Engl J Med* 333:588–589, 1995.
3. Giugliano D, Quatraro A, Consoli G, et al: Metformin for obese, insulin-treated diabetic patients: Improvement in glycaemic control and reduction in metabolic risk factors. *Eur J Clin Pharmacol* 44:107–112, 1993. (1994 YEAR BOOK OF MEDICINE, pp 638–639.)

The Efficacy of Acarbose in the Treatment of Patients With Non–Insulin-Dependent Diabetes Mellitus: A Multicenter Controlled Clinical Trial

Chiasson J-L, Josse RG, Hunt JA, Palmason C, Rodger NW, Ross SA, Ryan EA, Tan MH, Wolever TMS (Centre de Recherche/Hôtel Dieu de Montréal, Canada; Univ of Toronto, Ont, Canada; Vexco Labs Inc, Calgary, Alberta, Canada; et al)

Ann Intern Med 121:928–935, 1994 119-96-53–2

Background.—Acarbose, an α-glucosidase inhibitor, has been proposed as an alternative for the treatment of postprandial hyperglycemia in patients with non–insulin-dependent diabetes mellitus (NIDDM). The long-term efficacy of this agent was evaluated in 354 patients.

Patients and Methods.—Of the 354 patients enrolled, 77 were being treated with diet alone, 83 with diet and metformin, 103 with diet and sulfonylurea, and 91 with diet and insulin. The demographic characteristics of the groups were similar, except that the duration of diabetes was longer in the insulin-treated patients. Patients in each treatment group were randomly assigned to receive acarbose or placebo for 12 months. The initial dose was 50 mg at the start of each meal, and it was increased to 100 mg and then 200 mg unless the postprandial plasma glucose concentration was less than 180 mg/dL (10 mmol/L). The final dose was 100 mg three times daily in 60% of patients. Hemoglobin A_{1c} (HbA_{1c}) (Fig 3), fasting and postprandial (60, 90, and 120 min) plasma glucose, fasting and postprandial serum C-peptide, and fasting serum lipids were measured at baseline and at 3-month intervals thereafter.

Results.—A total of 316 patients were included in the final analysis (87% of the treatment and 92% of the placebo groups). The mean postprandial plasma glucose peak decreased in all 4 groups during acarbose treatment. As compared with the placebo group, the incremental areas under the curve of the postprandial plasma glucose concentrations in the acarbose groups were lower by 84 mg·h/dL (4.7 mmol·h/L) in the diet-only group, 38 mg·h/dL (2.1 mmol·h/L) in the metformin group, 46 mg·h/dL (2.6 mmol·h/L) in the sulfonylurea group, and 55 mg·h/dL (3.1 mmol·h/L) in the insulin group. The corresponding decreases in HbA_{1c} were 0.9% in the diet-only group, 0.8% in the metformin group, 0.9% in the sulfonylurea group, and 0.4% in the insulin group. The mean serum C-peptide

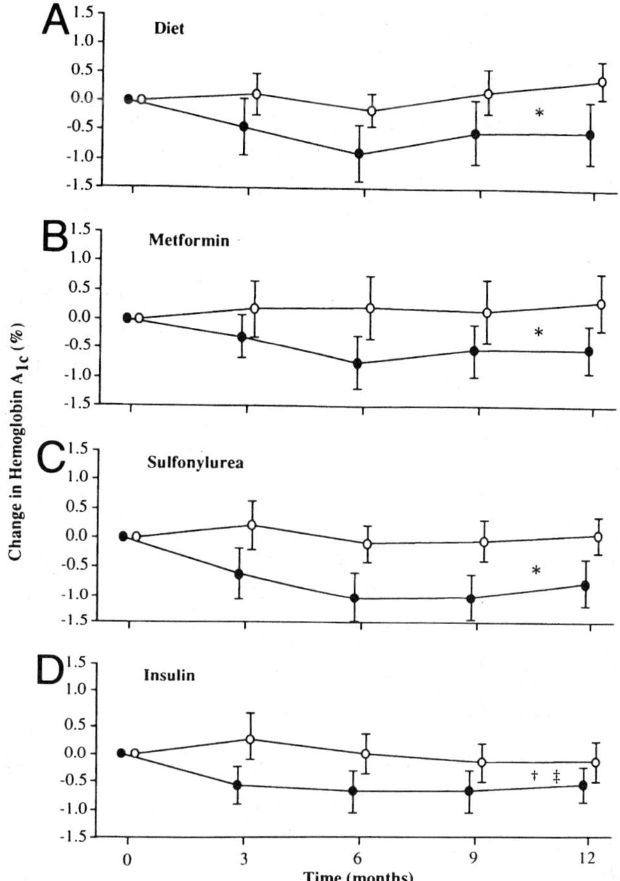

FIGURE 3.—The effects of acarbose (*filled circle*) and placebo (*open circle*) on hemoglobin A_{1c} levels throughout the 1-year study in groups of patients treated with diet alone (**A**), metformin (**B**), sulfonylurea (**C**), and insulin (**D**). Data are expressed as means with 95% confidence intervals. $*P \leq 0.010$, $\dagger P = 0.077$. The *P* values are for differences between changes from baseline (time 0) to end point (time 12 months) for acarbose and placebo. $\ddagger P = 0.01$ by covariance analysis. (Courtesy of Chiasson J-L, Josse RG, Hunt JA, et al: The efficacy of acarbose in the treatment of patients with non–insulin-dependent diabetes mellitus: A multicenter controlled clinical trial. *Ann Intern Med* 121:928–935, 1994.)

and serum lipid concentrations did not change during acarbose treatment. The dropout rates were 27% in the acarbose groups and 23% in the placebo group.

Conclusions.—Overall, 52% of the patients treated with acarbose responded to treatment, as compared with 26% of the placebo recipients. If dropouts were considered failures, 40% of the patients receiving acarbose and 18% of those receiving placebo responded. Acarbose thus provided improved long-term glycemic control in patients with NIDDM, regardless of concurrent antidiabetic treatment.

▶ Acarbose is another relatively new treatment for patients with NIDDM. It acts by inhibiting intestinal glucosidase activity, so that formation of monosaccharides from complex carbohydrates is diminished. When taken before eating, it minimizes the postmeal rises in blood glucose concentrations; however, it has little effect on fasting concentrations and does not impair the absorption of glucose itself.[1] This contrasts with the actions of other drugs (and insulin) used to treat diabetes, which affect fasting glucose concentrations as much as or more than postprandial glucose concentrations. Acarbose is equally effective in insulin-treated patients. The effect of acarbose on glycosylated hemoglobin values (Fig 3) is almost as great as that of metformin (see Abstract 119-96-53–1), but it has no effect on serum lipid concentrations.

Looked at in terms of individual patient responsiveness, 52% of the patients who received acarbose and 26% of those who received placebo had reductions in glycosylated hemoglobin of at least 15% or a value below 7.0% (or both). The acarbose-treated patients did not lose weight. Most completed the 1-year study, but the incidence of side effects, primarily flatulence, diarrhea, and abdominal cramps and discomfort, was high, and nonstudy patients might not be so willing to continue it.

I do not know which patients with NIDDM will benefit from acarbose, nor do I know how well it will be tolerated in practice, but it offers another option short of switching to insulin. Patients who may benefit include those who do not adequately respond to diet or to a sulfonylurea drug or metformin. So, too, might patients who are already taking maximal doses of both a sulfonylurea and metformin, and it could obviate the need for supplemental short-acting insulin before meals in patients treated with intermediate-acting insulin.

R.D. Utiger, M.D.

Reference

1. Hotta N, Kakuta H, Sano T, et al: Long-term effect of acarbose on glycemic control in non–insulin-dependent diabetes mellitus: A placebo-controlled double-blind study. *Diabetic Med* 10:134–138, 1993. (1994 YEAR BOOK OF MEDICINE, pp 640–641.)

United Kingdom Prospective Diabetes Study (UKPDS) 13: Relative Efficacy of Randomly Allocated Diet, Sulphonylurea, Insulin, or Metformin in Patients With Newly Diagnosed Non-Insulin Dependent Diabetes Followed for Three Years

United Kingdom Prospective Diabetes Study Group (Radcliffe Infirmary, Oxford, England)

BMJ 310:83–88, 1995 119-96-53-3

Background.—The United Kingdom Prospective Diabetes Study is an intervention trial that began in 1977 to investigate the ability of improved glycemic control in patients with non–insulin-dependent diabetes mellitus (NIDDM) to prevent diabetic complications and to determine whether any specific drug is more effective than treatment with diet alone. The relative efficacy of various treatments for NIDDM more than 3 years after diagnosis was evaluated in a multicenter, prospective, randomized, controlled study.

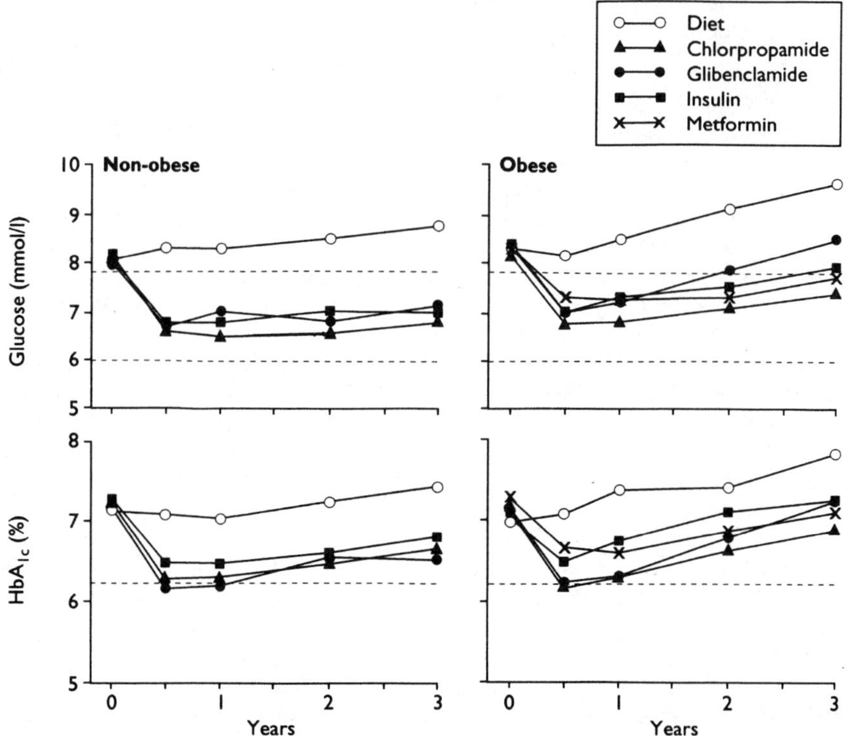

FIGURE 1.—Changes in median fasting plasma glucose and mean glycated hemoglobin concentrations in nonobese and obese research subjects, according to randomization group. (The *horizontal dashed lines* in the upper panels indicate 6.0 and 7.8 mmol/L and the *lower panels*, 6.2%). (Courtesy of the United Kingdom Prospective Diabetes Study Group: United Kingdom Prospective Diabetes Study (UKPDS) 13: Relative efficacy of randomly allocated diet, sulphonylurea, insulin, or metformin in patients with newly diagnosed non-insulin dependent diabetes followed for three years. *BMJ* 310:83–88, 1995.)

Methods.—The study subjects were 2,520 patients (mean age, 52 years), about half of whom were obese and half of whom were women, with newly diagnosed NIDDM. They were randomly assigned to treatment with diet alone or to treatment with diet and chlorpropamide, glyburide, insulin, or metformin, with the goal being to lower fasting plasma glucose concentrations to 6 mmol/L (108 mg/dL) or less.

Results.—At 3 years, the median fasting plasma glucose concentrations were significantly lower in patients receiving chlorpropamide, glyburide, or insulin as compared with those treated with diet alone (Fig 1); their mean glycated hemoglobin values were also lower. In patients treated with chlorpropamide, glyburide, or insulin, mean body weight increased significantly, but it did not increase in patients treated with diet alone. In the patients who were obese, metformin was as effective as the other drugs but mean body weight did not change. There were more episodes of hypoglycemia in the patients treated with a sulfonylurea drug or insulin than in those treated with diet or metformin.

Discussion.—The efficacy of the different drugs and insulin was similar in these patients with NIDDM, but most patients continued to have hyperglycemia.

► This ongoing study of patients with NIDDM was designed to determine the effect of different treatments not only on hyperglycemia but also eventually on diabetic complications. The study groups were well-matched, and the patients seem representative of patients with NIDDM who have moderate hyperglycemia and no complications of diabetes, except that only half were obese (more than 120% ideal body weight). About half had hypertension, but nothing is said about antihypertensive therapy, which can affect insulin secretion and sensitivity, except that thiazides were avoided.

It is evident from Figure 1 that the initial (1-year) response to therapy in the drug- and insulin-treatment groups was modest, with the fasting plasma glucose concentration falling about 1.6 mmol/L (30 mg/dL) and the glycosylated hemoglobin value falling about 1%; also, the improvement was not sustained, especially in the obese patients. From 74% to 79% of the patients in the diet and drug groups and 60% of the patients in the insulin group were still taking the assigned therapy after 3 years. The results in Figure 1 are those from an intention-to-treat analysis, but the changes were only slightly greater in those patients who received their assigned therapy for all 3 years. The tendency of fasting plasma glucose and glycosylated hemoglobin values to rise with time results from weight gain, the well-known decrease in action of sulfonylurea drugs, and probably also the natural tendency of NIDDM to worsen with time.[1] The percentage of patients having self-reported episodes of hypoglycemia in which they needed help by another person was less than 1.5% in all groups, not surprisingly being lowest in the diet and metformin groups.

The insulin and drug regimens clearly were more effective than diet, as would be expected. The treatments cannot be said to have had symptomatic benefit, because the patients had no symptoms at the start of the study.

Whether the different regimens reduce hyperglycemia enough to reduce the frequency of diabetic complications is yet to be determined. If the risk of complications varies little in patients who have glycosylated hemoglobin values below a threshold value of about 8% (see Abstract 119-96-53–6), then among these patients the risk would be high only in those in the diet group. If there is no threshold, then therapy should be more aggressive, if practicable. Since many of these patients are reluctant to begin insulin therapy, and since more sulfonylurea drug or metformin won't help, combination sulfonylurea and metformin therapy should be tried (see Abstract 119-96-53–1).

There is one other point to think about. Does how blood glucose concentrations are lowered, as well as how much they are lowered, have an effect on the risk of complications in patients with NIDDM? This study should provide some answers in a few more years.

R.D. Utiger, M.D.

Reference

1. Niskanen L, Karjalainen J, Siitonen O, et al: Metabolic evolution of type 2 diabetes: A 10-year follow-up from the time of diagnosis. *J Intern Med* 236:263–270, 1994.

Bedtime Insulin/Daytime Glipizide: Effective Therapy for Sulfonylurea Failures in NIDDM

Shank ML, Del Prato S, DeFronzo RA (Univ of Texas, San Antonio)

Diabetes 44:165–172, 1995 119-96-53–4

Background.—Many patients with non–insulin-dependent diabetes mellitus (NIDDM) have poorly controlled hyperglycemia despite taking maximal doses of a sulfonylurea drug. A combination of daytime treatment with a sulfonylurea drug and bedtime insulin therapy may be an effective way to treat patients with poorly controlled NIDDM. Bedtime insulin therapy alone was compared with bedtime insulin plus daytime sulfonylurea drug therapy and daytime sulfonylurea drug therapy alone in a study of these patients. The insulin was given as NPH insulin in a fixed dose of 20 units/1.73 m^2.

Methods.—The patients entered into the study had never been treated with insulin, had no other major illness, and had fasting plasma glucose concentrations no higher than 250 mg/dL (15.5 mmol/L) for 2 weeks while receiving no therapy. In phase I, they received 20 mg of glipizide twice daily for 2 months. In phase II, the 30 patients who completed phase I were randomly assigned to receive daytime sulfonylurea drug therapy (20 mg of glipizide twice daily), bedtime insulin alone, or a combination of daytime sulfonylurea drug therapy and bedtime insulin therapy for 3 months. In phase III, the bedtime insulin doses in both insulin-treated groups were titrated to keep the fasting plasma glucose concentrations below 120 mg/dL (6.7 mmol/L) for 3 months. Plasma glucose concentrations were

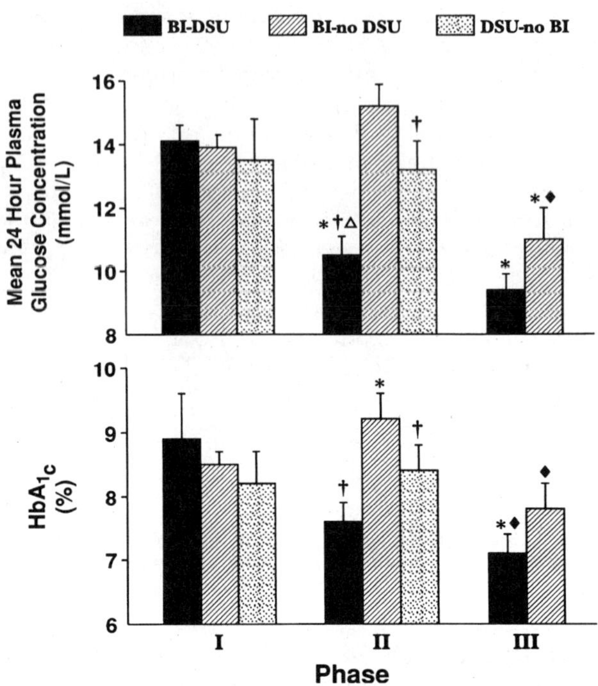

FIGURE 3.—Mean 24-hour in-hospital plasma glucose concentration (A) and HbA_{1c} (B) in the 3 groups of subjects who had non–insulin-dependent diabetes mellitus at the end of each treatment phase. *Asterisk,* $P < 0.05–0.001$ vs. phase I for same group; *solid diamond,* $P < 0.05–0.01$ vs. phase II for same group; *dagger,* $P < 0.05–0.001$ vs. bedtime insulin (BI) for same phase; and *open triangle,* $P < 0.025$ vs. glipizide alone for same phase. (Courtesy of Shank ML, Del Prato S, DeFronzo RA: Bedtime insulin/daytime glipizide: Effective therapy for sulfonylurea failures in NIDDM. *Diabetes* 44:165–172, 1995.)

measured every 30 to 60 minutes from 0730 to 2400 hours, and HbA_{1c} and 24-hour urinary glucose excretion were measured once at the end of each phase of the study.

Results.—In phase II, the patients receiving daytime sulfonylurea drug therapy and bedtime insulin therapy had substantial decreases in plasma glucose concentrations and HbA_{1c} values (Fig 3), as compared with those in phase I, whereas those in the other 2 groups had little change. In phase III, high-dose bedtime insulin improved these measurements to the same degree as did the combination of bedtime insulin therapy and daytime sulfonylurea drug therapy (mean insulin doses during this phase in the 2 groups, 38 and 20 units/day, respectively). The patients receiving combination therapy gained weight, which was attributed to decreased glucosuria.

Discussion.—Bedtime insulin therapy alone and a combination of bedtime insulin and daytime sulfonylurea drug therapy reduce hyperglycemia in patients who have failed sulfonylurea drug therapy. The bedtime insulin therapy/daytime sulfonylurea drug regimen is superior to bedtime insulin therapy alone and can provide prolonged glycemic control.

► In the past, patients with NIDDM who did not respond to therapy with a sulfonylurea drug or who became unresponsive during therapy were usually switched to insulin therapy alone. The key argument in favor of insulin monotherapy is that it made no sense (in terms of likelihood of good glycemic control, risk of side effects, or cost) to give 2 drugs when a larger daily dose of 1 (insulin) would be equally effective.[1] The argument for combined sulfonylurea-insulin therapy is that it deals with both of the pathophysiologic abnormalities of NIDDM: increased insulin resistance and decreased insulin secretion. As a result, less exogenous insulin is needed; therefore peripheral plasma insulin concentrations are lower, resulting in less adiposity and weight gain and perhaps less macrovascular disease.

The latter considerations have led to reexamination of the value of combined sulfonylurea-insulin therapy, particularly of regimens in which single doses of insulin are added to the sulfonylurea drug. Many patients with NIDDM resist the suggestion that they take insulin, particularly if they must take it 2 or 3 times daily, which is what most of them require to obtain reasonable glycemic control. An effective regimen of single-dose insulin, even if combined with continued sulfonylurea therapy, would be more acceptable. There has been particular interest in evening or bedtime as the time for administering the single dose of insulin. The rationale for insulin administration at this time is that it will inhibit nighttime hepatic glucose production and therefore lower fasting plasma glucose concentrations, thereby providing a lower base for meal-related increases in plasma glucose during the day.

This article and others[2, 3] demonstrate the efficacy and feasibility of this approach. The combination of a fixed dose of insulin and glipizide was associated with a very substantial decrease in fasting and 24-hour plasma glucose concentrations and in glycosylated hemoglobin values, both as compared with the preceding period of glipizide-only treatment in the same patients and the patients given the same dose of insulin alone. In this study, no patients received insulin in the morning, but in studies in which the effects of morning and evening insulin therapy were compared in sulfonylurea-treated patients with NIDDM, the improvements in glycemic control and glycosylated hemoglobin were comparable, although weight gain and hyperinsulinemia were less in the patients who received insulin in the evening.[2, 3] None of these studies lasted longer than 3 months. On balance, the evening regimen seems most attractive.

Another option for sulfonylurea-resistant patients is to add metformin or acarbose rather than insulin, and adding 1 of these drugs will undoubtedly become the preferred next step in sulfonylurea-resistant patients (see Abstracts 119-96-53–1 and 119-96-53–2).

R.D. Utiger, M.D.

References

1. Peters AL, Davidson MB: Insulin plus a sulfonylurea agent for treating type 2 diabetes. *Ann Intern Med* 115:45–53, 1991. (1992 YEAR BOOK OF MEDICINE, pp 521–523.)

2. Groop LC, Widen E, Ekstrand A, et al: Morning or bedtime NPH insulin combined with a sulfonylurea in treatment of NIDDM. *Diabetes Care* 15:831–834, 1992.
3. Yki-Jarvinen H, Kauppila M, Kujansuu E, et al: Comparison of insulin regimens in patients with non-insulin-dependent diabetes mellitus. *N Engl J Med* 327:1426–1433, 1992.

Variation in Office-Based Quality: A Claims-Based Profile of Care Provided to Medicare Patients With Diabetes

Weiner JP, Parente ST, Garnick DW, Fowles J, Lawthers AG, Palmer RH (Johns Hopkins Univ, Baltimore, Md; Brandeis Univ, Waltham, Mass; Park Nicollet Med Found, Minneapolis; et al)

JAMA 273:1503–1508, 1995 119-96-53-5

Background.—For many insured populations, expenditures for nonhospital care exceed those for institutional services. The enormous volume of services provided makes it difficult to monitor the quality of ambulatory care. Medicare's recently upgraded computerized claims transaction system documents ambulatory patterns for a cohort of approximately 35 million patients. A cross-sectional study based on Medicare claims data was performed to evaluate office-based care of diabetes and to identify physician- and geographic-related factors affecting compliance with recommended guidelines.

Methods.—Using the National Claims History File, data were obtained on claims for services provided to Medicare beneficiaries living in Alabama, Iowa, and Maryland from July 1990 through June 1991. One hundred percent of Part A (institutional) and Part B (physician and other) Medicare claims were available for the study population. The approximately 80,000 patients whose care was reviewed were all those covered by Medicare seen at approximately 3,000 primary care practices (10,000 physicians) and assigned a diagnosis of diabetes during the study year.

Results.—The recommended services for older patients with diabetes were hemoglobin A_{1C} measurement, an ophthalmologic examination, and serum total cholesterol measurement; blood glucose measurements were also recorded. Overall, 84% of patients with diabetes did not receive the recommended hemoglobin A_{1c} test, 54% did not see an ophthalmologist, and 45% did not receive cholesterol screening in the ambulatory setting. Even after adjusting for patient care mix and physician characteristics, there were wide variations in practice patterns in the 3 states (Table 3). Patients of internists or family practitioners were more likely to have the recommended services than patients of general practitioners, and urban physicians were more likely to meet the recommended quality criteria than were rural physicians.

Conclusion.—Office-based care of elderly patients with diabetes was found to be lacking. A substantial proportion of the cohort did not receive care that met the guidelines of the American Diabetes Association. However, many patients had a blood glucose test, which is considered to be a service of limited use.

TABLE 3.—Services to Patients With Diabetes by State, Specialty, and Geographic Location*

	Recommended Use, %			Limited Use, %
Stratifying Characteristic	Hemoglobin A_{1C} Measurement	Ophthalmologic Examination	Cholesterol Measurement	Blood Glucose Measurement
Entire sample (unadjusted)	16.3	45.9	55.1	80.5
State				
Alabama	9.2†	37.1†	54.7†	88.2†
Iowa	14.3‡	50.5‡	46.4‡	73.1‡
Maryland	21.9†	48.7	60.8†	80.2†
Specialty				
Family practice	18.6	44.5†	56.4	84.0†
General practice	10.8†	45.1§	49.8†	78.9
Internal medicine	16.7‡	47.8‡	57.5‡	79.9‡
Multispecialty	17.2	44.1†	51.9†	77.9
Location				
Urban	17.2†	45.9	58.1†	81.6†
Rural	14.5‡	45.8‡	48.4‡	78.1‡

* Unless otherwise noted, figures represent the adjusted proportion of patients with diabetes who had the specified service at least once during the year from any source. Using indirect regression adjustment, the following characteristics have been held constant, as appropriate: state, specialty, patient age and sex, patient disease burden, and urban/rural location.

† $P = 0.001$, based on significance of independent variable in linear regression equation.

‡ Indicates reference category.

§ $P = 0.01$, based on significance of independent variable in linear regression equation.

(Courtesy of Weiner JP, Parente ST, Garnick DW, et al; Variation in office-based quality: A claims-based profile of care provided to Medicare patients with diabetes. *JAMA* 273:1503–1508, 1995. Copyright 1995, American Medical Association.)

► There are considerable regional variations in medical care not only for patients with diabetes (non–insulin-dependent diabetes [NIDDM], given the age of the patients in this study) but also those who have coronary artery disease, cancer, and no doubt many other disorders. These differences are probably as much cultural as medical. Studies of this type, in which the quality of care provided to patients with a particular disorder (in this instance, diabetes) is judged from physicians' use of indicators or specific guidelines prepared by various expert groups[1, 2] and from administrative (claims) databases, should be evaluated in several ways.

How good are the data in the administrative databases? I confess to being skeptical, but the authors reviewed the medical records of about 5,000 of the patients and found good agreement with the claims data with respect to both diagnosis and tests. Are there justifiable reasons not to do the tests? One would be the presence of 1 or more other disorders that overshadow the diabetes, especially if the latter is mild. These patients were all aged 65 years or older, and more than half had 3 or more other "medical conditions" in addition to their diabetes. Could a lot of the patients have their yearly tests just before and just after the 1-year study? I doubt it. Are the recommended tests indicators of the quality of care, and is care suboptimal if they are not done? I am not sure. An order for the tests (excluding the ophthalmologic examination for the moment) means that the patient's diabetes has not been forgotten, but are the results used? The tests could have been ordered by an assistant from an algorithm for diabetes care, and the result could have been filed. Assuming the best case scenario (that the information was used), does treatment that lowers a high glycosylated hemoglobin value or serum cholesterol concentration in an older patient with NIDDM alter quality of life or outcome? Presumably so, but largely by analogy with younger patients rather than any direct evidence. Although blood glucose measurement is considered a limited use, nonroutine test, its more frequent use is not surprising. It may be more valuable than a glycosylated hemoglobin value in deciding whether to initiate or change therapy in these patients, and it is also useful in corroborating the results of home blood glucose measurements.

Whatever the value of these blood tests, the uniformly low frequency of ophthalmologic examinations is very distressing. This examination is unequivocally valuable. Diabetes is an important cause of blindness in older persons,[3] and there are many other reasons why an older person should have regular eye examinations.

R.D. Utiger, M.D.

References

1. American Diabetes Association, Committee of Professional Practice: Standards of medical care for patients with diabetes mellitus. *Diabetes Care* 17:616–622, 1994.
2. American Diabetes Association: Screening for diabetic retinopathy. *Diabetes Care* 16:16–18, 1993.
3. Tielsch JM, Sommer A, Witt K, et al: Blindness and visual impairment in an American urban population. *Arch Ophthalmol* 108:286–290, 1990.

Glycosylated Hemoglobin and the Risk of Microalbuminuria in Patients With Insulin-Dependent Diabetes Mellitus

Krolewski AS, Laffel LMB, Krolewski M, Quinn M, Warram JH (Joslin Diabetes Ctr, Boston; Harvard Medical School, Boston)
N Engl J Med 332:1251–1255, 1995 119-96-53-6

Background.—Diabetic nephropathy, the chief cause of premature mortality in patients with insulin-dependent diabetes mellitus (IDDM), is characterized by the sequential occurrence of microalbuminuria, overt albuminuria, and renal failure. Good glycemic control may delay or prevent the onset of microalbuminuria and other complications of diabetes, but a quantitative correlation has not yet been identified. In this study, the relationship between the degree and duration of hyperglycemia and the prevalence of microalbuminuria was examined in a large group of patients with IDDM.

Methods.—Urinary albumin excretion was measured in 1,613 patients (mean age, 29 years) with IDDM by analysis of 3 random urine samples collected at least 1 month apart. Microalbuminuria was defined as urinary albumin (in μg) to creatinine (in mg) ratios of between 17 and 299 in men and between 25 and 299 in women. Values of 300 or greater in either sex indicated overt albuminuria. The mean of all available glycosylated hemoglobin (hemoglobin A_1) values determined during the 4-year period before testing served as the index of hyperglycemia.

Findings.—Overt albuminuria was detected in 12 patients who were then excluded from the study. Eighteen percent of the patients with IDDM had microalbuminuria. The patients in both of these groups had longer postpubertal histories of diabetes and higher hemoglobin A_1 values over time than did the normoalbuminuric patients. The prevalence of microalbuminuria increased nonlinearly with the hemoglobin A_1 value within each 6-year interval of disease duration. The slope of the observed relationship was almost flat at mean hemoglobin A_1 values of less than 10.1%, but it rose sharply for values above that level (Fig 1).

Discussion.—For patients with IDDM, both the duration of diabetes and the degree of hyperglycemia are strongly related to the risk of microalbuminuria. The effect of the duration of diabetes was independent of the relationship between hemoglobin A_1 values and microalbuminuria. The latter relationship was nonlinear; the contrast in risk between patients with hemoglobin A_1 values less than and greater than 10.1% suggests that diabetes damages the kidneys through several mechanisms. At high hemo-

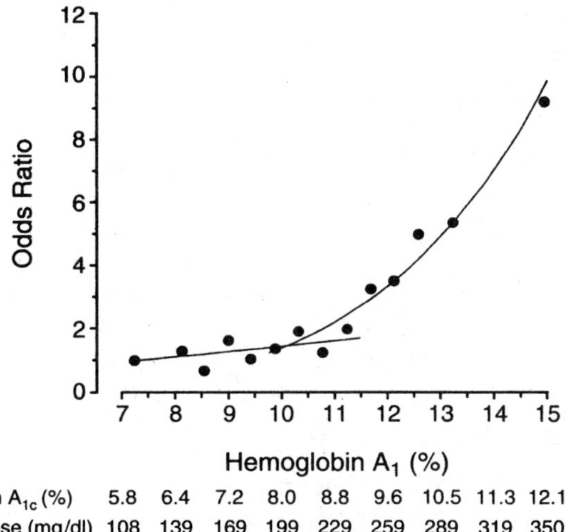

FIGURE 1.—Relationship between mean hemoglobin A_1 values and the risk of microalbuminuria in patients with insulin-dependent diabetes mellitus (*IDDM*). Hemoglobin A_1 values were grouped into small intervals of equal width (0.45% or 0.90% in the tails) and modeled with indicator variables in a logistic regression model of the prevalence of microalbuminuria with covariates to adjust for the age at onset of diabetes, the duration of diabetes, and sex. The reference group for the adjusted relative odds (*circles*) was the group of patients with hemoglobin A_1 values ranging from 5.9% to 7.9%. A changepoint model, including the same covariates, was fitted to the logarithm of hemoglobin A_1 as a continuous variable to estimate the location of the changepoint and the regression slopes below and above the changepoint (*continuous line*). The horizontal axis shows hemoglobin A_{1c} and the blood glucose profile. In the Diabetes Control and Complications Trial, the blood glucose profile was determined by measuring the capillary blood glucose concentration 7 times in a 24-hour period (before and 90 minutes after each of the 3 major meals and before bedtime). The results of quarterly determinations of the blood glucose profile over a 1-year period were averaged, and the line of regression was determined on the basis of the average of quarterly determinations of hemoglobin A_{1c} during the same year. To convert values for blood glucose to mmol/L, multiply by 0.05551. (Reprinted by permission of *The New England Journal of Medicine.* Krolewski AS, Laffel LMB, Krolewski M, et al: Glycosylated hemoglobin and the risk of microalbuminuria in patients with insulin-dependent diabetes mellitus. *N Engl J Med* 332:1251–1255, 1995. Copyright 1995, Massachusetts Medical Society.)

globin A_1 values, microalbuminuria is probably a result of the injurious effects of hyperglycemia on cell functions and extracellular structures such as the basement membrane and mesangial matrix. Ascribing high priority to maintaining hemoglobin A_1 values less than 10.1% may result in a decreased incidence of albuminuria and end-stage renal disease.

► Now that there is general agreement that hyperglycemia is associated with the microvascular complication of diabetes, the question has changed: What is the relationship between the severity of hyperglycemia and these complications? Is it more or less linear, with the risk increasing progressively as the mean blood glucose concentration or its proxy, the glycosylated hemoglobin (HbA_{1c}) value, increases, or is there a threshold below which the increase is small but above which the risk increases rapidly? The practical implications of the distinction are large. If there is a threshold, then treatment need not be aimed at lowering blood glucose and HbA_{1c} values as much; the patient need not be treated so intensively and the risk of hypoglycemia will be lower.

In this study, HbA_{1c} (actually, HbA_1, of which about 80% is HbA_{1c}) values were compared with urinary albumin excretion measured later. The results (Fig 1) do suggest the existence of a threshold for microalbuminuria (although measured as μg albumin/mg creatinine in this study, the lower limit of albumin excretion taken to indicate microalbuminuria is equivalent to an albumin excretion rate of 30 μg/min or about 400 mg/day). The strengths of this study are that many patients were studied and that both HbA_1 and urinary albumin excretion were measured repeatedly. There are, however, several weaknesses. The HbA_1 was measured well before urinary albumin excretion and not necessarily in the interval when microalbuminuria might have developed. There is no information about other factors that might have affected the appearance or progression of microalbuminuria, such as family history of diabetic nephropathy, smoking, and hypertension, or that might have protected against it, such as treatment with an angiotensin-converting enzyme inhibitor (one of these drugs would not have been given in the absence of hypertension). There is also the question of the relationship between microalbuminuria and macroalbuminuria (and end-stage renal disease). Suffice it to say that the latter does not invariably follow the former.[1] Finally, because this HbA_1-microalbuminuria study was not prospective, it is possible to argue that the relationship between higher blood glucose concentrations (manifested by higher HbA_1 values) and microalbuminuria was not causal but was simply the result of another, underlying abnormality.

In a letter to the editor published at the same time, several of the same authors analyzed data from 2 studies of diabetic retinopathy that led them to the conclusion that there is also a threshold HbA_{1c} value, about 8.5%, above which the risk of diabetic retinopathy rises sharply.[2]

On the other hand, the authors of the Diabetic Control and Complications Trial, which was a prospective study, concluded that there was no threshold above which the benefits of intensive therapy of diabetes were especially great.[3] I don't know who is correct, but practically speaking, one has to take

1 step at a time. The first steps should be to lower HbA_{1c} values to below the threshold (8.0% is a reasonable value, but keep in mind that there is a good deal of interlaboratory variation in HbA_{1c} assays), which should be possible with relatively little risk of hypoglycemia, and to deal with any other risk factors for nephropathy and retinopathy. If these efforts are successful, then it is reasonable to try to lower the blood glucose further. Should microalbuminuria appear anyway, treatment with an angiotensin-converting enzyme inhibitor is indicated. I would manage the much greater numbers of patients with non–insulin-dependent diabetes in much the same way, recognizing, however, that they are often insulin-resistant and that hypoglycemia may be more dangerous in them.

R.D. Utiger, M.D.

References

1. Almdal T, Norgaard K, Feldt-Rasmussen B, et al: The predictive value of microalbuminuria in NIDDM. *Diabetes Care* 17:120–125, 1994.
2. Warram JH, Manson JA, Krolewski AS: Glycosylated hemoglobin and the risk of retinopathy in insulin-dependent diabetes mellitus. *N Engl J Med* 332:1305–1306, 1995.
3. The Diabetes Control and Complications Trial Research Group: The effect of intensive treatment of diabetes on the development and progression of long-term complications in insulin-dependent diabetes mellitus. *N Engl J Med* 329:977–986, 1993.

Natural History of Peripheral Neuropathy in Patients With Non–Insulin-Dependent Diabetes Mellitus

Partanen J, Niskanen L, Lehtinen J, Mervaala E, Siitonen O, Uusitupa M
(Univ of Kuopio, Finland)
N Engl J Med 333:89–94, 1995 119-96-53-7

Introduction.—Up to 7.5% of patients with non–insulin-dependent diabetes mellitus (NIDDM) have clinical neuropathy at the time of diagnosis, and the likelihood of its occurrence increases with time. Little, however, is known about the incidence or natural history of this condition. To determine the long-term risk of diabetic polyneuropathy and the factors affecting that risk, a cohort of patients with NIDDM and normal subjects were followed for 10 years with regular evaluation of peripheral nerve function.

Methods.—The normal subjects and patients were examined at baseline (shortly after diagnosis of diabetes mellitus) and after 5 and 10 years. The examinations included assessments of pain and paresthesias and measurements of nerve conduction velocity and response-amplitude values. Eighty-six patients with NIDDM and 121 normal subjects survived to the end of the follow-up period.

Results.—The prevalence of definite or probable polyneuropathy at baseline was 8.3% among patients with NIDDM and 2.1% among the normal subjects. Paresthesias and lack of an Achilles tendon reflex were more common in patients with NIDDM (Fig 1); the patients also had

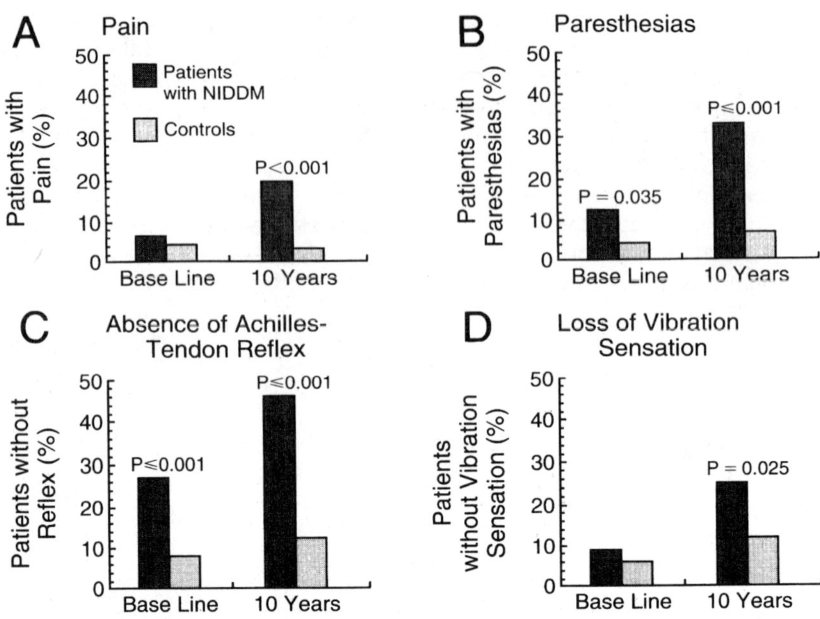

FIGURE 1.—Prevalence of clinical symptoms and signs in patients wtih non–insulin-dependent diabetes mellitus (*NIDDM*) and control subjects at baseline and after 10 years. Panel **A** shows the proportion of patients with bilateral pain in the legs and feet. Panel **B** shows the proportion with bilateral paresthesias of the legs and feet. Panel **C** shows the proportion with no Achilles tendon reflexes, and panel **D** the proportion with loss of vibration sensation on the medial malleoli. The comparisons of the groups at baseline have been previously reported. The *P* values for the comparisons between patients and controls were derived with McNemar's test. (Reprinted by permission of *The New England Journal of Medicine.* Partanen J, Niskanen L, Lehtinen J, et al: Natural history of peripheral neuropathy in patients with non–insulin dependent diabetes mellitus. *N Engl J Med* 333:89–94, 1995. Copyright 1995, Massachusetts Medical Society.)

slower nerve conduction velocity in sensory and motor nerves. After 10 years, the prevalence of polyneuropathy among the patients with NIDDM increased to 41.9%, whereas that among the normal subjects was 5.8%. Patients with NIDDM whose glycemic control was poor were more likely to have polyneuropathy than were those with better glycemic control. Regardless of the degree of glycemia, low serum insulin concentrations before and after oral glucose administration at baseline were associated with polyneuropathy.

Conclusion.—As the trial progressed, the frequency of polyneuropathy in the patients with NIDDM but not the normal subjects increased, suggesting a cumulative effect of neuropathic factors. Poor glycemic control appears to be an important risk factor for development or worsening of polyneuropathy. Axonal degeneration (as indicated by decreasing sensory amplitude values) appeared more important than demyelination (as indicated by the slowing of nerve conduction velocities) as a cause of diabetic polyneuropathy in these patients.

► At baseline, when their diabetes was diagnosed, the patients' mean age was 56 years, most were obese, many were hypertensive, their mean fasting and postprandial blood glucose concentrations were 216 and 353 mg/dL (12.0 and 19.8 mmol/L), respectively, and a few already had symptomatic polyneuropathy. They were, in short, typical of patients with NIDDM, as was their treatment (not done by the investigators). That more of them developed polyneuropathy during the 10-year follow-up is not surprising, but the results are enhanced by the results of the parallel follow-up of normal subjects (Fig 1). As is always the case in studies of diabetic polyneuropathy, more of the patients had abnormalities in nerve conduction than symptoms.

The risk factors for the development of polyneuropathy were higher blood glucose concentrations and higher glycosylated hemoglobin values (9.6% vs. 8.9%) after both 5 and 10 years of follow-up (no surprises there) and, curiously, lower serum insulin concentrations, seemingly independent of the blood glucose values. Glucose uptake by nerves is not dependent on insulin, and I don't know why less insulin would be worse for nerves than more. Age, alcohol consumption, and blood pressure were not risk factors.

Treatment is not mentioned in this article, but it is worth noting that the pain and parenthesias can often be ameliorated by amitriptyline and other antidepressant drugs and by capsaicin cream.[1] Also worth noting is the need for foot care and education about preventing foot injuries. The only way to prevent or delay diabetic polyneuropathy is to use intensive insulin therapy; in the Diabetes Control and Complications Trial, half as many patients who received intensive treatment as compared with conventional treatment had polyneuropathy after 5 years (5% vs. 13%).[2] Presumably, patients with NIDDM would have the same benefit, but intensive treatment with multiple daily doses of insulin is unrealistic for most of them. As I noted in the introduction to this section, new drugs that reduce hyperglycemia in different ways are becoming available, offering more opportunities for better glycemic control and, hence, less polyneuropathy and other complications of diabetes.

R.D. Utiger, M.D.

References

1. Clark CM Jr, Lee DA: Prevention and treatment of the complications of diabetes mellitus. *N Engl J Med* 332:1210–1217, 1995.
2. The Diabetes Control and Complications Trial Research Group: The effect of intensive diabetes therapy on the development and progression of neuropathy. *Ann Intern Med* 122:561–568, 1995.

Bone Density in Non–Insulin-Dependent Diabetes Mellitus: The Rotterdam Study

van Daele P, Stolk RP, Burger H, Algra D, Grobbee DE, Hofman A, Birkenhäger JC, Pols HAP (Erasmus Univ, Rotterdam, The Netherlands)

Ann Intern Med 122:409–414, 1995 119-96-53–8

Objective.—Low bone density is a known complication in patients with insulin-dependent diabetes mellitus, but the findings in those with non–insulin-dependent diabetes are conflicting. A prospective investigation of the relationship of non–insulin-dependent diabetes and bone density was performed.

Methods.—Using dual-energy x-ray absorptiometry, bone mineral density was measured in the lumbar spine and proximal femur of 5,931 subjects aged 55 years and older, including 243 men and 335 women with non–insulin-dependent diabetes mellitus. The subjects' glucose tolerance and bone density were assessed at the same time, and diabetes was diagnosed if the 2-hour postglucose value was 11.1 mmol/L (200 mg/dL) or if the subject was taking an antidiabetic drug or insulin.

Results.—Both men and women with non–insulin-dependent diabetes mellitus had substantially higher bone mineral density at all sites measured than did the nondiabetic subjects. The increases did not correlate with age, weight, medications affecting bone metabolism, smoking, osteoarthritis, renal function, or impairment in activities of daily living. Women with non–insulin-dependent diabetes mellitus had a lower incidence of nonvertebral fractures (mostly wrist, forearm, ankle, and foot fractures) than women without diabetes, but there were no differences between the diabetic and nondiabetic men.

Conclusion.—Both women and men with non–insulin-dependent diabetes have higher bone mineral density than their nondiabetic counterparts, and women with non–insulin-dependent diabetes mellitus have a lower incidence of nonvertebral fractures.

► Is there really some benefit from having NIDDM? The mean lumbar spine and femoral bone density was higher by about 3% in both men and women with NIDDM in this study, and the frequency of self-reported nonvertebral fractures was lower in the women with NIDDM. A similar study of 627 persons (about 40% of whom had impaired glucose tolerance or NIDDM) in a retirement community in California revealed higher bone density in the lumbar spine, femur, and wrist in the glucose intolerant or diabetic women, as compared with normal women, but there were no differences among the men.[1] In both studies, the results were similar among subjects with known NIDDM and those in whom it was newly diagnosed. There are many possible confounding factors in studies such as these, e.g., age, age of menopause, weight, physical activity, smoking, estrogen and thiazide therapy, and other illness. Although most of these factors were taken into account in the analyses, there is always concern that either the adjustments were inadequate or other confounding factors were overlooked. Notwithstanding these caveats, the answer seems to be that hyperglycemia does somehow slow bone loss in older persons. (Many of the subjects in both studies were not known to have hyperglycemia previously, and very few were taking insulin [such subjects were excluded in the California study].) In contrast, patients with insulin-dependent diabetes may lose bone at a very slightly increased rate.[2]

The results seem to suggest that hyperglycemia need not be severe or prolonged to have a beneficial effect on bone, which implies that it can be treated without abolishing the effect. What is the mechanism(s) responsible for the increase in bone density? I know of no evidence that hyperglycemia per se has any effect on bone formation or resorption. Hyperinsulinemia, which was likely present in many of the hyperglycemic subjects in these studies, has direct anabolic actions on bone, and it may act indirectly to increase serum free estrogen concentrations by reducing serum sex hormone–binding globulin concentrations (via the liver) or by stimulating production of sex steroids by the gonads.

The fracture data obtained by van Daele et al. suggest the increased bone density in older hyperglycemic subjects is clinically important. However, in 2 studies of risk factors for hip fracture in women, diabetes was not associated with fracture in one[3] and was not mentioned in the other.[4] The conclusion seems to be that in older persons hyperglycemia may limit bone loss, but its effect is small and should not be relied on to overcome other risk factors.

R.D. Utiger, M.D.

References

1. Barrett-Connor E, Holbrook TL: Sex differences in osteoporosis in older adults with non–insulin-dependent diabetes mellitus. *JAMA* 268:3333–3337, 1995.
2. Krakauer JC, McKenna MJ, Buderer NF, et al: Bone loss and bone turnover in diabetes. *Diabetes* 44:775–782, 1995.
3. Cummings SR, for the Study of Osteoporotic Fractures Research Group: Risk factors for hip fracture in white women. *N Engl J Med* 332:767–773, 1995. (Abstract 119-96-51–7.)
4. Grisso JA, Kelsey JL, Strom BL, et al: Risk factors for hip fracture in black women. *N Engl J Med* 330:1555–1559, 1994. (1995 Year Book of Medicine, pp 655–656.)

Hypoglycaemia Associated With Use of Inhibitors of Angiotensin Converting Enzyme

Herings RMC, de Boer A, Stricker BHC, Leufkens HGM, Porsius A (Utrecht Univ, The Netherlands; Erasmus Univ, Rotterdam, The Netherlands)

Lancet 345:1195–1198, 1995 119-96-53–9

Introduction.—Previous studies have linked angiotensin-converting enzyme (ACE) inhibitors to increased insulin sensitivity in patients with diabetes mellitus. This effect might be beneficial; however, it might also lead to hypoglycemia. The risk of hypoglycemia associated with ACE inhibitors was assessed among diabetic patients taking insulin and oral antidiabetic drugs.

Methods.—The nested case-control study was performed using data from the Dutch PHARMO record-linkage system. Using this database, a base cohort of patients who had been treated with insulin or oral antidiabetic drugs for at least 1 year from 1986 to 1992 was identified. From this cohort, 94 patients who had been hospitalized with a primary diagnosis of hypoglycemia and 654 patients who had been hospitalized for other reasons were selected. A possible association between hypoglycemia and ACE inhibitor therapy was sought, with adjustment for a wide range of potential confounders.

Results.—Among the case and control groups, 19% and 9%, respectively, of the patients were taking an ACE inhibitor. Current ACE inhibitor use was significantly associated with hypoglycemia, odds ratio of 2.8. The risk of hospital admission for hypoglycemia was increased both for patients taking insulin, odds ratio 2.8, and for patients taking oral antidiabetic drugs (odds ratio, 4.1). Up to 13.8% of the hospital admissions for hypoglycemia may have resulted from ACE inhibitor therapy.

Conclusions.—There is a significant association between hospitalization for hypoglycemia and ACE inhibitor therapy in patients with diabetes.

► The ability of ACE-inhibiting drugs to increase insulin sensitivity is modest,[1, 2] and it is clinically important only in patients with diabetes who are receiving sulfonylurea drug or insulin therapy. Both forms of antidiabetic therapy raise serum insulin concentrations, but they do not allow for their rapid reduction when serum glucose concentrations fall. The risk of hypoglycemia in all other patients—diabetic or otherwise—taking ACE inhibitor drugs must be very, very low, because any increase in insulin sensitivity results in decreased insulin secretion.

One might expect that younger patients receiving larger doses of insulin would be more at risk for hypoglycemia induced by a drug that increased insulin sensitivity. However, 58% of the patients in this study were aged 60 years or older. While more of the case patients than control patients were taking insulin, there was little difference among the insulin-treated patients in terms of the insulin concentration of the preparation being used. The paper contains no information about daily insulin dose, home blood glucose concentrations, or glycosylated hemoglobin values. The odds ratios for an increased risk of hypoglycemia were increased for all ACE inhibitors, but the 95% confidence interval did not overlap 1.0 only for captopril, the most commonly used of the drugs. Another useful bit of information from this study is that β-adrenergic antagonist drugs, often considered to be contraindicated in diabetic patients because of their ability to block the sympathoadrenal symptoms of hypoglycemia, were not associated with admission for hypoglycemia.

Angiotensin-converting enzyme inhibitor drugs have several beneficial effects in diabetic patients. Not only do they lower blood pressure, but they also reduce urinary albumin excretion and slow the progression of diabetic nephropathy, even in the absence of hypertension.[3, 4] Their ability to increase insulin sensitivity may also be considered a benefit, because it should be attended by lower serum insulin concentrations, regardless of whether the insulin is secreted or injected, and insulin is incriminated in weight gain and atherogenesis. In contrast, thiazide drugs decrease insulin sensitivity.[1] Overall, therefore, the benefits of ACE inhibitor drugs in patients with diabetes are hardly counterbalanced by a small risk of an increase in hypoglycemic episodes, an increase that should be easily managed by a small reduction in sulfonylurea drug or insulin therapy.

R.D. Utiger, M.D.

References

1. Pollare T, Lithell H, Berne C: A comparison of the effects of hydrochlorothiazide and captopril on glucose and lipid metabolism in patients with hypertension. *N Engl J Med* 321:868–873, 1989.
2. Paolisso G, Gambardella A, Verza M, et al: ACE inhibition improves insulin sensitivity in aged insulin-resistant hypertensive patients. *J Human Hypertens* 6:175–179, 1992.
3. Viberti G, for the European Microalbuminuria Captopril Study Group: Effect of captopril on progression to clinical proteinuria in patients with insulin-dependent diabetes mellitus and microalbuminuria. *JAMA* 271:275–279, 1994. (1994 YEAR BOOK OF MEDICINE, pp 675–676.)
4. Ravid M, Savin M, Jutrin I, et al: Long-term stabilizing effect of angiotensin-converting enzyme inhibition on plasma creatinine and on proteinuria in normotensive type II diabetic patients. *Ann Intern Med* 118:577–581, 1993.

54 Obesity and Lipid Metabolism

Changes in Energy Expenditure Resulting From Altered Body Weight

Leibel RL, Rosenbaum M, Hirsch J (Rockefeller Univ, New York)

N Engl J Med 332:621–628, 1995 119-96-54–1

Introduction.—Obese subjects who lose weight are often unable to maintain weight loss, suggesting the presence of some metabolic resistance to lower weight. Two groups of men and women—one of obese subjects and the other of subjects who had never been obese—were evaluated for the components of energy expenditure during the maintenance of usual and altered body weight.

Methods.—Eighteen obese subjects, 11 women and 7 men, mean age 29 years, and 23 normal-weight subjects, 7 women and 16 men, mean age 26 years, who had never been obese, were studied. All had normal physical and laboratory findings. Obesity was defined as a body mass index greater than 28 kg/m^2. All the subjects were studied at their usual body weight and after losing 10% to 20% of their body weight by underfeeding or gaining 10% by overfeeding (Fig 1). The measurements obtained were 24-hour total energy expenditure, resting and nonresting energy expenditure, and the thermic effect of feeding.

Results.—Both the obese and nonobese subjects had changes in their rates of energy expenditure after changes in body weight. An increase or decrease of 10% in usual weight was accompanied by a disproportionate 16% increase or a 15% decrease, respectively, in 24-hour total energy expenditure. The obese subjects had a significantly higher total energy expenditure and resting energy expenditure but a lower thermic effect of feeding. With stabilization of body weight after a 10% gain, total and resting energy expenditure and the thermic effect of feeding were significantly increased in both weight groups. At weights 10% or 20% below the initial weight, total energy expenditure and nonresting and resting energy expenditure were significantly lower. Adipose tissue and fat-free body mass increased with the 10% gain in weight and decreased with the 10% loss.

Conclusion.—When either a reduced or increased body weight is maintained, compensatory changes in energy expenditure occur. These changes

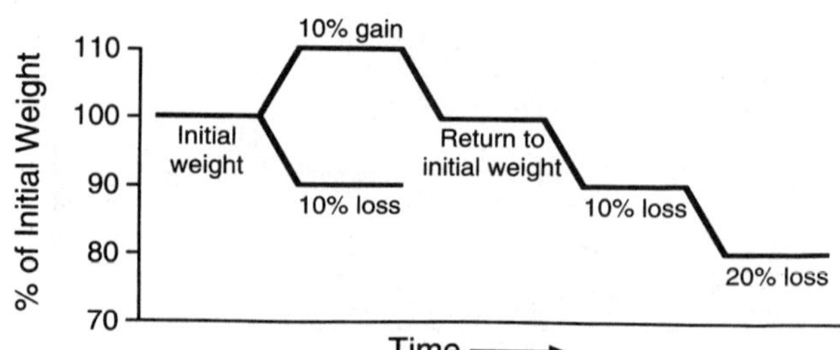

FIGURE 1.—Study design. All research subjects were studied at their initial weight and after at least 1 change in weight. (Reprinted by permission of *The New England Journal of Medicine.* Leibel RL, Rosenbaum M, Hirsch J: Changes in energy expenditure resulting from altered body weight. *N Engl J Med* 332:621–628, 1995. Copyright 1995, Massachusetts Medical Society.)

tend to cause the subjects to return to their initial weight, whether they were normal or obese at baseline. The occurrence of these metabolic alterations in obese subjects who lose weight may make it difficult for them to maintain the lower weight, despite the health benefits of a reduced body weight.

Metabolic Predictors of Obesity: Contribution of Resting Energy Expenditure, Thermic Effect of Food, and Fuel Utilization to Four-Year Weight Gain of Post-Obese and Never-Obese Women

Weinsier RL, Nelson KM, Hensrud DD, Darnell BE, Hunter GR, Schutz Y (Univ of Alabama, Birmingham; Baptist Med Ctr, Birmingham, Al; Mayo Clinic, Rochester, Minn; et al)

J Clin Invest 95:980–985, 1995 119-96-54–2

Objective.—The relationship between various metabolic factors, such as energy expenditure and substrate utilization and predisposition to obesity, was evaluated prospectively.

Methods.—The study subjects were 24 postmenopausal, moderately obese women with an average age of 59 years. They were evaluated when obese, after reduction to normal body weight, and again an average of 4 years later. The control subjects were 24 never-obese, age-matched women who had no family history of obesity. None of the study subjects were receiving hormone replacement therapy or taking any drug known to affect metabolic parameters and none had diabetes.

Results.—After the obese women had achieved normal weight, by losing an average of 12.9 kg, all measurements were similar to those of the never-obese women, including mean resting energy expenditure, thermic effect of food, and fasting and postprandial substrate oxidation and insulin-glucose metabolism. The previously obese women were followed for an average of 50 months and the normal women for an average of 48 months. The average weight gain at follow-up was 10.9 kg in the previously obese women and 1.7 kg in the never-obese women (Fig 1). Only 4 of the women who were initially obese maintained a normal body mass index of less than

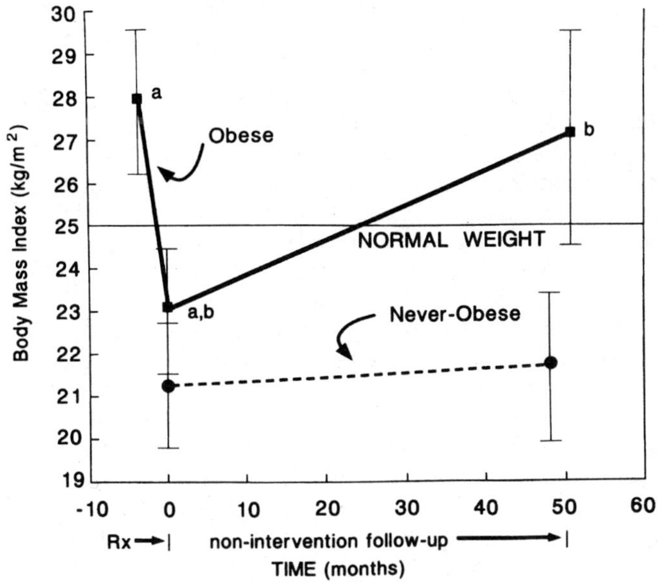

FIGURE 1.—Weight gain pattern (as body mass index, mean ± SD) of 24 obese women after being reduced to normal body weight, compared with 23 never-obese women. Corresponding letters indicate differences between means at $P < 0.001$. (Reproduced from *The Journal of Clinical Investigation,* 1995, 95, pp 980–985, by copyright permission of The American Society for Clinical Investigation.)

25 kg/m^2. The body fat pattern did not change in the obese group during the obese, post-obese, and follow-up states. No correlations were found between 4-year weight changes and energy expenditure or fuel oxidation, but self-reported physical inactivity was associated with greater weight gain. The 5 previously obese women who exercised regularly gained a mean of 6.0 kg, whereas those who never exercised gained a mean of 12.8 kg.

Conclusion.—None of the metabolic measurements that might have explained a predisposition to obesity differed between these previously obese and never-obese women studied at the same weight. Thus, weight gain in women with a family history of obesity may result from excess energy intake or physical inactivity rather than from an inherent set-point of reduced energy requirements.

▶ The first of these 2 studies (Abstract 119-96-54–1) indicates that weight gain and loss induced by changes in food intake in both obese and normal-weight persons are accompanied by increases and decreases, respectively, in caloric expenditure that make it difficult to maintain either higher or lower weight. In the second study (Abstract 119-96-54–2), which concerned only weight loss and spontaneous regain in obese persons, weight loss and regain were not accompanied by a decrease and increase, respectively, in caloric expenditure, and the regain was attributed to spontaneous changes in food intake and decreased physical activity. These differences may be more apparent than real, and they may mainly reflect the difficulties in measuring small changes in resting and total energy expenditure and in substrate utilization.

Both studies provide evidence for a regulatory mechanism that serves to make it difficult to deviate from the baseline fat stores and, therefore, baseline weight, e.g., there is a set point for body fat stores. The regulatory center for this set-point mechanism is presumably located somewhere in the hypothalamus. In simplistic terms, its input is from signals from adipose tissue (and probably from higher brain centers and the environment), and its output adjusts metabolic efficiency, food intake, and physical activity to maintain that amount of adipose tissue.[1]

This is all well and good for normal-weight persons, but it is not for obese persons, because it makes it much more difficult for them to lose weight and then to maintain the lower weight. With respect to obesity, the question then becomes, what happened to raise the set point? The problem could be in the signaling ability of the adipose tissue, the hypothalamic regulatory center, or any of the effector mechanisms. Current interest has focused on leptin, the product of the *ob* gene. Mice with a mutated *ob* gene (ob/ob mice) are polyphagic, obese, and inactive. If injected with leptin, they eat less, have increased energy expenditure, and lose weight, whereas leptin is inactive in mice with diet-induced obesity and in another strain (db) of obese mice.[2–4]

Variations in the production of leptin, whether inherited or resulting from an acquired disorder of adipose tissue, could well determine the set point about which weight is regulated. So far, however, no mutations have been detected in the *ob* gene in obese humans, and in fact its expression in adipose tissue was increased in a small group of them,[5] suggesting resistance of the set point mechanism to the protein. There are, of course, many other ways in which the operation of this system could be changed, including variations in other inputs from adipose tissue or other sites and variations in any of the components of the effector systems that govern metabolic efficiency or eating behavior. Needless to say, the physiologic and therapeutic ramifications of the discovery of leptin have already led to intense commercial activity and many premature headlines.[6]

R.D. Utiger, M.D.

References

1. Bennett WI: Beyond overeating. *N Engl J Med* 332:673–674, 1995.
2. Pelleymounter MA, Cullen MJ, Baker MB, et al: Effects of the *obese* gene product on body weight regulation in *ob/ob* mice. *Science* 269:540–543, 1995.
3. Halaas JL, Gajiwala KS, Maffei M, et al: Weight-reducing effects of the plasma protein encoded by the *obese* gene. *Science* 269:543–546, 1995.
4. Campfield LA, Smith FJ, Guisez Y, et al: Recombinant mouse ob protein: Evidence for a peripheral signal linking adiposity and central neural networks. *Science* 269:546–549, 1995.
5. Considine RV, Considine EL, Williams CJ, et al: Evidence against either a premature stop codon or the absence of obese gene mRNA in human obesity. *J Clin Invest* 95:2986–2988, 1995.
6. Barinaga M: "Obese" protein slims mice. *Science* 269:475–476, 1995.

Efficacy of Low-Dose Cholesterol-Lowering Drug Therapy in Men With Moderate Hypercholesterolemia

Denke MA, Grundy SM (Univ of Texas Southwestern Med Ctr, Dallas; Veterans Affairs Med Ctr, Dallas)

Arch Intern Med 155:393–399, 1995 119-96-54-3

Objective.—Three low-dose cholesterol-reducing drug regimens were evaluated sequentially in 26 men 31–70 years of age who had moderate hypercholesterolemia, with plasma low-density lipoprotein (LDL) cholesterol concentrations of 160–220 mg/dL (4.14–5.69 mmol/L) and plasma triglyceride concentrations less than 200 mg/dL (2.3 mmol/L). Several of the men had a history of coronary heart disease, but none were symptomatic when entered into the study.

Management.—After following of a Step-One cholesterol-lowering diet for 3 months, the men were treated with cholestyramine alone in a daily dose of 8 g; the same dose combined with 5 mg daily of lovastatin; and lovastatin alone in a dose of 20 mg daily. Each regimen was given for 3 months, with 1-month intervals of dietary treatment alone. Blood was sampled for lipid measurements on 5 days in the last 2 weeks of each regimen.

Results.—Compliance with drug treatment exceeded 90%. Plasma LDL cholesterol concentrations decreased significantly, by 9%, during initial dietary treatment. The mean concentration decreased further—by 22 mg/dL (0.6 mmol/L)—with cholestyramine alone. The addition of 5 mg of lovastatin resulted in an additional decrease of 20 mg/dL (0.5 mmol/L) to

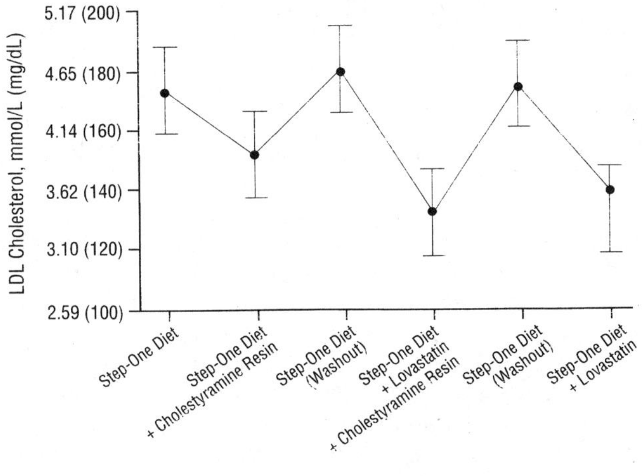

FIGURE 1.—Mean ± low-density lipoprotein (*LDL*) cholesterol level for the 26 men achieved during each study period. Each Step-One Diet period was 1 month long, and each drug period was 3 months long. The LDL cholesterol values returned to Step-One diet levels only during each washout period. (Courtesy of Denke MA, Grundy SM: Efficacy of low-dose cholesterol-lowering drug therapy in men with moderate hypercholesterolemia. *Arch Intern Med* 155:393–399, 1995.)

131 mg/dL (3.4 mmol/L), a decrease comparable to that achieved with the high dose of lovastatin. Between drug periods, the plasma LDL cholesterol concentrations returned to those associated with dietary treatment alone (Fig 1). Well over half the men achieved a plasma LDL cholesterol concentration less than 160 mg/dL (4.1 mmol/L) with cholestyramine alone, and 80% reached this point when the 5-mg dose of lovastatin was added.

Implications.—Hypercholesterolemic patients who do not respond adequately to dietary treatment may respond well to a low dose of cholestyramine plus a very low dose of lovastatin. This regimen should minimize the side effects of cholestyramine and lower the overall cost of therapy.

▶ Among patients with hypercholesterolemia, a so-called Step-One Diet (30% of calories from fat, 10% from saturated fat, and less than 300 mg of cholesterol), exercise, and, if appropriate, weight reduction usually reduce the plasma (or serum) cholesterol concentration by about 5% to 8%. While the fat and cholesterol intake can be restricted further, compliance is poor, so at this point drug therapy is often recommended.

The options for drug therapy are well-known; they are a 3-hydroxy-3-methylglutaryl coenzyme A (HMG-CoA) reductase inhibitor (lovastatin and related drugs), a bile acid sequestrant (cholestyramine or colestipol), or niacin. The efficacy of these drugs is roughly similar, except that niacin causes a greater rise in serum high-density lipoprotein (HDL) cholesterol concentrations, but their side effects are quite different, as are rates of discontinuation (see Abstract 119-96-54-4). The HMG-CoA–inhibiting drugs have few side effects, whereas bile acid–sequestering drugs are not very palatable and often cause constipation, flatulence, and nausea, and niacin often causes flushing, paresthesias, pruritus, and gastrointestinal symptoms.

As evidence grows that reduction in plasma cholesterol concentrations not only lowers the risk of myocardial infarction and death in patients with evident cardiovascular disease (secondary prevention) but also prevents their occurrence (primary prevention),[1] the need for simpler, less expensive treatments with few or no side effects increases. This is particularly the case for primary prevention, for which treatment will necessarily be prolonged. This study was designed with these points in mind. The low-dose 2-drug regimen was as effective as 4 times more lovastatin alone. (The 8-g dose of cholestyramine is about half the usual dose and the 5-mg dose of lovastatin is about one quarter its usual dose.) Not much is said about side effects, except that many patients had gastrointestinal symptoms (indigestion, bloating, and constipation) for the first 6 weeks of the 2 cholestyramine treatment periods and that compliance was good.

The fall in plasma LDL cholesterol concentrations to about 135 mg/dL (3.48 mmol/L), representing a fall of about 25%, during the cholestyramine–lovastatin therapy and lovastatin-only treatment periods may not seem large, but it would be enough to reduce the risk of coronary heart disease appreciably. One wonders what a small dose of lovastatin alone would accomplish, because the dose response for doses above 20 mg daily is flat.[2]

R.D. Utiger, M.D.

References

1. Havel RJ, Rapoport E: Management of primary hyperlipidemia. *N Engl J Med* 332:1491–1498, 1995.
2. Illingworth DR, Erkelens DW, Keller U, et al: Defined daily doses in relation to hypolipidaemic efficacy of lovastatin, pravastatin and simvastatin. *Lancet* 343:1554–1555, 1994.

Discontinuation of Antihyperlipidemic Drugs: Do Rates Reported in Clinical Trials Reflect Rates in Primary Care Settings?

Andrade SE, Walker AM, Gottlieb LK, Hollenberg NK, Testa MA, Saperia GM, Platt R (Harvard School of Public Health, Boston; Harvard Community Health Plan, Brookline, Mass; Brigham and Women's Hosp, Boston; et al)

N Engl J Med 332:1125–1131, 1995 119-96-54–4

Background.—The rates of discontinuation for drugs used to treat chronic conditions affect the success of therapy. Clinical trials of antihyperlipidemic drugs report discontinuation rates of from 4% to 15% in the first year of treatment to about 11% to 30% in the fifth year or more. However, discontinuation rates in clinical trials may not reflect those in primary care settings.

Study Design.—In a retrospective cohort study, computerized files and medical records of 2,369 new users of antihyperlipidemic drugs at 2 HMOs from 1988 to 1990 were reviewed. The rates of drug discontinuation in these primary care settings were compared with the rates reported in 17 randomized and 13 open-label clinical trials published from 1975 to 1993.

Findings.—Overall, 32% of the 3,223 courses of antihyperlipidemic treatment in the HMOs were discontinued at a median of 190 days (range, 1-1,093) after the start of treatment. The major reasons for discontinuation were adverse effects in 18%; therapeutic ineffectiveness, 10%; and noncompliance, 2%. The 1-year probability of drug discontinuation in the patients treated in the HMOs was 15% for lovastatin, 37% for gemfibrozil, 41% for bile acid sequestrants, and 46% for niacin. Except for lovastatin, each drug was discontinued at higher rates in the HMOs than in the randomized clinical trials, with estimates of 31% for the bile acid sequestrants, 15% for gemfibrozil, and 4% for niacin for clinical trials of 1 year or longer. The rates of drug discontinuation in open-label trials were similar to those in HMOs.

Conclusions.—The discontinuation rates for antihyperlipidemic drugs in randomized clinical trials do not reflect the rates actually observed in primary care settings.

► The results of this study serve as a reminder of what most everyone already knows—that an ordinary patient being treated with a particular drug is considerably more likely to discontinue that drug than is a patient receiving the same drug who is participating in a clinical trial. The major reasons for discontinuation of all the drugs in this study were adverse effects and, about half as often, lack of efficacy. Not surprisingly, both are more frequent in patients taking bile acid–sequestering drugs and niacin; the frequency of noncompliance was low—about 2% for each drug. The only drug for which the frequency of discontinuation was similar to that of clinical trials was lovastatin, which attests to its lack of side effects and its efficacy. The patients' physicians were clearly involved in the decisions to discontinue the drugs, because among the discontinued courses of treatment, 56% were followed by changes to another lipid-lowering drug; 11%, by addition of another drug; and 3%, by continuation of one of a combination of drugs.

It is surely no surprise that a drug is discontinued more often in practice than in clinical trials. The patients are not so carefully selected, have not volunteered to take medication, and are not usually followed so closely or solicitously. They are more likely to be taking other drugs and, therefore, be at risk for drug interactions. Their drugs are not supplied for them. The patients in this study were attending an HMO and had prescription drug coverage; noncompliance for personal and financial reasons would undoubtedly be higher in other situations.

Note that the rates cited in the abstract were for 1-year courses of therapy. These drugs are likely to be needed for prolonged periods, and they surely will be discontinued by additional patients in later years. While efficacy may not wane, and some patients may gradually adapt to some drug side effects, other patients may find persistent side effects increasingly intolerable. Hence, the cumulative rates of discontinuation of therapy will surely increase. The conclusion is obvious: The need for therapy should be unequivocal, and the most efficacious drug with the fewest side effects should be given.

R.D. Utiger, M.D.

PART SEVEN

KIDNEY, WATER, AND ELECTROLYTES

FRANKLIN H. EPSTEIN, M.D.

Introduction

This year's chapter on glomerular diseases includes an interesting abstract on the use of fish oil for patients with IgA nephritis and heavy proteinuria. (Patients with less than 1 g of protein per day who have this condition and who do not have hypertension generally have an excellent prognosis, so they do not need to be treated.) Over a 2-year period, fish oil appeared to retard the rate at which renal function was lost. Prospective trials are currently being carried out on the use of angiotensin-converting enzyme (ACE) inhibitors in nondiabetic glomerular disease, and one such study is summarized in the chapter on Chronic Renal Failure. These agents have already been shown to have a beneficial effect in diabetic nephropathy, as reported in the 1995 YEAR BOOK OF MEDICINE.

Glomerulonephritis accounts for a high proportion of adults seen with hematuria—46% in a large series reported from Leicester General Hospital in England. Even one red cell cast in the urinary sediment is enough to suggest the diagnosis, which can be confirmed by renal biopsy.

The treatment of membranous nephropathy remains controversial, but Abstract 119-96-55–3 suggests that if the patient with membranous glomerulopathy is progressively deteriorating, a trial of cyclosporine is indicated. Cyclosporine is also useful, together with prednisone, for the treatment of membranous nephropathy caused by lupus. On the other hand, cyclosporine is contraindicated when glomerulonephritis is caused by the hepatitis virus. In such cases, high-dose interferon-α may help. Finally, attention is called to the possible involvement of a deficiency of factor H (a glycoprotein that normally inhibits activation of complement) in cases of membranoproliferative glomerulonephritis.

The chapter on other diseases of the kidney leads off with an excellent review of HIV-associated nephropathy. This condition should now be at the top of the diagnostic list in urban hospitals in patients with nephritis who have leukopenia, especially if they have heavy proteinuria without edema, and in those with little hypertension or hematuria. In patients with diabetes mellitus, intensive insulin therapy designed to keep blood sugar as close to normal as possible retards the appearance and progression of albuminuria, though it has not yet been shown to change the rate of deterioration of the glomerular filtration rate or the appearance of hypertension. The use of expandable metal stents, common practice at present for the treatment of coronary artery occlusion, has improved the possibility of successful angioplasty of obstructed renal arteries and has lowered the occurrence of restenosis. In patients with the rare condition of primary hyperoxaluria, progressive loss of renal function can be slowed by treatment with oral phosphate and pyridoxine. Finally, I have included 2 papers dealing with preeclampsia, possibly the most common disorder of the kidneys in the world. Confirming an earlier report, dietary supplements of calcium appear to have lowered the incidence of preeclampsia in a group of pregnant women predisposed to this complication.

The chapter on acute renal failure leads off with an excellent clinical study on the best way to prevent radiocontrast-induced nephropathy. The key seems to be generous hydration with half-normal saline. Surprisingly, saline hydration alone turned out to be even better than supplementation of the hydration regimen with mannitol or furosemide in a population of patients who already had some degree of renal insufficiency and many of whom had diabetes. While "nonionic, low osmolar" (and more expensive) radiocontrast agents may have a very slight advantage in patients with underlying renal insufficiency, diabetes, or congestive heart failure, the edge is small and does not justify the use of the more expensive materials in patients who are not predisposed to radiocontrast-induced renal failure because of these preexisting disorders. Once acute renal failure has been established, there are at present no therapies that clearly improve prognosis in human patients, though several do so in animals. "Renal-range dopamine" does not improve renal function in patients with acute renal failure, although it may have a small diuretic effect as a proximal tubular diuretic. However, hemodialysis using cuprophane membranes, which activate complement and encourage neutrophil adhesion and sequestration, is clearly worse for patients with acute renal failure than hemodialysis against biocompatible membranes. These results, reported in an important study by Dr. Raymond Hakim and his associates, should change the standard of practice in the dialysis of patients with acute renal failure.

The chapter on chronic renal failure reports one of the first of many similar studies to come—a randomized controlled trial of enalapril and β-blockers in nondiabetic chronic renal failure. Treatment with an ACE inhibitor was more effective than treatment with β-adrenergic blockers, even though both modes of therapy controlled hypertension to about the same degree. The mechanism of this effect may involve the action of angiotensin II to promote the growth of fibroblasts and collagen synthesis. Another interesting paper deals with the mechanism for loss of concentrating ability in chronic renal failure. Collecting duct cells of partially nephrectomized rats appear to be resistant to the action of vasopressin even when grown in culture because the messenger RNA message for the receptor for antidiuretic hormone is downregulated.

The chapter on hypertension opens with 2 papers based on the idea that the local production of angiotensin II in the walls of blood vessels is likely to play a key role in some vascular diseases, including hypertension. The first paper provides evidence for a direct local effect of angiotensin in vascular hypertrophy. In the second, an epidemiological study of older hypertensive individuals suggests that the inheritance of a gene which increases the activity of ACE in tissues may predispose to high blood pressure. A new class of drugs has been developed that operate by blocking the receptor for angiotensin II rather than by inhibiting the formation of angiotensin II. These agents appear to be at least as useful as ACE inhibitors in the treatment of hypertension. Another study makes the sensible suggestion that a combination of low doses of several antihypertensive medications may prove effective while diminishing the likelihood of at least some drug-related side effects. In patients with a renal transplant, a calcium-channel blocker was more effective than an ACE inhibitor in controlling hypertension; in this situation, certain calcium-blocking agents (like diltiazem) have an added bonus because they decrease the dose of cyclosporine necessary to maintain adequate blood levels of this immunosuppressive drug. In other papers in this section, activation of the sympathetic nervous system by obesity is demonstrated directly, and the effect of coffee drinking on blood pressure is examined (it increases blood pressure in caffeine-naive or nontolerant persons, but not in regular coffee drink ers).

The chapter on transplantation reports a new immunosuppressant drug, mycophenolate mofetil, that inhibits the proliferation of T and B lymphocytes, the formation of antibodies, and the generation of cytotoxic T cells. It is effective in reducing rejection in recipients of renal transplants and thus decreases the need for antilymphocyte therapy, although there are some adverse side effects including gastrointestinal upset and leukopenia. Because of the increased efficacy of immunosuppressive treatments, it is now possible to undertake kidney transplants from spousal and living-unrelated donors, with a survival rate quite comparable to that of well-matched cadaveric renal transplants. For cadaveric transplants, however, a national program to ensure the best HLA match possible still appears to offer advantages in long-term survival. As patients are now living longer after renal transplantation, the risk of neoplasia because of chronic immunosuppression appears to be greater than previously thought. Skin cancer is the most common complication, and the risk of developing some form of cancer is as much as 40% by 20 years.

The chapter on dialysis reflects some changes that are taking place in the kind of patients who receive dialytic therapy. More and more very old patients (older than 80 years) now benefit from chronic hemodialysis, but common complications are hypertension during the procedure and problems with vascular access. Severe abdominal pain in a chronic dialysis patient (at any age) should raise the suspicion of mesenteric infarction as the most likely diagnosis. Extensive surgery can now be carried out successfully in patients with heart and vascular disease, but incurs the risk of acute renal failure. Continuous arteriovenous hemodiafiltration (CAVHD) is a convenient way to treat such patients, but it requires a trained team, necessitates anticoagulation, and has not yet been shown to reduce the high mortality (62%) that attends high-risk surgical acute renal failure. Dialysis, unfortunately, has its downside—it transiently worsens the defective platelet aggregation of uremia (even if "biocompatible" membranes are used), and if carried out in a dialysis unit where other patients may be infected, it increases the risk of acquiring hepatitis B or C.

The Water, Electrolytes, and Acid-Base chapter starts with a practical reminder about the adverse consequences of vigorous hydration, using normal saline, of patients who have been taking lithium for manic-depressive disorders. Because of the common occurrence (10%) of lithium-induced nephrogenic diabetes insipidus, such well-meant hydration may result, paradoxically, in net losses of water into the urine, leading to hypernatremia. Another article deals with the unusual syndrome described by Gitelman that is characterized by chronic hypokalemia, hypomagnesemia, alkalosis, and hyperreninemic hypoaldosteronism. Far more common these days is the syndrome of pentamidine-induced hyperkalemia, seen in patients with AIDS in whom pentamidine has been given prophylactically to prevent *Pneumocystis carinii* pneumonia. Like amiloride, pentamidine inhibits potassium secretion in the collecting duct and thus predisposes to a high serum potassium. The final abstract reminds us of the powerful effects of acidosis on serum phosphorus. In patients with uremia, acidosis increases serum phosphorus and the treatment of acidosis always tends to reduce serum phosphorus by accelerating its incorporation into organic phosphates inside cells.

In the Calcium, Phosphorus, and Bone chapter the effects of dietary sodium added either as bicarbonate or chloride are discussed. Although a high intake of sodium chloride always encourages hypercalciuria, the same amount of sodium given as the bicarbonate does not. This means that it is possible to prescribe sodium bicarbonate in patients with uric acid or cystine stones who also have hypercalciuria, to alkalinize the urine without incurring the risk of increasing urinary calcium. Alendronate, a new drug that decreases bone absorption by inhibiting the action of osteoclasts, is shown to reduce calcium mobilization from the skeleton that normally occurs during bed rest. It will probably find its greatest use in the treatment and prevention of postmenopausal osteoporosis. Finally, an interesting syndrome is described that occurs in patients after renal transplantation, consisting of severe pain in the legs beginning in the first few months after the transplant. Radiographs and bone scans are normal, however, ruling out a vascular necrosis or epiphyseal impaction, and the pain usually responds to nifedipine.

Franklin H. Epstein, M.D.

55 Glomerular Diseases

A Controlled Trial of Fish Oil in IgA Nephropathy

Donadio JV Jr, for the Mayo Nephrology Collaborative Group (Mayo Clinic and Found, Rochester, Minn)

N Engl J Med 331:1194–1199, 1994 119-96-55–1

Purpose.—No effective treatment is available for idiopathic IgA nephropathy, the most common glomerular disease. Fish oil might prevent immunologic renal injury in patients with IgA nephropathy, because the n-3 fatty acids in fish oil may limit the production or actions of cytokines and eicosanoids, thus altering renal hemodynamics and inflammation. This hypothesis was tested in a multicenter, randomized, placebo-controlled trial.

Methods.—In 106 patients with IgA nephropathy and persistent proteinuria, 68% had elevated serum creatinine concentrations, i.e., > 1.2 but ≤ 3.0 mg/dL. The patients were randomized to receive 12 g/day of either fish oil or, as a placebo, olive oil. Treatment continued for 2 years,

TABLE 2.—Effect of 2 Years of Treatment With Fish Oil or Placebo on the Occurrence of the Primary End Point in Patients With IgA Nephropathy, According to the Stratification Factors

Factor	Fish-Oil Group		Placebo Group		*P* Value
	Total No.	% Reaching End Point*	Total No.	% Reaching End Point*	
Hypertension					
Present	31	3	31	35	0.010
Absent	24	9	20	34	0.045
Elevated serum creatinine					
Present	36	9	32	42	0.010
Absent	19	0	19	19	0.035
Urinary protein excretion					
≥3.5 g/24 hr	15	14	15	65	0.030
1.0–3.4 g/24 hr	40	3	36	20	0.035

Note: The primary end point was an increase of 50% or more in the serum creatinine concentration.

* The percentages are estimated on the basis of Kaplan-Meier curves at 2.2 years.

(Reprinted by permission of *The New England Journal of Medicine*. Donadio JV Jr, for the Mayo Nephrology Collaborative Group: A controlled trial of fish oil in IgA nephropathy. *N Engl J Med* 331:1194–1199, 1994. Copyright 1994, Massachusetts Medical Society.)

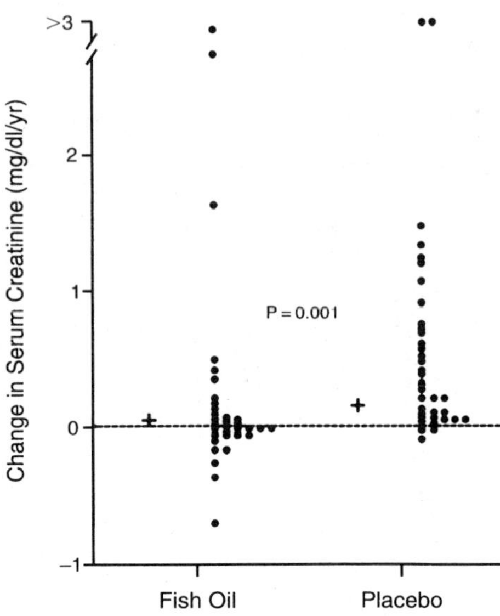

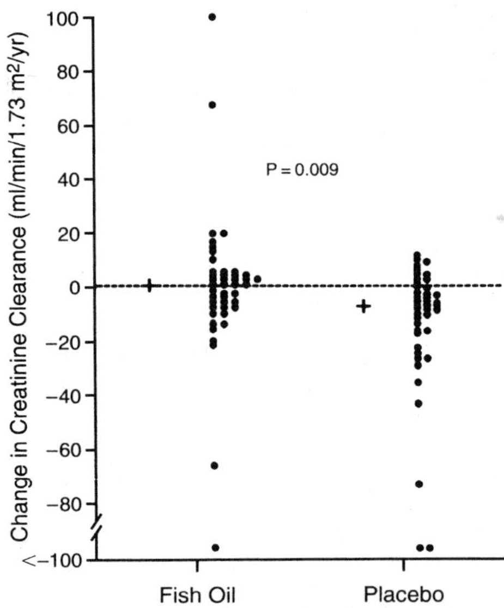

FIGURE 3.—Annualized rate of change in renal function in patients with IgA nephropathy treated with fish oil or placebo. The annual rates of change (slopes) for serum creatinine and creatinine clearance were computed for each patient by linear regression analysis with all results up to and including the 2-year findings. The annualized median change in the serum creatinine concentration was 0.03 mg/dL (2.7 μmol/L in the fish-oil group and 0.14 mg/dL (12.4 μmol/L) in the placebo group (P = 0.001). The annualized median change in creatinine clearance was −0.3 mL/minute per 1.73 m^2 of body-surface area in the fish-oil group and −7.1 mL/minute per 1.73 m^2 in the placebo group (P = 0.009). *Zero* represents no change; the median values are indicated by *plus signs.* (Reprinted by permission of *The New England Journal of Medicine.* Donadio JV Jr, for the Mayo Nephrology Collaborative Group: A controlled trial of fish oil in IgA nephropathy. *N Engl J Med* 331:1194–1199, 1994. Copyright 1994, Massachusetts Medical Society.)

during which serum creatinine concentrations and creatinine clearance were measured. The main study end point was a 50% or greater increase in serum creatinine concentration.

Results.—This end point was met during treatment in 6% of the fish-oil group vs. 33% of the placebo group, according to Kaplan-Meier estimates (Table 2). The fish-oil group had an annual median change in the serum creatinine concentration of 0.03 mg/dL, compared with 0.14 mg/dL in the placebo group (Fig 3). Both groups had slight reductions in proteinuria and comparable control of hypertension. At 4 years, 10% of the fish-oil group had died or progressed to end-stage renal disease compared with 40% of the placebo group. No adverse effects necessitated discontinuation of fish-oil treatment.

Conclusions.—In patients with IgA nephropathy, 2 years of dietary fish-oil supplementation can significantly reduce the rate of loss of renal function. The observed benefits are independent of the presence of hypertension and the baseline degree of elevated serum creatinine and urinary protein excretion. This is the largest study to date of fish-oil treatment for IgA nephropathy.

► These results are interesting enough to make me want to prescribe fish oil for patients with IgA nephritis and heavy proteinuria (excretion over 1 g of protein daily). If proteinuria is slight or absent and blood pressure is normal, the prognosis in this disease is so good that long-term treatment is not warranted. Some residual skepticism seems in order. Other investigators have not obtained as encouraging results with fish oil.[1-3] Note that Dr. Donadio and his colleagues did not treat patients whose serum creatinine was 3 mg/dL or higher. As you will see from the Figure 3, the outcome in some four fifths of the placebo-treated patients was identical to that in the bulk of those given fish oil, but 5 of the 51 who got placebo had a greater than 30% decline in creatinine clearance over the 2 years of the study vs. 2 of 55 who received fish oil. Incidentally, at this dose (12 g/day), no patient complained of fishy taste or odor from the capsules.

F.H. Epstein, M.D.

References

1. Bennett WM, Walker RG, Kincaid-Smith P: Treatment of IgA nephropathy with eicosapentaenoic acid (EPA), a two-year prospective trial. *Clin Nephrol* 31:128–131, 1989.
2. Cheng IKP, Chan, PCK, Chan, MK: The effect of fish-oil dietary supplement on the progression of mesangial IgA glomerulonephritis. *Nephrol Dial Transplant* 5:241–246, 1990.
3. Petterson EE, Rekola S, Berglund L, et al: Treatment of IgA nephropathy with omega-3 unsaturated fatty acids: A prospective, double-blind, randomized study. *Clin Nephrol* 41:183–190, 1944.

Glomerular Disease as a Cause of Isolated Microscopic Haematuria

Topham PS, Harper SJ, Furness PN, Harris KPG, Walls J, Feehally J (Leicester Gen Hosp, England)

Q J Med 87:329–335, 1994 119-96-55–2

Introduction.—Although the prevalence of glomerular abnormalities is high in patients with hematuria, there is no consensus among nephrologists on the indication of renal biopsy. Biopsy findings in 165 patients with isolated hematuria were investigated.

Methods.—Medical records were retrospectively reviewed for results of renal imaging, cystourethroscopy, renal history, and referral source. Patients met the following entry criteria: microscopic hematuria lasting more than 3 months, absence of hypertension or systemic disease, normal renal function, proteinuria of less than 300 mg/24 hrs, and availability of renal biopsy sample.

Results.—The mean patient age of the 94 males and 71 females was 37.5 years. Microscopic hematuria alone was observed in 112 patients, and 53 patients had additional episodes of macroscopic hematuria. Erythrocytes were seen in the urine of 118 patients. A positive dipstick reaction was accepted as sufficient evidence of hematuria, even in the absence of erythrocytes on microscopy. Four patients had abnormal findings on renal tract imaging. Two patients had duplex collecting systems, 1 had renal cysts, and 1 had an irregular ureteral outline. None of these findings could provide sufficient evidence to establish a cause of hematuria. In 7 of 103 cystoscopies, the findings were abnormal: 1 of the findings was bladder stone; 3 cystitis; 2, blood from ureteral orifice; and 1, urethral stricture. All patients younger than 45 years had cystoscopy. Biopsy findings were abnormal in 78 patients. The most common finding was IgA nephropathy (49 patients). Mesangial proliferative glomerulonephritis was present in 12 patients (7.3%) and thin basement membrane nephropathy in 7 (4.3%). In 2 of the 87 normal biopsy specimens, underlying causes were detected on cystoscopy. The detection of erythrocytes had no greater predictive value than dipstick testing.

Conclusion.—Cystoscopy in all patients older than 45 years of age is recommended. If the results are normal, the patients should be followed by renal biopsy from ages 45–70 years of age. Patients younger than age 45 years should have a renal biopsy and do not need cystoscopy. Patients younger than 45 years with isolated hematuria should be referred to a nephrologist. Those older than 45 years should see a urologist.

► All the 165 patients in this study had been referred to the Department of Nephrology at Leicester General Hospital in England, so they might not be entirely representative of other populations of patients with hematuria. Seventeen percent were referred by urologists after a negative cystoscopic examination. I was struck by 2 statistics. First, in more than half of the patients, no abnormality was found even after careful urologic examination and renal biopsy. Second (and not unexpectedly), the largest single diagnostic category, present in 49 patients, was IgA nephropathy. The importance of careful examination of a fresh urine sediment by the physician needs to be emphasized. Even a single red blood cell cast forecloses the necessity for cystoscopy and makes the diagnosis of some form of nephritis most probable.

F.H. Epstein, M.D.

A Controlled Trial of Cyclosporine in Patients With Progressive Membranous Nephropathy

Cattran DC, for the Canadian Glomerulonephritis Study Group (Univ of Toronto)

Kidney Int 47:1130–1135, 1995 119-96-55–3

Background.—The combination of a cytotoxic drug plus corticosteroids has been shown to be beneficial in the treatment of idiopathic membranous glomerulopathy. However, concerns about the long-term risk of this combination, coupled with the recognition that up to one third of patients will undergo spontaneous remission, has limited the widespread application of this regimen. An alternative approach is to treat only those patients at high risk of progression. Cyclosporine treatment was compared with placebo in patients with progressive membranous nephropathy in a randomized, placebo-controlled study.

Study Design.—In part 1 of the study, 64 patients with membranous glomerulopathy were assigned to follow a restricted-protein diet ($\leq$ 0.9 g/kg) and were followed closely for 12 months. Of these, 17 were considered at high risk for progression, with an absolute loss in creatinine clearance $\geq$ 8 mL/min and persistent nephrotic-range proteinuria. In part 2 of the study, these patients were assigned to receive either cyclosporine or placebo therapy for 12 months. Cyclosporine dose was started at 3.0 mg/kg/day in 2 divided doses and was adjusted to achieve a 12-hour trough level of 110–170 µg/L.

Results.—There were no significant differences between the cyclosporine- and placebo-treated patients at entry to part 2. After 12 months, the cyclosporine-treated patients showed an overall 88% slowing in the rate of decline of creatinine clearance compared with 23% in the placebo group. When expressed as a function of the concurrent creatinine clearance, the cyclosporine-treated patients showed a significant improvement in both the time to and the number of patients who halved their proteinuria (Fig 3). At a mean of 21 months after treatment was discontinued, 7 (88%) of 8 patients treated with cyclosporine maintained their improved creatinine clearance, whereas 7 of 8 patients treated with placebo deteriorated with 4 requiring dialysis (Fig 4). Patients who received cyclosporine showed a trend toward worse hypertension and an increase in the number of transient rises in serum creatinine.

Conclusion.—With careful monitoring, cyclosporine is safe and often effective in slowing the rate of renal deterioration and improving pro-

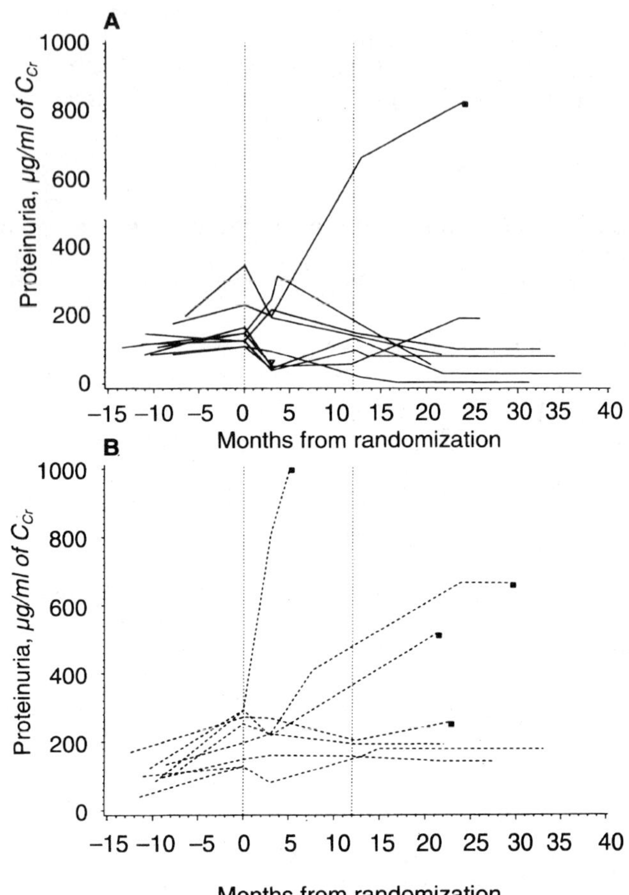

FIGURE 3.—Daily proteinuria expressed as a function of patients' concurrent glomerular filtration rate (μg per mL of C_{cr}) in the 2 treatment groups. Plots begin during the part 1 observation (months with minus sign) and continue during test medication (0–12 months) and to censor point, death (*open triangle*) or dialysis (*closed square*), in both groups. Patients given cyclosporine are in (**A**), *solid lines,* and placebo patients are in (**B**), *broken lines. Abbreviation:* C_{cr}, creatinine clearance. (Courtesy of Cattran DC, for the Canadian Glomerulonephritis Study Group: A controlled trial of cyclosporine in patients with progressive membranous nephropathy. *Kidney Int* 47:1130–1135, 1995. Reprinted by permission of Blackwell Science, Inc.)

teinuria in patients with proven progressive membranous nephropathy. These benefits extend for up to 2 years after treatment is stopped.

▶ This is a small series of patients—17 in all—out of a total of 64 with membranous disease, emphasizing that progressive deterioration is the exception rather than the rule in the natural history of membranous nephropathy. Four of 8 who received placebo deteriorated further, whereas only 1 of 9 who received cyclosporine got worse. No patient had a complete remission. I'd call these results interesting and suggestive, but not exactly

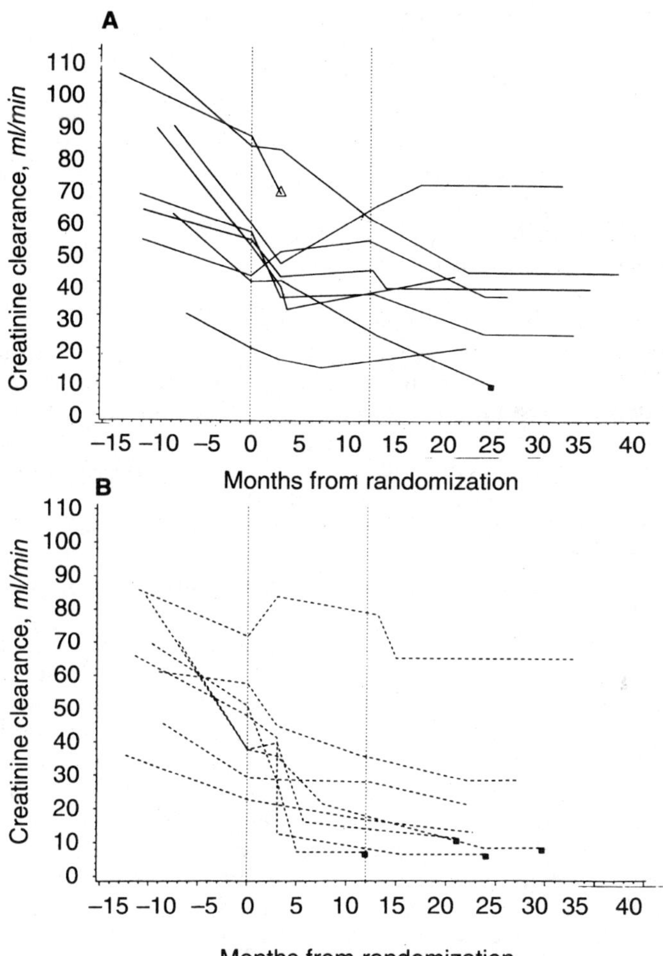

FIGURE 4.—Creatinine clearance measurements in all patients in the 2 treatment groups. Plots begin during the part 1 observation period (months with minus sign), continue during test medications (0–12 months) and postmedication to censor point, death (*open triangle*) or dialysis (*closed square*), in both groups. Cyclosporine patients are in (**A**), *solid lines,* and placebo patients are in (**B**), *broken lines.* (Courtesy of Cattran DC, for the Canadian Glomerulonephritis Study Group: A controlled trial of cyclosporine in patients with progressive membranous nephropathy. *Kidney Int* 47:1130–1135, 1995. Reprinted by permission of Blackwell Science, Inc.)

overwhelming. They illustrate how hard it is, under the best of circumstances, to find enough patients to prove therapeutic benefit in a disease that does not uniformly progress downhill. Nevertheless, they are enough to convince me that if my patient with membranous nephropathy had persistent heavy proteinuria and a progressive rise in serum creatinine, I would try cyclosporine.

F.H. Epstein, M.D.

Cyclosporine Treatment of Lupus Membranous Nephropathy

Radhakrishnan J, Kunis CL, D'Agati V, Appel GB (Columbia Univ, New York)

Clin Nephrol 42:147–154, 1994 119-96-55–4

Introduction.—Lupus membranous nephropathy accounts for 8% to 22% of renal biopsy diagnoses in patients with systemic lupus erythematosus, and few studies have described the treatment of this condition. Cyclosporine has been used to treat patients with nephrotic syndrome and those with systemic lupus. In a pilot study, the safety and efficacy of low-dose, long-term cyclosporine therapy in 10 patients with lupus membranous nephropathy were assessed.

Treatment.—Seven patients with pure membranous lupus nephropathy and 3 patients with membranous lupus nephropathy with superimposed mild proliferative lesions were treated with cyclosporine, starting at 2–3 mg/kg/day and increasing up to 4–5 mg/kg/day, in divided doses, for a mean of 21.2 months. Eight patients also received low-dose corticosteroids. The mean duration of follow-up was 29.7 months.

Outcome.—All patients experienced symptomatic improvement of their nephrotic syndrome. Six patients had a nadir of 24-hour urinary excretion of protein of 1 g or less at a mean of 9.6 months during cyclosporine therapy, 2 had a decline in urinary excretion of protein to 1–2 g/day, and 2 continued to excrete more than 2 g/day. The serum creatinine did not increase significantly. During cyclosporine treatment, 3 patients with superimposed mild proliferative lesions experienced renal and systemic lupus flares that required additional immunosuppressive therapy. Except for 1 patient with a transient increase in serum creatinine and another with drug-related hepatitis, the side effects were minor. Remission was maintained in 3 of 4 patients after discontinuing cyclosporine therapy. In 5 patients, repeat renal biopsies after at least 10 months of cyclosporine therapy showed a decrease in the lupus activity index and an increase in the chronicity index. In all cases, there was an increase in the stage of membranous nephropathy, with a reduced number of fresh subepithelial electron dense deposits. The increased interstitial fibrosis was usually proportional to the degree of glomerular sclerosis. None of the biopsy specimens showed the characteristic features of cyclosporine toxicity.

Summary.—Low-dose cyclosporine therapy effectively reduces proteinuria, causes clinical remission of the nephrotic syndrome, and possibly prevents formation of new immune deposits in patients with lupus membranous nephropathy. Not all patients respond to cyclosporine therapy; some may experience serious side effects. Despite an initial response, renal and systemic relapse of lupus activity was noted in 3 of these patients. The use of cyclosporine in lupus membranous nephropathy should be further evaluated in controlled clinical trials.

► The natural history of untreated lupus membranous nephropathy is not yet clear. The short-term course is relatively benign and indolent in comparison with the rapidly progressive course of untreated diffuse proliferative lupus glomerulonephritis. However, some patients with persistent heavy proteinuria develop progressive renal insufficiency, especially when hypertension is present. It would seem advantageous to produce a complete or partial remission in proteinuria if this can be done without toxic side effects. Prednisone and cyclophosphamide do not appear to help. In this study of 10 patients with membranous lupus nephropathy, on the other hand, cyclosporine and prednisone substantially decreased proteinuria in almost all patients, and the remission was sustained in many for months after cyclosporine was stopped. Unlike cyclosporine treatment of minimal-change disease, where proteinuria is usually reduced within a month after treatment is started, the nadir of protein excretion in these patients was reached only after 6–12 months of treatment with cyclosporine.

F.H. Epstein, M.D.

Membranoproliferative Glomerulonephritis Associated with Hepatitis C Virus Infection Responsive to Interferon-α

Yamabe H, Johnson RJ, Gretch DR, Osawa H, Inuma H, Sasaki T, Kaizuka M, Tamura N, Tsunoda S, Fujita Y, Sato A, Onodera K (Hirosaki Univ, Japan; Univ of Washington, Seattle)

Am J Kidney Dis 25:67–69, 1995 119-96-55–5

Introduction.—Glomerulonephritis with hepatitis C virus (HCV) infection has been reported. The long-term follow-up and repeat biopsy results in 1 patient with membranoproliferative glomerulonephritis (MPGN) with HCV infection were described.

Case Report.—Man, 42, with the nephrotic syndrome and liver dysfunction since 1989 was hospitalized with exacerbation of pretibial edema. Results of virologic studies indicated the following: hepatitis B surface antigen (HBsAg) and antibody to HBsAg were negative, antibody to HBcAg was positive, hepatitis C virus (HCV) antibody was positive, and HCV RNA was detected in serum and cryoprecipitates. Treatment with interferon-α, 10 million units subcutaneously daily for 2 weeks, followed by the same dose 3 times per week for 6 additional weeks, was initiated 1 month after admission. One week after treatment began, 24-hour urine protein excretion was reduced and total serum protein levels were increased. The patient lost 10 kg and his edema resolved. Liver function was normal, and HCV RNA was negative in serum and cryoprecipitates. Comparison of baseline and determinations of laboratory findings after 1 year of therapy showed the following: urine protein excretion of 12.3 g/day to 0.5 g/day; serum protein levels of 3.6 g/dL to 7.4 g/dL; blood urea nitrogen levels of 19 mg/dL to 20 mg/dL, serum creatinine levels of 0.8 mg/dL both times, serum aspartate aminotransferase levels of 199 IU/L to 22 IU/L; C3 levels of 49 mg/dL to 86 mg/dL, and C4 levels of 7 mg/dL to 8 mg/dL. Examination of an initial biopsy specimen showed marked mesangial hypercellularity in a lobular pattern in all glomeruli. Double contours of the basement membrane were observed. Deposition of IgG, IgM, and C3 was detected. Biopsy specimens in 1993 showed considerably milder mesangial cell proliferation. Glomerular IgG deposition was negative, but IgM and C3 deposition remained positive.

Conclusion.—A patient with HCV-induced MPGN treated with interferon-α had sustained elimination of HCV viremia and complete clinical remission of the nephrotic syndrome. These findings suggest that the dosage and duration of treatment in patients with HCV-associated MPGN needs to be reevaluated.

► Prompt remission of hepatitis C glomerulonephritis was obtained in this patient by treatment with a high dose of α-interferon—10 million units given daily for 2 weeks, followed by 10 million units given 3 times weekly for another 6 weeks. The usual dose, reported earlier by these authors in similar patients, has consisted of 3 million units given subcutaneously 3 times weekly for 6–12 months.[1] Standard doses are said to be associated with a high relapse rate. Although one swallow doesn't make a summer, this case report encourages a prospective controlled trial of high-dose α-interferon in glomerulonephritis associated with HCV.

F.H. Epstein, M.D.

Reference

1. 1994 Year Book of Medicine, pp 666–667.

Inherited Factor H Deficiency and Collagen Type III Glomerulopathy

Vogt BA, Wyatt RJ, Burke BA, Simonton SC, Kashtan CE (Rainbow Babies and Children's Hosp, Cleveland, Ohio; Univ of Tennessee, Memphis; Univ of Minnesota, Minneapolis; et al)
Pediatr Nephrol 9:11–15, 1995 119-96-55–6

Objective.—This is the first report of an association of inherited recessive factor H deficiency with collagen type III glomerulopathy, a newly recognized nonimmune complex-mediated chronic glomerulonephritis. Deficiency of factor H, a control glycoprotein, leads to chronic uncontrolled activation of the alternative complement pathway with consumption of C5–C9 and assembly of the membrane attack complex.

Case Report.—Boy, 6 years, had hypertension and congestive heart failure that began at age 13 months as acute mesangiocapillary glomerulonephritis that initially improved but did not disappear. He had progressive renal insufficiency with hematuria and proteinuria. He had no detectable factor H and had low serum C3 and low factor B. Both parents had low factor H levels, which is consistent with autosomal recessive transmission. Light microscopy of renal biopsy specimens showed capillary loop thickening with prominent double contours, endothelial proliferation, and mesangial hypercellularity. Ultrastructural studies revealed prominent mesangial interposition and subendothelial and mesangial deposition of flocculent material. Indirect immunofluorescence showed strong, diffuse deposition of type III collagen in the mesangium and glomerular capillary walls.

Discussion.—In 7 previously reported families with autosomal recessive factor H deficiency, associated renal disease included hemolytic uremic syndrome, atypical dense deposit disease, and membranoproliferative glomerulonephritis. In the present patient, the clinical course and pathologic findings are consistent with collagen type III glomerulopathy. It is not clear, however, whether there is a direct association between factor H deficiency and type III glomerulopathy. None of the previously reported patients with collagen type III glomerulopathy have hypocomplementemia or significant glomerular complement deposition. It is possible that factor H deficiency may facilitate glomerular deposition of collagen type III independently of complement activation, although there is no evidence that factor H deficiency is involved in collagen metabolism. On the other hand, this case may represent a chance association of unrelated recessive diseases.

► Factor H, a glycoprotein present in normal individuals, inhibits activation of complement by the alternative pathway. In its absence, complement activation is uncontrolled, levels of serum complement plunge, and patients are susceptible to mesangiocapillary (also called membranoproliferative) glomerulonephritis (MPGN). Two children deficient in factor H who had MPGN type II were reported earlier,[1] and hereditary MPGN has recently been described in piglets as being caused by factor H deficiency.[2] The detection of collagen type III in scarred glomeruli in the case described in this abstract above does not, in my opinion, make this a unique disease, because type III collagen has also been demonstrated in a variety of other glomerular diseases.[3] Membranoproliferative glomerulonephritis with hypocomplementemia is unusual in adults and more common in children and adolescents. The message of this paper is that when MPGN is found on renal biopsy, factor H deficiency may be responsible.

F.H. Epstein, M.D.

References

1. Levy M, Halbwachs-Mecarelli L, Gubber C, et al: H deficiency in two brothers with atypical dense intramembranous deposit disease. *Kidney Int* 30:949–956, 1986.

2. Hogasen K, Jansen JH, Molines TE, et al: Hereditary porcine membranoproliferative glomerulonephritis Type II is caused by Factor H deficiency. *J Clin Invest* 95:1054–1067, 1995.
3. Yoshioka K, Takemura T, Tohda M, et al: Glomerular localization of type II collagen in human kidney disease. *Kidney Int* 35:1203–1211, 1989.

56 Other Diseases of the Kidney

Human Immunodeficiency Virus-Associated Glomerulosclerosis
Humphreys MH (Univ of California, San Francisco)
Kidney Int 48:311–320, 1995 119-96-56–1

Introduction.—A distinct pattern of structural renal disease in patients infected with HIV has been termed HIV-associated nephropathy (HIVAN). Patients with this disorder show proteinuria, which may be massive, and renal insufficiency that often progresses to end-stage renal disease within 3–6 months. Affected patients frequently will also have kidneys that are highly echogenic on ultrasound but are normal to increased in size, an absence of peripheral edema, and a low incidence of hypertension and hematuria. Although a diagnosis of HIVAN is usually made for patients with other AIDS-related diagnoses, changes consistent with HIVAN have also been reported in asymptomatic patients infected with HIV.

Epidemiologic and Pathologic Characteristics.—Mode of transmission of the HIV virus does not appear to be a determining factor for risk of acquiring HIVAN. Black race may confer partial susceptibility to HIVAN; prevalence of the disease is higher among blacks than among whites. Whether male sex is an independent risk factor for HIVAN remains to be determined. Pathologically, the renal lesions involve focal sclerosis of glomerular tufts, with a distribution pattern progressing from segmental to global. Characteristic tubuloreticular inclusions occur commonly in invading leukocytes in the interstitium and in glomerular and peritubular capillary endothelial cells. The combination of histopathologic changes associated with HIVAN is considered unique.

Pathogenesis and Treatment.—Although the mechanism by which infection with HIV leads to HIVAN has not been established, one theory proposes that renal infection with HIV-1 causes increased production of transforming growth factor–beta (TGF-β) and other cytokines. Unchecked synthesis of TGF-β then leads to fibrotic disease. The progression of HIVAN has not yet been successfully halted with therapeutic intervention. Some evidence exists, however, that patients with HIVAN may benefit from steroid therapy. Therapy with zidovudine has also been suggested to temporarily ameliorate the progress of HIVAN. Most patients with HIVAN will progress to having end-stage renal disease and will require dialysis.

Conclusion.—A task force from the National Kidney Foundation and the National Institutes of Health concluded in 1990 that AIDS-associated renal diseases will develop in 10,000–15,000 persons. Many of these individuals will reach end-stage renal disease and require complex management. Decisions regarding biopsy and dialysis must be carefully formulated, given that alternative lesions or pathologic processes with better prognoses could be mistaken for HIVAN in patients with HIV-1 infection.

► Human immunodeficiency virus–associated nephropathy is now a familiar diagnosis in urban hospitals. Together with lupus nephritis, it should be a leading diagnostic consideration in any patient with proteinuria and leukopenia. Nephropathy may be the first clinical manifestation of HIV infection, appearing even before the usual parade of opportunistic infections have begun to debilitate the patient. In a few patients with elevated serum creatinine, prednisone given for 1–5 months has been reported to decrease renal insufficiency without, however, greatly altering proteinuria.[1] It is not clear to me how much of this effect should be ascribed to the known pharmacologic action of adrenal steroids in most patients to elevate the glomerular filtration rate. In patients with HIV infection treated with zidovudine, half of those who were noncompliant and stopped their medication rapidly lost renal function and went on to have end-stage renal failure, whereas none of those who faithfully continued the zidovudine progressed.[2] However, we all know that for a multitude of reasons, noncompliant patients with a variety of illnesses tend to do worse than those who are so constituted as to follow doctors' orders.

F.H. Epstein, M.D.

References

1. Smith MC, Pawar R, Carey JT, et al: Effect of corticosteroid therapy on human immunodeficiency virus-associated nephropathy. *Am J Med* 97:145–151, 1994.
2. Onyekachi I, Sreepada Rao TK, Tam CC, et al: Zidovudine is beneficial in human immunodeficiency virus-associated nephropathy. *Am J Nephrol* 15:217–221, 1995.

Effect of Intensive Therapy on the Development and Progression of Diabetic Nephropathy in the Diabetes Control and Complications Trial

The Diabetes Control and Complications Trial (DCCT) Research Group (DCCT Research Group, Bethesda, Md)

Kidney Int 47:1703–1720, 1995 119-96-56–2

Background.—The Diabetes Control and Complications Trial (DCCT), a multicenter, randomized clinical trial, compared the efficacy of intensive diabetes treatment, which sought to keep glucose levels as consistently

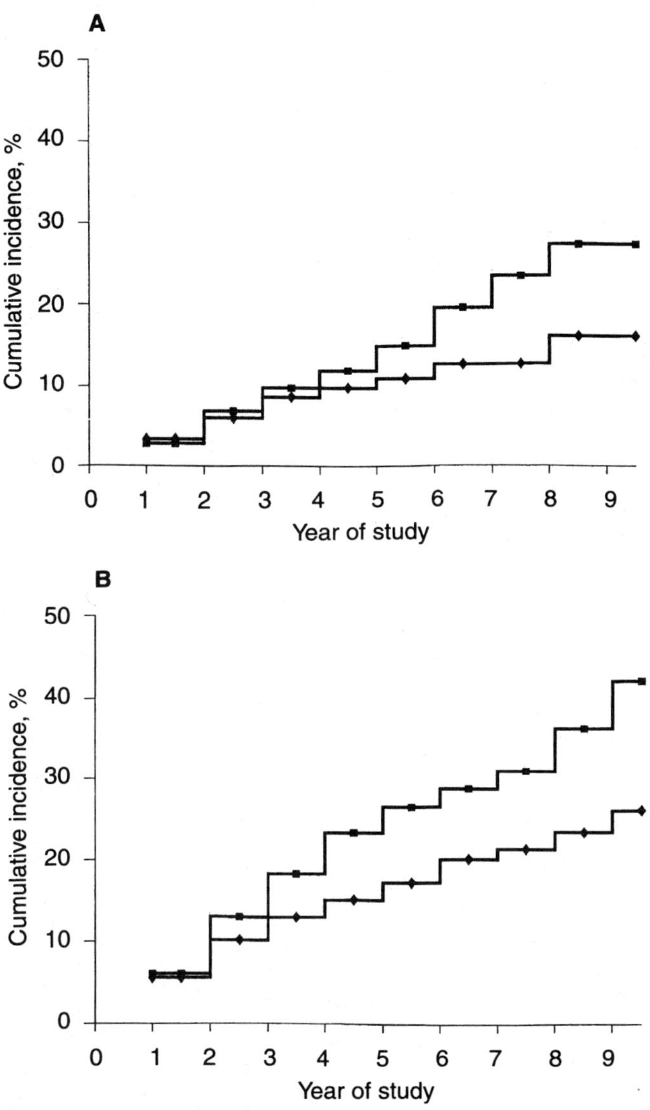

FIGURE 2.—Cumulative incidence of development of microalbuminuria (albumin excretion rate [*AER*] > 28 µg/min) in the intensive (*diamonds*) and conventional (*filled squares*) treatment groups. **A,** primary prevention cohort ($P = 0.04$); **B,** secondary intervention cohort (among those with baseline AER < 28 µg/min; $P = 0.001$). (Courtesy of the Diabetes Control and Complications Trial (DCCT) Research Group: Effect of intensive therapy on the development and progression of diabetic nephropathy in the Diabetes Control and Complications Trial. *Kidney Int* 47:1703–1720, 1995. Reprinted by permission of Blackwell Science, Inc.)

close to normal as possible, with conventional diabetes treatment on the development and progression of long-term complications in patients with insulin-dependent diabetes mellitus (IDDM). Previous reports have documented the superior efficacy of intensive diabetes therapy in delaying the

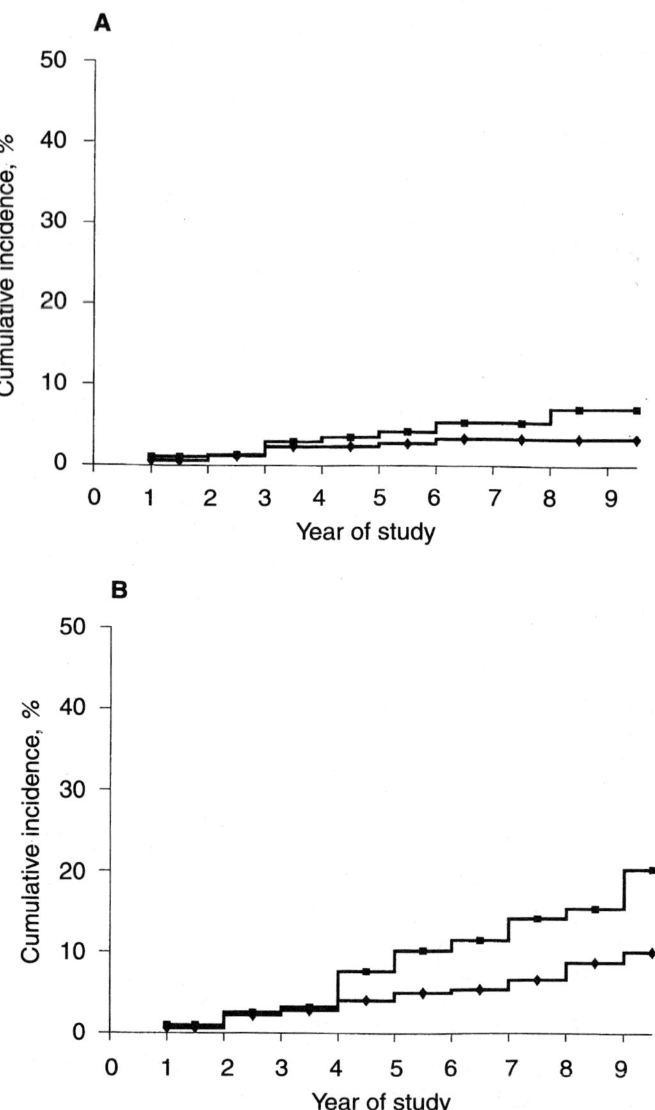

FIGURE 3.—Cumulative incidence of development of albumin excretion rate (*AER*) > 70 μg/min in the intensive (*diamonds*) and conventional (*filled squares*) treatment groups. **A**, primary prevention cohort ($P = 0.219$); **B**, secondary intervention cohort (among those with baseline AER < 28 μg/min; $P = 0.002$). (Courtesy of the Diabetes Control and Complications Trial (DCCT) Research Group: Effect of intensive therapy on the development and progression of diabetic nephropathy in the Diabetes Control and Complications Trial. *Kidney Int* 47:1703–1720, 1995. Reprinted by permission of Blackwell Science, Inc.)

onset or progression of retinopathy, microalbuminuria, and overt nephropathy. Changes in renal function were also studied in relation to the 2 treatment protocols in primary prevention and secondary intervention cohorts. Patients were followed for a mean of 6.5 years, with a range of

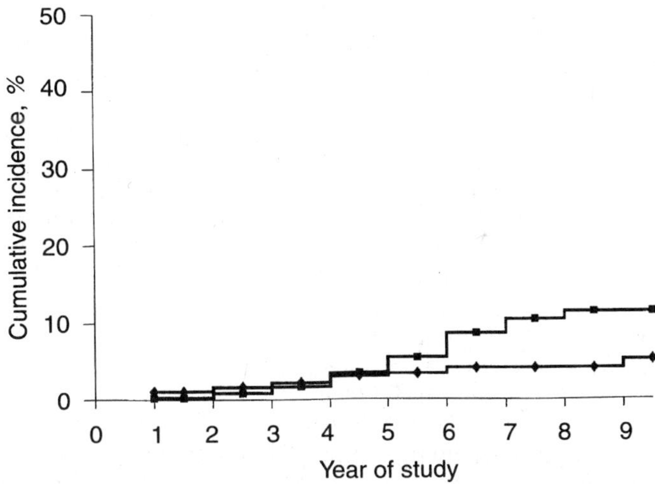

FIGURE 4.—Cumulative incidence of development of clinical albuminuria (albumin excretion rate (AER) > 208 µg/min) among all subjects in the intensive (*diamonds*) and conventional (*filled squares*) treatment groups in the secondary intervention cohort ($P = 0.01$). (Courtesy of the Diabetes Control and Complications Trial (DCCT) Research Group: Effect of intensive therapy on the development and progression of diabetic nephropathy in the Diabetes Control and Complications Trial. *Kidney Int* 47:1703–1720, 1995. Reprinted by permission of Blackwell Science, Inc.)

3–9 years. At baseline, mean HbA_{1c} levels were similar in both treatment groups, but after 3 months mean HbA_{1c} fell in the intensive treatment group. This difference was maintained throughout the study (7.2 vs. 9.1%, $P < 0.001$).

Methods.—At baseline, the 726 patients in the primary prevention cohort had IDDM for 1–5 years, a stimulated serum C-peptide level below 0.5 pmol/mL, no retinopathy, and a urinary albumin excretion rate (AER) below 28 µg/min. The 715 patients in the secondary intervention cohort had IDDM for 1–15 years, stimulated C-peptide levels below 0.2 pmol/L in those with IDDM for at least 5 years, minimal or moderate retinopathy, and urinary AER levels below 139 µg/min. Serum creatinine was measured after breakfast and the morning dose of insulin. Four-hour urine collections were analyzed for urine albumin and creatinine. The glomerular filtration rate (GFR) was measured after 3 years and at the end of the study. Associations were examined between treatment assignment and albuminuria, renal insufficiency, and hypertension.

Results.—The incidence of microalbuminuria ≥ 28 µg/min was 16% after 9 years of intensive therapy and 27% after 9 years of conventional therapy in the primary prevention cohort. Intensive treatment resulted in a 34% reduction in risk of having microalbuminuria. In the secondary intervention cohort, the 9-year incidence of microalbuminuria of ≥ 28 µg/min was 26% in the intensive therapy group and 42% in the conventional therapy group (Fig 2). Intensive therapy resulted in a 43% reduction in risk in this cohort. In the primary prevention cohort, the 9-year incidence of microalbuminuria of ≥ 70 μg/min was 3.3% with intensive treatment and 7% with conventional treatment, whereas it had a 9-year incidence of 10% with intensive treatment and 20.2% with conventional treatment in the secondary intervention cohort (Fig 3). The 9-year incidence of clinical albuminuria of ≥ 208 μg/min was 2.6% with intensive therapy and 2.3% in the conventional therapy group in the primary prevention cohort and 5.3% with intensive therapy and 11.3% with conventional therapy in the secondary intervention cohort (Fig 4). Intensive therapy reduced the risk of developing sustained elevations of urinary AER by 51% to 67%. Treatment assignment did not affect creatinine clearance or the development of hypertension. Glomerular filtration rate was nonsignificantly lower with intensive therapy.

Conclusions.—Intensive therapy was associated with a 39% reduction in the risk of microalbuminuria and a 54% reduction in the risk of clinical albuminuria. In the secondary intervention, AER levels increased 6.5% per year with conventional therapy but did not change significantly with intensive therapy. The use of intensive therapy is therefore recommended for most patients with IDDM.

▶ Intensive insulin therapy designed to keep blood sugar as close to normal as possible clearly seems to reduce the incidence of retinopathy, although the risk of unwanted hypoglycemic reactions is increased. As this study shows, the appearance and progression of albuminuria are also retarded (though not eliminated) by intensive insulin treatment of patients with childhood-type diabetes. An effect on glomerular filtration rate or hypertension was *not* shown in this trial, even though patients were followed for up to 9 years. (The efficacy of angiotensin-converting enzyme inhibitors in slowing renal deterioration[1] is more convincing.) Intensive treatment lowers the concentration of glycosylated hemoglobin and, presumably, other glycated proteins. A clue to the mechanism of the decrease in microalbuminuria may be that the administration of glycated proteins to mice increased the amount of extracellular matrix in their glomeruli and upregulated the glomerular expression of genes associated with renal scarring in experimental diabetes.[2]

F.H. Epstein, M.D.

References

1. 1995 Year Book of Medicine, pp 718–720.
2. Yang C-W, Vlassara H, Peten EP, et al: Advanced glycation and products upregulate gene expression found in diabetic glomerular disease. *Proc Natl Acad Sci USA* 91:9436–9440, 1994.

The Use of Expandable Metal Stents in Transplant Renal Artery Stenosis

Newman-Sanders APG, Gedroyc WG, Al-Kutoubi MA, Koo C, Taube D (St Mary's Hosp, London)

Clin Radiol 50:245–250, 1995 119-96-56–3

Background.—Transplant renal artery stenosis (TRAS) causes resistant hypertension as well as allograft dysfunction and failure. Despite the increasing success of percutaneous balloon dilatation angiography (PTA) for TRAS, a significant proportion will stenose again, usually within 6 months. The management of TRAS that recurs after 2 or more attempts of PTA is not clear. Expandable metallic vascular stents, as an adjunct to PTA, reduce the incidence of restenosis in the coronary and peripheral circulation as well as native renal arteries, providing a basis for their use in severe TRAS as an alternative therapeutic option.

Management.—Four patients who received cadaveric renal transplants with end-to-side external iliac anastomoses had TRAS that recurred 2–3 times, despite immediate success with PTA. The Wallstent-endoprosthesis was used in 3 patients, with an additional Palmaz stent in 1. The fourth patient had a Wiktor stent.

Outcome.—The stents were successfully deployed in all 4 patients. All patients demonstrated an arrest or slowing of previously aggressive recurrent TRAS. One patient had an acute stent thrombosis that responded to immediate thrombolysis. Two patients required repeat stenting; one demonstrated normal transplant artery and the other had a proximal stenosis despite 2 stents. At 4–24 months after stenting, all patients had adequate stable allograft function and satisfactory control of blood pressure, including the patient with significant residual stenosis.

Conclusion.—This early experience on the use of expandable metallic endoprostheses for recurrent TRAS is encouraging. Further studies are needed to define the long-term complications and patency rates after their use.

▶ The use of expandable metal stents, now the rage in interventional cardiology for treatment of obstructed coronary arteries, has opened new vistas for the treatment of renal artery stenosis. Ostial atherosclerotic renal artery stenosis was treated by stenting in 24 hypertensive patients in The Netherlands, for example, with restenosis at 6 months in only 16%.[1] Hypertension improved in 62% (this lesion, you recall, is normally resistant to ordinary balloon angioplasty, after which restenosis is the rule). In another report of stent replacement for atherosclerotic renal artery stenosis,[2] restenosis occurred in 25% by 6 months. Chronic rejection may accelerate stenosis, causing the renal artery to become critically narrowed in a transplanted kidney; in such patients, stent placement may be a way to avoid the morbidity of surgery in an immunocompromised patient.

F.H. Epstein, M.D.

References

1. van de Ven PJ, Beutler JJ, Kaatee R, et al: Transluminal vascular stent for ostial renal artery stenosis. *Lancet* 346:672–674, 1995.
2. Dorros G, Jaff M, Jain A, et al: Follow-up or primary Palmaz-Schatz stent placement for atherosclerotic renal artery stenosis. *Am J Cardiol* 75:1051–1055, 1995.

Association of Pregnancy-Induced Hypertension With Duration of Sexual Cohabitation Before Conception

Robillard P-Y, Hulsey TC, Périanin J, Janky E, Miri EH, Papiernik E (Univ Hosp of Pointe à Pitre, Guadeloupe, French West Indies, France; Med Univ of South Carolina, Charleston; Maternité Port Royal, Paris)
Lancet 344:973–975, 1994 119-96-56-4

Background.—It is thought that pregnancy-induced hypertension (PIH) occurs mainly in primigravidas and seldom recurs in later pregnancies. Some studies have, however, suggested that recurrent PIH may be related to a change in paternity, and that multigravidas and primigravidas are at similar risk when bearing a child by a new father. The father's genes code for early placental development, and imprinted paternal antigens initiate immune responses that sustain placental growth. It has been proposed that PIH represents a maternal reaction against antigenic sites in the placenta that are immunologically incompatible with maternal tissues.

Objective.—A relationship between PIH and the duration of sexual cohabitation before conception was sought by questioning 1,011 consecutive women who delivered children in a 5-month period.

Findings.—Pregnancy-induced hypertension was diagnosed in 102 women, 19 of whom had preeclampsia, and 2, eclampsia. Another 54 women were chronically hypertensive. Pregnancy-induced hypertension developed in 12% of primigravidas, 5% of multigravidas who had retained their initial partner, and 24% of multigravidas who had a new partner. In both primigravidas and multigravidas, the length of sexual cohabitation preceding conception correlated inversely with the risk of PIH developing (Table 2). The association remained evident after controlling for race, educational level, maternal age, marital status, and the number of pregnancies. The risk of PIH was significantly increased for women who conceived within the first year of sexual cohabitation.

Implications.—Pregnancy-induced hypertension may actually be a problem of "primipaternity" rather than primigravidity. Extended sexual cohabitation before conception may reduce the risk of PIH developing.

▶ This report from Guadeloupe in the West Indies raises the interesting possibility that bearing a child *by a new father* might increase the risk for PIH, even in multiparous women. Traditionally, of course, PIH is thought to be far more common in the first than in subsequent pregnancies. But I'm worried about these data, because in this series, the incidence of PIH was actually greater in women who had previous pregnancies than in those

TABLE 2.—Duration of Sexual Cohabitation Before Conception

Duration of sexual cohabitation (months)	0–4	5–8	9–12	12+
Primigravidae (*n*=252)				
Proportion (%) with PIH	16/50 (32)	6/30 (20)	3/24 (13)	5/148 (3·0)
RR (95% CI)	9·2 (3·5–23·9)	5·8 (1·9–18)	3·6 (0·94–14·3)	1·0
Multigravidae (*n*=705)				
Proportion (%) with PIH	26/54 (48)	9/34 (26)	4/22 (18)	33/595 (6)
RR (95% CI)	8·6 (5·6–13·5)	4·7 (2·5–9·1)	3·2 (1·2–8·4)	1·0
All women (*n*=957)				
Proportion (%) with PIH	42/104 (40)	15/64 (23)	7/46 (15)	38/743 (5)
RR (95% CI)*	7·8 (5·3–11·5)	4·5 (2·6–7·8)	2·9 (1·4–6·2)	1·0

* Chi-square for linear trend 130·8, $P < 0.0001$.
Abbreviations: PIH, pregnancy-induced hypertension; *RR,* relative risk.
(Courtesy of Robillard P-Y, Hulsey TC, Périanin J, et al: Association of pregnancy-induced hypertension with duration of sexual cohabitation before conception. *Lancet* 344:973–975, 1994. Copyright 1994, by The Lancet, Ltd.)

bearing their first child, at every level of duration of sexual cohabitation (see Table 2). We know that a prior history of PIH in the first pregnancy strongly predisposes to recurrence in later pregnancies, but no information is given about the presence or absence of PIH in the first pregnancy of the multiparous women who were studied. Is it possible that, for some reason, a tendency to PIH, manifested in the first pregnancy, is statistically associated with a predisposition to switch marital partners later?

F.H. Epstein, M.D.

Prevention of Pregnancy-Induced Hypertension by Calcium Supplementation in Angiotensin II–Sensitive Patients

Sanchez-Ramos L, Briones DK, Kaunitz AM, Delvalle GO, Gaudier FL, Walker CD (Univ of Florida Health Science Ctr, Jacksonville)
Obstet Gynecol 84:349–353, 1994 119-96-56–5

Purpose.—Although the pathogenesis of pregnancy-induced hypertension remains unclear, some studies have suggested it may be associated with abnormal calcium metabolism. The ability of oral calcium supplementation to reduce the incidence of pregnancy-induced hypertension was assessed in a group of high-risk nulliparous patients—those who were angiotensin sensitive.

Methods.—Sensitivity to IV angiotensin infusion at 24–28 weeks' gestation was assessed in 281 nulliparous women with positive roll-over tests. Those who proved sensitive to angiotensin were randomly selected to receive oral elemental calcium, 2 g/day, or placebo. The double-blind trial assessed compliance through the use of serially numbered computerized pill bottles. Some of the women underwent another angiotensin sensitivity test at 34–36 weeks' gestation.

Results.—Of the 67 angiotensin-sensitive nulliparas studied, 63 were assessable. Preeclampsia developed in 14% of the calcium group vs. 44% of the placebo group, for a relative risk of 0.37. Any type of hypertension developed in 31% of the calcium group vs. 65% of the placebo-treated group, for a relative risk of 0.46. In the 23 women who underwent a second angiotensin sensitivity testing, the mean effective pressor dose was significantly greater in the calcium group. Compliance was good in both groups.

Conclusions.—For nulliparous women at high risk of pregnancy-induced hypertension, calcium supplementation can reduce the risk of preeclampsia and other hypertensive complications. Calcium supplementation may reverse the postulated changes leading to hypocalciuria, thus lowering blood pressure and reducing the risk of pregnancy-induced hypertension. In this study, it showed no benefits in terms of overall perinatal morbidity.

▶ This study confirms an earlier report that dietary calcium supplementation is effective in reducing the incidence of pregnancy-induced hypertension, especially in a subset of women whose daily excretion of calcium was below normal.[1] If these preliminary reports are supported by large-scale trials, oral calcium would appear to be a useful way (together with low-dose aspirin) to decrease the risk of hypertension and preeclampsia in susceptible pregnant women. The mechanism of such an effect is obscure at present, but it may be related to the tendency of circulating 1,25-hydroxyvitamin D to be low in preeclampsia.[2, 3] If this is indeed the case, the consequent fall in serum ionized calcium and secondary stimulation of parathyroid gland secretion might trigger a rise in blood pressure.

F.H. Epstein, M.D.

References

1. Belizan JM, Villar J, Gonzalez L, et al: Calcium supplementation to prevent hypertensive disorders of pregnancy. *N Engl J Med* 325:1399–1405, 1991.
2. Seely EW, Wood RJ, Brown EM, et al: Lower serum ionized calcium and abnormal calciotropic hormone levels in pre-eclampsia. *J Clin Endocrinol Metab* 74:1436–1440, 1992.
3. August P, Marcaccio B, Gertner JM, et al: Abnormal 1,25 dihydroxyvitamin D metabolism in pre-eclampsia. *Am J Obstet Gynecol* 166:1295–1299, 1992.

Results of Long-Term Treatment With Orthophosphate and Pyridoxine in Patients With Primary Hyperoxaluria

Milliner DS, Eickholt JT, Bergstralh EJ, Wilson DM, Smith LH (Mayo Clinic and Found, Rochester, Minn)

N Engl J Med 331:1553–1558, 1994 119-96-56-6

Objective.—Because patients with primary hyperoxaluria have a poor prognosis without treatment, the long-term value of orthophosphate and pyridoxine was studied in 25 such patients who were treated for an average of 10 years, starting at a mean age of 12 years. Type I primary hyperoxaluria was confirmed in 9 patients and type II disease in 5. Most of the patients had symptoms or signs of urolithiasis.

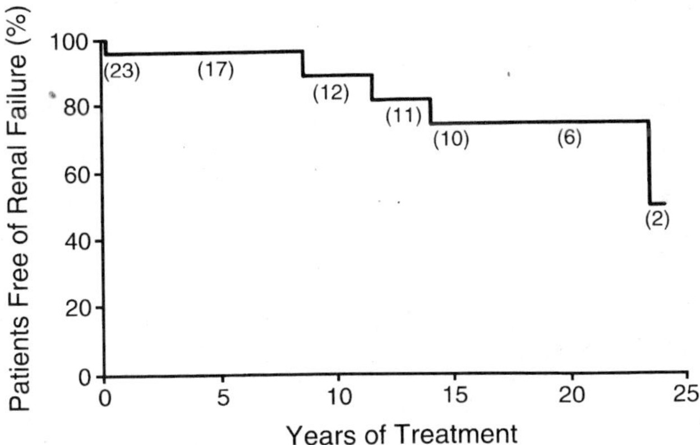

FIGURE 3.—Survival free of end-stage renal disease during treatment with orthophosphate and pyridoxine in 25 patients with primary hyperoxaluria. *Values in parentheses* are numbers of patients at risk. (Reprinted by permission of *The New England Journal of Medicine*. Milliner DS, Eickholt JT, Bergstralh EJ, et al: Results of long-term treatment with orthophosphate and pyridoxine in patients with primary hyperoxaluria. *N Engl J Med* 331:1553–1558, 1994. Copyright 1994, Massachusetts Medical Society.)

Results.—In 2 patients, urinary oxalate excretion became normal, or nearly so, shortly after the start of treatment. In 7 other patients, the urinary oxalate excretion decreased gradually over a period of years. Calcium oxalate supersaturation and crystal formation decreased, and inhibition of calcium oxalate formation increased during treatment. No patient had evidence of metabolic bone disease. Urinary phosphorus excretion nearly doubled during treatment. Eight of 23 assessable patients had new stones or showed the growth of preexisting stones during long-term follow-up. In 9 patients, the stone mass decreased. Five patients progressed to end-stage renal disease after 7–23 years of treatment (Fig 3). Four of them had renal transplantation. Two transplantation procedures were initially successful, and 1 patient did well after retransplantation.

Conclusion.—Combined treatment of primary hyperoxaluria with orthophosphate and pyridoxine at an early stage effectively reduces calcium oxalate crystallization in the urine and seemingly preserves renal function.

► Primary hyperoxaluria is an autosomal recessive disorder caused by defects in hepatic enzymes that catalyze the metabolism of glyoxylate, the major oxalate precursor. If untreated, by their third decade 80% of patients will have end-stage renal failure from the deposition of calcium oxalate crystals in the renal parenchyma and as stones in the collecting system. Treatment with oral phosphate (30–40 mg/kg/day) and pyridoxine (2–4 mg/kg/day) constitutes a 2-pronged attack designed to reduce the supersaturation of calcium oxalate in the urine. Phosphate depresses the renal excretion of calcium in everyone. Pyridoxine, a cofactor in the alanine-glycosylate transaminase pathway, may induce an increase in the activity of this enzyme, and reduces oxalate excretion modestly in about one third of patients.

Calcium oxalate supersaturation in the urine and crystalluria decreased in all 12 patients in whom these were measured. Prolonged treatment, starting when the diagnosis is first made, does not necessarily prevent progressive loss of renal function, but it certainly seems to slow that process.

F.H. Epstein, M.D.

57 Acute Renal Failure

Effects of Saline, Mannitol, and Furosemide on Acute Decreases in Renal Function Induced by Radiocontrast Agents

Solomon R, Werner C, Mann D, D'Elia J, Silva P (New England Deaconess Hosp, Boston; Joslin Diabetes Ctr, Boston; Harvard Med School, Boston)

N Engl J Med 331:1416–1420, 1994 119-96-57–1

Background.—Acute radiocontrast-induced reductions in renal function are an important cause of nosocomial renal insufficiency. Various prophylactic approaches have been recommended, such as saline hydration and the administration of mannitol or furosemide, to decrease the risk for this complication of the administration of radiocontrast agents. However, no randomized studies have directly compared these approaches.

Methods.—Seventy-eight patients with chronic renal insufficiency having cardiac angiography were prospectively studied. By random assignment, the patients received 0.45% saline alone at 1 mL/kg/hr for 12 hours before and 12 hours after angiography, saline plus 25 g of mannitol, or saline plus 80 mg of furosemide. Mannitol and furosemide were administered immediately before angiography. An acute radiocontrast-induced reduction in renal function was defined as an increase in the baseline serum creatinine level of at least 0.5 mg/dL within 48 hours of radiocontrast injection.

Findings.—In 26% of the patients, the serum creatinine level increased at least 0.5 mg/dL after angiography. Eleven percent of the 28 patients in the saline group had such an increase in the serum creatinine level compared with 28% of the 25 in the mannitol group and 40% of the 25 in the furosemide group. The mean increase in the serum creatinine level 48 hours after angiography was significantly higher in patients given furosemide than in those given saline (Fig 1).

Conclusions.—The best protection against contrast nephropathy for patients with chronic renal insufficiency who undergo angiography is a constant infusion of 0.45% saline. No added protection was noted with the addition of mannitol or furosemide.

► The most important finding in this study is that hydration alone was associated with the lowest incidence of radiocontrast-induced renal dysfunction. This is consistent with the general rule, summarizing years of

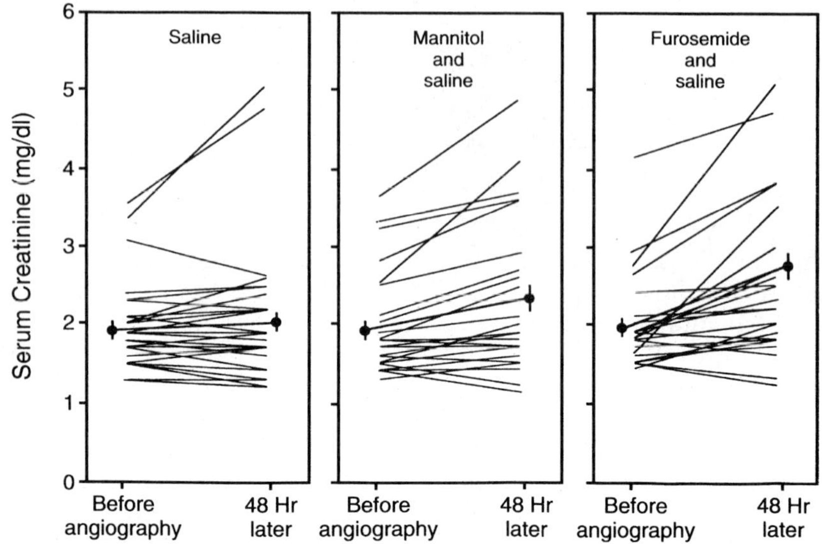

FIGURE 1.—Serum creatinine concentrations immediately before the administration of radiocontrast agent (after 12 hours of hydration) and 48 hours later in patients with chronic renal insufficiency. The mean ± 1 SE for each treatment group is indicated by the *heavy lines* and *circles*. The increase in serum creatinine was significantly greater in the furosemide group than in the saline group ($P < 0.01$) by *t*-test. To convert values for serum creatinine to micromoles per liter, multiply by 88.4. (Reprinted by permission of *The New England Journal of Medicine*. Solomon R, Werner C, Mann D, et al: Effects of saline, mannitol, and furosemide on acute decreases in renal function induced by radiocontrast agents. *N Engl J Med* 331:1416–1420, 1994. Copyright 1994, Massachusetts Medical Society.)

animal experiments and clinical experience, that generous prehydration reduces the incidence of severity of acute renal failure, whether toxic, ischemic, or postsurgical. A surprise was that neither mannitol nor furosemide added to the protection afforded by saline prehydration. In fact, patients given furosemide had significantly worse outcomes, even though they remained in positive fluid balance. The reason for this is not clear, but the authors speculate that it may be related to hemodynamic effects of furosemide, which is known to decrease systemic vascular resistance. Although some radiologists advocate immediate dialysis after a procedure involving the administration of radiocontrast material, on the grounds that the contrast agent might have late deleterious hemodynamic consequences, this does not appear to be necessary.[1]

F.H. Epstein, M.D.

Reference

1. Younathan CM, Kaude JV, Cook MD, et al: Dialysis is not indicated immediately after administration of non-ionic contrast agents in patients with end-stage renal disease treated by maintenance dialysis. *Am J Roentgenol* 163:969–971, 1994.

Nephrotoxicity of Ionic and Nonionic Contrast Media in 1196 Patients: A Randomized Trial

Rudnick MR, for the Iohexol Cooperative Study (Univ of Pennsylvania, Philadelphia)

Kidney Int 47:254–261, 1995 119-96-57–2

Background.—Nonionic contrast media have become more popular than ionic contrast media for radiographic procedures requiring intravascular contrast because the former agents are considered to be less nephrotoxic. Yet clinical experience has shown that nonionic contrast media are also capable of inducing acute renal failure. In a randomized prospective study, the incidence of contrast nephrotoxicity with iohexol, a nonionic agent, and diatrizoate, an ionic agent was compared.

Methods.—Patients were enrolled at 23 participating centers from July 1988 to March 1991. Eligible for recruitment were hemodynamically stable men and women who were referred for nonemergent diagnostic cardiac angiography. Patients were assigned at entry to 1 of 4 stratified study groups on the basis of diabetic or nondiabetic status and serum creatinine levels. The risk of contrast media–induced acute renal failure appears to be increased in patients with diabetes mellitus (DM) or preexisting renal insufficiency (RI), and the study population was intended to include both high- and low-risk patients. All received prophylactic hydration before and after angiography.

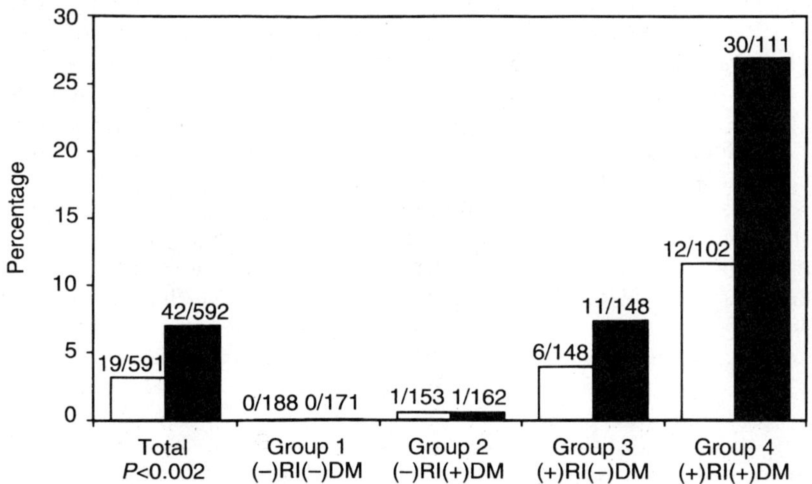

FIGURE 1.—Percent of assessable patients who had nephrotoxicity for each treatment and stratification group after cardiac angiography. Nephrotoxicity is defined as increase in serum creatinine of ≥ 1.0 mg/dL from baseline (0 hour) within 48–72 hours after contrast administration. Treatment groups: iohexol, *open squares*; meglumine/sodium diatrizoate, *filled squares*. *Abbreviations: RI,* renal insufficiency; *DM,* diabetes mellitus. (Courtesy of Rudnick MR, for the Iohexol Cooperative Study: Nephrotoxicity of ionic and nonionic contrast media in 1196 patients: A randomized trial. *Kidney Int* 47:254–261, 1995. Reprinted by permission of Blackwell Science, Inc.)

Results.—The randomized, double-blind trial enrolled 1,196 patients who received contrast, 364 with neither RI nor DM, 318 with DM only, 298 with RI only, and 216 with both RI and DM. Acute nephrotoxicity, defined as an increase in serum creatinine of ≥ 1 mg/dL 48–72 hours after contrast agent administration, occurred in 7% of those randomized to the ionic agent vs. 3% in the nonionic contrast group. Differences in nephrotoxicity, however, were confined to patients with RI alone or with both RI and DM (Fig 1). Multivariate analysis yielded 5 factors independently related to the risk of nephrotoxicity: baseline serum creatinine, male sex, DM, volume of contrast agent, and RI. There were only 15 clinically severe adverse renal events, 9 in the diatrizoate group and 6 in the iohexol group, not a significant difference. Of the 8 patients who ultimately required dialysis, 5 had received iohexol and 3 diatrizoate.

Conclusion.—In these patients who underwent cardiac angiography, the nonionic contrast agent iohexol was less nephrotoxic than the ionic contrast agent diatrizoate in those with preexisting RI alone or combined with DM. The 2 contrast agents did not differ in nephrotoxicity when given to patients with normal renal function, regardless of whether diabetes was present.

▶ This large randomized trial of ionic and nonionic radiocontrast agents generally confirms the impression gained from earlier, smaller comparisons. First, in previously well-hydrated patients without renal insufficiency or diabetes, the incidence of radiocontrast nephrotoxicity is low and is not affected by the choice of contrast agent. Second, those patients at greatest risk are those who have an elevated creatinine before the procedure, especially if they have diabetes (or, I would add, congestive heart failure). Third, nonionic, less hyperosmotic agents (in this case, iohexol), may have a slight edge over ionic, high-osmolar contrast agents (in this case, meglumine/sodium diatrizoate) in avoiding nephrotoxicity. Note, however, that the patients in this series were not prehydrated as much or as long as those in the preceding study, and that the frequency of serious renal failure requiring dialysis or its consideration was approximately the same with both types of radiocontrast agents. Generous prehydration remains the key to preventing radiocontrast nephropathy, and it seems possible to me that if there is any advantage of nonionic agents over the high-osmolar variety, it is because the latter is the more powerful diuretic and causes more dehydration.

F.H. Epstein, M.D.

Zaprinast Accelerates Recovery From Established Acute Renal Failure in the Rat

Guan Z, Miller SB, Greenwald JE (Washington Univ, St Louis, Mo)
Kidney Int 47:1569–1575, 1995 119-96-57–3

Background.—Some improvement in acute renal failure has occurred in response to administration of atrial natriuretic factor or nitric oxide, and the common denominator underlying this improvement may be the activation of cyclic guanosine monophosphate (cGMP). If so, zaprinast, which is a selective inhibitor of cGMP-specific phosphodiesterase, should mimic the biological action of atrial natriuretic factor and nitric oxide. By elevating intracellular cGMP, zaprinast could initiate a dose-dependent increase in renal blood flow and a significant natriuresis. Whether zaprinast is effective as therapy for established acute renal failure was investigated with rats as experimental models.

Methods.—The renal arteries were clamped bilaterally for 60 minutes to induce renal failure. Twenty-four hours later, the rats were administered either vehicle (5% dextrose), zaprinast (0.03 or 0.3 mg/kg/min), or atrial natriuretic factor (ANF24, 0.2 µg/kg/min) intravenously over 4 hours. Renal function was measured by daily serum creatinine measurements (days 1–7) and inulin clearance determination (day 2). A laser Doppler flowmeter was used to measure regional blood flow in the postischemic kidneys.

Findings.—Renal function was dramatically improved in rats receiving zaprinast, but not in those receiving ANF24 (Fig 1). In rats treated with zaprinast, the glomerular filtration rate 48 hours after renal ischemia measured 0.94 mL/min/100 g of body weight; whereas in rats receiving vehicle, the rate was only 0.14 mL/min/100 g of body weight. The effects on renal blood flow occurred only in rats receiving zaprinast; both doses of zaprinast produced an increase in cortical blood flow of about 17% and a much larger (40% to 60%) increase in outer medullary blood flow. Zaprinast also produced significant hypotension, which was more pronounced with the higher dose. The lower dose of zaprinast produced a 3-fold, and the higher dose a 12-fold, increase in urinary excretion of cGMP.

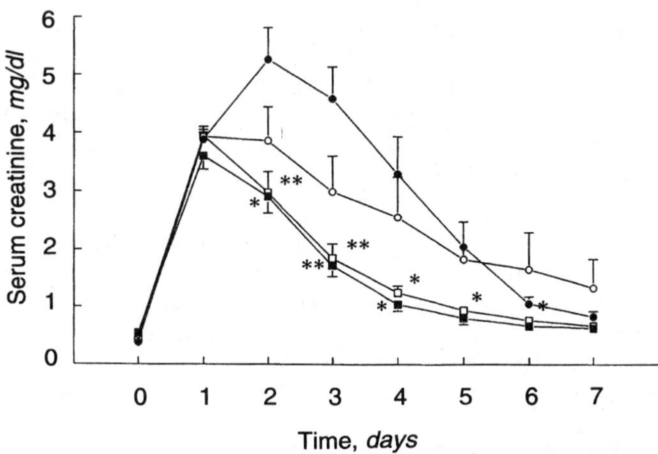

FIGURE 1.—Effect of zaprinast and atrial natriuretic factor (*ANF*) on established ischemic acute renal failure (*ARF*). Serum creatinine was determined daily after 60 minutes of bilateral renal arterial clamping. Drugs were infused for 4 hours only on day 1. *Filled squares,* zaprinast 0.3 mg/kg/min, $n = 4$; *open squares,* zaprinast 0.03 mg/kg/min, $n = 6$; *open circles,* ANF 200 ng/kg/min, n = 8; *filled circles,* D_5W, $n = 6$. Values are the mean ± 1 SEM of at least 4 determinations. * * $P < 0.01$, * $P < 0.05$ vs. D_5W group. (Courtesy of Guan Z, Miller SB, Greenwald JE: Zaprinast accelerates recovery from established acute renal failure in the rat. *Kidney Int* 47:1569–1575, 1995. Reprinted by permission of Blackwell Science, Inc.)

Discussion.—Inhibition of renal cGMP may be a reasonable strategy for therapy of established ischemic acute renal failure. Zaprinast shows a potency greater than that of ANF24 for stimulating recovery from renal failure at doses that are less hypotensive. Smaller, nonhypotensive doses of zaprinast may be equally effective; a full dose-response curve was not generated. Zaprinast alone may provide better therapy than the combination of atrial natriuretic factor with a peripheral vasoconstrictor, and may be less detrimental to intravascular volume and electrolyte balance. The increase in medullary circulation occurring with zaprinast administration may significantly contribute to renal synthesis of cGMP and to the kidney's regenerative capacity.

▶ I am impressed by this study in rats of a possible new therapy for acute renal failure for the following reasons: First, bilateral occlusion of the renal arteries for 60 minutes is a very severe insult in the rat, and anything that accelerates recovery should be taken seriously. Second, the therapeutic intervention (infusion of zaprinast) was not given until 24 hours after the initial insult—consonant with the need of the clinician to have something to give after the diagnosis of acute renal failure is made, rather than before. Third, the most marked effect on regional blood flow was seen in the outer medulla, where the major site of injury in most human acute postischemic renal failure is located. (This is also the site, as the authors point out, of the highest concentration of the inducible form of the enzyme that synthesizes nitric oxide, the actions of which are potentiated by zaprinast.) Systemic hypotension, the bugaboo of all attempts to treat acute renal failure with vasodilators, may prove to be a problem at the bedside. I would encourage the authors to press for clinical trials.

F.H. Epstein, M.D.

Mechanisms of Filtration Failure During Postischemic Injury of the Human Kidney: A Study of the Reperfused Renal Allograft

Alejandro V, Scandling JD Jr, Sibley RK, Dafoe D, Alfrey E, Deen W, Myers BD (Stanford Univ, Calif; Massachusetts Inst of Technology, Cambridge)

J Clin Invest 95:820–831, 1995 119-96-57–4

Rationale.—In animal models of postischemic filtration failure, a marked depression of glomerular filtration rate (GFR) lasts for a week or longer after the kidney is reperfused. This effect has been ascribed in large part to a decrease in the glomerular transcapillary hydraulic pressure difference (ΔP), a parameter that is not measurable clinically because hydraulic pressure cannot be determined in either the capillaries or Bowman's space.

Methods.—As an alternative approach, GFR and its determinants were measured in 12 renal allografts with normal filtration (group 1) and 11 allografts that subsequently exhibited persistent hypofiltration (group 2). The measurements were made at operation after 1–3 hours of reperfusion.

Results.—The GFR averaged 29 mL/min in group 1 kidneys and 6 mL/min in group 2 allografts. The respective values of renal plasma flow, determined by the Doppler flowmeter method, were 315 and 140 mL/min. The coefficient of glomerular ultrafiltration was comparable in the 2 groups, as were plasma oncotic pressures. Based on a mathematical model of glomerular ultrafiltration and sensitivity analysis, the estimated range of ΔP was 34–45 mm Hg in group 1 and 20–21 mm Hg in group 2 kidneys. Morphometric analysis suggested that the diameters of Bowman's space and the tubular lumens were similar in the 2 groups.

Implications.—It was concluded that a depressed transcapillary hydraulic pressure difference is the main cause of postischemic filtration failure and that afferent vasoconstriction is responsible. Increased segmental renovascular resistance probably is the proximate cause of filtration failure in newly transplanted kidneys.

▶ This careful study of postischemic acute renal failure in newly transplanted kidneys reinforces the generally held assumption that the chief factor responsible for the profound depression of GFR is constriction of the afferent arteriole. The pathogenesis of that selective vasoconstriction remains obscure, although some think it may be the result of tubuloglomerular feedback. It is noteworthy that the circulating levels of renin and of endothelin, 2 powerful endogenous vasoconstrictors, were only slightly higher in patients with renal failure than in those who escaped that complication. To my mind, the most important finding in this study was the *absence of any morphologic evidence for tubular obstruction,* which, by contrast, is usually prominent in animal models of postischemic acute renal failure.

F.H. Epstein, M.D.

Renal Support in Critically Ill Patients: Low-Dose Dopamine or Low-Dose Dobutamine?

Duke GJ, Briedis JH, Weaver RA (Preston & Northcote Community Hosp, Victoria, Australia)

Crit Care Med 22:1919–1925, 1994 119-96-57–5

Introduction.—Low-dose dopamine, because of its specific dopamine-receptor agonist properties, which can increase renal blood flow and diuresis, has been used to prevent renal dysfunction in critically ill patients. However, its benefit has not been clinically proven. A prospective, double-blind, randomized trial of low-dose dopamine and low-dose dobutamine examined the renal effects of these agents in critically ill patients.

Methods.—Eighteen stable patients with a critical illness associated with a significant risk of developing renal dysfunction were each given 3 sequential, randomized 5-hour infusions of low-dose dopamine, low-dose dobutamine, and placebo. Hemodynamic, arterial blood gas, glucose, lactate, serum creatinine, and electrolyte measurements were taken at baseline and just before completion of each infusion. Urine samples were collected during the last 4 hours of each infusion for analysis of urine volume, sodium, potassium, creatinine, creatinine clearance, and fractional excretion of sodium.

Results.—During the course of the 3 infusions, there were no changes in serum biochemistry values. There were no changes in central venous pressure, pulmonary artery occlusion pressure, or fluid balance. The dopamine infusion was associated with a significant increase in urine output, but no changes in the fractional excretion of sodium or creatinine clearance. Creatinine clearance was significantly increased during dobutamine administration, although urine output was only slightly increased. Side effects of dopamine included sinus tachycardia in 6 patients, hypertension in 4, and decreased peripheral oxygenation in 10. Side effects of dobutamine included sinus tachycardia in 4 patients and hypertension in 3.

Discussion.—In this group of critically ill patients, low-dose dopamine had a primary diuretic effect without improving creatinine clearance, whereas low-dose dobutamine improved creatinine clearance without changing urine output. These findings suggest that there is no benefit associated with the routine use of dopamine in critically ill patients.

▶ These conclusions agree with my own experience and are supported, I think, by a careful review of the literature. The small increase in glomerular filtration rate resulting from dobutamine in these studies probably reflects dobutamine's inotropic action on the heart. Low-dose dopamine has a tendency to increase glomerular filtration rate and renal blood flow in *normal* animals and humans, but that effect disappears when the circulation is compromised, as in dehydration, shock, or heart failure. It does not increase filtration rate or lower blood urea nitrogen or serum creatinine in patients with renal failure, whether incipient or full-blown. Because dopamine inhibits renal Na-K-ATPase, it has a diuretic action and may increase urine flow somewhat, as in this study. The best thing about "renal range dopamine" is its name, which is very reassuring to the doctor but is about as efficacious as prayer in altering the course of acute renal failure. Unfortunately, its prescription may lull the physician into neglecting careful attention to items like oxygenation, adequate blood pressure support, or treatment of sepsis or heart failure, which may be far more relevant than "renal-range dopamine" to prognosis in complicated patients with acute renal failure.

F.H. Epstein, M.D.

Ketorolac-Induced Acute Renal Failure and Hyperkalemia: Report of Three Cases

Haragsim L, Dalal R, Bagga H, Bastani B (St Louis Univ Health Sciences Ctr)
Am J Kidney Dis 24:578–580, 1994 119-96-57–6

Purpose.—Because the new nonsteroidal anti-inflammatory drug (NSAID) ketorolac tromethamine has potent analgesic effects without

CNS activity, it is widely used in the emergency department and postoperative settings. However, cases of ketorolac-related acute renal failure have been reported. Three additional cases of acute renal failure and hyperkalemia were seen after moderate doses of ketorolac.

Patients.—The patients were 2 women and 1 man aged 57–66 years. All received a moderate dose of ketorolac for the management of pain after surgery, followed by the development of acute renal failure and hyperkalemia. All patients had at least 1 risk factor predisposing them to NSAID-induced nephrotoxicity, such as congestive heart failure, chronic renal insufficiency, liver cirrhosis, or intravascular volume contraction.

All patients had a similar course of acute renal failure and hyperkalemia, but only 1 became oliguric. Acute renal failure and hyperkalemia began after 2–5 days of treatment, peaked 1–2 days after discontinuation of ketorolac therapy and resolved 5–7 days after discontinuation of therapy. Daily weight did not significantly change; no episodes of hypotension, skin rash, arthralgia or arthritis, fever, or pyuria developed; and none of the patients were taking any nephrotoxic drugs. These findings argue against the possibilities of acute interstitial nephritis, urinary tract obstruction, or infection.

Conclusions.—Acute renal failure and hyperkalemia may develop after treatment with moderate doses of ketorolac. The effects are transient, resolving after ketorolac therapy is discontinued. These potential side effects underscore the need to use ketorolac with caution, particularly in high-risk patients, such as those with renal hypoperfusion.

► Parenteral ketorolac is now widely used to relieve pain after surgical procedures because it is a potent analgesic but, unlike opiates, it does not depress respiration or cause addiction. Because it is a much more effective inhibitor of cyclooxygenase than indomethacin or other NSAIDs in common use, it is correspondingly more efficient in suppressing renal production of prostacyclin and prostaglandin E_2, which are first-line endogenous defenses against the renal vasoconstriction that causes acute renal failure. As a result, each year we now see several cases of acute renal failure induced by ketorolac in hospitalized patients. Sick, dehydrated, and elderly patients, or those with circulatory impairment or congestive heart failure, are most susceptible. The condition is usually reversible after several days, when ketorolac is discontinued.

F.H. Epstein, M.D.

Effect of the Dialysis Membrane in the Treatment of Patients With Acute Renal Failure

Hakim RM, Wingard RL, Parker RA (Vanderbilt Univ Med Ctr, Nashville, Tenn)
N Engl J Med 331:1338–1342, 1994 119-96-57–7

Introduction.—Despite the development of different methods of dialysis, mortality rates are persistently high among patients undergoing hemodialysis for acute renal failure. A prospective comparison was undertaken of survival associated with the use of 2 dialysis membranes with different degrees of biocompatibility—the cuprophane membrane, which activates complement and neutrophils, and the polymethyl methacrylate membrane, which activates complement and neutrophils to a more limited degree.

Methods.—Seventy-two consecutive adult patients requiring hemodialysis for acute renal failure were alternately assigned to dialysis treatment with either the cuprophane or the polymethyl methacrylate membrane. The patients were assessed with the Acute Physiology and Chronic Health Evaluation (APACHE II). Outcome measures, including survival, renal function recovery, the number of dialysis treatments given, the length of treatment, and the incidence of oliguria, were compared in the 2 treatment groups.

Results.—At the beginning of treatment, the 2 groups were comparable for age, sex, race, cause of acute renal failure, APACHE II score, and biochemical values. Renal function recovery occurred in 23 of 37 patients (62%) in the polymethyl methacrylate group and in 13 of 35 patients (37%) in the cuprophane group. The patients in the polymethyl methacrylate group recovered renal function with significantly fewer dialysis treatments than did the patients in the cuprophane group (Fig 1). The survival rate was higher in the polymethyl methacrylate group (57%) than in the cuprophane group (37%) (Fig 2), although this difference was not statistically significant ($P = 0.11$). Oliguria developed during treatment in 75% of the patients in the cuprophane group and in 40% of the patients in the polymethyl methacrylate group.

Discussion.—These data suggest that the use of a biocompatibility dialysis membrane may influence renal recovery, particularly in patients with

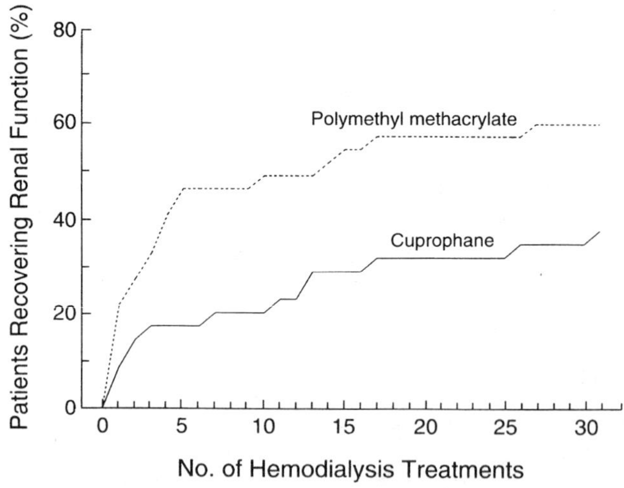

FIGURE 1.—Recovery of renal function in patients with acute renal failure undergoing dialysis with a polymethyl methacrylate or cuprophane membrane, according to the number of hemodialysis treatments. Not shown on the graph are the results for 1 patient in the group undergoing dialysis with the polymethyl methacrylate membrane, who recovered renal function after 72 treatments. (Reprinted by permission of *The New England Journal of Medicine.* Hakim RM, Wingard RL, Parker RA: Effect of the dialysis membrane in the treatment of patients with acute renal failure. *N Engl J Med* 331:1338–1342, 1994. Copyright 1994, Massachusetts Medical Society.)

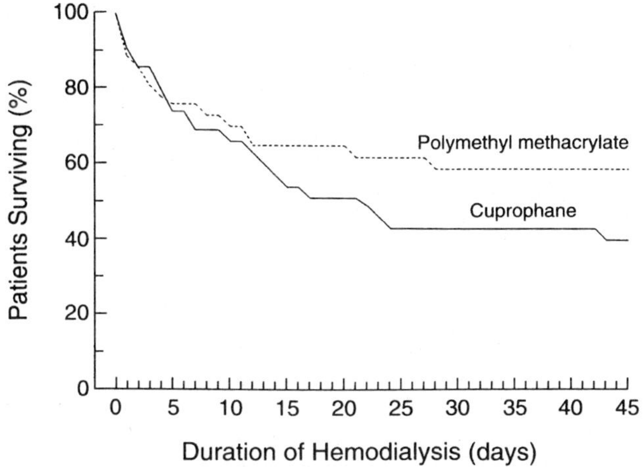

FIGURE 2.—Survival of patients with acute renal failure undergoing dialysis with a polymethyl methacrylate or cuprophane membrane. Not shown on the graph are the results for 1 patient in the group undergoing dialysis with the polymethyl methacrylate membrane, who died after 84 days, and 1 patient in the group undergoing dialysis with the cuprophane membrane, who died after 61 days. (Reprinted by permission of *The New England Journal of Medicine.* Hakim RM, Wingard RL, Parker RA: Effect of the dialysis membrane in the treatment of patients with acute renal failure. *N Engl J Med* 331:1338–1342, 1994. Copyright 1994, Massachusetts Medical Society.)

nonoliguric acute renal failure. Renal recovery may be delayed by both the direct and indirect vasoconstrictive effects of complement and neutrophil activation and by the toxic and inhibitory effects of the products of complement and neutrophil activation.

► These results strongly suggest that dialysis membranes like polymethyl methacrylate, which minimize the activation of complement and neutrophils, are better for patients with acute renal failure who require hemodialysis than is the more commonly used (and less expensive) cuprophane membrane. The data lend support to a growing sense that the most effective way to reduce mortality in acute renal failure—still close to 50% in the modern era—may be to turn our attention to the septic state and the systemic activation of cytokines that attend the demise of our sickest patients with acute renal failure. A similar prospective trial published in *The Lancet* came to the same conclusion and also noted that deaths from sepsis were reduced by dialysis with a biocompatible membrane.[1] Dr. Hakim tells me that a larger multicenter trial encompassing 156 patients that is now being analyzed confirms these results, and that with larger numbers the improvement in mortality now appears statistically significant.

F.H. Epstein, M.D.

Reference

1. Sdriffl H, Lang SM, Konig A, et al: Biocompatible membranes in acute renal failure: Prospective case-controlled study. *Lancet* 344:570–572, 1994.

58 Chronic Renal Failure

Randomised Controlled Trial of Enalapril and β Blockers in Non-Diabetic Chronic Renal Failure

Hannedouche T, Landais P, Goldfarb B, El Esper N, Fournier A, Godin M, Durand D, Chanard J, Mignon F, Suc J-M, Grünfeld J-P (Hôpital Necker, Paris; Hôpital Sud, Amiens, France; Hôpital de Bois-Guillaume, Rouen, France; et al)

BMJ 309:833–837, 1994 119-96-58–1

Purpose.—In insulin-dependent diabetic nephropathy, the rate of progression of renal failure is relatively rapid and uniform. Under these circumstances, antihypertensive therapy in the form of angiotensin-converting enzyme inhibitors and β-blockers is reportedly beneficial. Chronic renal failure caused by other diseases, however, develops by way of more diverse mechanisms and progresses at differing rates. The relative abilities of angiotensin-converting enzyme inhibitors and β-blockers to retard the development of end-stage renal failure in these patients were compared.

Patients and Methods.—A 3-year randomized multicenter trial was conducted wherein 100 nondiabetic patients with hypertension and chronic renal failure received therapy with furosemide in combination with either enalapril (52 patients) or a β-blocker (48 patients). Patients whose diastolic blood pressure exceeded 90 mm Hg were also given a calcium blocker or centrally acting drug.

Findings.—During the study, end-stage renal failure developed in 17 patients receiving conventional (β-blocker) therapy and in 10 patients receiving enalapril. The group of patients treated with enalapril showed a significantly better cumulative renal survival rate than did the patients treated conventionally (Fig p 835). Data from the conventionally treated patients also yielded a significantly steeper slope of the reciprocal serum creatinine concentration curve, although differences between the 2 groups in the rate of change if inulin clearance did not reach the level of statistical significance. The 2 groups did not differ significantly with regard to blood pressure control. Proteinuria diminished from 2.7 ± 1.85 g/24 hr to 1.85 ± 2.01 g/24 hr in patients receiving enalapril but did not change in the conventionally treated group.

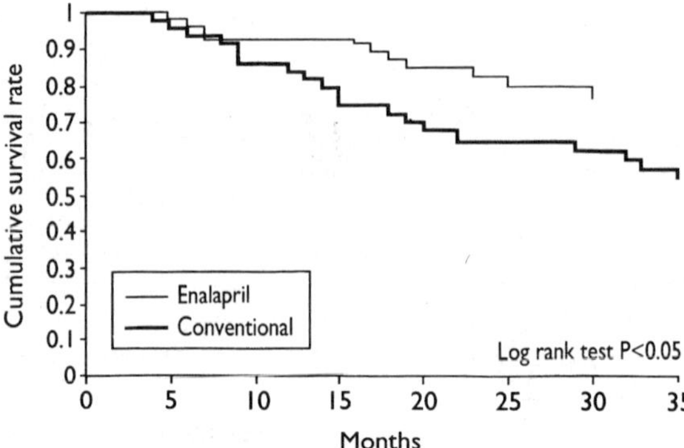

FIGURE p 835.—Survival rate in hypertensive patients treated with enalapril or conventional treatment. (Courtesy of Hannedouche T, Landais P, Goldfarb B, et al: Randomised controlled trial of enalapril and β blockers in non-diabetic chronic renal failure. *BMJ* 309:833–837, 1994.)

Conclusion.—Therapy with enalapril appears more effective than conventional therapy with β-blockers for treatment of nondiabetic patients with hypertension and chronic renal disease. Hypertension aggravates the progression of renal failure. However, because control of blood pressure was similar in both of these groups, the superior actions of angiotensin-converting enzyme inhibitors in slowing the progression of renal failure in these patients may be attributable at least partly to some other mechanism. Possibilities for other modes of action include better long-term reduction of intraglomerular hypertension by enalapril, or a favoring of enalapril by lack of restriction of protein intake. Other proposed protective effects of enalapril include reduced proteinuria, inhibition of the mitogenic action of angiotensin II, preservation of endothelial-cell structure and function, or promotion of local bradykinin activity. Converting-enzyme inhibitors should be used with caution in patients with moderate renal failure, and until further studies have addressed their use for specific forms of nondiabetic renal disease, wide use for all patients with chronic renal failure is not indicated.

► Angiotensin-converting enzyme (ACE) inhibitors appear to have a small edge over other methods of reducing blood pressure in the treatment of hypertensive patients with moderate renal insufficiency—not because they are more effective hypotensive agents, but because over the long term they may reduce the likelihood of progressive scarring of the kidneys. The mechanism of the latter effect is not yet clear, but it is being studied intensively. In addition to being a vasoconstrictor, angiotensin-II (A-II) promotes the growth of fibroblasts and smooth muscle, stimulates the release of endothelin, and increases the synthesis of transforming growth factor-β (TGF-β), which in turn enhances the deposition of extracellular matrix and collagen. Inhibiting the enzymatic synthesis or the action of A-II might therefore, in theory at least, reduce long-term renal scarring. Whether, over the long term, ACE inhibitors actually preserve glomerular filtration better than do other antihypertensive drugs given to patients with nondiabetic renal disease is still controversial.[1]

F.H. Epstein, M.D.

Reference

1. Liou HH, Huang TP, Campese VM: Effect of long-term therapy with captopril on proteinuria and renal function in patients with non–insulin-dependent diabetes and with non-diabetic renal diseases. *Nephron* 69:41–48, 1995.

Vasopressin Resistance in Chronic Renal Failure: Evidence for the Role of Decreased V_2 Receptor mRNA

Teitelbaum I, McGuinness S (Univ of Colorado, Denver)

J Clin Invest 96:378–385, 1995 119-96-58–2

Background.—The mechanism underlying the defect in urinary concentrating ability in chronic renal failure (CRF) is not clear. Studies suggest that the concentrating defect is, in part, attributable to impaired arginine vasopressin (AVP) responsiveness of the collecting duct at both pre- and post-cyclic adenosine monophosphate (cAMP) sites. Further studies were conducted to assess the nature of biochemical defect responsible for the impaired AVP-stimulated adenylyl cyclase activity in CRF.

Methods/Results.—Studies of cAMP accumulation were performed on cultured inner medullary collecting tubule cells from 5/6 nephrectomized rats as models of CRF and control animals. When stimulated with AVP, principal cells in uremic animals failed to accumulate cAMP, whereas control animals exhibited a dose-dependent response to AVP. The lack of responsiveness to AVP in CRF cells was not attributable to alterations in the catalytic unit function nor the stimulatory or inhibitory function of guanine nucleotide-binding proteins. Furthermore, AVP resistance was not restored by treatment with pertussis toxin, cyclooxygenase inhibition with flurbiprofen, or by inhibition or downregulation of protein kinase C. In contrast, CRF cells produced cAMP in response to other agonists of adenyl cyclase, including isoproterenol or prostaglandin E_2, indicating that the defect in CRF cells was unique to AVP. Inner medullary plasma membranes from animals with CRF exhibited a marked decrease in maximum AVP uptake without significant change in maximum uptake for β-adrenergic receptors. The latter observation indicates that the decrease in maximum uptake for the AVP receptor was not simply a consequence of cellular hypertrophy in the presence of CRF but was, indeed, specific to AVP. In support of this observation, reverse transcriptase-polymerase chain reaction of total RNA from the inner medullae of animals with CRF showed no detectable V_2 receptor messenger (mRNA), whereas mRNA for α_2 was present in normal abundance.

Implication.—Inner medullae of rats with CRF exhibit selective decrease in V_2 receptor message and protein product, suggesting that AVP resistance in CRF may be attributable, in part, to selective downregulation of the V_2 receptor.

► Polyuria and reduction in renal concentrating ability are well-known consequences of renal insufficiency. The classical explanation is that these phenomena are the result of an osmotic diuresis (with urea as the main osmotic solute) through the few remaining nephrons. However, this paper shows that the collecting duct cells of partly nephrectomized rats are actually resistant to the action of vasopressin when grown in culture—without being subjected to any diuresis—and that the mRNA message for the antidiuretic hormone receptor is severely downregulated. In this respect, partial renal ablation seems to induce a state not unlike lithium polyuria, which is also resistant to vasopressin but is characterized not by a deficiency of vasopressin receptors, but by downregulation of the apical water channel aquaporin-2.[1]

F.H. Epstein, M.D.

Reference

1. Marples D, Christensen S, Christensen EI, et al: Lithium-induced downregulation of aquaporin-2 water channel expression in rat kidney medulla. *J Clin Invest* 95:1838–1845, 1995.

59 Hypertension

Evidence for Direct Local Effect of Angiotensin in Vascular Hypertrophy: In Vivo Gene Transfer of Angiotensin Converting Enzyme

Morishita R, Gibbons GH, Ellison KE, Lee W, Zhang L, Yu H, Kaneda Y, Ogihara T, Dzau VJ (Stanford Univ, Calif; Osaka Univ, Japan)

J Clin Invest 94:978–984, 1994 119-96-59–1

Introduction.—Vascular remodeling and locally produced biologically active substances contribute to the pathogenesis of vascular diseases. Angiotensin may be an independent factor in vascular pathobiology. An in vivo gene transfer technique allows for the comparison of adjacent transfected and untransfected vessels. This technique was used on intact carotid arteries of the rat permitting study of the biochemical and physiologic results of the overexpression of angiotensin-converting enzyme (ACE) within vessel walls.

Methods.—The human ACE vector was transfected into the carotid arteries of rats by the hemagglutinating virus of Japan–liposome method. Angiotensin-converting enzyme activity was detected in the artery 3 days after transfection. Immunoreactive ACE was localized in the vascular smooth muscle and intimal endothelial cells. A parallel increase in DNA synthesis occurred, which was inhibited by angiotensin II receptor–specific antagonist. Two weeks later, the wall-to-lumen ratio of the transfected vessels increased. The increases in protein and DNA were not accompanied by an increase in cell number. No systemic effects, such as increased heart rate or blood pressure, from the procedure were found.

Conclusion.—Vascular angiotensin system has a direct role in the vascular hypertrophy process of hypertension. These changes are independent of systemic changes. The local gene transfer technique has potential to examine complex pathophysiologic processes in vivo and to suggest the development of new therapeutic directions.

► The conversion of angiotensinogen to angiotensin-II (A-II) is catalyzed by ACE. This rate-limiting enzyme is present in (and produced by) the walls of blood vessels, so that local production of angiotensin-II is likely to play a key role in certain vascular phenomena, quite apart from the level of ACE or A-II in the circulating blood. Because A-II stimulates growth of smooth muscle and the deposition of extracellular matrix, an increase in tissue concentration of ACE might enhance vascular hypertrophy, remodeling, and arteriosclerosis. These speculations are given substance by the present study. Local transfection of the genetic message (cDNA) for ACE into the carotid artery of rats induced substantial medial hypertrophy, without altering systemic blood pressure or the concentration of ACE in peripheral blood. Thus, changes in the production of A-II in peripheral tissues might be important in the pathogenesis of vascular disease.

The next paper touches on the same question, using an epidemiologic approach.

F.H. Epstein, M.D.

Different Frequencies of Angiotensin-Converting Enzyme Genotypes in Older Hypertensive Individuals

Morris BJ, Zee RYL, Schrader AP (Univ of Sydney, Australia)

J Clin Invest 94:1085–1089, 1994 119-96-59–2

Introduction.—The main functions of angiotensin-I–converting enzyme (ACE) are the conversion of angiotensin I to angiotensin II and the inactivation of kinins with natriuretic and vasodilator activities. Angiotensin I–converting enzyme is found in widespread locations such as the endothelial cells of all major vascular beds, absorptive epithelia, the choroid plexus, and fluids such as plasma and CSF. Concentrations of ACE track with the deletion (D) allele of the insertion/deletion polymorphism. Plasma concentrations of ACE are higher in the DD than in the ID and II genotypes. The DD genotype seems to contribute to a variety of fatal cardiovascular events in Asians and Caucasians. If the DD genotype is a risk factor for premature death, then the frequency of the population with DD should decrease with age. The hypothesis was tested by studying a specially selected group of individuals at high risk because of genetic factors.

Methods.—The controls were 196 offspring of parents who were normotensive after the age of 50 years. The experimental group was comprised of 118 white people with hypertension (HT) who had parents who were both hypertensive. All HT individuals had diastolic pressures > 100 mm Hg; all the normotensive individuals had diastolic pressures < 90 mm Hg. The DD genotype and ACE activity were determined in all individuals.

Findings.—The frequency of the DD genotype in normotensive individuals was 0.42, whereas in the HT, the frequency decreased from 0.28 in those younger than 50 years to 0.26 in those 50–59 years to 0.10 in those older than 59 years. The DD genotype was only 14% of the expected in HT individuals older than 60 years of age. No relationship with body mass index, sex, or blood pressure was found. Plasma concentrations of ACE were similar in the normotensive and hypertensive patients.

Conclusion.—A group of specially selected patients with HT showed a decrease in the DD genotype with progression in age. It is possible that the DD genotype increases the risk of premature death in patients with HT and a strong family history of this disease.

► These results suggest the possibility that inheritance of a double dose of the D allele of the gene coding for angiotensin-converting enzyme would increase the effective concentration of angiotensin II (A-II) in peripheral blood vessels. This might predispose to vascular disease resulting in early death—so that fewer and fewer DD individuals would remain alive later in life. The argument sounds a bit overextended to me, but in conjunction with the previous abstract, this study emphasizes an important principle—the likelihood that the peripheral action of A-II, modulated by local production of all the members of the A-II cascade as well as A-II receptors, plays an important role in the pathophysiology of diseases of the blood vessels. Provocative contributory evidence includes: (1) linkage of the angiotensinogen gene, in some studies, to essential hypertension and preeclampsia,[1] and (2) implication of increased expression of the vascular A-II receptor in glucocorticoid-induced hypertension.[2]

F.H. Epstein, M.D.

References

1. 1995 Year Book of Medicine, pp 725–728.
2. 1995 Year Book of Medicine, pp 732–733.

Biochemical Effects of Losartan, a Nonpeptide Angiotensin II Receptor Antagonist, on the Renin-Angiotensin-Aldosterone System in Hypertensive Patients

Goldberg MR, Bradstreet TE, McWilliams EJ, Tanaka WK, Lipert S, Bjornsson TD, Waldman SA, Osborne B, Pivadori L, Lewis G, Blum R, Herman T, Abraham PA, Halstenson CN, Lo M-W, Lu H, Spector R (Thomas Jefferson Univ, Philadelphia; Clinical Pharmacology Ctr, New Bedford, Mass; Clinical Pharmacokinetics Lab, Buffalo, NY; et al)

Hypertension 25:37–46, 1995 119-96-59–3

Background.—Losartan potassium is an angiotensin II (A-II) type 1 (At_1)-selective, nonpeptide receptor antagonist that increases both plasma renin activity (PRA) and A-II levels. The biochemical responses of hypertensive patients to 6 weeks of treatment with losartan were compared with responses to placebo and enalapril in a multicenter, double-blind, placebo-controlled, parallel study.

Methods.—Fifty-one nonblack, otherwise healthy adult patients with essential hypertension and supine diastolic blood pressure of 95–110 mm Hg were enrolled. After a 2- to 4-week tapering/placebo run-in period, the patients were randomly allocated to 4 groups: placebo, 25 mg of losartan, 100 mg of losartan, or 20 mg of enalapril daily. Blood pressure, renin-angiotensin-aldosterone system mediators, and plasma drug concentrations were measured multiple times during an initial 4-day inpatient evaluation, and at 2 and 6 weeks after treatment.

Results.—After the first and last doses of losartan, the plasma drug levels were similar. The antihypertensive activities of 100 mg of losartan

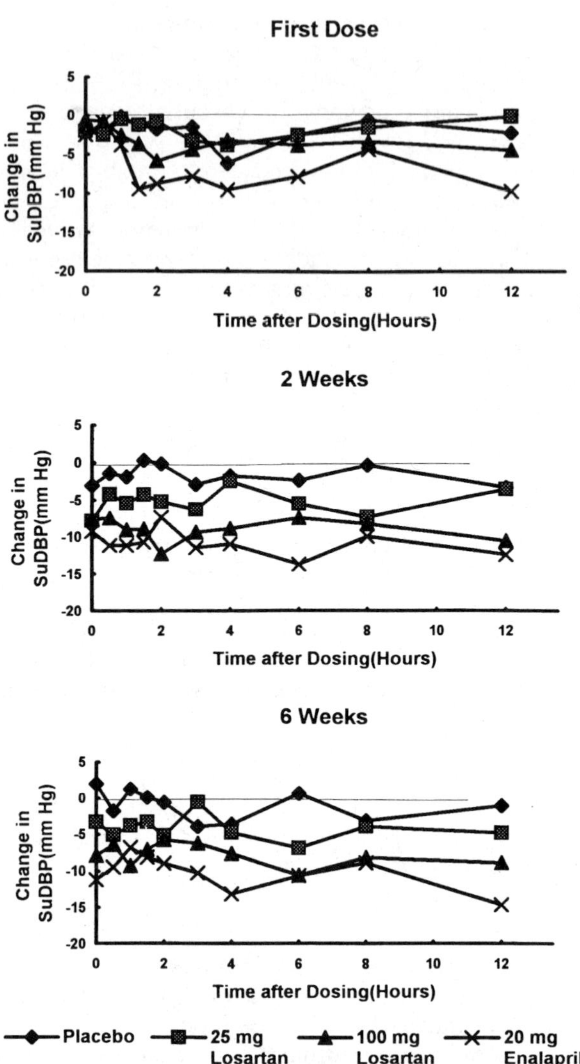

FIGURE 2.—Line graph showing changes from run-in day of supine diastolic blood pressure (*SuDBP*). Values are mean changes from the corresponding time relative to dosing at run-in of SuDBP to the same relative time after 6 weeks of double-blind therapy. Study drug was given at hour 0. Mean measurements at run-in did not differ among the groups. In the 100-mg losartan group, respective run-in measurements at 0, 1, 2, 3, 4, 6, 8, and 12 hours (n = 14) were 100.2, 99.6, 95.9, 92.5, 93.9, 91.0, 93.3, and 94.4 mm Hg (SD = 6.2–8.4 mm Hg). (Reproduced with permission. [*Hypertension.*] Copyright [1995] American Heart Association.)

and 20 mg of enalapril were similar at 6 weeks (Fig 2). The 25-mg dose of losartan had a smaller antihypertensive effect. Four hours after a dose, 100 mg of losartan increased PRA 1.7-fold and A-II 2.5-fold; enalapril increased PRA 2.8-fold and decreased A-II fourfold. Both losartan and enalapril decreased the plasma aldosterone concentration. Losartan-induced increases in PRA and A-II were greater at 2 weeks than at 6 weeks. The changes in PRA and plasma A-II level were similar to placebo changes within 36 hours of stopping losartan. One patient receiving 100 mg of losartan daily had symptomatic orthostatic hypotension.

Conclusions.—Losartan, a selective, orally active AT_1-receptor antagonist, is an effective antihypertensive agent at a dosage of 100 mg daily. Long-term (6 weeks) blockage of the feedback of the A-II receptors causes modest increases in plasma renin activity and A-II levels, but the antihypertensive response to the antagonist (losartan) is not affected.

► I selected this paper because it is typical of a number of descriptions of a new class of drugs that block A-II receptors and are now available for administration to patients. The A-II receptor antagonists can be expected to have the same general effects as inhibitors of angiotensin-converting enzyme (ACE); they lower blood pressure, protect rats with reduced renal mass against the progression of renal insufficiency,[1] and reduce plasma concentrations of aldosterone. They can be expected to predispose to hyperkalemia, especially in the elderly, and to renal failure in patients with renal artery stenosis. They may be a useful alternative for patients who have cough when receiving ACE inhibitors, because that symptom is thought to be the result of the unavoidable inhibition by those drugs of the enzyme kininase-2, responsible for bradykinin hydrolysis in the lung.[2] Losartan does not have that action. For the same reason, losartan and its congeners may not be effective hypotensive agents in patients with low-renin hypertension, even though ACE inhibitors (because they inhibit the destruction of vasodilatory kinins) may be able to lower blood pressure.

F.H. Epstein, M.D.

References

1. Mackenzie HS, Troy JL, Rennke HG, et al: TCV 116 prevents progressive renal injury in rats with extensive renal mass ablation. *J Hypertension* 12:11S–16S, 1994.
2. Lacourière Y, Brunner H, Irwin R, et al: Effect of modulators of the renin-angiotensin-aldosterone system on cough. *J Hypertension* 12:1387–1393, 1994.

Low-Dose Drug Combination Therapy: An Alternative First-Line Approach to Hypertension Treatment

Prisant LM, Weir MR, Papademetriou V, Weber MA, Adegbile IA, Alemayehu D, Lefkowitz MP, Carr AA (Med College of Georgia, Augusta; Univ of Maryland, Baltimore; Georgetown Univ, Washington, DC; et al)

Am Heart J 130:359–366, 1995 119-96-59–4

Background.—A remarkably poor blood pressure control rate at 21% has been recently reported in the United States. Single-drug therapy with several classes of antihypertensive agents lowers blood pressure through different mechanisms of action, but none of these agents are devoid of side effects, many of which are dose-dependent. An alternative approach is to combine low doses of 2 antihypertensive agents with different modes of action and additive effects.

Study Design.—In a randomized, double-blind parallel group, dose-escalation trial, the efficacy and safety of a low-dose combination of the β-blocker bisoprolol, and the diuretic hydrochlorothiazide (HCTZ) as initial treatment for mild-to-moderate hypertension (diastolic blood pressure between 95 and 114 mm Hg) was compared with the usual doses of the angiotensin-converting enzyme inhibitor enalapril and the calcium antagonist amlodipine. After a 4- to 5-week placebo washout period, 218 patients were treated either with amlodipine (2.5–10 mg), enalapril (5–20 mg), or the low-dose combination of bisoprolol (2.5–10 mg) with HCTZ 6.25 mg. All drugs were administered once daily, titrated to optimal response for 4 weeks, with the final titrated dose maintained for 8 weeks.

Results.—The response rates (diastolic blood pressure ≤ 90 mm Hg or a ≥ 10 mm Hg decrease from baseline) were 71% for bisoprolol–6.25 mg HCTZ, 69% for amlodipine, and 45% for enalapril. The mean decreases in systolic/diastolic blood pressure from baseline were 13.4/10.7 mm Hg for bisoprolol–6.25 HCTZ, 12.8/10.2 mm Hg for amlodipine, and 7.3/6.6 mm Hg for enalapril. The change with enalapril was significantly less than that with the other drugs, but the once-daily dosing of enalapril and the maximum dose of 20 mg might not have been optimal for this agent. The incidence of adverse experiences and early withdrawal from therapy tended to be lower with the low-dose bisoprolol-HCTZ combination. Side effects, such as fatigue and insomnia, and adverse metabolic effects often associated with diuretics and β-blockers were infrequent. Changes in the quality of life, as measured by the General Well-Being Index, did not deteriorate in any treatment group, with scores of +0.9 for bisoprolol-6.25 mg HCTZ, +0.5 for amlodipine, and −2.3 for enalapril, with a positive change indicating improvement.

Conclusion.—The combination of low doses of 2 antihypertensive agents with differing modes of action and additive effects is as effective as single-agent drugs without the adverse effects often associated with full-dose monotherapy. Low-dose combination therapy with bisoprolol–6.25 HCTZ appears to be a rational and effective alternative for the initial treatment of mild to moderate hypertension.

► The general approach exemplified by this paper deserves attention. Small doses of antihypertensive medications with differing mechanisms of action are likely to be synergistic. This may permit effective control of blood pressure without incurring the side effects associated with higher doses of either pharmacologic agent given alone. We've known for some time that 12.5 mg of hydrochlorothiazide daily would lower blood pressure almost as much as a dose 4 times as large, with less risk of potassium depletion. An even smaller dose, 6.25 mg, seemed effective in this study when given in combination with a small dose of β-adrenergic inhibitor. It's likely that similar combinations of thiazides with calcium-channel inhibitors or angiotensin-converting enzyme inhibitors would enhance the effect of these drugs and reduce their tendency to cause edema.

F.H. Epstein, M.D.

Sympathetic Activation in Obese Normotensive Subjects

Grassi G, Seravalle G, Cattaneo BM, Bolla GB, Lanfranchi A, Colombo M, Giannattasio C, Brunani A, Cavagnini F, Mancia G (Università di Milano, Italy; Centro Auxologico Italiano, Milano)

Hypertension 25:560–563, 1995 119-96-59–5

Objective.—It is not clear whether obesity is characterized by adrenergic activation. Microneurography, a technique that allows direct, precise, and reproducible measurement of sympathetic neural discharge from the human peroneal or brachial nerves, was used to determine whether muscle sympathetic nerve activity is modified by obesity.

Methods.—Ten young obese men with a mean body mass index of 40.5 kg/m^2 and normal blood pressure were studied. Eight age-matched lean normotensive men were also studied. All individuals underwent measurement of beat-to-beat arterial blood pressure (using the Finapres technique), heart rate, postganglionic muscle sympathetic nerve activity (with microneurography), and venous plasma level of norepinephrine under baseline conditions. Except for plasma norepinephrine, changes in these parameters were monitored during baroreceptor stimulation and deactivation caused by increases and reductions of blood pressure via IV infusions of phenylephrine and nitroprusside.

Results.—The baseline blood pressure, heart rate, and plasma levels of norepinephrine were similar in obese and control men, but muscle sympathetic nerve activity was about twice as high in obese individuals as in controls. Muscle sympathetic nerve activity and heart rate decreased during phenylephrine infusion and increased during nitroprusside infusion, but these changes were significantly smaller in obese individuals than in lean controls.

Implications.—Human obesity, even in the absence of any blood pressure elevation, is characterized by marked sympathetic activation, possibly because of an impairment of reflex sympathetic restraint. The pronounced sympathetic activation in obese normotensive individuals may facilitate, in the long term, the development of hypertension and other cardiovascular complications, including arrhythmias and sudden death. It will be important to determine whether a reduction in body weight may reverse the autonomic alterations associated with obesity.

► These observations in obese human subjects whose blood pressures were normal confirm an important hypothesis originally advanced by Landsberg and Young on the basis of animal experiments—that overeating activates the sympathetic nervous system.[1] Using direct electric recordings from the peroneal nerve, sympathetic discharges were found to be about twice as frequent in obese subjects as in nonobese controls. It is interesting that plasma norepinephrine—known to be an insensitive measure of peripheral sympathetic activity—was similar in the 2 groups. These data and those of others[2] provide strong pathophysiologic evidence for the role of weight gain in contributing to human hypertension.

F.H. Epstein, M.D.

References

1. Landsberg L, Young JB: Fasting, feeding and regulation of the sympathetic nervous system. *N Engl J Med* 298:1295–1301, 1978.
2. Troisi RJ, Weiss ST, Parker DR, et al: Relation of obesity to sympathetic nervous activity. *Hypertension* 17:669–677, 1991.

Prolonged Increase in Blood Pressure by a Single Oral Dose of Caffeine in Mildly Hypertensive Men

Sung BH, Whitsett TL, Lovallo WR, al'Absi M, Pincomb GA, Wilson MF (State Univ of New York, Buffalo; Univ of Oklahoma Health Sciences Ctr, Oklahoma City)

Am J Hypertens 7:755–758, 1994 119-96-59-6

Background.—Although previous reports have shown that acutely administered caffeine increases blood pressure in normotensive individuals, few studies have addressed cardiovascular effects in hypertensive populations. The blood pressure responses of patients with hypertension after ingestion of a single dosc of caffeine were investigated and compared with those of normotensive individuals.

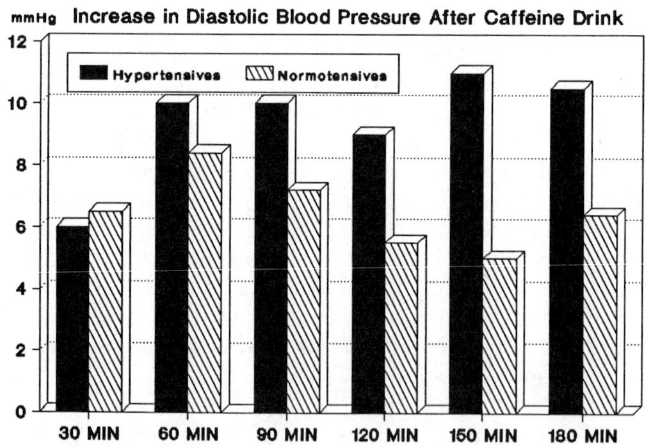

FIGURE 1.—Comparison of an increase in diastolic blood pressures in normotensive and hypertensive subjects after a single dose of caffeine. Values are net caffeine-placebo difference scores at each period. *Solid bar* represents hypertensive group and *hatched bar* represents normotensive group. (Reprinted by permission of Elsevier Science, Inc. Sung BH, Whitsett TL, Lovallo WR, et al: Prolonged increase in blood pressure by a single oral dose of caffeine in mildly hypertensive men. *Am J Hypertens* 7:755–758, 1994. Copyright 1994 by American Journal of Hypertension, Inc.)

Participants and Methods.—Thirty men aged 30–45 years were studied. Of these, 18 were hypertensive and 12 were normotensive. All men were well matched for age, height, body surface area, and daily caffeine consumption. The participants consumed a single oral dose of caffeine, 3.3 mg/kg (equal to 2–3 cups of coffee). Hemodynamic measurements were performed at baseline and at 30-minute intervals after caffeine ingestion for a total of 3 hours.

Results.—At baseline, the hypertensive men had a significantly higher heart rate, blood pressure, and peripheral vascular resistance than the normotensive men. Cardiac output and stroke volume were similar between groups. After caffeine ingestion, systolic blood pressures were significantly higher in both groups for the entire 3 hours. Hypertensive men demonstrated persistent elevation in diastolic blood pressure for 3 hours. In normotensive men, the increment of diastolic blood pressure became smaller at 90 minutes after caffeine intake (Fig 1).

Conclusions.—Caffeine consumption may affect both the diagnosis and treatment of hypertension. Abstinence from caffeine may be useful, particularly for individuals with hypertension.

▶ The effect of caffeine on blood pressure seems to depend on whether the individual is habituated to caffeine. Coffee increases blood pressure in caffeine-naive or nontolerant persons but not in regular coffee drinkers.[1] Thus, withdrawal of coffee from mildly hypertensive patients accustomed to drinking at least 3 cups a day had no discernible effect on blood pressure.[2, 3] In this study, however, the ingestion of caffeine in the morning appeared to increase blood pressure slightly, especially in hypertensive men, some of whom used coffee infrequently. The hypertensive effects of coffee, therefore, are probably variable and not as important in most patients as the effects of alcohol and obesity.

F.H. Epstein, M.D.

References

1. Sharp DS, Benowitz NL: Pharmacoepidemiology of the effects of caffeine on blood pressure. *Clin Pharmacol Ther* 47:57–60, 1990.
2. MacDonald TM, Sharpe K, Fowler G, et al: Caffeine restriction: Effect on mild hypertension. *BMJ* 303:1235–1238, 1991.
3. Eggersten R, Andreasson A, Hedner T, et al: Effect of coffee on ambulatory blood pressure in patients with treated hypertension. *J Intern Med* 233:301–305, 1993.

Hypertension After Renal Transplantation: Calcium Channel or Converting Enzyme Blockade?

van der Schaaf MR, Hené RJ, Floor M, Blankestijn PJ, Koomans HA (Univ Hosp Utrecht, The Netherlands)
Hypertension 25:77–81, 1995 119-96-59–7

Background.—Although cyclosporine A (CsA) has improved graft survival after renal transplantation, up to 70% of patients who receive CsA have hypertension. The immunosuppressive drug may also induce marked renal vasoconstriction. A double-blind crossover trial was designed to compare the effects on blood pressure and renal function of 4 weeks of a calcium-channel blocker (amlodipine) vs. those of an angiotensin-converting enzyme (ACE) inhibitor (lisinopril).

Patients and Methods.—Study participants were 20 renal transplant patients with CsA-induced hypertension. The group included 12 men and 8 women, had a mean age of 42.8 years, and was a mean of 3.3 years after transplant. Eighteen grafts were from cadaveric donors, and 2 were from related living donors. Nine patients had been hypertensive before transplantation. After at least 2 weeks devoted to tapering their hypertensive medication, patients received placebo for 2 weeks and were then randomly assigned to receive amlodipine or lisinopril, each at 5 mg once daily. The patients were switched to the other drug after 4 weeks of active treatment and a second washout placebo period of 4 weeks. During each active drug treatment period, the dose was doubled if blood pressure exceeded 150/95 mg Hg after 2 weeks.

Results.—After titration the average dosage of each drug was 8.5 mg/day. The calcium-channel blocker was significantly more effective than the same dose of ACE inhibitor in controlling hypertension. Although blood pressure during both treatments was lower than during placebo, amlodipine was associated with a significant increase in glomerular filtration rate and effective renal plasma flow and a decrease in renal vascular resistance. Lisinopril treatment did not alter renal hemodynamics. Proteinuria, noted in 13 cases, was similar during amlodipine, lisinopril, and placebo periods.

Conclusion.—Amlodipine, a calcium-channel blocker, had a somewhat more pronounced antihypertensive effect in these patients with CsA-induced hypertension after renal transplantation. This drug, unlike the ACE inhibitor lisinopril, led to an increase in glomerular filtration rate and effective renal plasma flow and a decrease in renal vascular resistance. It would appear that the renin-angiotensin system plays no more than a minor role in determining CsA-associated changes in renal hemodynamics and only a limited role in determining CsA-associated hypertension.

► These results are consistent with other data suggesting that calcium-channel blockade is more effective than ACE inhibition in controlling the hypertension of chronic renal disease while entailing less chance of simultaneously reducing the glomerular filtration rate.[1] Certain calcium-blocking agents (e.g., diltiazem) have an added bonus in renal transplant recipients because they interfere with the disposal of CsA. Co-administration of diltiazem to patients receiving cyclosporine not only tends to keep blood pressure normal, but also reduces the dose of cyclosporine necessary to achieve immunosuppressive levels in the circulating blood and therefore saves money.

F.H. Epstein, M.D.

Reference

1. 1993 Year Book of Medicine, pp 627–629.

60 Transplantation

Mycophenolate Mofetil for the Prevention of Acute Rejection in Primary Cadaveric Renal Allograft Recipients

Sollinger HW, for the US Renal Transplant Mycophenolate Mofetil Study Group (Univ of Wisconsin, Madison)

Transplantation 60:225–232, 1995 119-96-60–1

Background.—Mycophenolate mofetil (MMF) is a new immunosuppressive agent that reversibly inhibits inosine monophosphate dehydrogenases and selectively inhibits the proliferation of both T and B lymphocytes. Mycophenolate mofetil is more bioavailable when given orally than is mycophenolic acid.

Objective.—A randomized double-blind trial was designed to determine whether the risk of acute rejection—the major cause of loss of transplanted cadaveric kidneys—is lessened by treatment with MMF.

Methods.—A total of 499 adult patients at 14 centers in the United States who were scheduled to receive their first cadaveric kidney allograft were randomly assigned to receive MMF in a dose of 1.0 or 1.5 g twice daily or azathioprine in a dose of 1–2 mg/kg daily. Patients in all groups received additional immunosuppressive therapy including cyclosporine A, steroids, and antithymocyte globulin.

Efficacy.—The incidence of biopsy-proven acute rejection or treatment failure within 6 months of transplantation was 47.6% in azathioprine-treated patients and 31.1% in both MMF-treated groups, a significant reduction. The rate of graft loss or death without biopsy-proven rejection was 3.6% in the azathioprine group, 1.8% in patients given 2 g of MMF daily, and 1.2% in those given the higher dose of MMF. Patients in all groups received comparable amounts of steroids and cyclosporine in the maintenance phase. Patients prepared with azathioprine required more immunosuppressive therapy subsequently and had higher serum creatinine values.

Safety.—Anemia and hypertension were comparably frequent in all treatment groups, but diarrhea was more frequent in patients given MMF. There was no significant difference in the risk of opportunistic infection. Three MMF-treated patients had lymphoma or lymphoproliferative disorder.

Conclusions.—Mycophenolate mofetil is a very effective means of preventing acute rejection in recipients of primary cadaveric kidney allografts, and it appears to be acceptably safe. Whether this new immunosuppressive agent improves long-term graft survival remains to be established.

► Biopsy-proven acute rejection episodes or treatment failure occurred in 47.6% of patients in the azathioprine group compared with 31.1% (P = 0.0015) of the patients in the treatment group receiving 2 g of MMF. and 31.3% (P = 0.0021) of patients in the 3 g treatment groups. Time to first biopsy-proven rejection episode or treatment failure was significantly longer for 2 g of MMF vs. azathioprine (P = 0.0036) and 3 g of MMF vs. azathioprine (P = 0.0006). First biopsy-proven rejection alone occurred in 38.0% of patients who received azathioprine compared with 19.8% of patients who received 2 g of MMF and 17.5% of those who received 3 g. Patients in the azathioprine group received a greater number of full courses of antirejection treatment (44.5%) than did those receiving 2 g of MMF (24.8%) and 3 g of MMF groups (21.1%). The use of antilymphocyte agents to treat rejection was greater in the azathioprine group (20.1%) compared with the group receiving 2 g of MMF group (10.3%) and the group taking 3 g of MMF (5.4%). At 6 months after transplant, graft and patient survival were similar in all 3 treatment groups. The incidence and types of adverse events were similar among treatment groups, with the exception of a higher incidence of diarrhea, certain other infrequent gastrointestinal adverse events, clinically important leukopenia, and tissue-invasive cytomegalovirus disease in the MMF groups, particularly in the group taking 3 g. Three patients who received MMF had lymphoma/lymphoproliferative disorder. This study demonstrated that MMF administered at a dose of 2 g or 3 g daily, in combination with maintenance cyclosporine A and corticosteroids as triple therapy after ATGAM induction therapy, is more effective than an otherwise identical regimen that includes azathioprine instead of MMF in preventing acute allograft rejection in patients receiving a first cadaveric renal transplant. This regimen also has an acceptable adverse event profile. The 3-g dose of MMF was considered to be somewhat less well tolerated than the 2-g dose.

T.B. Strom, M.D.

Placebo-Controlled Study of Mycophenolate Mofetil Combined With Cyclosporin and Corticosteroids for Prevention of Acute Rejection

European Mycophenolate Mofetil Cooperative Study Group (Medizinische Hochschule Hannover, Klinik für Abdominal und Transplantationschirurgie, Germany)

Lancet 345:1321–1325, 1995 119-96-60–2

Objective.—Mycophenolate mofetil (MMF) is an immunosuppressant that was developed to prevent the important clinical problem of acute allograft rejection seen in 60% of renal transplant recipients. The efficacy of MMF when given with cyclosporine and corticosteroids was assessed in a 1-year, multicenter, double-blind, placebo-controlled study.

Patients and Study Design.—Four hundred ninety-one male and female recipients of first or second cadaveric renal allografts were divided into 3 groups: placebo (166 patients), MMF at 2 g/day (165 patients), and MMF at 3 g/day (160 patients). Daily doses of cyclosporine and corticosteroids were adjusted as needed. For 1 year, the patients were observed for allograft rejection or treatment failure and all adverse effects.

Results.—Significantly fewer patients in the 2 MMF treatment groups withdrew prematurely from the study or had biopsy-proven rejection. The frequency of acute rejection episodes was reduced 60% to 70% by the addition of MMF to corticosteroid and cyclosporine therapy. The relative risk of treatment failure was reduced to 0.535 for MMF 2 g and 0.65 for MMF 3 g, compared with placebo. Fewer patients in the MMF treatment groups required a full course of immunosuppressive treatment for rejection: 86 patients in the placebo group, 47 in the MMF 2-g group, and 39 in the MMF 3-g group. Also, there were fewer courses of treatment with antilymphocyte preparations, lower serum creatinine concentrations, and a lower percentage of patients needing dialysis for patients in the MMF treatment groups compared to those in the placebo group. Gastrointestinal adverse events, leukopenia, anemia, and cytomegalovirus tissue-invasive disease were more common in the MMF treatment groups than in the control group.

Conclusions.—The number of patients with a biopsy-proven rejection episode or treatment failure was significantly lower in the MMF treatment groups than in the placebo group. Although there was a greater frequency of gastrointestinal adverse effects and leukopenia in the MMF treatment groups, a clear clinical advantage of reduced need for antilymphocyte therapy for corticosteroid-resistant rejection with MMF treatment was noted.

▶ Mycophenolate mofetil, a newly developed metabolite, has been approved by the Food and Drug Administration (FDA) for use in patients receiving a kidney transplant. Mycophenolate mofetil is the 2-morpholinoethyl ester of mycophenolic acid. It is a reversible inhibitor of inosine monophosphate dehydrogenase and thereby inhibits the de novo pathway of purine synthesis. Lymphocytes, unlike most other cell types, rely on the de novo pathway more than the salvage pathway for purine synthesis. Another purine inhibitor, azathioprine, has long been used as part of the immunosuppressive regimen applied to many transplant patients. Thus, mycophenolate mofetil and azathioprine were directly compared as components of an aggressive quadruple drug protocol in a multicenter trial conducted in the United States (Abstract 119-96-60–1). The results proved that mycophenolate mofetil is an effective immunosuppressive agent. The incidence of early rejection episodes was diminished in patients receiving this drug, yet the outcomes at 1 year, as measured by the proportion of functioning grafts or the level of graft function, were not superior to that observed in the standard treatment group. It was surprising that the incidence of side effects in patients receiving mycophenolate mofetil—putatively more lymphocyte-specific in action—was not less than that noted in the control group. Overimmunosuppression, as detected through the occurrence of lymphoma/lymphoproliferative disease and cytomegalovirus infection, was noted in the mycophenolate mofetil group.

Another recent clinical trial of mycophenolate mofetil therapy was completed in Europe (Abstract 119-96-60–2), using a somewhat less aggressive immunosuppressive protocol. The results of the European trial were quite similar to those discerned in the American trial.

In this age of cost containment it will be interesting to observe the patterns of mycophenolate mofetil usage. The drug is far more costly than azathioprine and the outcome at 6 months was not substantially improved over the results achieved using azathioprine. Nonetheless, the additional treatments needed to treat rejection episodes in the azathioprine group are costly, and there is a strong statistical correlation between the occurrence of early rejection episodes and hastened chronic rejection. Is the mycophenolate mofetil cup half-filled or half-empty?

T.B. Strom, M.D.

High Survival Rates of Kidney Transplants From Spousal and Living Unrelated Donors

Terasaki PI, Cecka JM, Gjertson DW, Takemoto S (Univ of California, Los Angeles)

N Engl J Med 333:333–336, 1995 119-96-60–3

Introduction.—Because of the unexpectedly high survival rates of kidney grafts from spouses and other living unrelated donors, transplantations from living unrelated donors have been used increasingly in patients with end-stage renal disease. The survival rates of these grafts, although typically mismatched for HLA antigens, are significantly higher than those of mismatched cadaveric grafts. The factors contributing to the high survival rates of grafts from living unrelated donors were examined.

Methods.—The survival rates of kidney grafts from 368 spouses, 129 living unrelated donors, 3,368 parents, 1,984 HLA-identical siblings, 1,411 children, and 43,341 cadavers were compared using data from the United Network for Organ Sharing Renal Transplant Registry.

Results.—The grafts' 3-year survival rates were 85% for kidneys from spouses, 81% for kidneys from living unrelated donors, 82% for kidneys from parents, 91% from HLA-identical siblings, 84% for kidneys from children, and 70% for cadaveric kidneys. Preoperative transfusions improved the 3-year survival rate of grafts from spouses from 81% to 90%. Because HLA matching was better with cadaveric grafts than with grafts from spouses or other living donors, HLA matching does not account for the differences in graft survival. In addition, the improved graft survival with kidneys from spouses and other living unrelated donors could not be attributed to donor age or the duration of cold ischemia. However, the cadaveric grafts that functioned on the first day had significantly higher survival rates than those that did not function on the first day, regardless of HLA matching. Cadaveric grafts that functioned on the first day and had no HLA-a, B, or DR mismatches had survival rates similar to those of grafts from spouses.

Conclusions.—Kidney grafts from living unrelated donors have higher survival rates than cadaveric kidney grafts, even though they typically have more HLA mismatching. This is probably attributable to damage sustained in approximately 10% of cadaveric kidneys before removal.

► The development of end-stage renal failure and the attendant requirement for renal replacement therapy have a marked adverse effect on the quality of life of the spouse of the affected patient. Insofar as renal transplantation offers the best hope of rehabilitating the patient, the spouse of that patient has a vested interest in successful rehabilitation. For these reasons, a growing number of centers now consider ABO blood group–compatible spouses acceptable candidates for kidney transplant organ donation.

The frequency with which spousal donors will be approached for organ donation will probably increase as a consequence of this analysis, because the rate and duration of successful engraftment of spousal donor kidney transplants are excellent, perhaps surprisingly so. With the exception of the rare perfectly matched HLA transplant, the success achieved with transplanted organs obtained from genetically unrelated spousal donors is far superior to the results achieved using unrelated cadaver donor organs.

As compared with cadaver donor transplantation, the donor evaluation is far more complete. There is no need for split-second decision-making. The potential donor can be evaluated through measures of glomerular filtration, not just blood urea nitrogen and serum creatinine. Because normal or near normal levels of blood urea nitrogen and creatinine can be found in patients—especially small or elderly individuals—with abysmal glomerular filtration rate, the ability to evaluate the donor carefully is not a trivial advantage. In addition, in living donors, the requirement for prolonged extracorporeal preservation is obviated, along with its attendant problems.

These gratifying results have encouraged us to broaden the circle of potential kidney transplant donors. This article represents a very positive step in underlining the potential value of obtaining living donors for transplantation. The article, by implication, points to the pitfalls in our approach to evaluation of the cadaveric donor.

T.B. Strom, M.D.

The Impact of HLA Mismatches on the Survival of First Cadaveric Kidney Transplants

Held PJ, Kahan BD, Hunsicker LG, Liska D, Wolfe RA, Port FK, Gaylin DS, Garcia JR, Agodoa LYC, Krakauer H (Univ of Michigan, Ann Arbor; Univ of Texas, Houston; Univ of Iowa Hosp and Clinics, Iowa City; et al)

N Engl J Med 331:765–770, 1995 119-96-60–4

Background.—The survival of renal grafts and of patients with end-stage renal disease undergoing cadaveric renal transplantation has improved greatly in the past decade. Authorities continue to disagree on the importance of HLA mismatches in cadaveric transplantation. The effects of HLA-A, B, and DR mismatches on a large group of cadaveric implants and the potential impact of a national policy to maximize HLA matching for cadaveric grafts were investigated.

Methods.—Data on 30,564 Medicare patients receiving a first cadaveric kidney transplant between 1984 and 1990 were obtained for analysis. Graft survival was estimated by proportional-hazards methods, with adjustment for patient and donor characteristics. A simulated allocation of organs to 20,000 candidates for transplantation was analyzed to determine the effects of minimal achievable HLA mismatches and maximal matching on graft survival.

Findings.—For grafts with no mismatches, the adjusted 1-year graft survival was 84.3%. For grafts with 4 mismatches, it was 77%. Minimal mismatching and maximal matching achieved through national rationing of donor organs could reduce the mean number of HLA mismatches from 3.6 to 1.2, with a corresponding rise in the number of matches. Consequently, the projected 5-year graft survival may increase from 58.5% to 62.9%. However, the proportion of kidneys given to black recipients would decline from 22.2% to 15%.

Conclusions.—A maximal-matching program would probably improve the 5-year graft survival by about 2 percentage points. It is debatable whether this benefit is worth the economic and social cost involved. The adverse effects of ischemic injury suggest a potential advantage to shortening organ-storage times.

► There is no doubt that transplantation of histocompatible cadaveric donor grafts improves the rate and length of engraftment. This effect is particularly evident in the setting of HLA-identical donors and recipients. Nonetheless, a great deal of HLA typing is done nowadays, enabling a few HLA-identical matches to emerge.

There is a downside to this effort: time and cost. The quality of cadaveric donor organs deteriorates during the preservation period at a steady rate. Quality histocompatibility matching requires a large, geographically dispersed pool of donors and recipients. It requires time to ship these organs. The benefits of quick transplantation and HLA matching run at cross purposes. Although the "fine-print conclusions" of this report are subject to debate, the broad conclusions appear valid. This analysis—among other considerations—has stimulated Terasaki and others in the transplant community to try to identify less stringent markers for histocompatibility than the "fine" HLA specificities (e.g., broad, "public" specificities) in the hope that a smaller and geographically more compact pool of donors and recipients may suffice. In this way, we might work toward rapid engraftment of histocompatible organs. An effort to evaluate this approach is well under way.

T.B. Strom, M.D.

Risk of Neoplasia in Renal Transplant Patients

London NJ, Farmery SM, Will EJ, Davison AM, Lodge JPA (St James's Univ Hosp, Leeds, England)

Lancet 346:403–406, 1995 119-96-60–5

Purpose.—Renal transplant recipients are at increased risk of neoplasia. However, much of what is known about the extent of this risk is based on multicenter epidemiologic surveys, which are of questionable accuracy. Most patients with transplanted kidneys can be expected to live for many years, so the transplant unit must be able to estimate the relative risk in a particular region. A retrospective cohort study in 1 European transplant population was conducted.

Methods.—The study took place at a northern English transplant center that serves a population of 3.6 million. Nine hundred eighteen patients who received their first renal allograft from 1967 to 1991 were reviewed. Information on the prevalence of neoplastic disease in these patients was gathered from 6 different sources, including registries, hospital departmental records, and hospital notes.

Results.—At least 1 neoplastic lesion developed in 70 patients, a rate of 7.6%. Ten of the patients had more than 1 type of tumor. Fifty-three percent of the neoplasia were cutaneous, mainly squamous-cell carcinomas. Less common categories included urogenital, lymphoreticular, and gastrointestinal tumors. The patients' risk of neoplasia was calculated as 13.6% in the first 10 years and 40.0% by 20 years. These figures were much higher than the cumulative 6% risk of neoplasia in an age-matched control population. Age at transplantation and length of dialysis before transplantation were the only significant risk factors.

Conclusions.—The problem of neoplasia after renal transplantation appears to be greater than previously thought. Patients who are candidates for renal allografting need to be counseled about this risk, although most will probably find it acceptable. As transplant recipients live longer, they clearly need lifelong surveillance and closer investigation.

▶ The incidence of skin cancer among renal transplant recipients is alarmingly high, especially on areas of the skin exposed to sun. Genetic factors such as skin type (fair or dark) and HLA type, as well as past sun exposure, environment, and the intensity of immunosuppression, play important and often overlooked roles in predisposing renal transplant recipients to the development of skin cancer.

Renal transplant recipients need to be informed that the "sun is your enemy." I urge my patients to (a) apply industrial-strength sunscreens before going outside, throughout the year—winter as well as summer; (b) wear hats while outdoors; and (c) never, ever, lounge in the sun.

Ideally, preventive measures to avoid ultraviolet damage to skin should be initiated in every potential renal transplant recipient at the time the diagnosis of chronic renal insufficiency is established. Lifelong surveillance is required, as the risk of skin cancer after transplantation increases with time.

T.B. Strom, M.D.

61 Dialysis

High-Risk Surgical Acute Renal Failure Treated by Continuous Arteriovenous Hemodiafiltration: Metabolic Control and Outcome in Sixty Patients

van Bommel EFH, Bouvy ND, So KL, Vincent HH, Zietse R, Bruining HA, Weimar W (Univ Hosp Rotterdam 'Dijkzigt', The Netherlands)

Nephron 70:185–192, 1995 119-96-61–1

Background.—Acute renal failure (ARF) still carries a high mortality, particularly in the setting of several other failing organs. Continuous renal replacement therapy has become the treatment of choice for this complex and unstable patient population. Continuous arteriovenous hemodiafiltration (CAVHD) was developed to combine the advantages of continuous arteriovenous hemofiltration and intermittent hemodialysis. An experience of 60 consecutive patients with ARF treated with CAVHD in a surgical intensive care unit was evaluated.

Patients.—The patients all received CAVHD in 1 surgical ICU between 1986 and 1992. Eighty-three percent received mechanical ventilation, and 70% received vasopressor support. The mean number of organ system failures per patient was 3.

Outcomes.—Treatment with CAVHD was well tolerated and rapidly reduced serum urea and creatinine levels. There were no significant changes in cardiorespiratory measures during the first 24 hours of CAVHD. A significant net fluid loss of up to 5 L/day was possible with no significant decline in mean arterial pressure. Thereafter, controlled steady-state levels were achieved with serum urea levels maintained at less than 30 mmol/L. This result was obtained in the presence of full protein alimentation and frequently despite hypotension, surgery, and septicemia. Other than filter clotting, there were no major complications related to the extracorporeal circuit per se.

Forty-three percent of patients lived to ICU discharge, and 38% lived to hospital discharge. The chances of survival were unaffected by age or sex. Factors associated with a worse prognosis included the need for mechanical ventilation or vasopressor support, higher Acute Physiology and Chronic Health Evaluation II scores, and septicemia. The number of organ system failures was also related to a poor prognosis; however, one fourth of patients with 3 or more organ system failures lived to hospital discharge. There were no deaths among patients with nonoliguric ARF or isolated ARF. Seventy percent of deaths resulted from refractory septic shock and/or irreversible multiple organ failure.

Conclusions.—For critically ill patients with ARF, CAVHD is an efficient means of providing renal support. Overall mortality is 62% and is more affected by the patient's underlying disease than by uremia per se. The results of this series compare favorably with those of previous reports of patients with ARF treated by conventional dialysis. There is currently no way to determine which patients with ARF are likely to benefit from prolonged intensive treatment, nor which are likely to do poorly if additional organ system failures develop.

► The treatment of patients with ARF in ICUs is commonly complicated by severe fluid overload, cardiorespiratory failure, sepsis and/or multiorgan failure in addition to the metabolic disorders of ARF. Continuous arteriovenous (or venovenous) hemodiafiltration (CAVHD or CVVHD) combines the advantage of continuous hemofiltration to remove fluid without worsening hypotension with the superiority of intermittent hemodialysis to control uremia. The authors report that a consecutive series of 60 patients in a surgical ICU who had ARF treated with CAVHD had a survival rate of 38%. Treatment with CAVHD provided satisfactory control of fluid and metabolic parameters with minimal complications in this high-risk group of patients. The use of CVVHD has been advocated by Bellomo and Boyce[1] to provide results similar to those of CAVHD but to avoid the risk of arterial catheterization (which necessitated repair of 1 femoral artery pseudoaneurysm in the 60 patients of the above series). In a group of 72 critically ill elderly patients (older than 65 years of age), a survival rate of 42% was achieved using either CAVHD or CVVHD.[2] Though no randomized controlled study has proven a conclusive advantage of CAVHD or CVVHD over intermittent hemodialysis, the advantages of the continuous procedures to improve fluid balance, allow nutritional and drug infusion support, and maintain steady metabolic balance without hemodynamic instability make these techniques preferable in the majority of critically ill patients with ARF.

R.S. Brown, M.D.

References

1. Bellomo R, Boyce N: Continuous venovenous hemodiafiltration compared with conventional dialysis in critically ill patients with acute renal failure. *ASAIO J* 39:794M–797M, 1993.
2. Bellomo R, Farmer M, Boyce N: The outcome of critically ill elderly patients with severe acute renal failure treated by continuous hemodiafiltration. *Int J Intern Organs* 17:466–472, 1994.

Hemodialysis Therapy in the United States: What Is the Dose and Does It Matter?

Held PJ, Carroll CE, Liska DW, Turenne MN, Port FK (Univ of Michigan, Ann Arbor; Urban Inst, Washington, DC)

Am J Kidney Dis 24:974–980, 1994 119-96-61–2

Background.—The adequacy of hemodialysis in the United States has been of great concern to the dialysis community. Many believe that a large proportion of patients undergoing hemodialysis are receiving insufficient doses of dialysis, which result in deaths that could have been prevented. This possibility was explored.

Hemodialysis Treatment in the United States.—One way to assess the efficacy of hemodialysis treatment is to compare the experience in the United States with that of other countries. Recent research has indicated that the mortality among patients receiving chronic dialysis is greater in the United States than in Japan and Europe. Mortality differences between Japanese and US patients with end-stage renal disease (ESRD) do not appear to reflect underlying differences in mortality in the general populations without ESRD stratified by age and sex. When several sources of bias are considered, international comparisons may actually underestimate death rate differences between the United States and Japan and Europe.

Another way to determine treatment efficacy is to assess the prescription and delivery of dialysis therapy that patients in the United States receive. In general, it appears that patients in the United States do not receive the level of dialysis prescribed. The mean Kt/V prescribed for new patients in 1986 and 1987 was 1.00, compared with 1.07 Kt/V by 1990, which is a 7% increase. When delivered dialysis was analyzed, it appeared that a great proportion of patients were still receiving a low dose.

Conclusions.—Patients undergoing hemodialysis in the United States receive less treatment than their counterparts in Japan and Europe. Furthermore, patients in the United States generally do not receive the dialysis level prescribed. These findings are associated with an increased death rate among patients undergoing hemodialysis in the United States.

► There has been understandable concern about the apparently greater mortality of patients in the United States receiving hemodialysis compared with those in Japan and Europe. The authors argue that even when population sources of bias are considered, patients in the United States fare less well. Furthermore, the decreased dose of hemodialysis received by these patients compared with their Japanese and European counterparts may well explain the increased mortality. However, as pointed out by Keane and Collins,[1] differences in case mix and severity of illness may contribute to the increased mortality in the United States. The proportion of patients with ESRD who initiated dialysis in the United States was one third greater than that in Japan and 2½ times that in Europe. It's likely that the increased co-morbidity with such unselected patients accounts for part of the high death rate in the United States.[1] Nevertheless, the evidence supporting the argument to provide and deliver an adequate dose of dialysis has mounted enough to gain widespread acceptance in the renal community.

R.S. Brown, M.D.

Reference

1. Keane WF, Collins AJ: Influence of co-morbidity on mortality and morbidity in patients treated with hemodialysis. *Am J Kidney Dis* 24:1010–1018, 1994.

Incidence of and Risk Factors for Hepatitis B Virus and Hepatitis C Virus Infection Among Haemodialysis and CAPD Patients: Evidence for Environmental Transmission

Neto MC, Draibe SA, Silva AEB, Ferraz ML, Granato C, Pereira CAP, Sesso RC, Gaspar AMC, Ajzen H (Escola Paulista de Medicina, São Paulo, Brazil; Instituto Oswaldo Cruz, Rio de Janeiro, Brazil)

Nephrol Dial Transplant 10:240–246, 1995 119-96-61–3

Background.—In a previous study of Brazilian patients receiving hemodialysis and continuous ambulatory peritoneal dialysis (CAPD), the prevalence of hepatitis C virus (HCV) infection was reported to be high. Anti-HCV positivity was independently related to duration of renal replacement therapy (RRT), number of previous blood transfusions, and a history of hemodialysis. The findings for hepatitis B virus (HBV) infection were comparable. The risk factors associated with these viral infections in patients receiving dialysis were further investigated.

Methods and Findings.—One hundred eighty-five patients receiving hemodialysis and 124 receiving CAPD between 1987 and 1990 were enrolled in the prospective study. Sixty-nine patients receiving hemodialysis and 70 receiving CAPD were susceptible to HBV. There were 17 HBsAg seroconversions with hemodialysis and 1 with CAPD among these patients. According to a Cox proportional hazards model, hemodialysis treatment was the only risk factor significantly correlated with HBV infection, which suggests transmission through the environment. Eighteen seroconversions to HCV occurred among 83 initially anti-HCV-negative patients receiving hemodialysis and 2 seroconversions to HCV among 46 patients receiving CAPD. The only risk factor significantly related to a greater risk of HCV infection was hemodialysis. Four patients with HCV seroconversions were not transfused during the study and 3 of these had never been transfused. Compared with CAPD patients, hemodialysis patients had a hazard ratio of 5.7 for HCV infection. For the 2 patients receiving CAPD, the likely source of HCV infection was prior blood transfusions in 1 and previous hemodialysis in the other.

Conclusions.—The hemodialysis environment appears to have played a role in the transmissions of HBV and HCV in these patients, despite the existence of prophylactic measures. The high incidence of HBV observed may be attributable to blood leaks, a delay between collection of blood samples for HBsAg and isolation of newly infected patients, and even low staff compliance to prophylactic measures. Further research is needed to determine the exact mechanisms of environmental HCV transmission to attain effective prevention.

► It has been well recognized that hepatitis B infection can occur by patient-to-patient transmission in hemodialysis units, as well as by blood transfusions. Contamination with HBV has been documented on environmental surfaces in dialysis units. Furthermore, combining isolation of HBV-positive patients with universal precautions has lowered the incidence of HBV in patients receiving hemodialysis.[1] In this paper, the authors offer additional evidence for the environmental transmission of HBV infection in hemodialysis patients by statistical analysis and by HBV serotyping; furthermore, 4 of the 17 patients with HBV seroconversion had never been transfused. These observations were extended to hepatitis C infections in which the transmission of HCV was also statistically correlated to hemodialysis.

Similar to the finding for HBV seroconversion, 3 of the 18 HCV seroconversions were in patients who had never been transfused. For patients receiving CAPD, only prior hemodialysis or blood transfusions were associated with HBV or HCV seroconversions. Uncontrolled studies appear to show that techniques designed to diminish patient-to-patient contamination, such as universal precautions, may be effective in decreasing the incidence of HCV seroconversion without isolation of HCV-positive patients[2] or with the use of a dedicated area and dialysis equipment, but not a separate room for HCV-positive patients.[3] However, since many dialysis units might have difficulty isolating HCV-positive patients and most do not do so, controlled studies of techniques to prevent environmental transmission of HCV in hemodialysis units would be desirable.

R.S. Brown, M.D.

References

1. Tokars JI, Alter MJ, Favero MS, et al: National surveillance of dialysis associated diseases in the United States 1991. *ASAIO J* 39:966–975, 1993.
2. Fabrizi F, Lunghi G, Guarnori I, et al: Incidence of seroconversion for hepatitis C virus in chronic haemodialysis patients: A prospective study. *Nephrol Dial Transplant* 9:1611–1615, 1994.
3. Blumberg A, Zehnder C, Burckhardt JJ: Prevention of hepatitis C infection in haemodialysis units: A prospective study. *Nephrol Dial Transplant* 10:230–233, 1995.

Defective Platelet Aggregation in Uremia Is Transiently Worsened by Hemodialysis

Sreedhara R, Itagaki I, Lynn B, Hakim RM (Vanderbilt Univ, Nashville, Tenn; Toray Industries Inc, Kanagawa, Japan)

Am J Kidney Dis 25:555–563, 1995 119-96-61–4

Objective.—Bleeding is a significant problem in patients requiring hemodialysis (HD). In this prospective crossover study, the effects of different types of dialysis membranes on shear-induced platelet aggregation (SIPA) were compared in 8 patients undergoing chronic HD for longer than 1 year. Shear-induced platelet aggregation is a clinically relevant marker of platelet function that reflects the interaction of von Willebrand factor with glycoproteins in the platelet membrane.

Methods.—Studies were repeated during 2-week periods of HD using low-flux biocompatible polymethyl methacrylate, low-flux complement-activating cuprophane, and high-flux biocompatible polysulfone membranes. The expression of platelet membrane glycoproteins Ib and IIb-IIIa on the platelet surface was estimated by flow cytometric analysis using fluorescein isothiocyanate-conjugated monoclonal antibodies CD42b and CD41a, respectively.

Results.—The type of dialysis membrane used did not significantly influence SIPA, calcium flux, or the production of thromboxane B_2 by platelets. Shear-induced platelet aggregation was markedly reduced compared to that in normal control subjects before dialysis, and it decreased further after HD. At the same time the expression of both glycoprotein fractions was significantly decreased. Dialysis did not alter calcium flux or thromboxane B_2 production in response to shear stress. Shear-induced platelet aggregation correlated negatively with levels of platelet-bound von Willebrand factor.

Implications.—Hemodialysis in itself leads to a transient decrease in platelet aggregation, which apparently is mediated by a loss of surface receptor glycoproteins. This decrease could account for the increased bleeding sometimes noted during and just after dialysis. It may be best to avoid surgery immediately after a session of dialysis.

► Uremic coagulopathy with active bleeding is one of the commonly recognized indications for the initiation of hemodialysis therapy in patients with renal failure. However, several investigators have pointed out that platelet function and bleeding may be negatively impacted by the dialysis procedure. In this well-controlled study using a platelet aggregometry technique that is considered to be an effective surrogate for in vivo platelet function, Sreedhara et al. confirm that the defective platelet aggregation of patients with uremia was further worsened by hemodialysis, at least transiently. Moreover, the choice of dialysis membrane did not appear to influence the negative impact of hemodialysis on platelet function. Therefore, a prudent choice would be to treat uremic patients who are actively bleeding with one of the effective agents known to improve platelet function, i.e., desmopressin, cryoprecipitate, or estrogen, before the initiation of hemodialysis therapy. It is also common practice to perform a hemodialysis treatment to improve the metabolic status of patients with end-stage renal disease who are about to undergo an operative procedure. Because the authors didn't determine for how long after hemodialysis the platelet defect persists, one cannot speculate what the appropriate interval between hemodialysis and surgery might be. Until more data are known, we must balance the possible benefits of metabolic balance against the possible increased risk of bleeding in an operative procedure that need not be done immediately after dialysis.

R.S. Brown, M.D.

Acute Abdomen in the Hemodialysis Patient Population

Bender JS, Ratner LE, Magnuson TH, Zenilman ME (Johns Hopkins Bayview Med Ctr, Baltimore, Md; Johns Hopkins Univ, Baltimore, Md)

Surgery 117:494–497, 1995 119-96-61–5

Background.—The causes of abdominal pain in patients undergoing long-term hemodialysis have not been defined. To understand the frequency and causes of pain in this group of patients, the records of all 567 patients undergoing long-term hemodialysis at the Johns Hopkins Bayview Medical Center from July 1988 to June 1993 were reviewed.

Findings.—Of the initial group of 567 patients, only 12 were admitted during the study period for an acute abdominal problem. There were 6 men and 6 women with an average age of 60 years who had been receiving dialysis for an average of 6.6 years. Their average age, length of dialysis, and cause of kidney failure were no different from those who did not have acute abdomen. No patient experienced abdominal pain during dialysis. Patients were admitted several days after dialysis with abdominal pain; 4 were in shock. Of the 12 patients, 6 died. Only 1 patient had the correct diagnosis, pancreatitis, made on presentation. The other patients had mesenteric infarction, which was diagnosed at varying times, in 2 cases at autopsy.

Conclusions.—Although an acute abdomen is not common among the long-term hemodialysis population, it is associated with a high morbidity and mortality because the most common cause of acute abdomen in this population is bowel infarction. Therefore, in patients who have received long-term hemodialysis who are seen with acute abdominal pain or unexplained sepsis, mesenteric infarction should be the presumptive diagnosis.

► In this retrospective review, the authors point out that bowel ischemia was the source of hospitalization for 11 of 12 hemodialysis patients with acute abdominal signs. Despite recent reports of mesenteric ischemia and/or infarction in patients receiving hemodialysis, the diagnosis was made only later in the course of 9 of the 11 and at autopsy in 2. The delay in diagnosis may be explained, in part, because abdominal pain was the chief complaint in only 7 of the 12 patients. The authors stress that physicians should recognize that mesenteric ischemia is the overwhelming cause of acute abdominal pain and sepsis in patients receiving hemodialysis.

R.S. Brown, M.D.

Chronic Haemodialysis for Very Old Patients

Neves PL, Sousa A, Bernardo I, Anunciada AI, Pinto I, Bexiga I, Aniceto J, Amorim JP (Hosp Distrital de Faro, Portugal; Hosp Distrital de Euora, Portugal)

Age Ageing 23:356–359, 1994 119-96-61–6

Background.—As the population continues to age, more and more elderly patients will be admitted to chronic renal failure treatment programs. However, some practitioners have questioned whether chronic hemodialysis treatment of the very old is ethical, given the current limitation of available resources. Few studies have examined the effects of chronic hemodialysis among patients older than 80 years of age. An experience with dialysis treatment among very old patients with end-stage renal disease was therefore evaluated.

Patients and Methods.—Fifty patients older than 80 years of age—all of whom had been admitted to a chronic hemodialysis program in Portugal during a 10-year period—were included in the study. All patients underwent 3- to 4-hour dialysis sessions 3–4 times per week. Medical records were reviewed to determine age at initiation of dialysis, etiologic basis of renal disease, the presence of co-morbid conditions, time on dialysis, number of hospitalization days, reasons for hospitalization, and causes of death.

Results.—The mean patient age at initiation of hemodialysis treatment was 83 years, and the mean time of treatment was 20 months. The etiologic basis of renal disease was interstitial nephritis in 26%, hypertensive nephrosclerosis in 14%, chronic glomerulonephritis in 8%, diabetes in 8%, and adult polycystic renal disease in 2% of the patients. Disease etiology was not known in the remaining 42%. Intradialytic hypotension was the most common co-morbid disease, noted in 82% of the patients. Cardiovascular disease also was observed in 74%, gastrointestinal disease in 64%, cerebrovascular disease in 26%, and hypertension in 24%. The main reasons for hospitalization were associated with vascular access and vascular and gastrointestinal disease. There were 78 hospital admissions, corresponding to 765 hospitalization days. Cardiac and cerebral vascular diseases were the leading causes of death among this patient population, followed by infection and neoplasia. At 6 months, actuarial survival was 89%. Corresponding figures at 12 months were 78%; at 24 months, 56%; and at 36 months, 48%.

Conclusions.—Very old patients with chronic renal failure can be effectively treated with hemodialysis, which presently remains the best therapeutic alternative for such patients. Additional studies should focus on means by which quality of life can be improved for this particular population.

► The authors describe the morbidity and mortality in a relatively unselected group of 50 octogenarians who started hemodialysis in Portugal between 1982 and 1992. The very high frequency of hemodialysis-induced hypotension may be caused, in part, by the acetate dialysate used; current techniques with volumetric monitoring of ultrafiltration and bicarbonate dialysate are likely to improve this problem. Moreover, despite the high incidence of co-morbid conditions to be expected in this age group, the survival of almost four fifths at 1 year and one half at 3 years is surprisingly high. The hospitalization rate in this group of patients aged 80 years and older (9.8 days per admission and 15.3 days per patient) compares favorably with that noted for patients 65 years and older receiving hemodialysis in the United States,[1] using data from the United States Renal Data System's 1993 Annual Data Report (19.8 days per patient year). With relatively low initial expense of initiating hemodialysis in patients with progressive chronic renal disease, the authors' findings argue strongly to plan for and offer hemodialysis as an effective therapy for the very old.

R.S. Brown, M.D.

Reference

1. Habach G, Bloembergen WE, Mauger EA, et al: Hospitalization among United States dialysis patients: Hemodialysis *versus* peritoneal dialysis. *J Am Soc Nephrol* 5:1940–1948, 1995.

62 Water, Electrolytes, and Acid-Base

Nephrogenic Diabetes Insipidus Secondary to Lithium Therapy in the Postoperative Patient: A Case Report

Johnson MA, Ogorman J, Golembiewski GH, Paluzzi MW (Keesler Med Ctr, Keesler Air Force Base, Miss)

Am Surg 60:836–839, 1994 119-96-62–1

Introduction.—Nephrogenic diabetes insipidus (NDI) is a recognized complication of long-term lithium treatment. Although NDI rarely occurs in the perioperative period, it can pose challenging fluid management problems. A case of previously undiagnosed NDI caused by lithium treatment was encountered in a surgical patient with perforated duodenal ulcer.

Case Report.—Man, 42, with a history of schizophrenia and mild hypertension underwent surgery for a perforated duodenal ulcer. He received the standard preoperative and postoperative regimen of hydration with normal saline solution. By 36 hours after surgery, his urine output had increased gradually and his serum sodium level had risen to 161 mEq/L, despite conversion to hypotonic saline. Because of hypernatremia and hyperosmolality, aggressive hypotonic fluid replacement was needed to restore preoperative values. By 10 days after surgery, the patient was taking liquids by mouth and was restarted on hydrochlorothiazide; lithium was not restarted. The suspected diagnosis of NDI was confirmed by the patient's low baseline urine osmolality and its failure to rise with 1-desamino-8-D-arginine-vasopressin (dDAVP) administration. Serum AVP level when serum sodium was 162 mEq/L and urine osmolality was 144 mosm/kg, was 19 pcg/mL, an extraordinarily high value. The patient had a long history of polydipsia and had been receiving lithium therapy for about 12 years.

Conclusions.—Nephrogenic diabetes insipidus may cause difficult fluid management problems in postoperative patients. This condition is refractory to dDAVP; thiazide diuretics and nonsteroidal anti-inflammatory drugs can be used in selected patients. Successful perioperative management relies on careful fluid and electrolyte management.

▶ About 10% of patients taking lithium have polydipsia and polyuria as a result of the development of NDI. Because the kidneys' ability to concentrate urine is greatly restricted, a solute load excreted by the kidneys necessarily drags out lots of water into a hypotonic urine. Saline infusions paradoxically, therefore, result in rapid dehydration with rising serum sodium. The hypernatremia is exaggerated if, as in most hospital situations, the patient cannot drink at will to satisfy thirst.

F.H. Epstein, M.D.

Correction of Hypokalemia With Antialdosterone Therapy in Gitelman's Syndrome

Colussi G, Rombolà G, De Ferrari ME, Macaluso M, Minetti L (Niguarda-Ca'Granda Hosp, Milan, Italy)

Am J Nephrol 14:127–135, 1994 119-96-62–2

Introduction.—Gitelman's syndrome (GS), also known as a hypocalciuric variant of Bartter's syndrome, is an inherited primary renal tubular disorder characterized by chronic hypokalemia, hypomagnesemia, alkalosis, hyperreninemic hyperaldosteronism and normal renal function. It is a rather benign condition not uncommonly detected in asymptomatic adults because of hypokalemia. The long-term effects of antialdosterone therapy, using spironolactone or amiloride, were evaluated in 6 patients with GS.

Methods.—Six patients aged 26–57 years were treated for symptoms related to hypokalemia. They received spironolactone or amiloride. Venous and arterial blood and urine were obtained at follow-up, which was 1 month after start of therapy and every 3–6 months thereafter.

Results.—Significant increases in serum potassium concentration were observed during treatment, particularly treatment with spironolactone. Changes in potassium concentration were associated with a significant decrease in clearance of potassium and fractional excretion of potassium. No significant changes were noted in daily potassium or sodium excretion before or after treatment. Arterial blood PH and bicarbonate levels were not significantly changed. A significant increase in serum magnesium concentration was associated with a significant decrease in clearance of magnesium and fractional excretion of magnesium, but no change in urine magnesium excretion. A significant decrease was observed in creatinine clearance during treatment, with plasma renin activity and aldosterone levels significantly increased, suggesting extracellular fluid volume contraction. Mean arterial blood pressure decreased from 92.9 mm Hg before treatment to 85.9 mm Hg after treatment and body weight decreased from 61.5 kg before treatment to 59.7 kg after treatment.

Conclusion.—These findings suggest that hypokalemia in patients with GS is a consequence of increased tubular secretion in the cortical collecting tubule. Inhibitors of potassium secretion like amiloride or spironolactone were effective in reversing hypokalemia and raising serum magnesium.

► The familial syndrome described by Gitelman[1] is best thought of as a variant of Bartter's syndrome (potassium wasting, hyperreninemia with normal blood pressure, alkalosis) in which hypomagnesemia is prominent, hypercalciuria (a usual feature of Bartter's syndrome) is absent, and prostaglandin E_2 excretion (elevated in Bartter's syndrome) is normal. Prostaglandin synthetase inhibitors, which are generally helpful in Bartter's syndrome in reducing renin secretion and improving hypokalemic alkalosis, are not effective in patients with Gitelman's syndrome, because renal synthesis of prostaglandins is not abnormally elevated.[2] Blockade of potassium secretion can be accomplished, however, with spironolactone or amiloride.

F.H. Epstein, M.D.

References

1. Gitelman HJ, Graham JB, Welt LG: A new familial disorder characterized by hypokalemia and hypomagnesemia. *Trans Assoc Am Phys* 79:221–235, 1966.
2. Lüthy C, Betinelli A, Iselin S, et al: Normal prostaglandinuria E_2 in Gitelman's syndrome, the hypercalciuric variant of Bartter's syndrome. *Am J Kidney Dis* 25:824–828, 1995.

A Mechanism for Pentamidine-Induced Hyperkalemia: Inhibition of Distal Nephron Sodium Transport

Kleyman TR, Roberts C, Ling BN (Univ of Pennsylvania, Philadelphia; Veterans Affairs Med Ctr, Philadelphia; Emory Univ and Veterans Affairs Med Ctr, Atlanta, Ga)
Ann Intern Med 122:103–106, 1995 119-96-62–3

Introduction.—When patients with AIDS are treated with pentamidine for more than 6 days for *Pneumocystis carinii* pneumonia, hyperkalemia is observed in as many as 100% of patients. Hyperkalemia is usually out of proportion to the extent of coexisting renal insufficiency and is frequently associated with hyperchloremic metabolic acidosis. To determine whether pentamidine directly affects renal tubular K^+ secretion, cultured kidney cells were studied.

Methods.—Transepithelial and single-channel measurement techniques were applied to 2 well-established models of cortical collecting tubule ion transport. The models were the A6 amphibian cell line and primary cultured rabbit cortical tubules. The short-circuit current was measured under voltage-clamp conditions. Amiloride was added to the luminal bath after each experiment to determine the amiloride-sensitive component of the short-circuit current, because it is a measure of the net Na^+ transport across the renal epithelium. Varying concentrations of pentamidine were added to the solution.

Results.—Luminal exposure to pentamidine inhibited Na^+ reabsorption in the distal nephron cells in both models. At concentrations greater than 50 μM, luminal pentamidine inhibited amiloride-sensitive, macroscopic short-circuit currents; a similar effect was seen at concentrations greater than 1 μM for individual Na^+ channels.

Conclusion.—At concentrations found clinically in urine, pentamidine directly and reversibly blocks apical Na^+ channels in a way similar to "potassium-sparing" diuretics. This results in a decrease in the electrochemical driving force for both K^+ and H^+ secretion in the cortical collecting tubule.

► The organic cation pentamidine resembles amiloride in structure. Like amiloride, it binds to and inhibits Na^+ channels on the apical surface of collecting tubules, thus reducing the lumen-negative voltage across the collecting duct and impairing K^+ movement into the urine. Because pentamidine is excreted in the urine, it reaches a high concentration in the collecting duct, where it can effectively interfere with K^+ secretion. For similar reasons, trimethoprim (commonly prescribed for patients with AIDS in combination with sulfa) also predisposes to hyperkalemia.[1] Both drugs are secreted into the urine in the proximal tubule via a cation transporter that also transports creatinine. By competing with creatinine for secretion, they may be responsible for a rise in serum creatinine that does not necessarily reflect a fall in glomerular filtration rate.

F.H. Epstein, M.D.

Reference

1. 1994 Year Book of Medicine, 734–735.

Metabolic Acidosis Is a Potent Stimulus for Cellular Inorganic Phosphate Generation in Uraemia

Bevington A, Brough D, Baker FE, Hattersley J, Walls J (Leicester Gen Hosp, England)

Clin Sci 88:405–412, 1995 119-96-62–4

Objective.—Inorganic phosphate (P_i) is known to fluctuate between cellular and extracellular fluid during metabolic acidosis. The P_i in erythrocytes from 16 patients receiving regular hemodialysis therapy was measured before and after treatment, and correlated with plasma pH (acidosis), plasma P_i (hyperphosphatemia), and cellular organic phosphate concentrations. Findings obtained using uremic erythrocytes were compared with those of normal erythrocytes acidified in vitro.

Findings.—An inverse correlation between the ratio of cellular to extracellular P_i concentration and plasma pH was observed before dialysis, with a 2.5-fold increase observed as pH decreased from 7.4 to 7.2. After the in vitro addition of acid to normal erythrocytes, an increase in cellular P_i was noted within 90 minutes, comparable to that observed in uremic patients.

A 25% increase in the total P_i cell suspension content, accompanied by a net efflux of P_i into plasma, was observed when pH fell from 7.4 to 7.2. This was attributed to the production of P_i from 2,3-bisphosphoglycerate in the cells. Furthermore, the increase in steady-state cellular P_i concentration was 50% higher at pH 7.2 than at 7.4 when adding a constant extracellular P_i load. Thus, changes in regulation of the transmembrane P_i gradient also may lead to the increased cellular P_i noted at low pH. When pH was lowered from 7.4 to 7.2, glycolytic flux (lactate production) was inhibited by 20% at normal plasma P_i concentrations. This inhibition was obstructed, however, when cellular P_i was increased by the in vitro addition of P_i to the plasma.

Conclusions.—Metabolic acidosis acts as a powerful stimulus for P_i production in erythrocytes. Glycolysis, which typically is suppressed by low pH, may be activated by P_i. Additional studies are needed to clarify further the interactions between acidosis, P_i, and glycolysis.

► Acidosis and alkalosis have potent and opposite effects on serum inorganic phosphate. The reason is that the rate-limiting enzyme for glycolysis, phosphofructokinase, is extremely sensitive to intracellular pH. Enzymatic activity is enhanced by alkalosis and inhibited by an acid pH. Hence, intracellular alkalosis stimulates the formation of phosphorylated intermediates of glucose metabolism, sucking inorganic phosphate into cells from the extracellular pool of phosphate, whereas acidosis reduces glycolysis and diminishes the intracellular concentration of glycolytic 2-carbon and 3-carbon phosphorylated compounds, liberating inorganic phosphate to leave cells and increase plasma level of phosphate. Correction of uremic acidosis will usually lower serum phosphorus even though urinary excretion of phosphate is not increased. Respiratory (and, to a lesser extent, metabolic) alkalosis, on the other hand, is often attended by a serum phosphorus level that is depressed below normal.

F.H. Epstein, M.D.

63 Calcium, Phosphorus, and Bone

Dietary Chloride and Urinary Calcium in Stone Disease

Muldowney FP, Freaney R, Barnes E (Univ College, Dublin, Ireland)

Q J Med 87:501–509, 1994 119-96-63–1

Introduction.—Several well-defined abnormalities, including hypercalciuria, hyperuricosuria, and cystinuria, can cause renal stone disease, and in some patients 2 or more of these abnormalities may be present. Salt restriction is known to decrease hypercalciuria as well as cystinuria. Although the ideal treatment should be capable of managing all risk factors, a potential conflict may develop when traditional methods for preventing cystine and uric acid stones, such as alkalinization of the urine with oral sodium bicarbonate, are prescribed together with salt restriction for patients with stones of mixed composition. Sodium chloride and $NaHCO_3$ may affect urinary Ca excretion quite differently. The effect of interchanging NaCl, $NaHCO_3$, and KCl was studied in patients with combination stone disease.

Methods.—Six patients with stone disease of mixed etiology underwent a series of dietary tests to determine the effect on urinary Ca (UCa) of sodium or chloride deprivation or addition.

Results.—Chloride deprivation after high NaCl intake showed that UCa decreased significantly during $NaHCO_3$ substitution and increased with equivalent NaCl loading, even though urine Na remained fairly constant (Fig 1). In 3 patients, plasma bicarbonate levels rose slightly during $NaHCO_3$ ingestion. Changing between equimolar NaCl and KCl did not alter UCa, in spite of a sharp decrease in urine Na (Fig 6). When KCl was substituted for NaCl after a high NaCl intake, urine Na decreased and urine Cl and Ca remained fairly constant. The addition of 120 mM $NaHCO_3$ to a standard diet containing 80 mM NaCl did not alter urinary Ca. Body weight and creatinine clearance were stable in all patients.

Conclusions.—The results indicate the Cl rather than Na ions play the major role during sodium chloride–induced changes in UCa. In patients with mixed stone disease where alkalinization as well as reduction in UCa may be desirable, $NaHCO_3$ can be prescribed and normocalciuria maintained as long as dietary Cl is kept moderately low at 80–100 mmol/day.

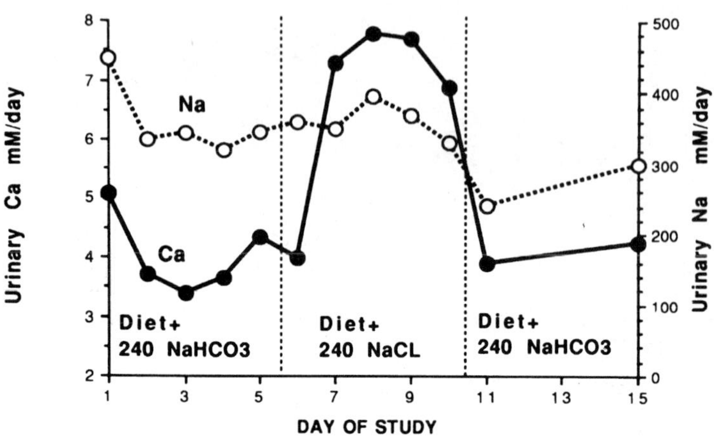

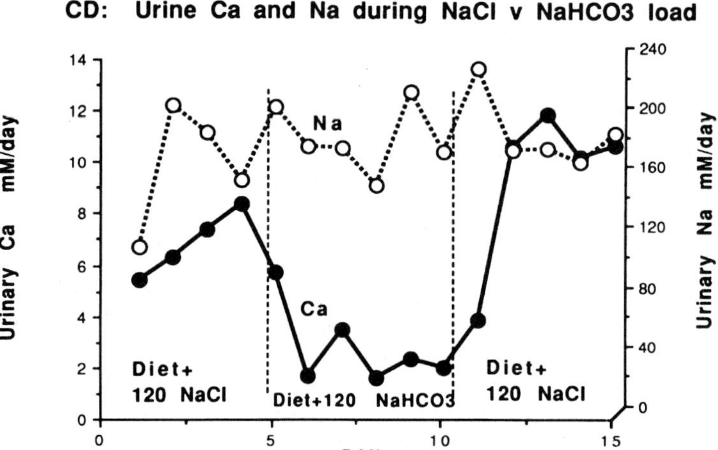

FIGURE 1.—Effect of interchanging equimolar NaCl and $NaHCO_3$ on urinary Na and Ca in patients PC and CD. Urinary Ca fell during $NaHCO_3$ and rose during NaCl ingestion, while urinary Na remained relatively stable. (Courtesy of Muldowney FP, Freaney R, Barnes E: Dietary chloride and urinary calcium in stone disease. *Q J Med* 87:501–509, 1994. By permission of Oxford University Press.)

If these data are confirmed in larger studies, patients with combined stone disease can receive alkali treatment, no matter what the Na content is, provided that Cl intake is reduced.

► Earlier studies showed that a diet low in NaCl (80 mM/day) could reduce urinary calcium to normal in hypercalciuric patients. These new results

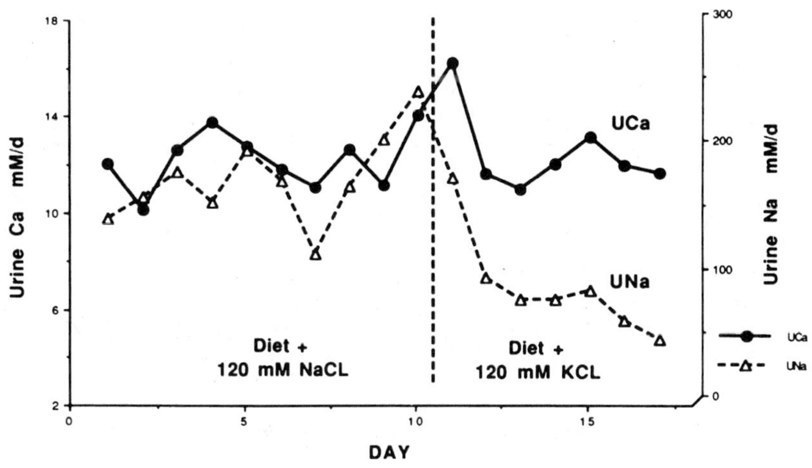

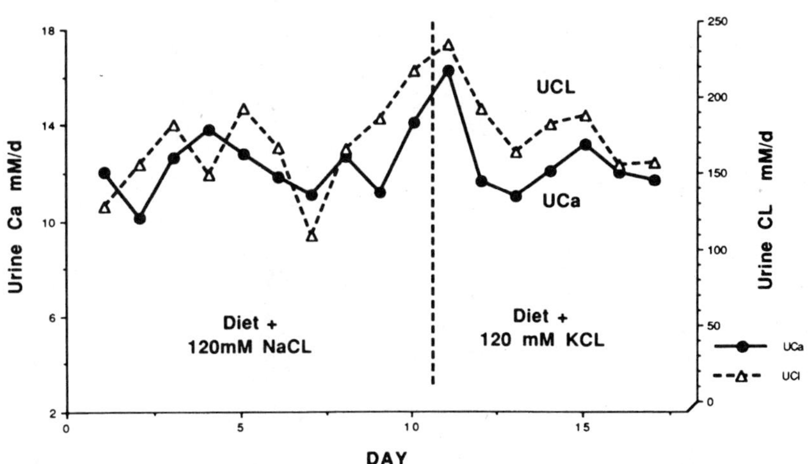

FIGURE 6.—Effect of substituting equimolar KCl for NaCl on urinary Ca, Na, and Cl in patient JM. Urinary Ca and Cl remained essentially constant, despite falling urinary Na. (Courtesy of Muldowney FP, Freaney R, Barnes E: Dietary chloride and urinary calcium in stone disease. *Q J Med* 87:501–509, 1994. By permission of the Oxford University Press.)

indicate that urinary calcium may (at least under some circumstances) be influenced more by the intake and excretion of Cl^- than of Na^+. The addition of $NaHCO_3$ to a basal 60-mM NaCl diet did not affect urinary Ca, while the addition of KCl raised urinary Ca substantially. The physiologic explanation for this is not yet clear; the authors believe firmly that changes in acid-base balance have nothing to do with it, but I think that's hard to assess. In any case, the facts should encourage the use of sodium bicarbonate in patients with uric acid or cystine stones who also have hypercalciuria. Adding $NaHCO_3$ to a low-salt diet won't increase calcium excretion in such cases.

F.H. Epstein, M.D.

Prevention of Hypercalciuria and Stone-Forming Propensity During Prolonged Bedrest by Alendronate

Ruml LA, Dubois SK, Roberts ML, Pak CYC (Univ of Texas Southwestern Med Ctr, Dallas)

J Bone Miner Res 10:655–662, 1995 119-96-63–2

Introduction.—It is well established that loss of bone mineral occurs during immobilization or with decreased gravitational forces of space. This loss increases the risk of formation of calcium-containing kidney stones by producing hypercalciuria and hyperphosphaturia. Inhibitors of

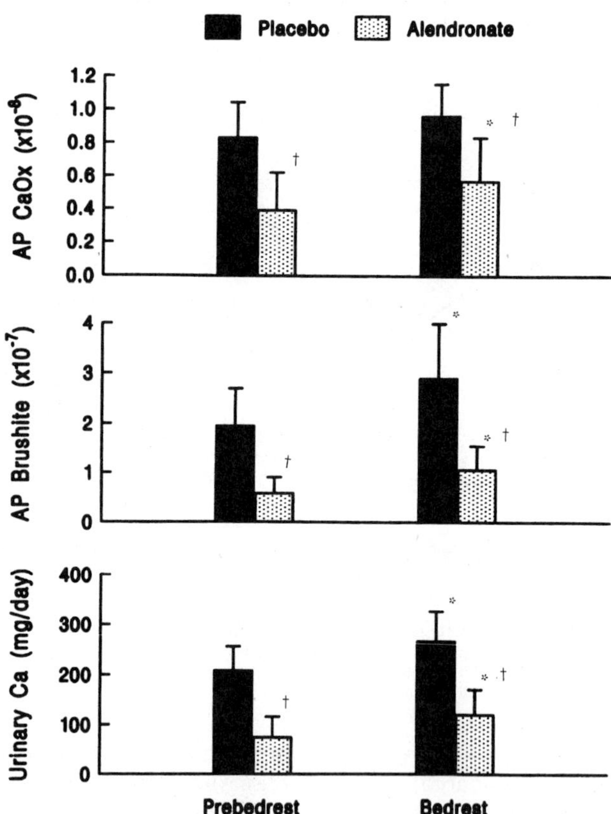

FIGURE 2.—Parameters of urinary crystallization of calcium-containing, stone-forming salts during period before bed rest (week 2) and during period of bed rest (week 5). Values presented are mean ± SD. *Asterisk,* before bed rest vs. bed rest within the same group; $P < 0.01$. *Dagger,* placebo vs. alendronate for the corresponding phase; $P < 0.01$. *Abbreviation: AP,* activity product. (Courtesy of Ruml LA, Dubois SK, Roberts ML, et al: *J Bone Miner Res* 10:655–662, 1995.)

osteoclast resorption may have a therapeutic potential in inhibiting bone loss of immobilization. Using a model of bed rest immobilization, the efficacy of a potent inhibitor of osteoclast action, the aminobisphosphonate alendronate, was evaluated for preventing the hypercalciuria and increased propensity for crystallization of stone-forming calcium salts in urine.

Study Design.—In a double-blind, placebo-controlled study, 16 healthy men were randomly assigned to receive either alendronate, 20 mg/day, or placebo 2 weeks before and during 3 weeks of strict bed rest. Parameters of bone and calcium metabolism and urinary crystallization of stone-forming salts were monitored.

Results.—In the placebo group, urinary calcium and saturation of calcium phosphate increased significantly after 3 weeks of bed rest; saturation of calcium oxalate also increased, but not significantly. Before bed rest, the alendronate group had significantly lower serum calcium and phosphorus, and significantly higher serum parathyroid hormone and $1,25(OH)_2D$ than the placebo group (Fig 2). In addition, the alendronate group had significantly lower urinary calcium and saturation of calcium oxalate and calcium phosphate. These effects of alendronate were sustained during 3 weeks of bed rest. Intestinal absorption of calcium was similar in both groups. After bed rest, urinary calcium increased in the alendronate group at a level lower than that in the placebo group before or during bed rest. Urinary saturation of calcium oxalate and calcium phosphate increased during bed rest in the alendronate group but remained below the values found in the placebo group before or during bed rest. Alendronate was well tolerated.

Conclusion.—Alendronate effectively blocks bone resorption that occurs during strict bed rest and averts the hypercalciuria and increased propensity for crystallization of stone-forming calcium salts.

► Alendronate is one of a family of diphosphonates that decrease bone reabsorption by inhibiting the action of osteoclasts. These compounds have been shown to diminish the progression of postmenopausal osteoporosis[1] and to reduce calcium and phosphorus excretion in normal subjects, presumably by increasing their net deposition in bone. The effectiveness of alendronate in reducing the calcium mobilization of bed rest suggests that it might also prove useful in avoiding or delaying the osteoporosis that too often attends the administration of high-dose adrenal steroids. That, however, remains to be seen.

F.H. Epstein, M.D.

Reference

1. 1995 Year Book of Medicine, pp 653–655.

Bone Pain in Transplant Recipients Responsive to Calcium Channel Blockers

Gauthier VJ, Barbosa LM (Univ of Washington, Seattle)

Ann Intern Med 121:863–865, 1994 119-96-63–3

Introduction.—A small fraction of patients receiving transplants experience a bone pain syndrome that is localized to the epiphyseal regions. The only patients who reported the pain received a combination of cyclosporine and corticosteroids; it was not found in patients who received azathioprine and prednisone. The pain seemed to be related to an increase in cyclosporine levels, which was relieved with decreasing the dose and resumed with resumption of the dosage.

Methods.—Fifteen consecutive patients who received transplants also had bone pain syndrome. The pain was severe and unexplained, typically bilateral in the lower limbs, and increased with recumbency. Calcium-channel blockers were used to control hypertension or the recurrent bone pain. In some cases, calcium-channel blockade relieved pain within minutes.

Results.—Thirteen of the patients had no history of bone or joint problems. Twelve of the patients reported pain within 2.5 months of transplantation. The pain increased at night and was slightly relieved by elevation of the legs. The pain was different from the pain associated with osteonecrosis or microfractures in patients receiving renal transplants. However, the pain was similar to that from intraosseous hypertension. The pain could either disappear as rapidly as it developed or could take hours to dissipate. The administration of calcium-channel blockers relieved pain in all the patients.

Conclusion.—The purposeful modification of intraosseous pressures by medication has not been systematically studied in humans. In the meantime, calcium-channel blockers will be beneficial in the treatment of transplant recipients with bone pain. Future work will define the pathophysiology of the pain and whether intraosseous hypertension is the source of the pain.

► Severe pain in the legs that begins in the first few months after transplantation should raise the suspicion of avascular necrosis or epiphyseal impaction, associated with immunosuppressive regimens and especially with prednisone. Those 2 conditions can usually be diagnosed by bone scan and MRI; the pain is often worse with weight-bearing, and serum alkaline phosphatase is often elevated. In contrast, the bone pain described here is worse at night and in most patients, MRI, limb radiographs, and bone scans showed no abnormality. Nifedipine, given either as 10 mg orally/sublingually or as an extended-release tablet at night, was remarkably effective in relieving pain.

F.H. Epstein, M.D.

PART EIGHT

RHEUMATOLOGY

STEPHEN E. MALAWISTA, M.D.

64 Rheumatoid Arthritis

Introduction

This year we learn that low-dose corticosteroids given over 2 years can substantially reduce the rate of radiologic progression of early, active rheumatoid arthritis (Abstract 119-96-64–1); that the combination of cyclosporine and methotrexate can produce clinical improvement in patients with severe rheumatoid arthritis whose response to previous therapy with methotrexate alone was only partial (Abstract 119-96-64–2); that minocycline given over 48 weeks is safe and moderately effective treatment for patients with mild-to-moderate rheumatoid arthritis (Abstract 119-96-64–3); that folic acid over a broad dosage range protects patients with rheumatoid arthritis from methotrexate toxicity without interfering with efficacy (Abstract 119-96-64–4); that misoprostol reduces serious gastrointestinal complications in patients with rheumatoid arthritis receiving nonsteroidal anti-inflammatory drugs (Abstract 119-96-42–6); and that most African-American patients with rheumatoid arthritis do not have the so-called rheumatoid antigenic determinant (epitope) (Abstract 119-96-64–5).

Noted in passing: For clinical studies, the American College of Rheumatology has issued a preliminary definition of improvement in rheumatoid arthritis[1]; and there was further validation[2, 3] of last year's report[4] of the use of reduced joint counts (28, instead of 60-odd) for assessment of rheumatoid inflammatory activity. Also, pre-existing lung disease characterized by radiographic interstitial infiltrates may predispose patients with rheumatoid arthritis to develop methotrexate pneumonitis.[5]

Stephen E. Malawista, M.D.

References

1. Felson DT, Anderson JJ, Boers M, Bombardier C, Furst D, Goldsmith C, Katz L, Lightfoot R Jr, Paulus H, Strand V, Tugwell P, Weinblatt M, Williams HJ, Wolfe F, Kieszak S: American College of Rheumatology preliminary definition of improvement in rheumatoid arthritis. *Arthritis Rheum* 38:727–735, 1995.
2. Smolen JF, Breedveld FC, Eberl G, Jones I, Leeming M, Wylie GL, Kirkpatrick J: Validity and reliability of the twenty-eight-joint count for the assessment of rheumatoid arthritis activity. *Arthritis Rheum* 38:38–43, 1995.
3. Prevoo MLL, van'T Hof MA, Kuper HH, van Leeuwen MA, van de Putte LBA, van Riel PLCM: Modified disease activity scores that include twenty-eight-joint counts. *Arthritis Rheum* 38:44–48, 1995.

Fuchs HA, Pincus T: Reduced joint counts in controlled clinical trials in rheumatoid arthritis. *Arthritis Rheum* 37:470–475, 1994.
Golden MR, Katz RS, Balk RA, Golden HE: The relationship of preexisting lung disease to the development of methotrexate pneumonitis in patients with rheumatoid arthritis. *J Rheumatol* 22:1043–1047, 1995.

The Effect of Glucocorticoids on Joint Destruction in Rheumatoid Arthritis

Kirwan JR, and the Arthritis and Rheumatism Council Low-Dose Glucocorticoid Study Group (Bristol Royal Infirmary, England)
N Engl J Med 333:142–146, 1995 119-96-64–1

Background.—Oral glucocorticosteroids are widely prescribed for patients with rheumatoid arthritis (RA), even though their role and value in this disease is still debated. The effect of these agents on joint destruction, as determined by radiography, has not been established. Use of a fixed daily dose of prednisolone, 7.5 mg, combined with other treatments, was evaluated in a randomized, double-blind, placebo-controlled trial.

Methods.—One hundred twenty-eight adults with active rheumatoid arthritis of less than 2 years' duration were studied. They were allowed other treatments as well, except for systemic corticosteroids. The Larsen index was used to measure the progression of damage noted on hand radiographs after 1 and 2 years. A statistical analysis of radiologic changes was performed on the 106 patients for whom such films were taken at baseline and 2 years later.

Findings.—The patients receiving prednisolone had a mean increase in Larsen scores of 0.72 units after 2 years, indicating very little change. By contrast, patients given placebo had a mean change of 5.37 units, indicating marked joint destruction (Fig 1). Of the total of 212 affected hands, 147, or 69.3%, showed no erosions at the beginning of the study. At 2 years, 15 of 68 of these hands in the prednisolone group and 36 of the 79 in the placebo group showed erosions. The respective percentages were 22.1 and 45.6. Compared with patients receiving placebo, those receiving prednisolone had greater decreases in scores on an articular index and for pain and disability at 3 months; for pain at 6 months; and for disability at 6, 12, and 15 months. Standardized scores for the acute-phase response did not differ between groups (Fig 2).

Conclusions.—Prednisolone, 7.5 mg daily, given for 2 years along with other treatment can greatly decrease the rate of radiologic disease progression in patients with early, active RA. These data also showed that the development of erosions, clinical symptoms, and to some degree the acute-phase response can occur independently of one another after glucocorticoid therapy. Thus these RA features should not be combined in a single measure. Further research is needed to identify their different control mechanisms.

► In this randomized, double-blind trial comparing oral prednisolone (7.5 mg daily for 2 years) with placebo in 128 adults with active RA of less than 2

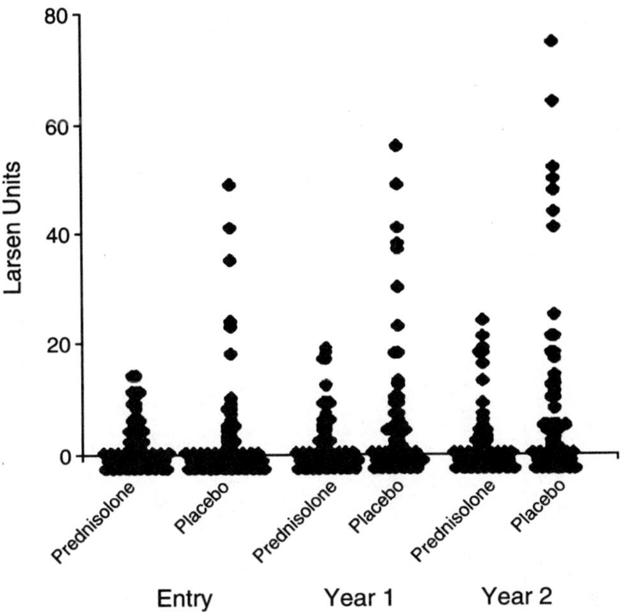

FIGURE 1.—Scores on Larsen index during treatment, according to study group. The mean values at study entry and 1 and 2 years thereafter, expressed in Larsen units, were as follows: prednisolone group, 2.65, 3.38, and 3.37, respectively; placebo group, 6.23, 9.86, and 11.60; difference between groups, 3.58, 6.48, and 8.23. $P = 0.479$, $P = 0.033$, and $P = 0.002$ for the respective group differences as calculated from log-transformed scores. The mean changes after 1 and 2 years were as follows: prednisolone group, 0.73 and 0.72, respectively; placebo group, 3.63 and 5.37; difference between groups, 2.90 and 4.65. $P = 0.052$ and $P = 0.004$ for the respective group differences as calculated from log-transformed scores. (Reprinted by permission of *The New England Journal of Medicine*. Kirwan JR, and the Arthritis and Rheumatism Council Low-Dose Glucocorticoid Study Group: The effect of glucocorticoids on joint destruction in rheumatoid arthritis. *N Engl J Med* 333:142–146, 1995. Copyright 1995, Massachusetts Medical Society.)

years' duration in relation to radiologic alterations, there was very little change in the corticosteroid group in contrast to the substantial joint destruction that occurred in controls ($P = 0.004$; see Fig 1). These were patients with active disease, defined by the presence of 6 or more painful joints, 3 or more joints with active synovitis, and early-morning stiffness for more than 20 minutes, and an erythrocyte sedimentation rate of greater than 28 mm/hr, a plasma viscosity greater than 1.72, or a level of C-reactive protein greater than 10 mg/L. Most patients in both groups had clinical improvement, apparently accelerated at first by prednisolone (Fig 2), but that additional symptomatic benefit did not persist into the second year of treatment. It is important to note that these were patients with early disease; it is likely that the anti-inflammatory properties of prednisolone operate to better advantage at a time when most patients do not yet have radiologic evidence of destruction than when such deterioration is well under way. Although in an editorial[1] it was pointed out that it is not known how closely radiologically detected damage of the hands is related to functional deterioration, I think it's a safe bet that function will eventually follow structure.

Adding prednisolone early to other second-line agents represents an approach more aggressive than the classic one[1] on the grounds that much of the damage to joints occurs early. In doing so, we will have to address the association of long-term, low-dose (≥ 5 mg/day) prednisolone therapy with the development of specific adverse events (e.g., fracture, gastrointestinal events, infection).[2] As for which patients are most likely to benefit from early combined therapy, strategies are emerging to predict severity of subsequent disease at the onset of RA (see Abstract 119-96-64–5).[3] In the meantime, we will hope that any severity subgroups were equally distributed between the experimental and control groups in the current study, whose results are crystal clear.

S.E. Malawista, M.D.

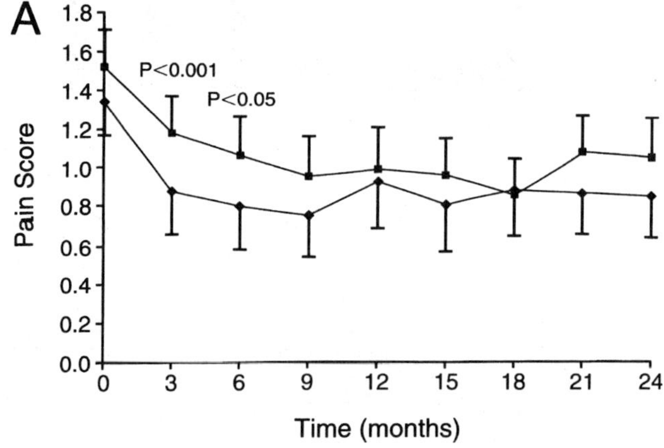

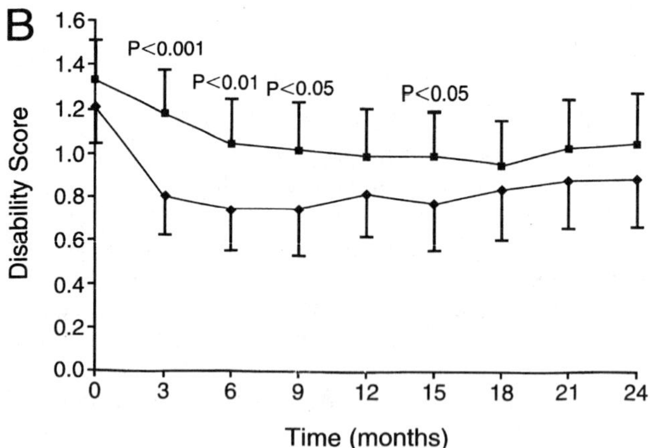

(Continued.)

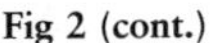
Fig 2 (cont.)

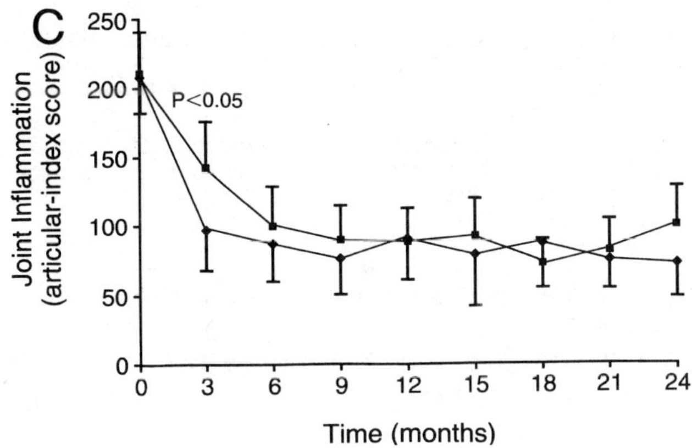

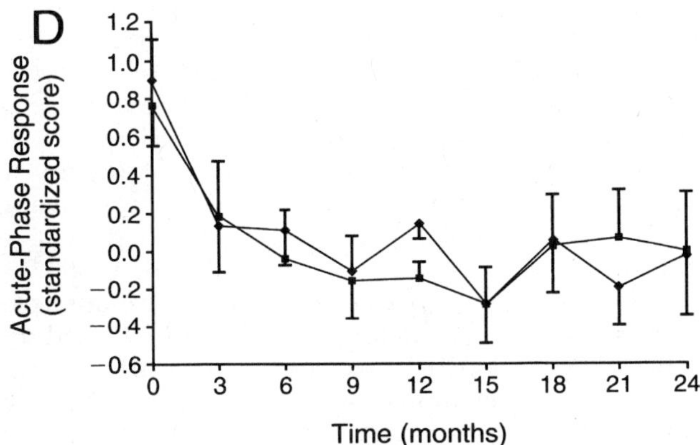

FIGURE 2.—Changes in clinical variables during treatment, according to study group. The group means and 95% confidence intervals are shown for the prednisolone (*filled diamonds*) and placebo (*filled squares*) groups. Pain scores (**A**) were derived from a visual-analogue scale that recorded severity of pain over previous 24 hours on a scale ranging from 0 (no pain) to 3.0 (worst possible pain). Disability scores (**B**) were derived from the disability scale of the Health Assessment Questionnaire and were expressed on a scale ranging from 0 (no disability) to 3.0 (inability to perform most activities of daily living). Scores for joint inflammation (**C**) were assessed by an articular index of inflamed joints and were expressed on a scale ranging from 0 (no joint inflammation) to 534 (all joints of hands and wrists inflamed). Acute-phase response (**D**) was reported as a standardized score (number of SDs from mean) for each patient to allow a variety of methods to be used to measure overall acute-phase response for the group. (Reprinted by permission of *The New England Journal of Medicine*. Kirwan JR, and the Arthritis and Rheumatism Council Low-Dose Glucocorticoid Study Group: The effect of glucocorticoids on joint destruction in rheumatoid arthritis. *N Engl J Med* 333:142–146, 1995. Copyright 1995, Massachusetts Medical Society.)

References

1. Breedveld FC: New perspectives on treating rheumatoid arthritis. *N Engl J Med* 333:183, 1995.
2. Saag KG, Koehnke R, Caldwell JR, Brasington R, Burmeister LF, Zimmerman B, Kohler JA, Furst DE: Low dose long-term corticosteroid therapy in rheumatoid arthritis: An analysis of serious adverse events. *Am J Med* 96:115–123, 1994.
3. Weyand CM, Goronzy JJ: HLA-DRB1 alleles as severity markers in RA. *Bull Rheum Dis* 43:5–8, 1994.

Combination Therapy With Cyclosporine and Methotrexate in Severe Rheumatoid Arthritis

Tugwell P, for the Methotrexate-Cyclosporine Combination Study Group (Univ of Ottawa, Ont, Canada; Vanderbilt Univ, Nashville, Tenn; Univ of Arizona, Tucson; et al)

N Engl J Med 333:137–141, 1995 119-96-64–2

Objective.—The traditional approach to drug treatment for rheumatoid arthritis has been stepped use of 1 medication at a time. However, dissatisfaction with side effects has led some to question the use of monotherapy for rheumatoid arthritis. Combination therapy has attracted more and more attention. For patients with severe rheumatoid arthritis, methotrexate therapy often yields only partial improvement. Combination therapy with cyclosporine and methotrexate was evaluated in patients with severe rheumatoid arthritis.

Methods.—A multicenter, placebo-controlled, randomized trial included 148 patients with rheumatoid arthritis. All had had a substantial but partial response to previous treatment with methotrexate and were now left with residual inflammation and disability. The patients were randomly assigned to receive 6 months of treatment with cyclosporine, 2.5–5.0 mg/kg/day, plus methotrexate at the maximal tolerated dose, or with methotrexate plus placebo. The primary treatment outcome was the tender joint count.

Results.—Patients in the combination therapy group had a net improvement of 25%, or 4.8 joints, in the tender joint count. There was also an improvement of 25%, or 3.8 joints, in the swollen joint count. Improvement in overall disease activity, as assessed by the physician and the patient; in joint pain; and in degree of disability were all significantly greater for the patients receiving methotrexate plus cyclosporine. The 1993 criteria for improvement of the American College of Rheumatology were met by 48% of the patients receiving cyclosporine vs. 16% of those receiving methotrexate (Fig 1). The mean increase in the serum creatinine concentration was 0.14 vs. 0.05 mg/dL, respectively.

Conclusions.—The combination of methotrexate and cyclosporine can produce clinical improvement in patients with severe rheumatoid arthritis who had only a partial response to previous treatment with methotrexate

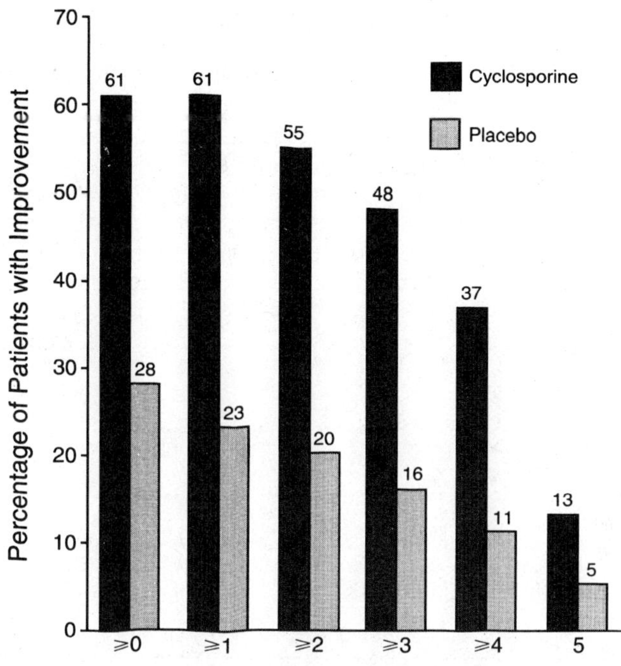

FIGURE 1.—Percentage of patients with rheumatoid arthritis who had 20% improvement in the number of tender and swollen joints and improvement in other variables. The American College of Rheumatology defines improvement as improvement in at least 3 of 5 variables (degree of disability, pain, patient's global assessment, physician's global assessment, and erythrocyte sedimentation rate) in addition to 20% improvement in the number of tender and swollen joints. (Reprinted by permission of *The New England Journal of Medicine.* Tugwell P, for the Methotrexate-Cyclosporine Combination Study Group: Combination therapy with cyclosporine and methotrexate in severe rheumatoid arthritis. *N Engl J Med* 333:137–141, 1995. Copyright 1995, Massachusetts Medical Society.)

only. Combination therapy causes no substantial increase in side effects. Further follow-up is needed to determine the long-term results.

► Unlike the patient population described in Abstract 119-96-64–1, those who took part in this study had had rheumatoid arthritis for about a decade on average and had severe disease insufficiently controlled by as much as 15 mg of methotrexate per week. In this 6-month, randomized, double-blind trial, those who received additional low-dose cyclosporine (2.5–5 mg/kg of body weight per day) did better than those who remained on methotrexate alone. Figure 1 shows the proportions of patients in each group who met the preliminary criteria of the American College of Rheumatology for improvement in rheumatoid arthritis. Thirty-six patients (48%) in the cyclosporine group satisfied the overall criteria for improvement, compared with 12 (16%) in the placebo group ($P < 0.001$).

In using more than 1 second-line agent at a time, one hopes that therapeutic effects will be additive or synergistic, but that toxic effects will not be.[1] That seems to have been the case in this study. Much progress has been made in the use of cyclosporine in rheumatoid arthritis while avoiding its (especially renal) toxicity.[2, 3] However, keep in mind that this was only a 6-month study and that the use of cyclosporine for rheumatoid arthritis is not yet approved by the Food and Drug Administration. While its longer-term effects are becoming established, either alone or in combination with other drugs, cyclosporine is best viewed, I think, as an experimental agent whose use should probably be overseen by the special expertise of rheumatologists.

S.E. Malawista, M.D.

References

1. Breedveld FC: New perspectives on treating rheumatoid arthritis. *N Engl J Med* 333:183, 1995.
2. Stein CM: Cyclosporine in the treatment of rheumatoid arthritis. *Bull Rheum Dis* 44:1–4, 1995.
3. Forre O, and the Norwegian Arthritis Study Group: Radiographic evidence of disease modification in rheumatoid arthritis patients treated with cyclosporine. *Arthritis Rheum* 37:1506–1512, 1994.

Minocycline in Rheumatoid Arthritis: A 48-Week, Double-Blind, Placebo-Controlled Trial

Tilley BC, for the MIRA Trial Group (Henry Ford Health Sciences Ctr, Detroit; Univ of Alabama, Birmingham; Natl Inst of Arthritis and Musculoskeletal and Skin Diseases, Bethesda, Md; et al)

Ann Intern Med 122:81–89, 1995 119-96-64–3

Introduction.—Although there are numerous pharmacologic agents for treating rheumatoid arthritis (RA), no agent has been completely effective. Based on the assumption that *Mycoplasma* may cause RA, courses of tetracycline have been attempted with some success, whereas a 1-year clinical trial failed to show benefits for patients with RA. Tetracyclines, like minocycline, inhibit collagenase activity in fibroblasts of diabetic rats. Twice daily doses of minocycline, 100 mg/day for 10 days, reduced collagenase activity in patients with RA. Tetracyclines also inhibit protein synthesis and lymphocyte proliferation, and they have anti-inflammatory effects. These are most likely the result of the antioxidant activity of tetracyclines. The induction of RA in rats is suppressed by minocycline. The effects of minocycline in the treatment of patients with RA were studied.

Methods.—A total of 219 patients with RA were randomly assigned to receive a placebo or minocycline (200 mg/day) for 48 weeks. Six medical centers participated. Tenderness and swelling were evaluated in 60 diarthrodial joints. Grip strength was also determined. Activities of daily living were assessed by the Modified Health Assessment Questionnaire

(MHAQ). A variety of RA-specific laboratory tests were obtained. Adverse drug reactions and compliance were determined.

Findings.—Randomization resulted in similar demographic, clinical, and laboratory results between the groups, and all had mild-to-moderate disease. At week 48, 79% of the patients in the minocycline group and 78% of those in the placebo group still received the study medication. Compared with the placebo group, more patients in the minocycline group had improvement in swelling (54% vs. 39%) and tenderness (56% vs. 41%). For patients in the minocycline group, improvements in joint swelling and tenderness continued through week 48, but reached a plateau at week 24 for patients in the placebo group (Fig 1). The experimental group

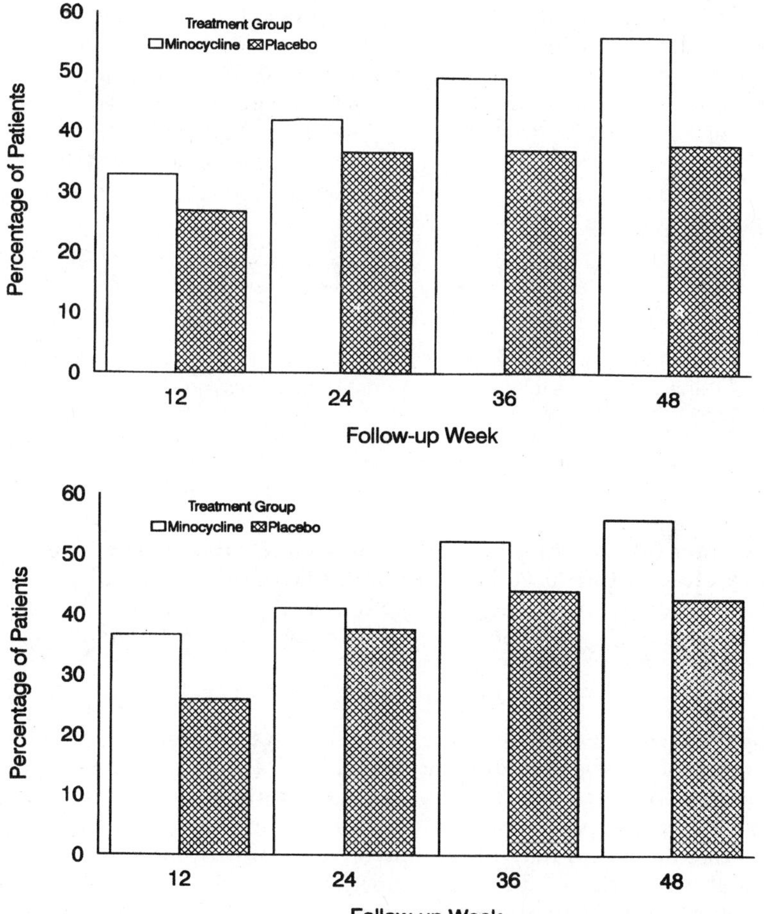

FIGURE 1.—**Top,** proportion of patients with 50% or greater improvement in joint swelling, by visit. **Bottom,** proportion of patients with 50% or greater improvement in joint tenderness, by visit. (Courtesy of Tilley BC, for the MIRA Trial Group: Minocycline in rheumatoid arthritis: A 48-week, double-blind, placebo-controlled trial. *Ann Intern Med* 122:81–89, 1995.)

showed significant improvements in selected laboratory tests. There were more patients with laboratory results in the normal range in the minocycline group than the placebo group. Grip strength was improved in the experimental group, but subjective measures (e.g., MHAQ, disease activity scores, morning stiffness) were not different between the groups.

Conclusion.—Minocycline is effective treatment for patients with mild-to-moderate RA. Side effects were mild and few. The majority of outcomes improved with the treatment. The mechanisms, long-term effectiveness, and potency are yet to be determined.

► Two double-blind, placebo-controlled studies, this one and another from Holland,[1] published 1 year ago, showed minocycline to be moderately effective in the treatment of RA and to have generally fewer side effects than most of the second-line agents currently in use. Patients in the latter study had more severe disease than those in the current group (arthritis for an average of 12–14 years vs. 8 years; joint erosions in 95% of patients vs. 57%), and they were treated for 26 weeks instead of for 48 weeks. The mechanism of action of this drug is unknown and may have nothing to do with its antibacterial properties.[2] We can look forward to studies of its longer-term effects.

S.E. Malawista, M.D.

References

1. Kloppenburg M, Breedveld FC, Terwiel JP, Mallee C, Dijkmans AC: Minocycline in active rheumatoid arthritis: A double-blind, placebo-controlled trial. *Arthritis Rheum* 37:629–636, 1994.
2. Paulus HE: Minocycline treatment of rheumatoid arthritis. *Ann Intern Med* 122:147–148, 1995.

Supplementation With Folic Acid During Methotrexate Therapy for Rheumatoid Arthritis: A Double-Blind, Placebo-Controlled Trial

Morgan SL, Baggott JE, Vaughn WH, Austin JS, Veitch TA, Lee JY, Koopman WJ, Krumdieck CL, Alarcón GS (Univ of Alabama, Birmingham)
Ann Intern Med 121:833–841, 1994 119-96-64–4

Purpose.—Low-dose methotrexate is useful in the treatment of chronic inflammatory diseases, including rheumatoid arthritis. There is some evidence that impaired folate status is related to methotrexate toxicity, and that folic acid supplementation can lessen such toxicity. However, high doses of folinic acid may negate the efficacy of methotrexate. The effects of different doses of folic acid on methotrexate toxicity and efficacy are unknown. Two different weekly doses of folic acid were assessed for their effects on the toxicity and efficacy of low-dose methotrexate therapy in patients with rheumatoid arthritis.

Methods.—A total of 79 adult patients with rheumatoid arthritis, as diagnosed by the American Rheumatism Association criteria, were stud-

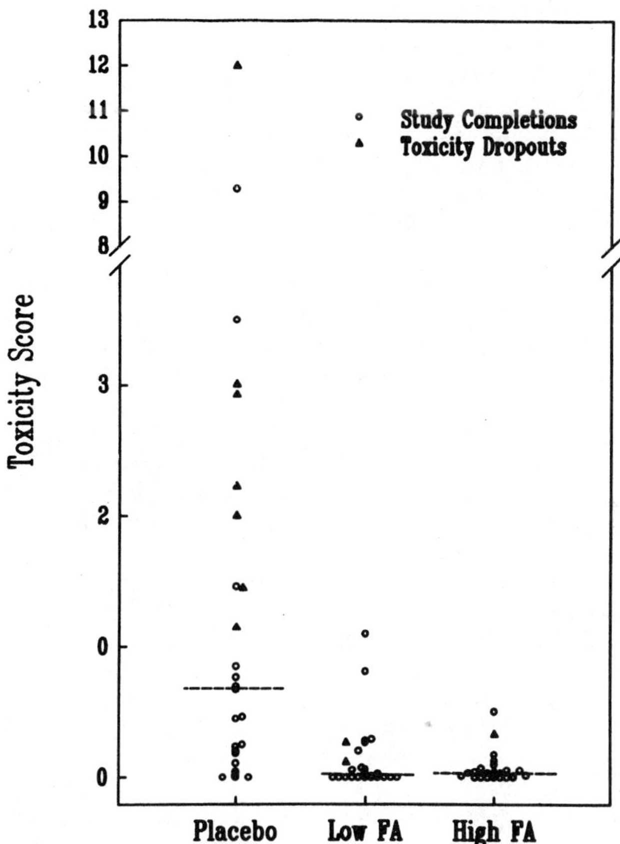

FIGURE 2.—Median toxicity scores in the 3 study groups. The placebo group had a statistically higher toxicity score ($P = 0.001$) than folic acid supplementation groups. The toxicity score was not significantly different between low-dose folic acid and high-dose folic acid groups ($P = 0.71$). *Solid triangles,* patients withdrawn from the trial because of toxic effects; *open circles,* patients who completed the trial. (Courtesy of Morgan SL, Baggott JE, Vaughn WH, et al: Supplementation with folic acid during methotrexate therapy for rheumatoid arthritis: A double-blind, placebo-controlled trial. *Ann Intern Med* 121:833–841, 1994.)

ied. The patients were randomly assigned to receive either placebo or folic acid at a dose of 5.0 or 27.5 mg/week. At the same time, they started receiving oral methotrexate, beginning at a median oral dose of 16.5 µmol/week and increasing in 5.5-µmol increments at the rheumatologist's discretion. Before the start of methotrexate treatment and a mean of 13, 26, 39, and 53 weeks afterward, the patients were evaluated for the duration, intensity, and severity of toxic events; efficacy, assessed by indices of joint tenderness and swelling and grip strength; and laboratory variables including plasma and erythrocyte folate levels.

Results.—The 3 groups were not significantly different in terms of the percentages of patients in different outcome categories; thus, neither dose of folic acid appeared to affect the efficacy of methotrexate therapy. Some form of toxicity was noted in 89% of patients in the placebo group, 48% in the low-dose folic acid group, and 65% in the high-dose folic acid group. The median toxicity scores were 0.685, 0.016, and 0.031, respectively, with the score in the placebo group significantly higher than those in the folic acid supplementation groups (Fig 2). Laboratory findings associated with substantial methotrexate toxicity were low blood folate levels and increased mean corpuscular volumes. Patients with dietary intakes of folic acid exceeding 900 nmol/day had very little methotrexate toxicity.

Conclusions.—Folic acid supplementation at a broad range of doses can decrease the toxicity of methotrexate without compromising its efficacy. The mechanism of its protective effect is unknown. Safety and cost considerations suggest that folic acid is preferable to folinic acid.

▶ Methotrexate has become the most widely prescribed of the newer slow-acting antirheumatic agents. It has the highest probability of any second-line agent of being continued for as long as 10 years of use. The current authors have built upon earlier work[1] on the apparent ability of oral folic acid supplementation to prevent methotrexate toxicity. In this year-long, double-blind, placebo-controlled trial using low (5 mg/week) or high (27.5 mg/week) doses of folic acid, either dosage appeared to be protective, without interfering with the efficacy of methotrexate. Folinic acid (leucovorin, citrovorum factor), a one-carbon–substituted, fully reduced folate (which runs around the methotrexate block of the enzyme dihydrofolate reductase), has also been used successfully to prevent methotrexate toxicity, but at higher doses it also reverses therapeutic efficacy, and it costs (in Birmingham, at least) 43 times as much as folate.

The authors have constructed a thoughtful toxicity score in which various components are weighted for quality and intensity so as to distinguish marginal toxic symptoms (e.g., alopecia) from severe and medically important ones (e.g., cytopenias).[1] The most frequently reported toxicities were nausea and indigestion (31 patients), diarrhea (11 patients), stomatitis (9 patients), and rash (9 patients). Elevated mean corpuscular volume is a predictor of hematologic toxicity due to methotrexate therapy.[2] Because large doses of folic acid can mask and exacerbate vitamin B_{12} deficiency, it would be wise to establish adequate B_{12} status before beginning folic acid supplementation.

See Abstract 119-96-42–6 for Dr. Greenberger's discussion of an interesting paper by Silverstein and associates entitled "Misoprostol reduces serious gastrointestinal complications in patients with rheumatoid arthritis receiving nonsteroidal anti-inflammatory drugs: A randomized, double-blind, placebo-controlled trial," which was published in the *Annals of Internal Medicine*, and its provocative accompanying editorial by Levine.

S.E. Malawista, M.D.

References

1. 1991 YEAR BOOK OF MEDICINE, p 681.

2. Weinblatt ME, Fraser P: Elevated mean corpuscular volume as a predictor of hematologic toxicity due to methotrexate therapy. *Arthritis Rheum* 32:1592–1596, 1990.

Most African-American Patients With Rheumatoid Arthritis Do Not Have the Rheumatoid Antigenic Determinant (Epitope)

McDaniel DO, Alarcón GS, Pratt PW, Reveille JD (Univ of Alabama, Birmingham; Univ of Texas Health Science Ctr, Houston)
Ann Intern Med 123:181–187, 1995 119-96-64–5

Purpose.—Alleles associated with rheumatoid arthritis share a common sequence known as the "rheumatoid epitope" and defined by a sequence motif in the HLA-DRB1 alleles. It has been suggested that the severity of rheumatoid arthritis and the extent of destructive arthropathy might depend on the dose of the rheumatoid epitope and whether it is encoded by an HLA-DR4 allele. The association between the rheumatoid epitope and disease severity was evaluated in African-Americans with rheumatoid arthritis.

Methods.—The cross-sectional study included 86 African-American patients with rheumatoid arthritis from 2 rheumatology outpatient clinics. Of these patients, 66 were seropositive for the rheumatoid factor and 20 were seronegative. In each patient, HLA-DRB1 allele determination was made by restriction fragment length polymorphism and by allele-specific oligonucleotide typing of polymerase chain reaction–amplified HLA-DRB1 second exons. Eighty-eight healthy African-Americans also were studied.

Results.—The frequency of HLA-DRB1*04 alleles was 27% in the seropositive patients with rheumatoid arthritis vs. 13% in controls. Oth-

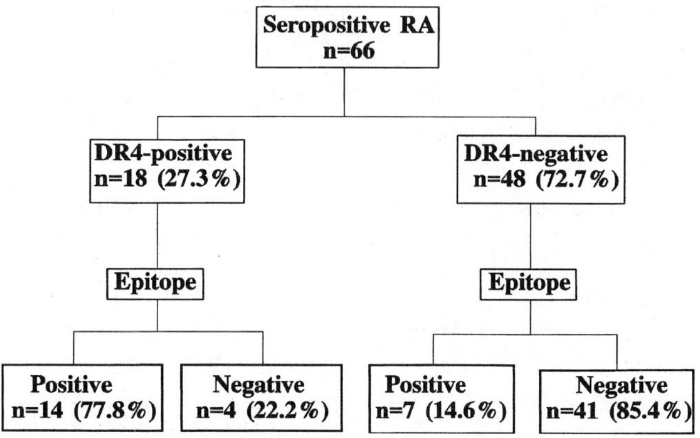

FIGURE 1.—Frequencies of rheumatoid epitope and HLA-DRB1 alleles in seropositive African-American patients with rheumatoid arthritis (RA). (Courtesy of McDaniel DO, Alarcón GS, Pratt PW, et al: Most African-American patients with rheumatoid arthritis do not have the rheumatoid antigenic determinant (epitope). *Ann Intern Med* 123:181–187, 1995.)

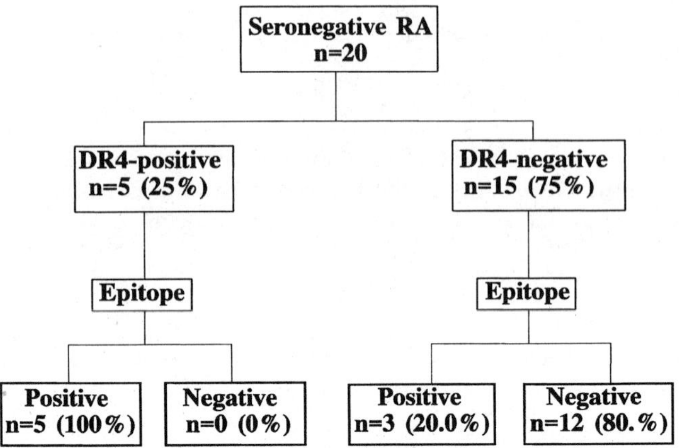

FIGURE 2.—Frequencies of rheumatoid epitope and HLA-DRB1 alleles in seronegative African-American patients with rheumatoid arthritis (RA). (Courtesy of McDaniel DO, Alarcón GS, Pratt PW, et al: Most African-American patients with rheumatoid arthritis do not have the rheumatoid antigenic determinant (epitope). *Ann Intern Med* 123:181–187, 1995.)

erwise, the patients and controls showed no differences in the frequencies of HLA-DRB1 alleles (Fig 1). Approximately three fourths of both seropositive and seronegative patients were HLA-DR4 negative. However, 15% of seropositive patients and 20% of seronegative patients studied inherited the rheumatoid epitope on a non-DR4 allele (Fig 2). There were no differences in disease severity or other disease features for patients with vs. without the epitope or for those with a single or double dose of an epitope-positive allele. There was a weak association between disease severity and rheumatoid factor positivity but not rheumatoid epitope.

Conclusions.—Expression of the rheumatoid epitope is not found in most African-American patients with rheumatoid arthritis. The racial predisposition to, and severity of, rheumatoid arthritis among African-Americans does not seem to depend on the presence and dose of the shared rheumatoid epitope. Thus, HLA-DRB1 typing alone cannot be used to predict the occurrence of destructive arthropathy among African-Americans with rheumatoid arthritis.

► The rationale for early, aggressive therapy with multiple antirheumatic agents is that much of the damage to joints occurs early, and that the addition, one at a time, of progressively more powerful (and generally more toxic) drugs is likely to represent too little, too late. On the other hand, it is becoming increasingly clear that many patients do not experience this early relentless course,[1, 2] and that pulling out all the therapeutic stops early in the courses of such patients may be subjecting them to unnecessary risk of toxicity. The dream is that we can recognize at onset of disease those patients who are at greatest risk for rapid progression and can concentrate the more aggressive therapeutic approaches on them. This seemed to be the case in the apparent correlation of disease severity with single or double doses of a "rheumatoid epitope," a particular sequence motif in the HLA-DRB1 alleles.[3, 4]

We now learn that expression of the rheumatoid epitope is not found in most African-American patients with rheumatoid arthritis. This complicates matters, but I do not see it as more than a temporary setback. Susceptibility and severity of rheumatoid arthritis are likely to be governed by multiple genes[5]; indeed, its causes may be diverse, and particular etiologies may be handled differently by different hosts. The job will be to identify genetic and environmental factors that contribute to severity in particular populations. That's not easy, but we seem to be well under way.

S.E. Malawista, M.D.

References

1. Suarez-Almazor ME, Soskolne CL, Saunders LD, Russell AS: Outcome in rheumatoid arthritis: A 1985 inception cohort study. *J Rheumatol* 21:1438–1446, 1994.
2. van Zeben D, Hazes MW, Zwinderman AH, Vandenbroucke JP, Breedveld FC: The severity of rheumatoid arthritis: A six-year followup study of younger women with symptoms of recent onset. *J Rheumatol* 21:1620–1625, 1994.
3. 1994 YEAR BOOK OF MEDICINE, pp 755–758.
4. Weyand CM, Goronzy JJ: HLA-DRB1 alleles as severity markers in RA. *Bull Rheum Dis* 43:5–8, 1994.
5. Harris J, Edward D: Excitement—and Confusion—about HLA and Rheumatoid Arthritis. *Ann Intern Med* 123:232–233, 1995.

65 Systemic Lupus Erythematosus

Introduction

This chapter deals with the management of thrombosis in the antiphospholipid-antibody syndrome (Abstract 119-96-65–1); long-term, treatment-free remissions in severe systemic lupus erythematosus (SLE) after synchronization of plasmapheresis with subsequent pulse cyclophosphamide (Abstract 119-96-65–2); the risk of postmenopausal estrogen therapy for developing SLE (Abstract 119-96-65–3); and the causes of death in SLE (Abstract 119-96-65–4).

Noted in passing: A major review of the treatment of various manifestations of SLE[1, 2]; a 10-year follow-up of 100 patients with anti-Ro (SS-A) antibody positivity (outcomes were diverse)[3]; and the outcome of children referred to a pediatric rheumatology clinic with a positive antinuclear antibody test but without an autoimmune disease (the vast majority did not develop an autoimmune disease).[4]

Stephen E. Malawista, M.D.

References

1. Boumpas DT, Austin HA III, Fessler BJ, Balow JE, Klippel JH, Lockshin MD: Systemic lupus erythematosus: Emerging concepts: Part 1. Renal, neuropsychiatric, cardiovascular, pulmonary, and hematologic disease. *Ann Intern Med* 122:940–950, 1995.
2. Boumpas DT, Fessler BJ, Austin HA III, Balow JE, Klippel JH, Lockshin MD: Systemic lupus erythematosus: Emerging concepts: Part 2. Dermatologic and joint disease, the antiphospholipid antibody syndrome, pregnancy and hormonal therapy, morbidity and mortality, and pathogenesis. *Ann Intern Med* 123:42–53, 1995.
3. Simmons-O'Brien E, Chen S, Watson R, Antoni C, Petri M, Hochberg M, Stevens MB, Provost TT: One hundred anti-Ro (SS-A) antibody positive patients: A 10-year follow-up. *Medicine* 74:109–130, 1995.
4. Deane PMG, Liard G, Siegel DM, Baum J: The outcome of children referred to a pediatric rheumatology clinic with a positive antinuclear antibody test but without an autoimmune disease. *Pediatrics* 95:892–895, 1995.

The Management of Thrombosis in the Antiphospholipid-Antibody Syndrome

Khamashta MA, Cuadrado MJ, Mujic F, Taub NA, Hunt BJ, Hughes GRV
(Rayne Inst, London; Guy's Hosp, London; St Thomas's Hosp, London)
N Engl J Med 332:993–997, 1995 119-96-65–1

Background.—The antiphospholipid-antibody syndrome is a thrombophilic disorder in which venous thrombosis, arterial thrombosis, or both may occur in patients with antiphospholipid antibodies. Although the prevention of thrombosis in this syndrome is important, there is no consensus on the duration and extent of prophylactic treatments. The efficacy of several different methods of antithrombotic treatment was assessed in the antiphospholipid-antibody syndrome: warfarin, low-dose aspirin, or a combination of both.

Method.—A total of 147 patients were classified into 3 groups: 62 patients in which the syndrome was primary; 66 in which the syndrome was associated with systemic lupus erythematosus; and 19 in which it was associated with lupus-like disease. The antithrombotic treatment history of these patients with either warfarin, low-dose aspirin, or both was retrospectively reviewed, and the rates of recurrent thrombosis were analyzed.

Results.—One hundred one patients (69%) had 186 episodes of recurrent thrombosis. The median time between the initial thrombosis and the first recurrence was 12 months. Treatment with high-intensity warfarin (producing an international normalized ratio of 3 or above), with or without low-dose aspirin (75 mg/day), was significantly more effective in preventing thrombosis than treatment with low-intensity warfarin (international normalized ratio of less than 3) with or without low-dose aspirin, or aspirin alone (recurrence rates per patient-year were 0.013, 0.23, and 0.18, respectively) (Fig 1). The first 6 months after the cessation of warfarin therapy were associated with the highest rate of recurrence of thrombosis. Nonfatal complications of treatment included bleeding in 29 patients during warfarin treatment, with severe symptoms in 7 patients.

Conclusions.—A high risk of recurrent thrombosis exists in patients with the antiphospholipid-antibody syndrome. Long-term anticoagulation therapy with or without low-dose aspirin, in which an international normalized ratio of 3 or above is maintained, is recommended for these patients.

► This important retrospective study of 147 patients with the antiphospholipid-antibody syndrome seen over a 10-year period establishes as the treatment of choice long-term anticoagulation therapy with warfarin, in which the international normalized ratio is maintained at or above 3. In those who received this treatment, with or without low-dose aspirin, the probability that there would be no new thrombotic event over a 5-year period was 90% (Fig 1). After cessation of warfarin therapy (16.2 patient-years), the first 6 months were associated with the highest rate of recurrence: 1.30 thrombotic events

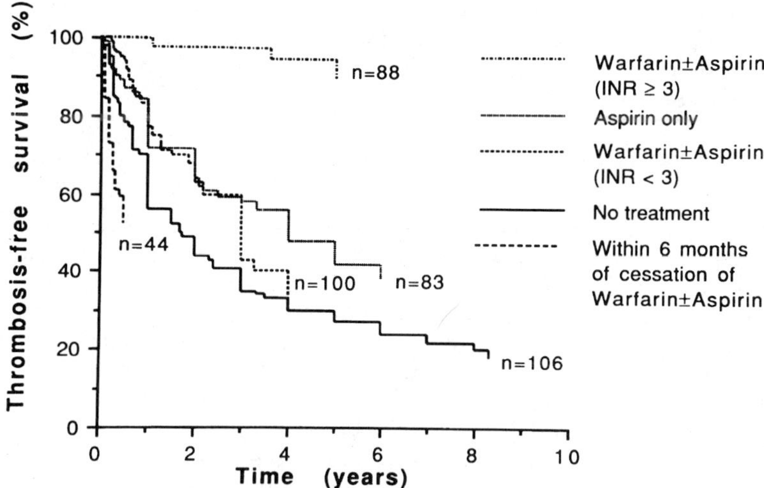

FIGURE 1.—Kaplan-Meier analysis of the interval from each episode of thrombosis or change in treatment to the next episode of thrombosis or censoring event in the same patient, throughout the follow-up, according to antithrombotic treatment. The total number of such intervals for patients while they were receiving each treatment is shown after each *curve*. *Abbreviation: INR,* international normalized ratio. (Reprinted by permission of *The New England Journal of Medicine*. Khamashta MA, Cuadrado MJ, Mujic F, et al: The management of thrombosis in the antiphospholipid-antibody syndrome. *N Engl J Med* 332:993–997, 1995. Copyright 1995, Massachusetts Medical Society.)

per year, a higher rate than that of the untreated patients ($P < 0.001$). The median time to recurrence after cessation of warfarin was 2 months (range, 0.5–6 months). When all consecutive pairs of thromboses in the same patient were analyzed, an arterial thrombosis was followed by an arterial thrombosis in 89 of 96 cases (93%); a venous thrombosis was followed by a venous thrombosis in 68 of 90 cases (76%).

The risk that warfarin in this range will cause hemorrhage (which occurred in 29 patients) was 1 in 14 per year; the risk of serious hemorrhage (7 patients) was 1 in 50. These risks compare favorably with the annual risk for new thrombosis of 1 in 3 for untreated patients, and 1 in 5 in patients treated with aspirin alone or with warfarin at lower doses.[1]

Note that inclusion in this study required positive tests for lupus anticoagulant, anticardiolipin antibodies, or both, as well as a history of thrombosis (venous, arterial, or both). That is because up to 2% of apparently normal individuals have detectable antiphospholipid antibodies.[1] Most of them may never have the syndrome (we worry most about the 0.2% of "normals" in whom the titers are high). Also excluded were pregnant women with a history of spontaneous abortion, because of the teratogenic properties of warfarin. Some of them do well with a combination of heparin and aspirin.

S.E. Malawista, M.D.

Reference

1. Lockshin MD: Answers to the antiphospholipid-antibody syndrome (editorial)? *N Engl J Med* 332:1025–1027, 1995.

Treatment-Free Remission in Severe Systemic Lupus Erythematosus Following Synchronization of Plasmapheresis With Subsequent Pulse Cyclophosphamide

Euler HH, Schroeder JO, Harten P, Zeuner RA, Gutschmidt HJ (Christian Albrecht Univ, Kiel, Germany; Municipal Hosp, Kiel, Germany)

Arthritis Rheum 37:1784–1794, 1994 119-96-65–2

Introduction.—Severe cases of systemic lupus erythematosus (SLE) have been treated by corticosteroids with azathioprine and/or cyclophosphamide (CYC). The administration of CYC as repeated IV pulse doses has yielded better results with fewer side effects. An intensified, experimental protocol was designed in which plasmapheresis, a promising therapeutic strategy in SLE, was combined with subsequent high-dose pulse CYC. The goal of this protocol was to schedule all aspects toward maximal clonal deletion, using the antibody rebound kinetics.

Patients and Methods.—Fourteen consecutive patients, all women, were prospectively enrolled in the treatment protocol. All had severe, active SLE unresponsive to at least 2 standard drugs. The mean age of the group was 29 years, and the average duration of disease was 48 months. Patients had a mean score of 28.4 on the Systemic Lupus Activity Measure (SLAM). Immunosuppression was withdrawn before treatment, consisting of plasmapheresis (3 × 60 mL/kg) and subsequent high-dose pulse CYC (total

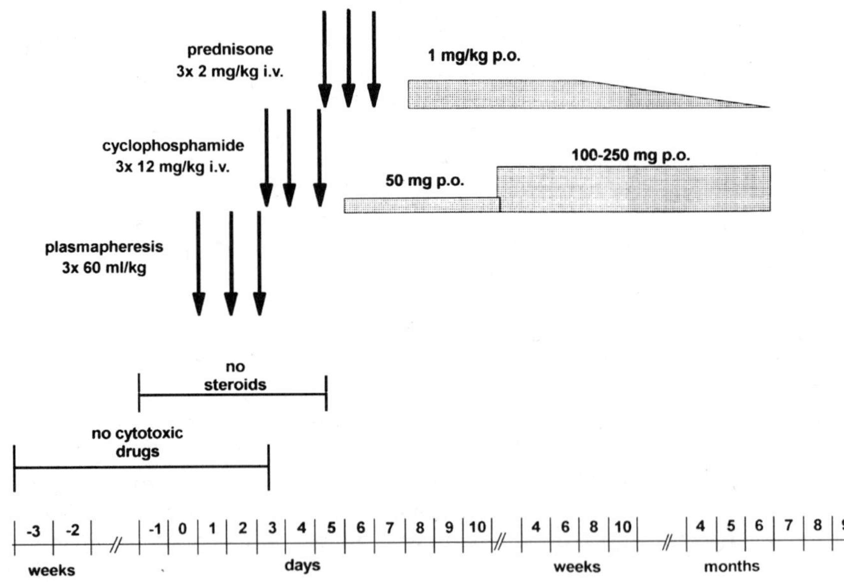

FIGURE 1.—Schedule of synchronized treatment with plasmapheresis and subsequent pulse IV cyclophosphamide, followed by 6 months of peroral (p.o.) cyclophosphamide and prednisone. (Courtesy of Euler HH, Schroeder JO, Harten P, et al: Treatment-free remission in severe systemic lupus erythematosus following synchronization of plasmapheresis with subsequent pulse cyclophosphamide. *Arthritis Rheum* 37:1784–1794, 1994.)

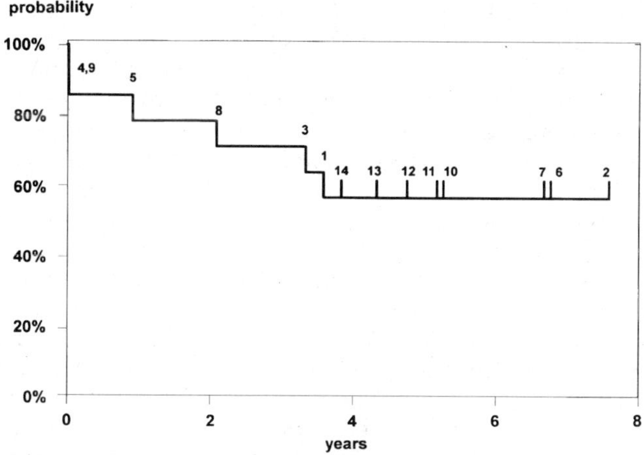

FIGURE 3.—Kaplan-Meier plot of the probability of a treatment-free course after synchronization of plasmapheresis with subsequent pulse cyclophosphamide in 14 patients with severe systemic lupus erythematosus. *Numbers* are the individual patient numbers. (Courtesy of Euler HH, Schroeder JO, Harten P, et al: Treatment-free remission in severe systemic lupus erythematosus following synchronization of plasmapheresis with subsequent pulse cyclophosphamide. *Arthritis Rheum* 37:1784–1794, 1994.)

dose 36 mg/kg) followed by 6 months of peroral CYC and prednisone (Fig 1). The overall hospital time averaged 31 days.

Results.—All 14 patients showed rapid clinical improvement and a marked decrease in the mean SLAM score to 14.7 at 4 weeks and 8.9 at 6 months after treatment. The mean hemoglobin levels increased from 97 g/L at entry to 114 g/L at 6 months. Improvements were also observed in thrombocytopenia and proteinuria, and in symptoms of arthritis and arthralgia. Twelve of 14 patients had achieved clinical remission after 6 months of peroral treatment with CYC and prednisone and were able to discontinue immunosuppressants. The mean SLAM score in these patients decreased further to 3.3 at 1 year. Eight patients (57%) remained in treatment-free clinical remission without relapse after a mean follow-up of 6 years (Fig 3). There were 4 cases of treatment-induced amenorrhea; other side effects included fever and reversible alopecia.

Conclusion.—The rationale of the protocol employed for these cases of severe SLE is based on a feedback between circulating antibodies and their clones. Long-term, treatment-free clinical remission was achieved in a substantial proportion of patients, but the protocol requires extended inpatient surveillance and close follow-up. The dose of CYC is lower than that associated with an increased risk of malignancy in patients treated for rheumatoid arthritis, but the potential risk for induction of malignancy cannot be excluded.

► Some years ago,[1] I described a study in which 2 patients with severe SLE had prolonged treatment-free remissions after therapy designed to induce the proliferation of pathogenic clones (by plasmapheresis), followed by partial clonal deletion (from cyclophosphamide, given during the assumed period of increased B-cell vulnerability). Subsequently, an oft-cited controlled trial suggested that plasmapheresis therapy in severe lupus nephritis did not improve upon standard therapy with cyclophosphamide and prednisone.[2] The earlier authors persisted, however, and they have now enlarged their series to 14 consecutive patients with severe SLE, all of whom improved in the short-run, and 8 of whom have been in treatment-free clinical remission for a mean observation of 67 months (range, 46–91 months). The treatment schedule is shown in Figure 1, and a Kaplan-Meier plot of the probability of a treatment-free course in Figure 3.

The authors stress that their treatment regimen is aggressive and experimental. With 36 mg of cyclophosphamide per kg of body weight (corresponding to ~1.2–1.4 g/m^2), the dosage of pulse cyclophosphamide therapy was 20% to 40% higher than previously used in patients with rheumatic diseases (up to 1.0 g/m^2), approaching dosages used in oncologic protocols. The patients were treated in a university clinic with extensive oncologic experience and a well-coordinated, experienced ICU. The utmost care was taken to ensure the complete exclusion of infections during the pretreatment and post-treatment periods, extended in patient surveillance, strict adherence to the protocol, and close subsequent follow-up by the original investigators. The authors believed that more traditional treatment approaches were indicated if any of these conditions could not be met. They recognize the need for controlled trials and cite as a first step in that direction the randomization of 6 cycles of pulse cyclophosphamide alone vs. 6 cycles of plasmapheresis with subsequent pulse cyclophosphamide in a multicenter trial being conducted by the International Lupus Plasmapheresis Study Group.

S.E. Malawista, M.D.

References

1. 1989 YEAR BOOK OF MEDICINE, pp 650–651.
2. 1993 YEAR BOOK OF MEDICINE, pp 591–592.

Postmenopausal Estrogen Therapy and the Risk for Developing Systemic Lupus Erythematosus

Sánchez-Guerrero J, Liang MH, Karlson EW, Hunter DJ, Colditz GA (Harvard Med School, Boston; Brigham and Women's Hosp, Boston; Harvard School of Public Health, Boston)

Ann Intern Med 122:430–433, 1995 119-96-65–3

Objective.—Data from the Nurses' Health Study were used to determine whether the risk for development of systemic lupus erythematosus was increased in women taking hormone supplements after menopause. There is strong evidence linking sex steroid hormones to the pathogenesis of this disease.

Methods.—The Nurses' Health Study cohort, assembled in 1976, included all female, married registered nurses aged 30–55 years living in 11 states. Biennial questionnaires completed by the cohort from 1976 onward sought information on various diagnoses and health practices, including the use of postmenopausal estrogen therapy. From 1976 to 1990, a total of 69,435 postmenopausal women had been followed. Included in the study were women with systemic lupus erythematosus whose condition was diagnosed during this 14-year period. These women were classified as never-users or ever-users of estrogen therapy.

Results.—Forty-five definite cases of systemic lupus erythematosus were confirmed during the study. Fifteen cases were in women who never used hormones and 30 were in women who used hormones currently or were past users. The incidence of systemic lupus erythematosus was 4.5 per 100,000 women among never-users and 9.9 per 100,000 women among ever-users. Women who used postmenopausal hormones for more than 5 years had a greater risk for the disease than those who took the hormones for 1–4 years. The age-adjusted relative risk was 2.1 for ever-users and 3.5 for women who received estrogen therapy for more than 11 years. After adjustment for smoking, the age-adjusted relative risk was similar for that seen after adjustment for age only.

Conclusion.—The use of postmenopausal hormone therapy was associated with an increased risk for systemic lupus erythematosus. This finding is in keeping with the results of other studies that report evidence of a strong association between sex steroid hormones and the disease. Current users had a higher risk than past users, and longer duration of hormone replacement therapy was associated with an even greater risk for the development of systemic lupus erythematosus.

► During 631,551 person-years of follow-up among 69,435 postmenopausal women in the Nurses' Health Study, the authors found that the use of postmenopausal hormone therapy was associated with an increased risk for systemic lupus erythematosus (SLE) compared with no use of such hormones, and that among ever-users, the risk for SLE was higher in current users than in past users. In all, 45 definite cases of SLE were confirmed, 15 among patients who never used hormones and 30 among women who had or were currently using them. The incidences of SLE per 100,000 women were 4.5 and 9.9, respectively.

This study represents another link between sex steroid hormones and the propensity to develop SLE, but should it affect our treatment of postmenopausal women? Such questions are properly decided individually, but the authors suggest, and I agree, that the changes in the absolute risks imposed by this therapy on other major illnesses and comforts should in general take precedence over the increase in the relative risk for SLE.

S.E. Malawista, M.D.

Mortality Studies in Systemic Lupus Erythematosus. Results From a Single Center: I. Causes of Death

Abu-Shakra M, Urowitz MB, Gladman DD, Gough J (Univ of Toronto)
J Rheumatol 22:1259–1264, 1995 119-96-65–4

Background.—Since the 1950s, there have been significant improvements in the survival of patients with systemic lupus erythematosus (SLE). Previous studies have suggested that mortality in SLE follows a bimodal pattern: most early deaths result from active SLE and/or intercurrent infection, whereas most late deaths result from reactivated SLE and non–SLE-related causes, such as atherosclerosis and infection. The causes of death in a cohort of 665 patients with SLE were analyzed.

Methods.—The patients were prospectively followed in a single lupus center, in which they were enrolled from 1970 to 1993. Information was drawn from hospital files, autopsy reports, and death certificates to determine causes of death. Kaplan-Meier estimates of survival probabilities were calculated by means of nonparametric life-table models.

Results.—Nineteen percent of the patients died during follow-up. In this group of 124 patients, the primary cause of death was active SLE in 16%, infection in 32%, an acute vascular event in 15%, sudden death in 8%, organ failure in 5%, cancer in 7%, other causes in 7%, and unknown causes in 11%. Patients who died within 5 years after their diagnosis of SLE were more likely to die of active SLE than those who died later. For patients who died after 5 years, death from vascular causes and from end-organ failure was more frequent. Overall survival was 93% at 5 years, 85% at 10 years, 79% at 15 years, and 68% at 20 years. Compared with the general population, the risk of death for patients with SLE was increased by nearly fivefold.

Conclusions.—Survival has improved for patients with SLE. The causes of death vary at different stages of the disease, but infection occurs throughout the course of illness. Future management of patients with lupus may be aided by understanding the prognostic factors associated with death.

► The authors point out that over the past 40 years, the survival of patients with SLE has increased significantly. A study in 1955 reported a survival rate of less than 50% at 5 years; most recent studies find survival rates greater than 90% at 10 years. The difference has been attributed to earlier diagnosis, more appropriately used antilupus therapies (recall that corticosteroids were introduced as therapeutic agents in the early 1950s), and advances in medical therapy in general. Therefore, although work in the 1960s and 1970s attributed more than half of all deaths to active SLE, the current analysis found active SLE to be the primary cause of death in only 16%, whereas complications of therapy and disease-related morbidity are becoming increasingly important.

A bimodal pattern of causes of death apparent in recent years is again seen, with active SLE and/or intercurrent infection leading the causes of death in patients who died within 5 years of diagnosis; later on, death tends to result from complications of atherosclerosis (the latter perhaps encouraged by corticosteroid therapy), end-organ failure, major infection, and occasionally from reactivation of SLE. Note that major infections were the primary cause of death in 40 (32%) patients, contributed to death in another 12 (9.7%), and occurred both early and late. Concurrent active SLE was seen in 67% of the 54 patients who died with infection, suggesting that infections were more likely to develop in patients with active disease receiving high doses of corticosteroids and/or immunosuppressive therapy.

In an accompanying paper,[1] predictor values for mortality were unsurprising: renal damage, thrombocytopenia, lung involvement, an SLE disease activity index (SLEDAI) 20 or greater at presentation, and age 50 years or older at diagnosis.

S.E. Malawista, M.D.

Reference

1. Abu-Shakra M, Urowitz MB, Gladman DD, Gough J: Mortality studies in systemic lupus erythematosus: Results from a single center: II. Predictor variables for mortality. *J Rheumatol* 22:1265–1270, 1995.

66 Spondyloarthropathy and Reactive Arthritis

Introduction

In this chapter, we examine the use of sulfasalazine in the treatment of spondyloarthropathy (Abstract 119-96-66–1) and learn that the germ-free state prevents the development of gut and joint inflammatory disease in HLA-B27 transgenic rats (Abstract 119-96-66–2).

Noted in passing: A review of the treatment of psoriasis.[1]

Stephen E. Malawista, M.D.

Reference

1. Greaves MW, Weinstein GD: Treatment of psoriasis. *N Engl J Med* 332:581–588, 1995.

Sulfasalazine in the Treatment of Spondylarthropathy: A Randomized, Multicenter, Double-Blind, Placebo-Controlled Study

Dougados M, van der Linden S, Leirisalo-Repo M, Huitfeldt B, Juhlin R, Veys E, Zeidler H, Kvien TK, Olivieri I, Dijkmans B, Bertouch J, Brooks P, Edmonds J, Major G, Amor B, Calin A (Université René Descartes, Paris, France; Academisch Ziekenhuis Maastricht, The Netherlands; Helsinki Univ Central Hosp; et al)

Arthritis Rheum 38:618–627, 1995 119-96-66–1

Background.—The spondyloarthropathies are a heterogenous group of arthritic disorders that are usually treated symptomatically with nonsteroidal anti-inflammatory drugs (NSAIDs). However, NSAIDs are ineffective in preventing progression of these disorders, and the addition of other therapeutic agents is often necessary. Because of the success of sulfasalazine (SSZ) in the therapy of inflammatory bowel disease, a disorder often accompanying the spondyloarthropathies, the efficacy and safety of SSZ were assessed in the treatment of spondyloarthropathies.

Methods.—The 6-month study was multicenter (8 sites, including Australia and 7 European countries), randomized, double-blind, and placebo-controlled. Patients were subgrouped into 3 categories depending on their underlying disease: ankylosing spondylitis, psoriatic arthritis, and symmetrical peripheral arthritis. The degree of arthritic involvement was graded on the basis of clinical and laboratory findings. Patients were randomly assigned to receive placebo or SSZ, administered in 500-mg increments until a total of 3 g/day was attained. The primary efficacy end points were the physician's and the patient's overall assessments of pain and morning stiffness. Secondary efficacy endpoints were changes in biological markers of inflammation.

Results.—A series of 351 patients (179 randomly assigned to receive SSZ and 172 to receive placebo) constituted the intent-to-treat group. During the study, 88 patients withdrew prematurely. Of these, 17 (5 SSZ and 12 placebo) withdrew because of lack of efficacy; 37 because of side effects (28 SSZ and 9 placebo); and 34 for reasons unrelated to treatment (20 SSZ and 14 placebo). Thus, 263 (126 SSZ and 137 placebo) constituted the protocol-completed group. The 2 groups were comparable as far as demographic data and baseline clinical and laboratory findings. In the intent-to-treat group, there was a statistically significant

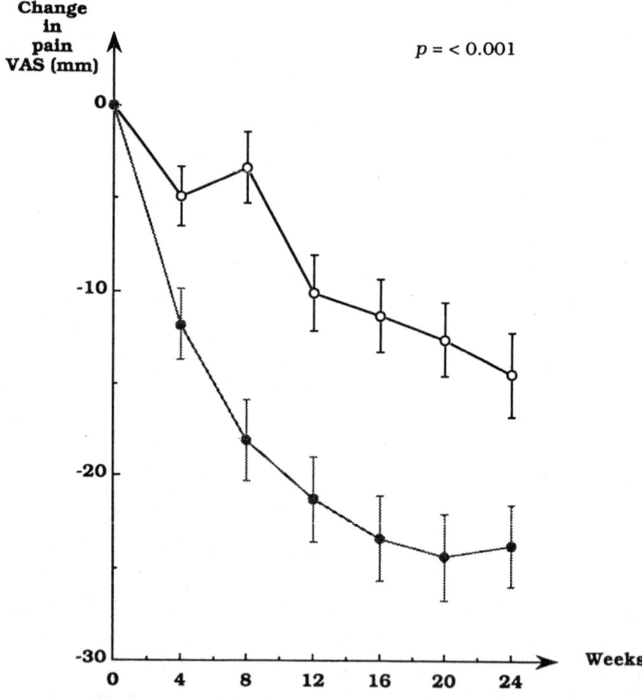

FIGURE 1.—Mean ± SEM change in pain (measured on a visual analogue scale [*VAS*]) over time in 137 patients given placebo (*open circles*) and 126 patients given sulfasalazine (*filled circles*) who completed the 6 months of the trial. The *P* value is the statistical significance of difference between treatment groups in time course of effect, determined by repeated-measures analysis of variance. (Courtesy of Dougados M, van der Linden S, Leirisalo-Repo M, et al: Sulfasalazine in the treatment of spondylarthropathy: A randomized, multicenter, double-blind, placebo-controlled study. *Arthritis Rheum* 38:618–627, 1995.)

TABLE 6.—Type and Frequency of the Main Reported Adverse Effects in the 351 Spondyloarthropathy Patients, by Treatment Group*

Side effect	Treatment group Placebo (n = 172)	Sulfasalazine (n = 179)
Gastrointestinal disorders		
Nausea	13 (3)	36 (4)
Abdominal pain	15 (1)	14 (4)
Diarrhea	10	9 (1)
Stomatitis	2 (2)	1 (1)
Duodenal ulcer	0	1 (1)
Skin disorders		
Pruritus	4 (1)	6 (2)
Eruption	7	11 (8)
CNS disorder		
Dizziness	10	8
Headache	8	24 (1)
Neuropathy	0	1 (1)
Hematologic disorders		
Hemoglobin decrease of at least 2 gm/dl	10	28
WBC $\leq 3.5 \times 10^9$/liter	6	6 (3)
Liver disorders		
Increase in hepatic enzyme levels (at least twice the normal range)	0	2 (2)
Other		
Myalgia	1 (1)	0
Anxiety	1 (1)	0

* Values are number of patients with the adverse event (number who dropped out of trial because of the adverse event).

Abbreviation: WBC, white blood cells.

(Courtesy of Dougados M, van der Linden S, Leirisalo-Repo M, et al: Sulfasalazine in the treatment of spondylarthropathy: A randomized, multicenter, double-blind, placebo-controlled study. *Arthritis Rheum* 38:618–627, 1995.)

difference favoring SSZ-treated patients in the patients' overall assessments (P = 0.007), and a strong tendency favoring SSZ in pain and physicians' overall assessments. In the protocol-completed group, there were significant differences favoring the SSZ-treated group in 3 of the 4 primary efficacy end points and in the secondary end points representing biological markers of inflammation. The plateau of maximal efficacy of SSZ appeared to occur after 16 weeks of treatment (Fig 1). All 3 patient subgroups participated in these efficacy results, but the most notable improvement occurred in patients with psoriatic arthritis. At least 1 adverse event was reported in 108 SSZ-treated patients (60%), compared with 93 in the placebo-treated group (48%). Withdrawals resulting from adverse events occurred in 28 patients in the SSZ group and in 9 in the placebo group (P = 0.002) (Table 6). All adverse events were reversible on drug withdrawal.

Conclusions.—Sulfasalazine was superior to placebo in the treatment of 3 groups of spondyloarthropathies—ankylosing spondylitis, psoriatic arthritis, and symmetrical peripheral arthritis. Although the incidence of adverse events was significantly higher with SSZ than with placebo, all events were reversible on drug withdrawal.

► The spondyloarthropathies comprise several disorders: reactive arthritis, psoriatic arthritis, arthritis related to inflammatory bowel disease, a subgroup of juvenile chronic arthritis, and ankylosing spondylitis, the last being the prototype of this group of interrelated and often HLA-B27–associated disorders. Classification within this group may be based either on the clinical diagnosis (e.g., ankylosing spondylitis, psoriatic arthritis) or on the presenting symptoms (axial disease, peripheral articular disease, or extra-articular manifestations). Some believe that monitoring and treatment are better related to presenting symptoms than to clinical diagnosis. This study, from centers in 8 countries on 2 continents, was designed to evaluate the efficacy of SSZ in the treatment of the group of spondyloarthropathies as a whole, and the relationships between patient characteristics and the effects of SSZ on the course of these illnesses.

In addition to the positive findings noted in the abstract and in Figure 1, the results suggest a clear beneficial effect in the reduction of synovitis in patients with polyarticular involvement, but not in spinal mobility in patients with axial involvement. However, the mean duration of disease in these patients (~9 years) was rather long, and some axial lesions may have been fixed. The incidence of uveitis during the study was lower in the treated group (1 vs. 6), in accordance with previous work. Note that the improvement in placebo-treated patients (Fig 1) makes differences between them and the SSZ group more difficult to appreciate; this may reflect a relatively benign natural history of spondyloarthropathies, as well as their characteristic flares and remissions independent of treatment. The side effects of SSZ (Table 6) were reversible and generally acceptable.

S.E. Malawista, M.D.

The Germfree State Prevents Development of Gut and Joint Inflammatory Disease in *HLA-B27* Transgenic Rats

Taurog JD, Richardson JA, Croft JT, Simmons WA, Zhou M, Fernández-Sueiro JL, Balish E, Hammer RE (Univ of Texas Southwestern Med Ctr, Dallas; Univ of Wisconsin, Madison)

J Exp Med 180:2359–2364, 1994 119-96-66–2

Introduction.—Individuals with the human major histocompatibility complex class I allele HLA-B27 have a greatly increased frequency of various inflammatory disease states. In patients with B27-associated reactive arthritis, the disease may be triggered by infection with enteric or genitourinary bacterial pathogens. Although no pathogenetic role for bacteria has been shown for most types of B27-associated disease, intestinal inflammation is often present and sometimes makes up a large part of the clinical picture. The effects of living in a germ-free state on the development of inflammatory disease in B27 transgenic rats were assessed.

Methods and Results.—Rats transgenic for B27 were used because they have previously been shown to develop a disorder resembling B27-associated disease in humans. Manifestations in these animals include prominent intestinal, joint, skin, and male genital inflammatory lesions. When B27 transgenic rats were raised in a germ-free environment, the inflammatory intestinal and peripheral joint disease did not occur (Fig 1). In contrast, the

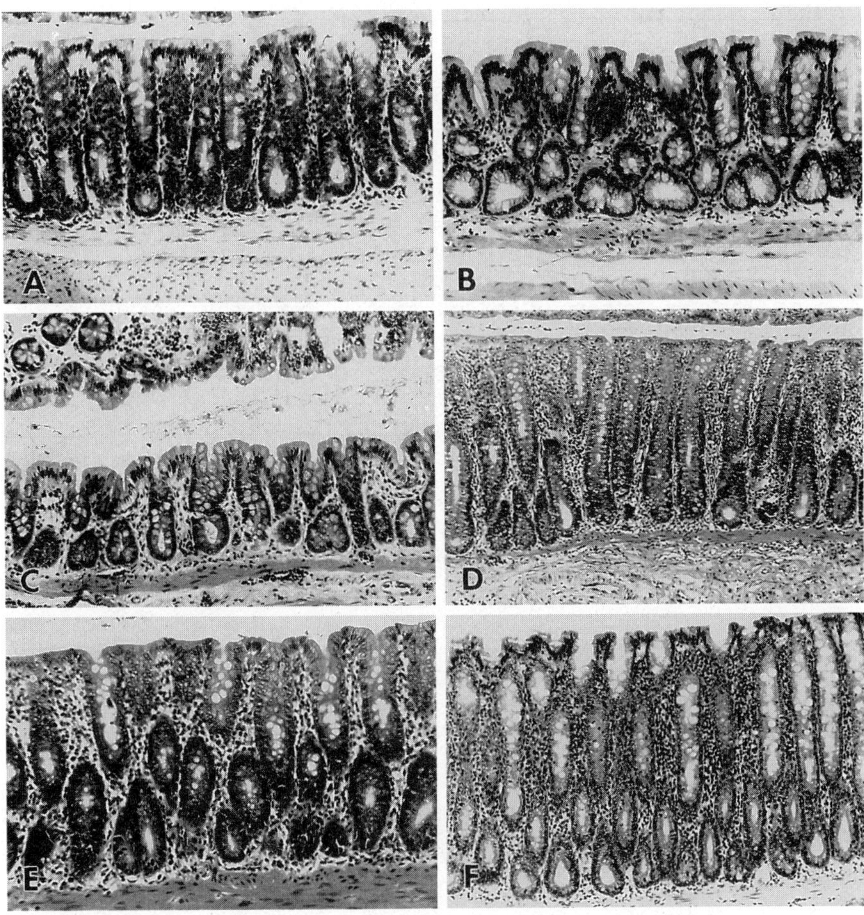

FIGURE 1.—Histology of distal colon in germ-free and non–germ-free rats. **A,** colon of a 52-week-old germ-free 21-4H male rat. The section shows shallow crypts with no inflammation. **B,** colon of a 39-week-old germ-free 33-3 male rat, with histology similar to that shown in **A. C,** colon of a 48-week-old germ-free nontransgenic male 21-4H littermate, with histology similar to that shown in **A. D,** colon of a 52-week-old 21-4H female rat born and raised in a barrier facility. The section shows typical chronic colitis, with crypt hyperplasia, loss of mucin-containing cells, and an inflammatory infiltrate in the lamina propria. **E,** colon of a 55-week-old 21-4H male rat germ-free until age 52 weeks and then housed in a conventional room for 23 days. The section shows early inflammatory changes. **F,** colon of a 52-week-old 21-4H male rat germ-free until age 8 weeks and then housed in a barrier facility for 44 weeks. The section shows changes similar to those shown in **D.** For **A–C,** and **E,** original magnification, ×130; for **D,** ×73; for **F,** ×100. (Reproduced from *The Journal of Experimental Medicine,* 1994, 180, pp 2359–2364, by copyright permission of The Rockefeller University Press.)

skin and genital inflammatory lesions did occur. When the transgenic rats were removed from the germ-free environment, suppression of gut inflammation was rapidly reversed.

Conclusions.—The pathogenesis of gut and joint inflammation in B27-related disease appears to be closely related. The commensal gut flora seems to play a key role in the development of B27-associated gut and joint inflammation. Further study will identify the bacterial components critical to the development of B27-related disease.

▶ This elegant paper speaks for itself. Because of the evidence for a potential role for intestinal flora in the pathogenesis of B27-associated disease, the authors investigated the effect of the germ-free state on the inflammatory disease resembling B27-associated human disease, which is expressed in B27 transgenic rats.[1] The germ-free animals did not develop either inflammatory intestinal or peripheral joint disease, linking these 2 lesions and tying them pathogenetically to the presence of commensal gut flora. The germ-free state did not protect the rats from typical skin and nail lesions. Their persistence is not immediately explainable, but the authors offer 2 possibilities: (1) the environment was germ-free but not antigen-free, and conceivably nonviable organisms may have played a role in the induction of these lesions; and (2) the skin and nail changes may be constant manifestations of transgene expression unrelated to environmental factors.

S.E. Malawista, M.D.

Reference

1. 1992 Year Book of Medicine, p 639.

67 Sclerosing Syndromes

Introduction

In this chapter we consider silicone breast implants and the risk of connective-tissue diseases and symptoms (Abstract 119-96-67–1), and the status of 205 patients with the eosinophilia-myalgia syndrome 2 years after onset (Abstract 119-96-67–2).

Noted in passing: A 12-year follow-up study of the epidemic toxic oil syndrome that occurred in Spain in 1981,[1] with more long-term morbidity noted than in a study discussed last year[2]; anti-topoisomerase I antibodies in patients with silica-associated systemic sclerosis, suggesting silica particles as the trigger to disease expression in genetically susceptible individuals[3]; and the relation of the modulation of collagen gene expression to fibrosis in systemic sclerosis and other disorders.[4]

Stephen E. Malawista, M.D.

References

1. Kaufman LD, Martinez MI, Serrano JM, Gomez-Reino JJ: 12-Year follow-up study of epidemic spanish toxic oil syndrome. *J Rheumatol* 22:282–288, 1995.
2. 1995 YEAR BOOK OF MEDICINE, pp 803–805.
3. McHugh NJ, Whyte J, Harvey G, Haustein UF: Anti-topoisomerase I antibodies in silica-associated systemic sclerosis: A model for autoimmunity. *Arthritis Rheum* 37:1198–1205, 1994.
4. Varga J, Jimenez SA: Modulation of collagen gene expression: Its relation to fibrosis in systemic sclerosis and other disorders. *Ann Intern Med* 122:60–62, 1995.

Silicone Breast Implants and the Risk of Connective-Tissue Diseases and Symptoms

Sánchez-Guerrero J, Colditz GA, Karlson EW, Hunter DJ, Speizer FE, Liang MH (Harvard Med School, Boston; Brigham and Women's Hosp, Boston; Harvard School of Public Health, Boston)

N Engl J Med 332:1666–1670, 1995 119-96-67–1

Introduction.—More than a million women in the United States and Canada have received silicone breast implants in the past 3 decades, either for reconstruction after removal of breast cancer or prophylactic mastectomy or for cosmetic reasons. Approximately 300 implant-bearing women

TABLE 2.—Age-Adjusted Relative Risk of Connective-Tissue Disease Among Women With Breast Implants as Compared With Women Without Implants

Case Type	No Implant (n = 86.318)	Breast Implant: any type (n = 1183)	Breast Implant: silicone-gel-filled* (n = 876)
Self-reported connective-tissue disease			
No. of cases	5,054	32	21
Age-adjusted relative risk	1.0	0.7	0.6
95% Confidence interval		0.5–1.0	0.4–0.9
Self-reported signs or symptoms of connective-tissue disease†			
No. of cases	1,277	17	11
Age-adjusted relative risk	1.0	1.5	1.2
95% Confidence interval		0.9–2.4	0.7–2.2
Documented signs or symptoms of connective-tissue disease‡			
No. of cases	898	6	4
Age-adjusted relative risk	1.0	0.7	0.6
95% Confidence interval		0.3–1.6	0.2–1.6
Definite connective-tissue disease			
No. of cases	513	3	1
Age-adjusted relative risk	1.0	0.6	0.3
95% Confidence interval		0.2–2.0	0.0–1.9
Duration of implant			
Mean (±SD) yr		9.9 ± 6.4	10.0 ± 6.2
Range		1 mo–40.5 yr	1 mo–37.5 yr

* This category is a subgroup of "any type" of implant.

† Signs and symptoms are those included in screening questionnaire on connective-tissue disease.

‡ Data were derived from medical record review. Documented signs and symptoms included proximal weakness, a high creatinine kinase concentration, positive electromyogram, positive muscle biopsy, proximal scleroderma, sclerodactyly, digital scars, bibasilar lung fibrosis, malar or discoid rash, photosensitivity, nasopharyngeal ulcers, nonerosive arthritis, pleuritis, pericarditis, proteinuria, renal casts, seizures, psychosis, hemolytic anemia, leukopenia, lymphopenia, thrombocytopenia, positive test for lupus erythematosus, antibodies to double-stranded DNA, biological false positive serologic test for syphilis, positive test for anticardiolipin antibody, positive antinuclear antibody test, Raynaud's phenomenon, morning stiffness for more than 1 hour, arthritis in 3 or more joint areas, arthritis in hand joints, rheumatoid nodules, positive rheumatoid factor tests, radiographic changes characteristic of rheumatoid arthritis, keratoconjunctivitis, xerostomia, salivary gland biopsy positive for Sjögren's syndrome, and anti-Ro, anti-La, anti–extractable-nuclear-antigen and anti–U1-RNP antibodies.

(Reprinted by permission of *The New England Journal of Medicine*. Sánchez-Guerrero J, Colditz GA, Karlson EW, et al: Silicone breast implants and the risk of connective-tissue diseases and symptoms. *N Engl J Med* 332:1666–1670, 1995. Copyright 1995, Massachusetts Medical Society.)

with connective-tissue disease or rheumatic disease have been reported in the English-language literature since 1982, and many more cases have been reported in abstract form.

Objective.—The relationship between silicone breast implants and connective-tissue disease was examined in follow-up data from the Nurses' Health Study cohort, which includes married female registered nurses aged 30–55 years.

Findings.—A definite diagnosis of connective tissue-disease was made in 516 of 87,501 eligible women. Breast implants were present in 1,183 participants; a majority were filled with silicone gel. Three women with implants had rheumatoid arthritis during an average follow-up of 10 years. One each had a silicone gel–filled, a saline-filled, and a double-lumen implant. The age-adjusted relative risk of definite connective-tissue disease being diagnosed in women with implants of any type was 0.6, and for those with silicone gel–filled implants, 0.3 (Table 2). When women with possible early, mild, or atypical connective-tissue disease and those having any symptom or sign of such disease were considered, the age-adjusted relative risk for those with breast implants was 0.7.

Conclusion.—This large cohort gives no evidence of a significant association between silicone breast implants and connective-tissue disease.

▶ In this large cohort study (1,181,244 person-years of follow-up), the authors did not find an increased risk of any connective-tissue disease or of 41 signs and symptoms of connective-tissue disease (Table 2) among women with any breast implant or with specific types of breast implants. Because connective-tissue diseases occur infrequently, their study cannot be considered definitively negative; they point out that the upper bound of the 95% confidence interval for the relative risk of definite connective-tissue disease (2.0) does not exclude minor associations that would still be of public health importance.

They found no association between breast implants and previously reported signs and symptoms, such as Raynaud's phenomenon, photosensitivity, arthritis, morning stiffness, xerostomia, dry eyes, sclerodactyly, positive antinuclear-antibody tests, and positive rheumatoid factor tests. They could not study subjective and largely unverifiable symptoms such as fatigue, decreased ability to sleep, frequent sore throats, cognitive deficits, arthralgias, lymphadenopathy, or dizziness, or diseases such as fibromyalgia.

Their results are consistent with other published results of epidemiologic studies of breast implants and rheumatic diseases, including the large population-based retrospective cohort study reported in these pages last year.[1] Meanwhile, women with implants who have any number of vague complaints continue to line up for large cash awards.[2]

S.E. Malawista, M.D.

References

1. 1995 Year Book of Medicine, pp 831–833.
2. Boot M: Rule of law. *The Wall Street Journal,* October 4, 1995.

The Eosinophilia-Myalgia Syndrome: Status of 205 Patients and Results of Treatment 2 Years After Onset

Hertzman PA, Clauw DJ, Kaufman LD, Varga J, Silver RM, Thacker HL, Mease P, Espinoza LR, Pincus T (Los Alamos Med Ctr, New Mexico; Georgetown Univ, Washington, DC; State Univ of New York, Stony Brook; et al)

Ann Intern Med 122:851–855, 1995 119-96-67–2

Objective.—There is little information about the treatment and status of patients with eosinophilia-myalgia syndrome. The symptoms, physical findings, laboratory data, and response to treatment at onset and 18–24 months later were reviewed in patients with eosinophilia-myalgia syndrome.

Methods.—A total of 205 patients (79% female, 98% white), aged 20–82 years, with eosinophil counts of 1,000 cells/mm^3 or greater; and with fasciitis, peripheral neuropathy, polyradiculopathy, interstitial pulmonary disease, pulmonary hypertension, or myocardial involvement; and with a history of L-tryptophan consumption; and an absence of other conditions that could account for symptoms, were studied.

Results.—A total of 98% of patients had used L-tryptophan for an average of 8 months, 47% on the advice of a health professional. The mean eosinophil count was 4,705 cells/mm^3. After 18–24 months, all symptoms except for cognitive changes had improved in more than 60% of patients. In 32% of patients, cognitive changes had worsened. Most symptoms had resolved or improved except for peripheral neuropathy, which was unchanged in 47% of patients. Nine patients died. Older age and ascending neuropathy were significant predictors of death. Prednisone effected improvement in 79% of patients. A variety of other drug treatments were effective in approximately 50% of patients.

Conclusion.—Eighteen to 24 months after onset, most symptoms had improved or abated in the majority of patients. Cognitive changes deteriorated in 32% of patients. Prednisone was effective in 79% of patients during the acute phase of the syndrome. No drug treatments were effective during the later stages of the disease.

▶ The eosinophilia-myalgia syndrome, associated with the ingestion of L-tryptophan, appeared in the fall of 1989; within 6 months almost 1,500 cases had been reported to the Centers for Disease Control and Prevention. This article represents the largest collection of data so far on the status of patients with this syndrome 2 years after onset, coming from 15 clinical settings and organized according to a predefined protocol. The outcomes are generally good—better than those from a smaller single-author group reported last year.[1] Eighteen to 24 months after onset, myalgia, fatigue, rash, respiratory symptoms, edema, muscle weakness, arthralgia, alopecia, weight loss, fever, weight gain, dry mouth, and oral ulcerations had resolved or improved in more than 60% of patients. The downside was persistent peripheral neuropathy and, in almost a third of patients, a worsening of cognitive changes (impaired memory, impaired concentration, or mood change). Other symptoms reported as worse in at least 10% of patients were muscle weakness (10%), weight gain (10%), and fatigue (11%). New symptoms developing in patients 1 year after onset were unusual: new cognitive changes in 15%, new muscle cramps in 10%, and new other symptoms in 5%.

S.E. Malawista, M.D.

Reference

1. 1995 Year Book of Medicine, pp 803–805.

68 Crystal-Associated Arthritis

Introduction

In this chapter, we examine the treatment of acute gouty arthritis with intramuscular ketorolac tromethamine (Abstract 119-96-68–1), and learn that it is formalin, not water, that is largely responsible for dissolving urate crystals in tophaceous tissue samples (Abstract 119-96-68–2).

Noted in passing: Treatment of severe colchicine overdose with colchicine-specific Fab fragments.[1]

Stephen E. Malawista, M.D.

Reference

1. Baud FJ, Sabouraud A, Vicaut E, Taboulet P, Lang J, Bismuth C, Rouzioux JM, Scherrmann J-M: Treatment of severe colchicine overdose with colchicine-specific fab fragments. *N Engl J Med* 332:642–645, 1995.

Treatment of Acute Gouty Arthritis With Intramuscular Ketorolac Tromethamine

Shrestha M, Chiu MJ, Martin RL, Cush JJ, Wainscott MS (Univ of Texas, Dallas; Parkland Mem Hosp, Dallas)

Am J Emerg Med 12:454–455, 1994 119-96-68–1

Background.—Both orally administered colchicine and nonsteroidal anti-inflammatory drugs (NSAIDs) require some time to relieve the symptoms of acute gouty arthritis. Parenteral colchicine or indomethacin yields a more rapid response but may have serious side effects. Ketorolac is a parenteral NSAID that reportedly is effective in treating perioperative pain.

Objective.—Intramusclar ketorolac was evaluated in 9 consecutive patients seen in the emergency department with an acute attack of gout. Eight patients had monarticular involvement, most often of the great toe or ankle.

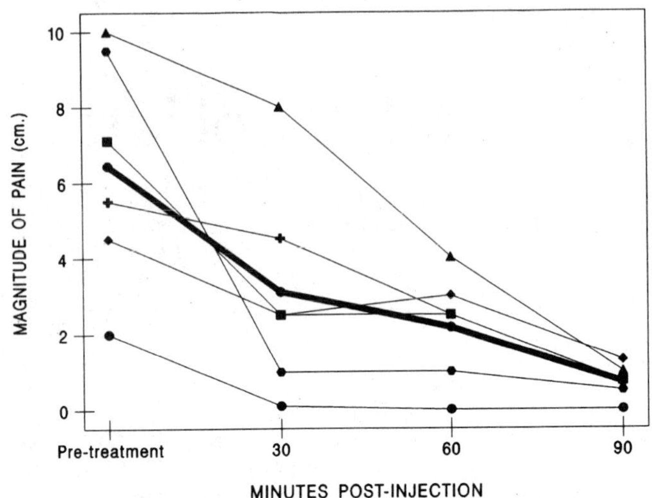

FIGURE 1.—Time course of pain scores for 6 patients (represented by *different symbols* connected with *thin lines*) before and 30, 60, and 90 minutes after administration of ketorolac, 60 mg IM. Mean pain-score progression is shown by the *bold line*. (Courtesy of Shrestha M, Chiu MJ, Martin RL, et al: Treatment of acute gouty arthritis with intramuscular ketorolac tromethamine. *Am J Emerg Med* 12:454–455, 1994.)

Management.—The patients received 60 mg of ketorolac intramuscularly, and their degree of pain was monitored serially for up to 90 minutes using a visual analogue scale as well as a descriptive scale.

Results.—In the 6 patients studied in detail, the mean pain score decreased from 6.4 to 1.0 after 90 minutes (Fig 1). The degree of subjective pain relief averaged 80%. The patients who were less closely observed also responded rapidly to treatment and were promptly discharged. No adverse effects were noted.

Conclusion.—Intramuscular ketorolac is a safe and rapidly effective means of treating attacks of acute gouty arthritis. A randomized, double-blind trial comparing this treatment with oral indocin has been instituted.

▶ The results of this emergency department study are impressive. The criteria for acute gouty arthritis were scrupulous; the treatment, simple; and the response over a mere 90 minutes, dramatic (Fig 1). None of the patients required crutches on discharge (8 of the 9 had had lower extremity involvement). The 4 patients reachable by telephone the following day were pain free and without adverse effects; the 5 without telephones did not return to that facility within the next 2 weeks. If these results are confirmed, this regimen may replace oral indomethacin as the treatment of choice in those patients who can tolerate NSAIDs (IV indoprofen has been used for some time in Europe, with resolution of gouty pain occurring within a few hours[1]).

S.E. Malawista, M.D.

Reference

1. Marcolongo R, Lucchese M, Caruso I: Intravenous indoprofen for prompt relief of acute gout: A regimen finding study. *J Intern Med Res* 8:326–331, 1980.

Not Water, But Formalin, Dissolves Urate Crystals in Tophaceous Tissue Samples

Simkin PA, Bassett JE, Lee QP (Univ of Washington, Seattle)
J Rheumatol 21:2320–2321, 1994 119-96-68–2

Purpose.—To preserve the urate crystals in tophaceous material for subsequent examination, biopsy specimens of suspected tophi are fixed in alcohol rather than in formalin. The reason given for this practice is that urate crystals dissolve in the aqueous base of formalin. The relative solubility of urate crystals was examined.

Methods.—Weighed triplicate aliquots of synthetic urate crystals were incubated in water, formalin, and ethanol for 72 hours at 4°C under constant agitation. At the end of the study period, the crystals were examined with a standard polarizing microscope.

Results.—Urate crystals did not dissolve in alcohol, dissolved somewhat in water, and dissolved in formalin (Table 1). However, urate crystals dissolve in formalin because of the formation of urate:formaldehyde addition products, rather than the weak solvent properties of water.

▶ Take away the crystals from a gouty tophus, and the pathologic landscape, as Professor Leon Sokoloff taught us some 35 years ago, can resemble a rheumatoid nodule. The simplest approach to such a mystery nodule is needle aspiration and microscopic examination of the aspirate in polarized light, seeking the strongly negatively birefringent crystals that will clinch the diagnosis. When that does not work, a biopsy specimen can be examined in cryostat sections or fixed for subsequent study. In the latter case, we have always abjured our fellows to fix the tissue in absolute alcohol, lest the aqueous media leech away the diagnostic crystals. The procedure was right, the reason, wrong; the formaldehyde in that media is a better urate solvent than water by 2 orders of magnitude (Table 1).

TABLE 1.—Qualitative Assessment of Visible Urate Crystals After 72 Hours in 10-mL Aliquots of 3 Different Solvents

	Urate Crystal Mass (mg)						
	0.5	2	5	20	50	200	500
Formalin	0	0	0	0	0	0	3+
Water	0	0	2+	4+	4+	4+	4+
Ethanol	3+	3+	4+	4+	4+	4+	4+

(Courtesy of Simkin PA, Bassett JE, Lee QP: Not water, but formalin, dissolves urate crystals in tophaceous tissue samples. *J Rheumatol* 21:2320–2321, 1994.)

We have long known that urate is only sparingly soluble in water. The solubility of urate in plasma at 37°C is roughly the same as the upper limit of normal as defined by 2 SDs above the mean of normal individuals (e.g., near 7 mg%); it is less so at cooler temperatures (The work in Table 1 was done at 4°C to discourage contamination during the 72-hour incubation). If the solubility of urate in vivo were much higher, we would never get the gout. Dissolution of urate in aqueous media was probably attributed to the relatively large volumes of fixative employed, but in fact that explanation does not survive examination. Simkin et al. have gently left us with a little egg on our faces for not having pursued this paradox further for all of these years.

S.E. Malawista, M.D.

69 Vasculitis

Introduction

This chapter deals with apparent fluctuations in a cyclic pattern in the incidence of giant-cell (temporal) arteritis in Olmsted County, Minnesota (Abstract 119-96-69-1); the increased incidence of aortic aneurysm and dissection in giant-cell arteritis in that same population (Abstract 119-96-69–2); tissue cytokine patterns in patients with polymyalgia rheumatica and giant-cell arteritis (Abstract 119-96-69–3); and an analysis of 42 patients with Wegener's granulomatosis treated with methotrexate and prednisone (Abstract 119-96-69–4).

Noted in passing: A review of 18 patients (by 17 authors!) with the hypocomplementemic urticarial vasculitis syndrome.[1]

Stephen E. Malawista, M.D.

Reference

1. Wisnieski JJ, Baer AN, Christensen J, Cupps T, Flagg DN, Jones JV, Katzenstein PL, McFadden ER, McMillen JJ, Pick MA, Richmond GW, Simon SR, Smith HR, Sontheimer RD, Trigg L, Weldon D, Zone JJ: Hypocomplementemic urticarial vasculitis syndrome. *Medicine* 74:24–41, 1995.

The Incidence of Giant Cell Arteritis in Olmsted County, Minnesota: Apparent Fluctuations in a Cyclic Pattern

Salvarani C, Gabriel SE, O'Fallon WM, Hunder GG (Mayo Clinic and Found, Rochester, Minn)

Ann Intern Med 123:192–194, 1995 119-96-69–1

Purpose.—The cause of giant-cell arteritis remains unknown, although environmental factors have been suggested to play a pathogenetic role. Trends in the incidence of giant-cell arteritis during 4 decades were analyzed in the hope of identifying some possible pathogenetic factors.

Methods.—The population-based incidence study included all incidence cases of giant-cell arteritis occurring between 1950 and 1991 among the residents of 1 Minnesota county. The cases were identified using a unified medical records linkage system. The number of incidence cases was used to calculate age- and sex-specific incidence rates of giant-cell arteritis. The

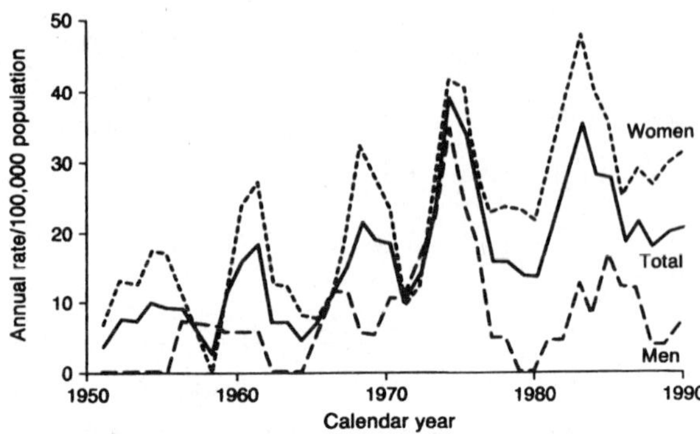

FIGURE 1.—Annual incidence rates of giant-cell arteritis in Olmsted County, Minnesota, per 100,000 persons 50 years of age or older. Rates were calculated using a centered 3-year moving average. (Courtesy of Salvarani C, Gabriel SE, O'Fallon WM, et al: *Ann Intern Med* 123:192–194, 1995.)

overall rates were age-adjusted and sex-adjusted to the 1980 United States white population, and the annual incidence rates were calculated using a centered 3-year moving average.

Results.—One hundred twenty-five incidence cases were identified during the 42-year study: 103 women and 22 men. Thirty-five percent of the patients also had polymyalgia rheumatica. Among people aged 50 years and older, the age- and sex-adjusted incidence of giant-cell arteritis was 17.8 per 100,000 persons. The incidence in women and men was 24.2 and 8.2 per 100,000, respectively. As age increased, so did the age-specific incidence rates. Annual incidence rates increased significantly with time, clustering in 5 peak periods that occurred approximately every 7 years. There was a significant calendar-time effect, which predicted an increase in incidence of 2.6% every 5 years (Fig 1).

Conclusions.—The incidence rates of giant-cell arteritis show a regular cyclic pattern over time. The findings are consistent with an infectious cause for giant-cell arteritis, perhaps in a genetically predisposed host. The findings must be confirmed in other populations.

▶ That giant-cell arteritis is more common in women and in those older than 70 years confirms earlier studies. A statistically significant increase in the incidence of giant-cell arteritis during the study is of interest but could result from heightened physician awareness and surveillance. The big-ticket item in this study, not reported previously, is an apparent cyclic fluctuation in the incidence over the 42-year study. Peaks appeared at intervals of about 7 years and lasted about 3 years. In 92% of cases, the diagnosis was confirmed by temporal artery biopsy, making overascertainment unlikely. Moreover, the patients were identified using the superb medical records linkage system of the Mayo Clinic, which ensures almost complete ascertainment of all cases of *any* disease diagnosed in Olmsted County dating back 75 years. As illnesses with cyclic frequencies are most often infectious, this is a provocative finding.

S.E. Malawista, M.D.

Increased Incidence of Aortic Aneurysm and Dissection in Giant Cell (Temporal) Arteritis: A Population-Based Study

Evans JM, O'Fallon WM, Hunder GG (Mayo Clinic, Rochester, Minn)

Ann Intern Med 122:502–507, 1995 119-96-69–2

Purpose.—Giant-cell, or temporal, arteritis of the large- and medium-sized arteries is one of the most common forms of vasculitis. It is occasionally complicated by aortic aneurysmal disease, and even death from aortic dissection. The frequency and clinical relevance of this purported association were examined in a population-based cohort study of patients with giant-cell arteritis.

Methods.—Ninety-six residents of 1 Minnesota county in whom the diagnosis of giant-cell arteritis was made between 1950 and 1985 were studied. Each patient's records were reviewed to obtain information about the presence of aortic aneurysm, with or without dissection, along with other factors. Aneurysm was diagnosed by CT, ultrasonography, angiography, or autopsy (Figs 1 and 2). The incidence of aortic aneurysm was assessed, as were the clinical features of giant-cell arteritis that might be associated with an increased risk of aneurysm formation.

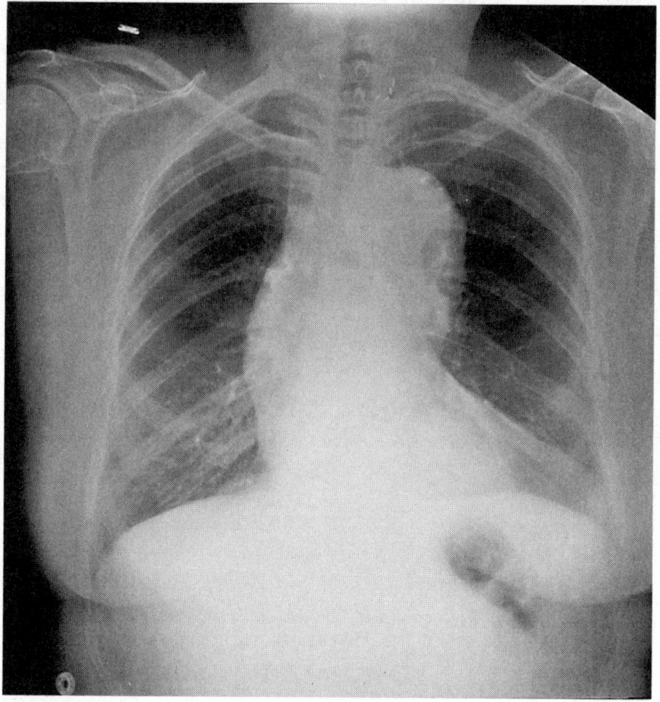

FIGURE 1.—Chest radiograph of patient 6 showing a thoracic aortic aneurysm found 7.5 years after diagnosis of giant-cell arteritis. (Courtesy of Evans JM, O'Fallon WM, Hunder GG: Increased incidence of aortic aneurysm and dissection in giant cell [temporal] arteritis: A population-based study. *Ann Intern Med* 122:502–507, 1995.)

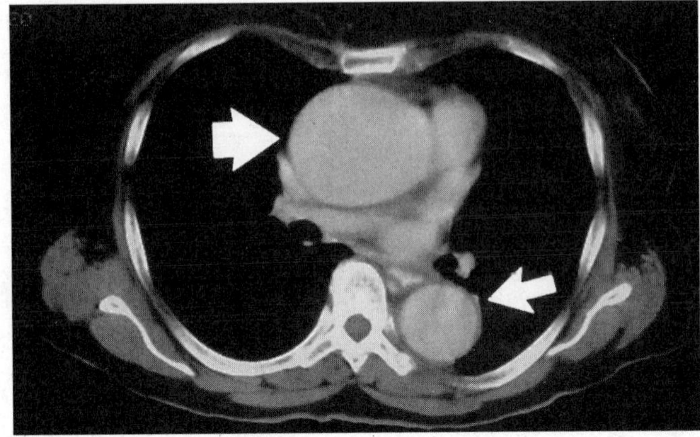

FIGURE 2.—Computed tomographic scan of chest of patient 8 showing section including a thoracic aortic aneurysm. Ascending portion of thoracic aorta (*large arrow*) is more dilated than descending portion (*small arrow*). (Courtesy of Evans JM, O'Fallon WM, Hunder GG: Increased incidence of aortic aneurysm and dissection in giant cell [temporal] arteritis: A population-based study. *Ann Intern Med* 122:502–507, 1995.)

Results.—Aneurysms of the thoracic aorta developed in 11 of 96 patients. Two cases of aneurysm were diagnosed at the same time as giant-cell arteritis. For the rest, the diagnosis of aneurysm was made a median of 6 years after that of giant-cell arteritis. In 6 cases, thoracic aortic dissection led to sudden death. In 5 patients without thoracic aortic dissection, isolated abdominal aortic aneurysms developed a median of 2½ years after the diagnosis of giant-cell arteritis. The incidence of aneurysms in patients with giant-cell arteritis was 999 per 100,000 person-years for thoracic aortic aneurysms and 555 per 100,000 person-years for abdominal aortic aneurysms. Compared with the age- and sex-matched population of the

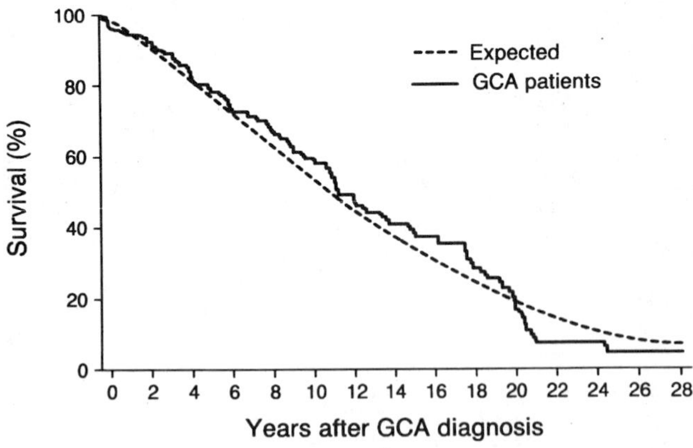

FIGURE 3.—Survival in 96 patients with giant-cell arteritis compared with expected survival rates among whites. Data obtained from United States life-table of 1980. *Abbreviation: GCA,* giant-cell arteritis. (Courtesy of Evans JM, O'Fallon WM, Hunder GG: Increased incidence of aortic aneurysm and dissection in giant cell [temporal] arteritis: A population-based study. *Ann Intern Med* 122:502–507, 1995.)

county, patients with giant-cell arteritis were 17 times more likely to have thoracic aortic aneurysm and more than twice as likely to have isolated abdominal aortic aneurysm. Survival for the cohort with giant-cell arteritis was not significantly different than that of the population (Fig 3). No significant risk factors were identified, beyond giant-cell arteritis itself.

Conclusions.—The risk of aortic aneurysm is markedly increased among patients with giant-cell arteritis. Abdominal and especially thoracic aortic aneurysms may occur as a late and potentially fatal complication. The findings suggest that patients with giant-cell arteritis should receive an annual assessment to detect aortic aneurysm, with palpation of the abdominal aorta and a radiograph of the chest, including a lateral view.

▶ As the authors point out, the most common clinical manifestations of giant-cell arteritis, such as headache, jaw claudication, and blindness, are related to inflammation in more distal branches of the extracranial carotid arteries. In about 15% of cases, ischemic neurologic or peripheral vascular symptoms are caused by major involvement of the carotid, vertebral, or subclavian arteries. In this population-based, retrospective cohort study, among 94 patients with giant-cell arteritis and no history of aneurysm followed for 901 person-years, a whopping 9 patients subsequently had thoracic aortic aneurysms, a figure 17 times expected of those of the same age and sex in the general population of the county. The diagnosis was confirmed pathologically, angiographically, by ultrasonography or echocardiography, or by CT. During the same follow-up, abdominal aortic aneurysms developed in 5 patients, 2.4 times the expected incidence in that general population. If aortitis is the inciting event leading to these complications, then aortitis occurs more frequently than was previously thought. Despite these potentially catastrophic events, the overall survival of these 96 patients was no different from age- and sex-matched controls, possibly because of the small number of patients and the relatively short overall life span in this age group.

No other risk factors for aneurysm other than arteritis were identified, again perhaps because of the relatively small number of patients in the study. Hence, there was no correlation with differences in corticosteroid therapy, uncontrolled hypertension, or congenital abnormalities of structural proteins. Given the uncertainty of which patients are likely to develop this complication, along with its relative frequency, the authors' recommendations of an annual physical examination, including palpation of the abdominal aorta, as well as an annual radiograph of the chest with lateral view, seem eminently reasonable.

S.E. Malawista, M.D.

Tissue Cytokine Patterns in Patients With Polymyalgia Rheumatica and Giant Cell Arteritis

Weyand CM, Hicok KC, Hunder GG, Goronzy JJ (Mayo Clinic, Rochester, Minn)

Ann Intern Med 121:484–491, 1994 119-96-69–3

Objective.—The pathology of giant-cell arteritis remains unclear. The inflammatory process observed in this condition may represent a local

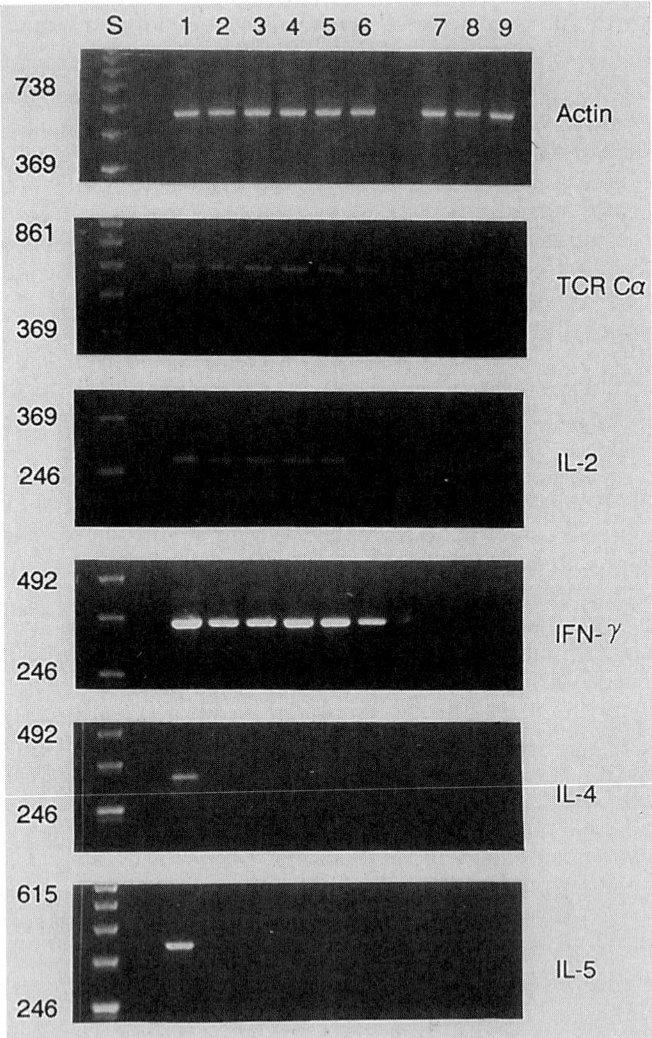

FIGURE 2.—Polymerase chain reaction amplification of lymphokine-specific sequences. *Lanes 2–6* represent specimens from patients with giant-cell arteritis: *lanes 7–9* represent control patients. *Lane 1* represents a positive control. *Abbreviations: IFN,* interferon; *IL,* interleukin; *S,* size marker; *TCR,* T-cell receptor. (Courtesy of Weyand CM, Hicok KC, Hunder GG, et al: Tissue cytokine patterns in patients with polymyalgia rheumatica and giant cell arteritis. *Ann Intern Med* 121:484–491, 1994.)

immune response to some unidentified antigen in the arterial walls, but this model does not explain the systemic features of the disease. Polymyalgia rheumatica is a closely related condition that affects many of the same patients as giant-cell arteritis, suggesting that the 2 conditions may represent a spectrum of disease. Temporal artery specimens of patients with giant-cell arteritis and polymyalgia rheumatica were analyzed for the presence of inflammatory cytokines to determine whether there is any specific cytokine pattern for the 2 conditions.

Methods.—The study included 48 specimens from 34 patients who underwent temporal artery biopsy procedures. There were 15 patients with giant-cell arteritis, 9 with polymyalgia rheumatica but no evidence of vasculitis, and 10 with neither polymyalgia rheumatica nor vasculitis. Polymerase chain reaction with cytokine-specific primer sets was performed to analyze each specimen for the in vivo presence of cytokine messenger RNA (mRNA).

Results.—In specimens from patients with giant cell arteritis, the vasculitic lesions were characterized by in situ production of interleukin-1β, interleukin-6, and transforming growth factor-β1 mRNA, indicating macrophage activation. There was also evidence of interferon-γ and interleukin-2 mRNA (Fig 2), indicating selective T-cell activation. However, specimens from patients with polymyalgia rheumatica also showed macrophage- and T-cell–derived cytokines. Distinctive lymphokine profiles were noted in tissue-infiltrating T cells in both conditions. Whereas two thirds of samples from patients with giant-cell arteritis showed interferon-γ, samples from patients with polymyalgia rheumatica showed only interleukin-2.

Conclusions.—In situ production of mRNA specific for macrophage-derived cytokines is common to patients with both polymyalgia rheumatica and giant-cell arteritis. In giant-cell arteritis, T cells recruited to vasculitic lesions produce mainly interleukin-2 and interferon-γ; in contrast, interferon-γ is not produced in polymyalgia rheumatica. Interferon-γ may therefore play a role in the progression to overt arteritis.

► Polymyalgia rheumatica is a syndrome characterized by pain and stiffness about the shoulder and hip girdles, an elevated erythrocyte sedimentation rate, and an often dramatic response to low doses of corticosteroids. Although this is quite different from the picture of giant-cell (temporal) arteritis (see previous editorial), a medical emergency requiring high doses of corticosteroids, the former syndrome may be a harbinger of the latter, and about 10% or 15% of patients with polymyalgia rheumatica will, on temporal artery biopsy, have vasculitic lesions already present.

The authors of this study have been developing the idea that these 2 illnesses form a spectrum of disease.[1] First, both syndromes are genetically associated with the same HLA-DRB1 alleles. Second, concentrations of the cytokine interleukin-6 are increased in both. Third, in both illnesses, patients share a high frequency of activated circulating monocytes. Finally, as seen in this paper, both groups of patients produce inflammatory cytokines in the temporal artery. What distinguishes the 2 is the lack of a histologically detectable granulomatous infiltrate in the arterial wall in polymyalgia rheumatica (despite there presumably being enough unseen cells present to generate the cytokine messages detectable by polymerase chain reaction; controls suggest that those amplifications are not false positives), and the lack of local detection of a particular cytokine mRNA, that for interferon-γ. This paper and its accompanying editorial[2] also constitute a useful primer to the world of inflammatory and anti-inflammatory cytokines lurking beneath our surfaces.

S.E. Malawista, M.D.

References

1. Weyand CM, Goronzy JJ, Hunder GG: Cytokines in polymyalgia and giant cell arteritis (letter). *Ann Intern Med* 122:634, 1995.
2. Getsy JA, Phillips SM: Cytokines in polymyalgia and giant cell arteritis (editorial). *Ann Intern Med* 121:536–537, 1994.

An Analysis of Forty-Two Wegener's Granulomatosis Patients Treated With Methotrexate and Prednisone

Sneller MC, Hoffman GS, Talar-Williams C, Kerr GS, Hallahan CW, Fauci AS (Natl Inst of Allergy and Infectious Diseases, Bethesda, Md)
Arthritis Rheum 38:608–613, 1995 119-96-69–4

Background.—For patients with Wegener's granulomatosis, daily treatment with low-dose cyclophosphamide (CYC) is a highly effective treatment. However, patients treated with this regimen over time are prone to repeated relapses, and prolonged courses of CYC carry serious long-term toxicity. Low-dose methotrexate (MTX) plus prednisone was evaluated as an alternative treatment of Wegener's granulomatosis (WG).

Methods.—The open-label study included 42 patients with active WG that was not immediately life-threatening. Fifteen were in their first episode of WG, and the rest were in relapse. All patients received oral MTX, 20–25 mg/wk, and prednisone, starting at 1 mg/kg/day. The results of treatment were assessed by the clinical, pathologic, laboratory, and radiographic findings.

Results.—Weekly MTX plus prednisone therapy led to disease remission in 71% of patients. The median time to remission was 4 months. After remission, the estimated median time to relapse was 29 months (Table 2). Of 8 patients with relapses who received a second course of MTX plus prednisone, 6 went into remission again. Treatment with MTX was fairly well tolerated, although 10 patients had persistent elevations of liver transaminase levels and 4 had opportunistic infection with *Pneumocystis carinii*.

Conclusions.—Weekly low-dose MTX plus prednisone is an effective treatment in selected patients with WG. Apart from *P. carinii* infection,

TABLE 2.—Clinical Response in 42 Patients With Wegener's Granulomatosis Treated With Methotrexate and Prednisone

No. (%) surviving	39 (93)
No. (%) achieving remission	30 (71)
No. (%) with relapse after achieving remission	11/30 (36)
Median months to remission	4.2
Median months to relapse in patients achieving remission	29
Median months to tapering to alternate-day prednisone therapy	3.1
Median months to discontinuation of prednisone	7

(Courtesy of Sneller MC, Hoffman GS, Talar-Williams C, et al: An analysis of forty-two Wegener's granulomatosis patients treated with methotrexate and prednisone. *Arthritis Rheum* 38:608–613, 1995.)

toxicity appears to be less than with daily CYC. The regimen described may be useful for patients with WG who do not have rapidly progressive renal or pulmonary disease or who have serious CYC-associated toxicity.

▶ This open-label study extends earlier work by this group[1] on the ability of MTX and prednisone to induce remission in patients with WG, and defines the relapse rate seen with this therapeutic regimen. Behind this effort is long-term dissatisfaction with the therapeutically effective but more toxic regimen of CYC and prednisone. The results in this study are again encouraging; disease remitted in 30 of the 42 patients (71%) within a median of 4.2 months, the estimated median time to relapse for those in remission was 29 months, and a second remission was induced in 6 of 8 patients who received the same regimen a second time. Exclusion criteria for this study were (1) the presence of immediately life-threatening disease, defined as acute renal failure resulting in a serum creatinine level of > 2.5 mg/dL (221 μmol/L), acute pulmonary hemorrhage with an arterial partial pressure of oxygen (PaO_2) value of < 70% of predicted; (2) the presence of chronic liver disease or history of excessive alcohol intake (> 14 oz of 100-proof liquor or equivalent per week); (3) pregnancy; (4) evidence of infection with HIV; (5) a recent increase (within 4 weeks) in immunosuppressive medication; or (6) the presence of chronic renal insufficiency, with a serum creatinine level of > 2.5 mg/dL. Nevertheless, these patients had significant disease, with 60% having 3 or more organ systems affected at study entry, including 21 patients with active glomerulonephritis. This new regimen is welcome.

S.E. Malawista, M.D.

Reference

1. 1994 Year Book of Medicine, pp 799–801.

70 Infectious Arthritis

Introduction

This chapter addresses long-term clinical outcomes of Lyme disease (Abstract 119-96-70–1); bloodstream invasion in early Lyme disease (Abstract 119-96-70–2); uveitis caused by *Tropheryma whippelii* (Whipple's bacillus) (Abstract 119-96-70–3); and the relationship of leukocytoclastic vasculitis and cryoglobulinemia to infection with hepatitis C (Abstract 119-96-70–4).

Noted in passing: The emergence of human granulocytic ehrlichiosis in Massachusetts, a rickettsial illness transmitted by *Ixodes dammini* (also known as *Ixodes scapularis*), the same tiny tick that transmits babesiosis and Lyme disease.[1]

Stephen E. Malawista, M.D.

Reference

1. Telford SR III, Lepore TJ, Snow P, Warner CK, Dawson JE: Human granulocytic ehrlichiosis in Massachusetts. *Ann Intern Med* 123:277–279, 1995.

The Long-Term Clinical Outcomes of Lyme Disease: A Population-Based Retrospective Cohort Study

Shadick NA, Phillips CB, Logigian EL, Steere AC, Kaplan RF, Berardi VP, Duray PH, Larson MG, Wright EA, Ginsburg KS, Katz JN, Liang MH (Harvard Med School, Boston; Brigham & Women's Hosp, Boston; Tufts Univ, Boston; et al)

Ann Intern Med 121:560–567, 1994 119-96-70–1

Background.—Lyme disease is now the most common vector-borne disease in the United States. The late consequences of Lyme disease include musculoskeletal and neurologic sequelae. Some of these sequelae are thought to be caused by persistent spirochetal infection and are amenable to antibiotic therapy. Other syndromes suggest a mechanism other than active infection. The prevalence of, and risk factors for, long-term sequelae from acute Lyme disease were determined by studying patients who contracted it while the clinical syndromes and optimal antibiotic treatments were still evolving.

Methods.—The patients were 38 residents of a coastal area of Massachusetts endemic for Lyme disease who were infected with *Borrelia burgdorferi* in the early 1980s. These patients were followed up for a mean of 6.2 years. Their findings on a standardized physical examination, health status measure, psychometric test battery, and serologic analysis were compared with those of 43 control individuals randomly selected from the same population.

Findings.—Arthralgias were found in 61% of the group with Lyme disease and in 16% of the control group; distal paresthesias in 16% and 2%, respectively; concentration problems in 16% and 2%; and fatigue in 26% and 9%. The group with Lyme disease also had poorer global health status scores, more abnormal joints, and more verbal memory deficits than the control group. Overall, 34% had long-term sequelae from Lyme disease. Compared with the control individuals, patients with long-term sequelae had higher IgG antibody titers to the spirochete and were given treatment later.

Conclusions.—Individuals with a history of Lyme disease had more musculoskeletal impairment and a greater prevalence of verbal memory impairment compared with those without a history of Lyme disease. Disseminated Lyme disease may be associated with long-term morbidity.

▶ Disseminated Lyme disease may indeed be associated with long-term morbidity. However, the critical statistic in this study appears in the following statement: "Compared with controls, patients who had long-term sequelae ...received treatment later (34.5 months compared with 2.7 months; $P < 0.0001$)." A total of 34.5 months! Imagine contracting syphilis and waiting almost 3 years to treat it; would residual morbidity in some patients be unexpected? A tribute to the *efficacy* of antibiotics is that even those *without* long-term sequelae did not get treated for a median of 2.7 months.

The best way to prevent long-term sequelae of Lyme disease is to identify and treat the illness early. That point would have been driven home more forcefully had the title of the current article been "The Long-Term Clinical Outcomes of Lyme Disease *After Inordinate Delay in Treatment.*"

S.E. Malawista, M.D.

Bloodstream Invasion in Early Lyme Disease: Results From a Prospective, Controlled, Blinded Study Using the Polymerase Chain Reaction

Goodman JL, Bradley JF, Ross AE, Goellner P, Lagus A, Vitale B, Berger BW, Luger S, Johnson RC (Univ of Minnesota, Minneapolis; Spooner Clinic, Wis; River Valley Med Ctr, St Croix Falls, Wis; et al)

Am J Med 99:6–12, 1995 119-96-70–2

Background.—Lyme disease is the most common tick-borne infection in North America. In many cases, laboratory testing is important to diagnosis because the typical accompanying skin rash does not occur or is not noted. In early Lyme disease, serologic results are negative in 50% of patients. Therefore, direct detection of spirochetes may be valuable to diagnosis.

The polymerase chain reaction (PCR) is highly sensitive in detecting Lyme disease spirochetes. Recent studies of this technique in detecting spirochetes have reported high and low frequencies of blood PCR positivity. There have been no prospective, blinded studies of the PCR technique. Optimal techniques for PCR in early Lyme disease were determined. The frequency and clinical correlates of blood-borne infection detected by PCR in the dissemination of Lyme disease were also determined prospectively.

Methods.—Blood samples were obtained from 76 patients with erythema migrans and 29 control individuals. Blood was fractionated and PCR, culture, and serologic studies were performed. Results of laboratory studies and clinical information were correlated.

Results.—Of the 76 patients with erythema migrans, 4 had positive cultures. In 14 of these 76 patients, spirochetemia was documented by PCR of their plasma. Of the 29 control individuals, none were culture or PCR positive. Spirochetemia documented by PCR correlated with clinical evidence of disseminated disease: of 33 patients with systemic symptoms, 10 were PCR positive; of 43 patients without evidence of disease, 4 were PCR positive. In patients with fever, arthralgia, myalgia, or headache, PCR positivity was more frequent; this was also true for patients with more total symptoms and presence of multiple skin lesions. The strongest independent predictor of PCR positivity was the number of systemic symptoms.

Conclusions.—Plasma testing with PCR is more sensitive than culture for detecting spirochetemia from *Borrelia burgdorferi*. The frequency of spirochetemia is significantly correlated with clinical evidence of disseminated infection. Spirochetemia may have an important role in the dissemination of Lyme disease.

▶ In this prospective, controlled, blinded study, 14 of 76 patients (18.4%) with erythema migrans were PCR positive for DNA of *B. burgdorferi,* whereas only 4 (5.3%) were culture positive; none of 29 control patients were PCR or culture positive. As might be expected, PCR positivity was more likely in those with systemic symptoms and multiple skin lesions. For PCR, the authors found best results with nucleic acids from 0.1 mL of a resuspended plasma pellet that had been concentrated 5 times; for culture, 0.1 mL of a plasma fraction. As they point out, although these findings are of pathogenetic interest, PCR of plasma is less sensitive for diagnostic purposes than serology (even this early in infection) or than culture or PCR of erythema migrans lesions (positive in up to 80% of samples). Moreover, plasma PCR positivity is most likely in those in whom the diagnosis is clinically most apparent. The best diagnostic use of PCR in Lyme disease would currently appear to be in Lyme arthritis, where positivity of synovial fluid from untreated patients approaches 100%.[1]

S.E. Malawista, M.D.

Reference

1. 1995 Year Book of Medicine, pp 821–824.

Brief Report: Uveitis Caused by *Tropheryma whippelii* (Whipple's Bacillus)

Rickman LS, Freeman WR, Green WR, Feldman ST, Sullivan J, Russack V, Relman DA (Univ of California, San Diego; Johns Hopkins Univ, Baltimore, Md; Stanford Univ, Calif)

N Engl J Med 332:363–366, 1995 119-96-70–3

Introduction.—Patients with the multisystem bacterial disease Whipple's disease typically have malabsorption, diarrhea, and polyarthritis. Ocular manifestations, such as blurred vision or visual loss, usually occur in patients who also have gastrointestinal or CNS involvement. A patient with chronic, bilateral uveitis but no gastrointestinal or CNS involvement who proved to have Whipple's disease was described.

Case Report.—Woman, 59, was referred for evaluation of bilateral uveitis (Fig 2). She had a long history of seronegative arthritis of the wrists, knees, and ankles. She had no clinical signs of gastrointestinal involvement, and duodenal biopsy specimens were negative on light microscopic examination. Vitreous aspiration and light microscopy led to a preliminary diagnosis of Whipple's disease. Bacilli resembling those of Whipple's disease, i.e., *Tropheryma whippelii*, were detected on electron microscopy (Fig 3). Polymerase chain reaction (PCR) identified 16S ribosomal RNA gene sequences corresponding to *T. whippelii* in the vitreous, confirming the diagnosis of Whipple's disease. A nearly identical gene sequence was detected in the duodenal mucosa.

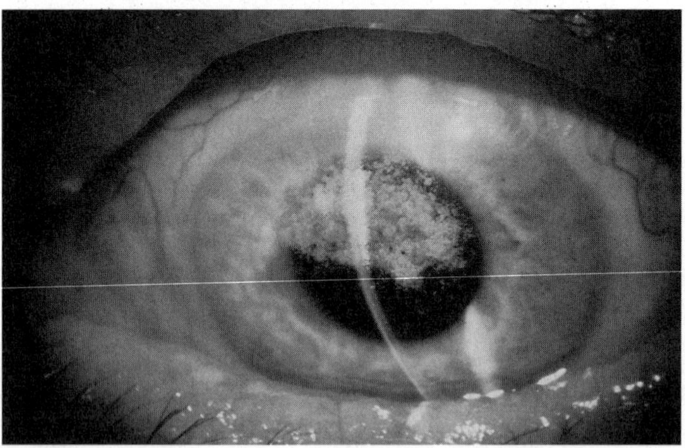

FIGURE 2.—Slit-lamp photograph of the right eye, revealing flocculent, inflammatory debris that adhered to the posterior corneal surface and eventually obscured the optical axis. (Reprinted by permission of *The New England Journal of Medicine*. Rickman LS, Freeman WR, Green WR, et al: Brief report: Uveitis caused by *Tropheryma whippelii* (Whipple's bacillus). *N Engl J Med* 332:363–366, 1995. Copyright 1995, Massachusetts Medical Society.)

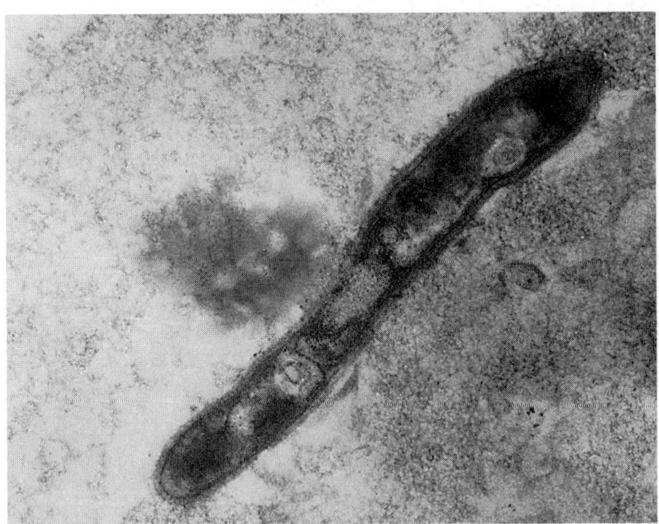

FIGURE 3.—Electron micrograph taken in March 1993, revealing a bacillary structure in the vitreous. The organism appeared to be undergoing cell division; original magnification, ×88,320. (Reprinted by permission of *The New England Journal of Medicine*. Rickman LS, Freeman WR, Green WR, et al: Brief report: Uveitis caused by *Tropheryma whippelii* (Whipple's bacillus). *N Engl J Med* 332:363–366, 1995. Copyright 1995, Massachusetts Medical Society.) Figure provided through the courtesy of Darlene J. Whitney, Stanford University.)

Discussion.—A case of uveitis caused by the bacillus associated with Whipple's disease was reported in a patient with few clinical signs of extraocular Whipple's disease. For patients with Whipple's disease and visual impairment, treatment should include antimicrobial agents that penetrate the vitreous. Polymerase chain reaction may be the most sensitive test for persistent bacilli in patients treated for Whipple's disease.

► Whipple's disease is a protean systemic infectious disorder characterized most commonly by fever, weight loss, diarrhea, polyarthritis, and adenopathy. Although the causative organism has never been grown in culture, it has often been seen in biopsy specimens of small bowel or lymph nodes, stained with the periodic acid–Schiff reagent, as small, intracytoplasmic, diastase-resistant, gram-positive rods. Whipple's disease experienced a renaissance recently[1] when, first with broad-range primers for DNA coding for bacterial 16S ribosomal RNA and then with specific primers, the bulk of the 16S rRNA gene was amplified by PCR and sequenced, revealing an amplicon that fit phylogenetically among the gram-positive actinomycetes, and resulting in the uncultured bacillus being named *Tropheryma whippelii.*

Polymerase chain reaction is proving useful in the diagnosis of Whipple's disease and in establishing its range.[2] In the current case, for example, a biopsy specimen of duodenal mucosa was PCR positive (as was a sample of vitreous) even though there was no clinical evidence of gastrointestinal disease, and light microscopy of repeated duodenal biopsy specimens was negative (in such cases one should also consider the possibility of false positive PCR). In another recent report,[3] 2 splenectomized patients with Whipple's disease had erythrocyte-associated gram-positive bacilli in smears of peripheral blood, which were PCR positive for *T. whippelii.*

S.E. Malawista, M.D.

References

1. 1993 Year Book of Medicine, pp 435–436.
2. Dobbins WO III: The diagnosis of Whipple's disease. *N Engl J Med* 332:390–392, 1995.
3. Lowsky R, Archer GL, Fyles G, Minden M, Curtis J, et al: Brief report: Diagnosis of Whipple's disease by molecular analysis of peripheral blood. *N Engl J Med* 331:1343–1346, 1994.

71 Other Topics

Introduction

Subjects of rheumatologic interest lying outside the 7 categorical chapters include choosing among bed rest, exercises, or ordinary activity in patients with acute low back pain (Abstract 119-96-71–1); the treatment of deep cartilage defects in the knee with autologous chondrocyte transplantation (Abstract 119-96-71–2); a multifactorial intervention to reduce the risk of falling among elderly people living in the community (Abstract 119-96-71–3); the risk of kidney failure associated with the use of acetaminophen, aspirin, and nonsteroidal anti-inflammatory drugs (Abstract 119-96-71–4); and the association of running with decreased development of disability with age (Abstract 119-96-71–5).

Noted in passing: The lack of efficacy of intra-articular injections of 750 kD hyaluronan in the treatment of osteoarthritis,[1] the use of parathyroid hormone for the prevention of bone loss induced by estrogen deficiency,[2] the long-term treatment of osteopetrosis with recombinant human interferon gamma,[3, 4] and immunologic contributions to understanding the cause, pathogenesis, and therapy of myositis.[5]

Stephen E. Malawista, M.D.

References

1. Henderson, EB, Smith EC, Pegley F, Blake DR: Intra-articular injections of 750 kD hyaluronan in the treatment of osteoarthritis: A randomised single centre double-blind placebo-controlled trial of 91 patients demonstrating lack of efficacy. *Ann Rheum Dis* 59:529–534, 1994.
2. Finkelstein JS, Klibanski A, Schaefer EH, Hornstein MD, Schiff I, Neer RM: Parathyroid hormone for the prevention of bone loss induced by estrogen deficiency. *N Engl J Med* 331:1618–1623, 1994.
3. Key LL Jr, Rodriguiz RM, Willi SM, Wright NM, Hatcher HC, Eyre DR, Cure JK, Griffin PP, Ries WL: Long-term treatment of osteopetrosis with recombinant human interferon gamma. *N Engl J Med* 332:1594–1599, 1995.
4. Whyte MP: Chipping away at marble bone disease (editorial). *N Engl J Med* 332:1639–1640, 1995.
5. Plotz PH, Rider LG, Targoff IN, Raben N, O'Hanlon TP, Miller FW: Myositis: Immunologic contributions to understanding cause, pathogenesis, and therapy. *Ann Intern Med* 122:715–724, 1995.

The Treatment of Acute Low Back Pain: Bed Rest, Exercises, or Ordinary Activity?

Malmivaara A, Häkkinen U, Aro T, Heinrichs M-L, Koskenniemi L, Kuosma E, Lappi S, Paloheimo R, Servo C, Vaaranen V, Hernberg S (Finnish Inst of Occupational Health, Helsinki; Natl Research and Development Ctr for Welfare and Health, Helsinki; City of Helsinki Occupational Health Care Ctrs)
N Engl J Med 332:351–355, 1995 119-96-71–1

Purpose.—Two competing strategies—bed rest and back-extension exercises—are commonly prescribed for patients with low back pain. Experts disagree as to which treatment is best for this extremely common and expensive problem. The 2 treatments were compared with usual activity for effectiveness and cost in a randomized, controlled trial.

Methods.—A total of 186 employees of the city of Helsinki who were evaluated at the city's occupational health centers for acute, nonspecific low back pain were studied. The patients were randomly assigned in roughly equal numbers to 3 groups. One group was assigned to 2 days of bed rest and another to perform light back-mobilizing exercises; the third group was told to continue ordinary activities as tolerated. The outcomes and costs of the 3 groups were evaluated at 3 and 12 weeks.

Results.—At both assessments, the control group demonstrated better recovery than either the bed rest or the exercise group. The findings in terms of duration of pain, pain intensity, lumbar flexion, subjective ability to work, Owestry back-disability index, and lost work days all favored the ordinary activity group to a significant degree. Patients in the bed rest group had the longest recovery times. There were no significant differences in cost between the 3 groups.

Conclusions.—In patients with acute low back pain, simply maintaining ordinary activity as tolerated leads to quicker recovery than either bed rest or back mobilization exercises. The advantages of ordinary activity are remarkably consistent across outcome variables. If widely used in clinical practice, this approach would likely yield considerable cost savings.

▶ Several years ago,[1] I reviewed evidence that 7 days of bed rest for acute low back pain, besides being almost impossible to carry out correctly, was no better therapeutically than 2 days. Now we learn that continuation of ordinary activities within the limits permitted by the pain leads to more rapid recovery than either 2 days of bed rest or back-mobilizing exercises. Note that we are addressing here patients with acute, nonspecific low back pain who required the services of a physician; the cause of the pain was presumably injury to muscles, ligaments, or facet joints. Excluded were patients with sciatica, defined by the presence of at least 1 neurologic deficit or a positive Lasègue's sign of 60 degrees or less. The physicians' natural urge to "do something" when confronted with a patient with nonspecific, acute low back pain should probably be limited to reassurance and to anti-inflammatory or analgesic drugs, which most patients in all 3 of the study groups received.

S.E. Malawista, M.D.

Reference

1. 1988 YEAR BOOK OF MEDICINE, p 759.

Treatment of Deep Cartilage Defects in the Knee With Autologous Chondrocyte Transplantation

Brittberg M, Lindahl A, Nilsson A, Ohlsson C, Isaksson O, Peterson L (Univ of Göteborg, Sweden)

N Engl J Med 331:889–895, 1994 119-96-71-2

Introduction.—Full-thickness defects of articular cartilage may progress to osteoarthritis and eventually require total knee replacement. Encouraged by the results of transplanted cultured autologous chondrocytes in focal patellar defects in rabbits, autologous chondrocyte transplantation was performed in 23 patients with isolated deep cartilage defects of the knee.

> *Technique.*—Cartilage slices are obtained from an uninvolved area of the injured knee during arthroscopy. The chondrocytes are isolated and cultured in the laboratory for 14–21 days. The cultured chondrocytes are injected into the area of defect and covered with a periosteal flap taken from the proximal medial tibia.

Patients.—Patients' ages ranged from 14 to 48 years. The full-thickness defects ranged in size from 1.6 to 6.5 cm^2. Thirteen patients had defects of the femoral condyle resulting from trauma, 3 had isolated femoral defects caused by osteochondritis dissecans, and 7 had defects of the patellar facet.

Outcome.—The mean follow-up period was 39 months (range, 16–66 months). Initially, all patients reported considerable reduction in knee pain, swelling, and crepitation, and elimination of knee locking. After 3 months, arthroscopy showed regenerated areas of cartilage with visible borders that were level with the surrounding articular surface. The transplants were spongy when probed. A second arthroscopic examination was performed at 12–46 months after the surgery. In many instances, the transplants had the same macroscopic appearance as the surrounding cartilage but were firmer when probed. Two years after transplantation, 14 of the 16 patients with femoral condylar transplants had either excellent or good results; the other 2 underwent a second operation for severe central wear in the transplants, with locking of the knee and pain. In patients with patellar transplants, 2 had excellent results, 3 had fair, and 2 had poor results during a mean follow-up of 36 months. Of these, 2 patients required a second operation because of severe chondromalacia. Biopsy specimens from the central part of the transplant showed an intact articular surface and a hyaline appearance with metachromatic staining in 11 of 15 femoral transplants and 1 of 7 patellar transplants. Immunohistochemical staining for type II collagen was positive in the biopsy specimens studied.

Conclusion.—Cultured autologous chondrocytes can be used to repair articular cartilage defects in the femorotibial surface of the knee. This treatment restores the function of the joint by forming predominantly hyaline-like cartilage containing type II collagen.

► As Dr. Mankin points out in the editorial accompanying this article,[1] we are still perplexed by the question posed by William Hunter in the 18th century: Why does hyaline articular cartilage not heal? (In today's terms, what can we do to make articular cartilage heal?) In one tentative answer to the latter question, the authors have found that autologous chondrocytes, harvested from the same joint, expanded in tissue culture, introduced into a knee-cartilage defect, and sealed over with a periosteal flap, can lead to the growth of material resembling and presumably behaving like normal cartilage. Of special importance is that this regenerated cartilage contained a metachromatically staining matrix and an abundance of type II collagen, critical for the macromolecular framework of the extracellular matrix that gives hyaline cartilage its unique biomechanical properties. Fourteen of 16 patients with distal femoral lesions had good-to-excellent clinical results, vs. clinical improvement in only 2 of 7 patients with patellar transplants, perhaps because of greater weight-bearing in the latter. We can look forward to further results with these techniques.

S.E. Malawista, M.D.

Reference

1. Mankin HJ: Chrondrocyte transplantation: One answer to an old question (editorial). *N Engl J Med* 331:940–941, 1994.

A Multifactorial Intervention to Reduce the Risk of Falling Among Elderly People Living in the Community

Tinetti ME, Baker DI, McAvay G, Claus EB, Garrett P, Gottschalk M, Koch ML, Trainor K, Horwitz RI (Yale Univ, New Haven, Conn; Yale–New Haven Hosp, Conn; Quinnipiac College, Hamden, Conn)

N Engl J Med 331:821–827, 1994 119-96-71–3

Purpose.—Falling is an important public health problem in the elderly that is associated with considerable morbidity and costs. Up to one third of community-dwelling elderly individuals fall each year. Although uncontrolled studies have suggested that interventions directed against known modifiable risk factors can reduce the incidence of falls, these results have not been confirmed in controlled trials. A multifactorial, targeted risk-abatement strategy to reduce the risk of falling among elderly individuals was assessed in a controlled trial.

Methods.—The study sample comprised 301 community-dwelling men and women aged 70 years or older. All had at least 1 known risk factor for falling, including postural hypotension; sedative use; at least 4 medication prescriptions; and impairment of arm or leg strength or range of motion, balance, transfer skills, or gait. Baseline assessments were performed in the individuals' homes by a nurse practitioner and a physical therapist. Patients were randomly assigned to an intervention group or a control group. The intervention group received a combination of adjustment in their medications, behavioral instructions, and exercise regimens designed to modify their risk factors (Table 1), whereas the control group received a matched number of home social work visits along with usual health care. The main outcome measure was the incidence of falls; all patients reporting falls were followed up by telephone.

Results.—Significantly fewer patients in the intervention group fell during 1 year of follow-up than in the control group, 35% vs. 47% (Fig 1). The adjusted incidence-rate ratio for falls in the intervention group was 0.69. When interventions for a specific risk factor were not performed, it was usually because of a higher priority risk factor or a contraindication to the intervention. On reassessment for risk factors a median of 4½ months after baseline, the mean number of risk factors present had declined by 1.1 in the intervention group vs. 0.6 in the control group. The total average cost per subject in the intervention group was about $900,

TABLE 1.—Targeted Risk Factors and Corresponding Interventions

Risk Factor	Intervention
Assessed by a nurse	
Postural hypotension: drop in systolic blood pressure ≥ 20 mm Hg or to < 90 mm Hg on standing	Behavioral recommendations, such as ankle pumps or hand clenching and elevation of head of bed; decrease in dosage, discontinuation, or substitution for medications that may contribute to hypotension*
Use of any benzodiazepine or other sedative-hypnotic agent	Education about the appropriate use of sedative-hypnotic agents; nonpharmacologic treatment of sleep problems, such as sleep restriction; tapering and discontinuation of medications*
Use of ≥ 4 prescription medications	Review of medications with primary physician*
Inability to transfer safely to bathtub or toilet	Training in transfer skills; environmental alterations, such as grab bars or raised toilet seats
Environmental hazards for falls or tripping	Appropriate changes, such as removal of hazards, safer furniture (correct height, more stable), installation of structures such as grab bars or handrails on stairs
Assessed by a physical therapist	
Any impairment in gait	Gait training; use of an appropriate assistive device; balance or strengthening exercises if indicated†
Any impairment in transfer skills or balance	Balance exercises; training in transfer skills if indicated; environmental alterations†
Impairment in leg or arm muscle strength or range of motion (hip, ankle, knee, shoulder, hand, elbow)‡	Exercises with resistive bands and putty; resistance was increased when the subject was able to complete 10 repetitions through the full range of motion†

* Primary physician made final decision on adjustments in medication.

† Balance exercises included performance of 4 levels of progressively more destabilizing maneuvers with decreasing amounts of support. Subjects were instructed to perform resistive and balance exercises twice daily for 15–20 minutes.

‡ Listed in descending order of priority. Subjects underwent no more than 3 programs to improve balance or of individual resistive exercise.

(Reprinted by permission of *The New England Journal of Medicine*. Tinetti ME, Baker DI, McAvay G, et al: A multifactorial intervention to reduce the risk of falling among elderly people living in the community. *N Engl J Med* 331:821–827, 1994. Copyright 1994, Massachusetts Medical Society.)

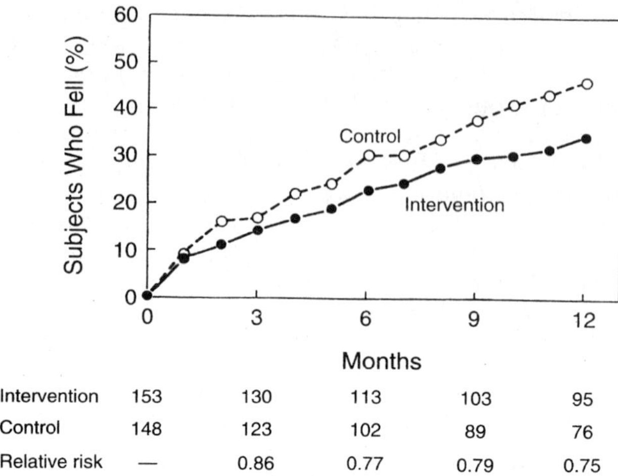

FIGURE 1.—Cumulative percentages of subjects in intervention and control groups who had 1 or more falls during 1 year of follow-up. The difference between groups was significant ($P = 0.05$, by log-rank test). The numbers still at risk for a fall at 3, 6, 9, and 12 months are shown below the figure. Only 10 of the subjects were lost to follow-up: 6 in the intervention group and 4 in the control group. Data on subjects were censored after a fall. The cumulative relative risks are shown for 3, 6, 9, and 12 months of follow-up. (Reprinted by permission of *The New England Journal of Medicine*. Tinetti ME, Baker DI, McAvay G, et al: A multifactorial intervention to reduce the risk of falling among elderly people living in the community. *N Engl J Med* 331:821–827, 1994. Copyright 1994, Massachusetts Medical Society.)

and the cost per fall prevented was $1,950. The cost for preventing 1 fall that required medical care was about $12,000, similar to the mean reported charge per hospitalization for injuries caused by falls.

Conclusions.—The multiple-risk-factor intervention strategy described can significantly reduce the risk of falls among community-dwelling elderly individuals. Individuals receiving targeted interventions have greater reductions in risk factors than controls, suggesting that risk factor modification explains at least some of their reduction in risk of falling. The interventions are also likely to improve functional independence among this population.

► This paper lines up some impressive facts about elderly people who fall. About 30% of individuals older than 65 years of age who live in the community fall each year. Unintentional injury, usually from a fall, is the sixth leading cause of death in this age group. The nonfatal results of falls include injury, fear, functional deterioration, and institutionalization. Although total costs associated with falls are unknown, costs of acute care from fall-related fractures are estimated at $10 billion per year. Falls and their consequences are the subject of considerable current attention[1–7] (see also Dr. Utiger's discussion of a paper on risk factors for hip fracture [Abstract 119-96-51–7]).

Until now, the evidence that modifying risk factors for falls actually reduces the risk of falling has been weak.[1] The authors report that assessment and intensive treatment to reduce several risk factors for falling (Table 1) decreased the risk of falling by 30% (Fig 1) and also reduced the fear of falling. Their program of gait, balance, and strength training, review of medications, education about sedatives, and environmental modification was conducted largely in the home by visiting nurses and physical therapists. The authors suggest that because many of the risk factors for falling also contribute to immobility and functional decline, their strategy could result in a reduction in the incidence of falls, as well as an improvement in functional independence among elderly patients.

S.E. Malawista, M.D.

References

1. Cummings SR, Nevitt MC: Falls. *N Engl J Med* 331:872, 1994.
2. Kaplan MS: Reducing the risk of falls among the elderly. *N Engl J Med* 332:268–269, 1995.
3. Rubenstein LZ, Josephson KR, Robbins AS: Falls in the nursing home. *Ann Intern Med* 121:442–451, 1994.
4. Guralnik JM, Ferrucci L, Simonsick EM, Salive ME, Wallace RB: Lower-extremity function in persons over the age of 70 years as a predictor of subsequent disability. *N Engl J Med* 332:556–561, 1995.
5. Cummings SR, Nevitt MC, Browner WS, Stone K, Fox KM, et al: Risk factors for hip fracture in white women. *N Engl J Med* 332:767–773, 1995.
6. Cooper C, Barker DJP: Risk factors for hip fracture. *N Engl J Med* 332:814–815, 1995.
7. Cauley JA, Seeley DG, Ensrud K, Ettinger B, Black D, et al: Estrogen replacement therapy and fractures in older women. *Ann Intern Med* 122:9–16, 1995.

Risk of Kidney Failure Associated With the Use of Acetaminophen, Aspirin, and Nonsteroidal Antiinflammatory Drugs

Perneger TV, Whelton PK, Klag MJ (Johns Hopkins Univ, Baltimore, Md; Univ of Geneva)

N Engl J Med 331:1675–1679, 1994 119-96-71–4

Background.—Although analgesic nephropathy was first described in the 1950s, evidence of nephrotoxicity from analgesic drugs is scanty and inconsistent. Of 4 case-control studies, none were population-based. Whether over-the-counter analgesic drugs are risk factors for end-stage renal disease was investigated in a population-based, case-control study.

Methods.—A total of 716 case patients with end-stage renal disease and 361 control subjects were interviewed by telephone about their lifetime use of 5 types of analgesic drugs. Average use and cumulative intake were examined for association with end-stage renal disease.

Results.—The sex and race of case patients and control subjects were significantly different. Age distribution was similar in the 2 groups. Heavier use of acetaminophen was associated with increased risk of end-stage renal disease in a dose-dependent fashion. Using a consumption of 0–104 pills per year as a reference, the odds ratio of end-stage renal disease was 1.4 for those who took 105–365 pills per year; the odds ratio was 2.1 for those who took 366 or more pills per year after adjusting for race, sex, age, and use of other analgesic drugs. Using a lifetime consumption of fewer than 1,000 pills containing acetaminophen as a reference, the odds ratio of end-stage renal disease was 2.0 for those who took 1,000–4,999 pills; the odds ratio was 2.4 for those who took 5,000 or more pills. Of the overall incidence of end-stage renal disease, 8% to 10% was attributable to use of acetaminophen. There was an association between a cumulative dose of 5,000 or more pills containing nonsteroidal anti-inflammatory drugs and an increased risk of end-stage renal disease; this association was not observed for aspirin.

Conclusions.—The risk of end-stage renal disease increases with use of acetaminophen. This risk does not increase with use of aspirin or lower doses of nonsteroidal anti-inflammatory drugs. The safety of long-term consumption of acetaminophen and consumption of large quantities of nonsteroidal anti-inflammatory drugs is questioned.

► Over 40 years ago,[1] we began to appreciate that chronic ingestion of analgesic drugs could lead to tubulointerstitial nephritis (analgesic nephropathy), a realization that led to the withdrawal of phenacetin from the market. Acetaminophen is a metabolite of phenacetin.[2] Its further metabolites, especially p-aminophenol, are concentrated in the hypertonic renal papillae, which may explain the occurrence of papillary necrosis as a hallmark of analgesic-induced nephropathy. Oxidized metabolites of *p*-aminophenol bind covalently to sulfhydryl-containing tissue macromolecules and deplete stores of reduced glutathione, leading to cell necrosis. Nonsteroidal anti-inflammatory agents (NSAIDs) administered chronically appear to injure the kidney by persistent inhibition of prostaglandin synthesis, leading to renal medullary ischemia.

In this study, we learn that heavy average use of acetaminophen—more than 1 pill per day—and medium-to-high cumulative acetaminophen intake—more than 1,000 pills in a lifetime—each doubled the odds of developing end-stage renal disease. There was also the suggestion of an association between end-stage renal disease and high lifetime intake—5,000 or more pills—of NSAIDs other than aspirin.

Consider that an estimated 15.8 million adults, or 12.1% of the United States population 24–74 years old, have signs and symptoms of osteoarthritis.[3] Recall that a recent and influential article[3] found that acetaminophen seemed as good as either high or low doses of ibuprofen for the *short-term* treatment of osteoarthritis of the knee (a study endlessly cited in advertisements for Tylenol). It will be important to ensure that such patients are not left on acetaminophen for the long-term.

S.E. Malawista, M.D.

References

1. Spühler, O, Zolinger HU: Die chronisch-interstitielle Nephritis. *Z Klin Med* 151:1–50, 1953.
2. Ronco PM, Flahault A: Drug-induced end-stage renal disease. *N Engl J Med* 331:1711–1712, 1994.
3. 1992 Year Book of Medicine, p 665.

Running and the Development of Disability With Age

Fries JF, Singh G, Morfeld D, Hubert HB, Lane NE, Brown BW Jr (Stanford Univ, Calif)

Ann Intern Med 121:502–509, 1994 119-96-71–5

Background.—Although physical activity is known to decrease mortality rates, its effects on morbidity and disability are less clear. An activity such as aerobic running might delay or prevent disability through increased fitness and training; however, it might also accelerate the development of disability as a result of osteoarthritis or cumulative trauma. The progression of disability scores between runners and nonrunners was studied longitudinally during an 8-year period.

Methods.—A total of 451 runners drawn from the membership of the 50+ Runners Association and 330 community controls were studied. The average history of running among the runners was 12 years. Both groups were aged 50–72 years in 1984 when they responded to a questionnaire concerning exercise, medical, and dietary history; musculoskeletal injuries; and other variables. They also responded to annual questionnaires during 8 years of follow-up. The main outcome measure was disability, as indicated by responses to the previously validated Health Assessment Questionnaire, which evaluates function in the areas of dressing and grooming, arising, eating, walking, hygiene, reach, grip, and activities.

Results.—At baseline, the runners—including control subjects with a history of running—were leaner, had less frequent joint symptoms, took fewer medications, had fewer medical problems, and had fewer and less severe instances of disability. These differences, which may have reflected either improved health because of running or self-selection bias, persisted after 8 years (Fig 1). One third of the runners' club members had stopped running; however, the frequency of other vigorous exercise increased in both groups, particularly among runners.

During follow-up, disability levels increased steadily from 0.026 to 0.071 for runners and from 0.079 to 0.242 for controls. The difference was significant and consistent between sexes. The lower rate of disability among runners' club members persisted after adjustment for age, sex, body mass, baseline disability, smoking history, history of arthritis, and other comorbid conditions. All age groups showed progressive increases in disability; the oldest groups showed an increase in the slope of the disability curve. Mortality was also lower in the runners' club members than in controls, 1.5% vs. 7%. The mortality differences remained after adjustment for age, sex, body mass, comorbid conditions, educational level, smoking history, alcohol intake, and mean blood pressure; conditional risk ratio for controls compared with runners was 4.27.

Conclusions.—Compared with community controls, older adults who engage in aerobic running and other vigorous exercise are significantly slower to develop disability. Mortality is lower in runners as well. The benefits of running most likely result from increased aerobic activity, strength, fitness, and organ reserve rather than from postponement of

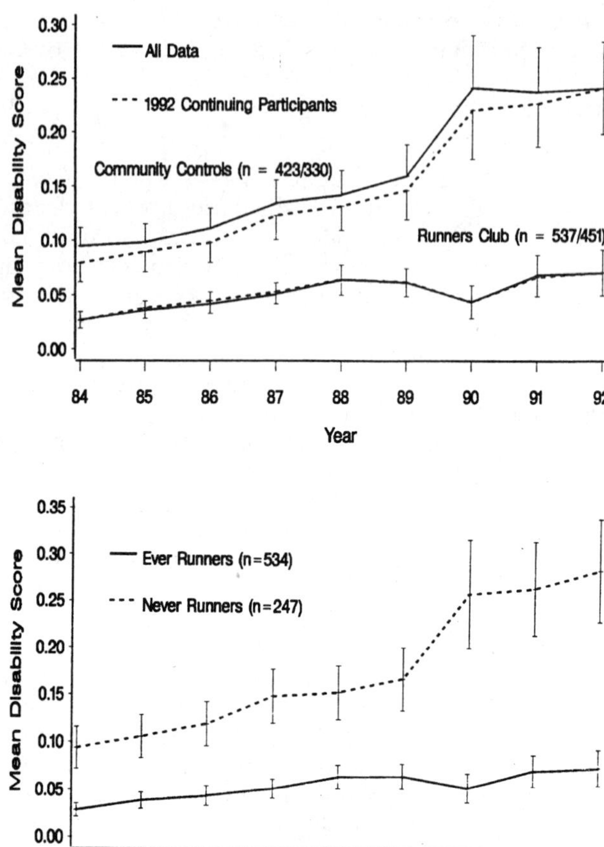

FIGURE 1.—Progression of disability over time. **Top,** runners' club members compared with community controls. Data from all patients and all data points were compared with data from continuing 1992 participants (completers). *Bars* represent 95% confidence limits. No significant differences existed between those completing 8 years of the study (1992 participants) and data including all data points, but significant differences between runners' club participants and community controls were observed at all time points ($P < 0.01$). **Bottom,** ever-runners compared with never-runners. Similar differences, significant at all time points, are seen when ever-runners, those who have ever run for 1 month or more, were compared with never-runners. *Bars* represent 95% confidence limits (1992 participants). (Courtesy of Fries JF, Singh G, Morfeld D, et al: Running and the development of disability with age. *Ann Intern Med* 121:502–509, 1994.)

osteoarthritis. The findings have important implications for efforts to increase regular physical exercise throughout the life span. It is difficult to remove the influence of self-selection bias, however, and there is no way to tell whether more rigorous exercise could make controls as healthy as runners.

▶ Do those who run "come apart" (i.e., develop disability) more readily than those who do not? Apparently not; in fact, they seem to develop less disability over time than controls. This advantage holds true even if one compares "ever runners" with "never runners" (Fig 1). The authors point out the inconclusiveness of cross-sectional studies on this subject, because increased physical activity could be the self-selected result of good health, rather than good health the result of the physical activity. However, this being a longitudinal study, they would expect that if a self-selection bias were present, a baseline difference in disability between exercising and nonexercising groups would narrow with time, and, if physical activity leads to the development of disability, that the trend lines eventually would converge. This has not happened over 9 years. In response to a call for prospective, controlled trials of exercise (difficult to do, even if someone were found to pay for them),[1] the authors are content to point out nondefensively how impressed they are "that a motivated group of persons exercised vigorously for 9 years at nearly 300 minutes a week while average ages increased from 59 to 68 years and that this group continues to be nearly free of disability through their seventh and eighth decades of life." That's enough to inspire me.

S.E. Malawista, M.D.

Reference

1. Venes D: Running and the development of disability with age. *Ann Intern Med* 122:475, 1995.

Drug Index

A

B

C

D

E

F

G

H

I

K

L

M

N

O

P

Q

T

U

V

W

Z

Subject Index

This cumulative index gives the volume (year) and page locations of subjects included in the five most recent annual editions of the YEAR BOOK. It will accumulate with each subsequent edition by deletion of the earliest year's references. The volumes (years) appear in *italic* type, preceding the page numbers and separated from them by a colon.

A

B

C

D

E

F

G

H

J

K

L

O

P

S

T

U

V

W

X

Y

Z

Author Index

A

B

C

D

E

F

G

H

I

J

K

L

M

N

O

P

Q

R

S

T

U

V

W

Y

Z